Care of the Fetus

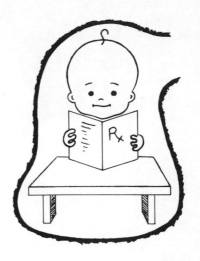

Care of the Fetus

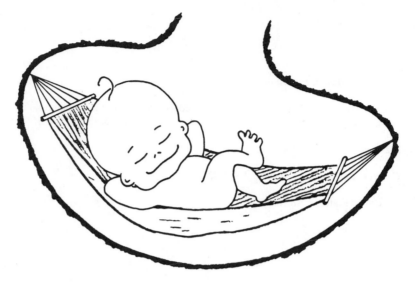

Robert C. Goodlin, M.D.

Professor of Obstetrics-Maternal-Fetal Medicine
Sacramento Medical Center
University of California, Davis
Sacramento, California

MASSON PUBLISHING USA, INC.

New York · Paris · Barcelona · Milan · Mexico City · Rio de Janeiro

TO MY WIFE
VELMA
AND TO OUR CHILDREN
JAMES, SARAH, BETH, and TOM
for their love, understanding
and efforts

Preface

Although obstetricians are accepted as being responsible for the care and welfare of the fetus (the *in utero* patient), there is a scarcity of writings describing obstetrical practice from the fetal point of view. In *Care of the Fetus*, clinical solutions are considered from the *in utero* patient's viewpoint, since it may be that only with this approach will a break with the dogma of the past occur, and perhaps better fetal health and development will be achieved. This is not to deny that maternal welfare is of concern to every obstetrician, but rather to suggest that we should consider and evaluate the fetus with every possible technique, and at every opportunity.

In order to achieve this goal, this textbook makes an effort to discuss in detail some of the common problems of fetal care, such as the fetal cardiovascular responses to stress and to distress, fetal nutrition, fetal infection, growth retardation, etc. In addition, the field of fetal health is expanded by including chapters relative to the fetus as a person, fetal learning, fetal evoked responses, fetal pain, fetal personality, and the fetal mirror syndrome.

Since many of the solutions for the problems in fetal medicine presented in the text are unconventional, in order to present a balanced viewpoint, there is included in most chapters, a section presenting "other points of view." In contrast to the free-wheeling and wide-ranging topic sections, the "Protocol" and "Data" sections are designed to provide concise, firm information sufficient for most any obstetrical problem.

The book, then, is designed to expand our horizons as concerns the care of the fetus, at the same time, it offers a practical and efficient guide for optimal obstetrical care.

Prologue

This monograph is not intended to be a substitute for a standard obstetrical textbook, but it is intended to be an expression of new and unusual viewpoints, with the necessary outlines and data, allowing for the practice of more innovative obstetrics.

I have attempted to present *Care of the Fetus* as I have practiced and studied fetology for the past 25 years: many of the chapters in the first section reflect my own interest (cardiovascular response), while other chapters represent areas that I regard as being filled with controversy and dogma (prenatal care). The second and third portions of this monograph (Protocols and Obstetrical Data) contain outlines of work-ups and of care for high-risk pregnancies, and a collection of antenatal and fetal data sufficient for most obstetrical problems. I hope that Mr. Hal Pullum's cartoons will inject a bit of humor into what some may consider as another dry collection of obstetrical dogma. Most chapters include a brief section, "Another Point of View," to emphasize that other viewpoints exist and usually prevail.

Despite containing more than 750 different references, excluding my own work, the various topics in the first section are under referenced. This reflects in part my fear of quoting out of context, as well as not wishing to pretend that this is an all-inclusive work. For the second and third sections, the 150 references are intended as only a starting point. However, I do hope that, for those interested, the bibliography is sufficient to allow further library work.

I am indebted to our department secretaries, LaVina Brasel and Karen Sullivan, for their efforts and to my wife, Velma, for her work and endurance during the time of this monograph's travail. Any comments concerning error, deletion, or contrasting views will be appreciated.

Contents

A. Topics

B. Protocols

C. Obstetrical Data D-1–D-209

Introduction

Throughout the Topics section frequent reference is made to the various tables and charts in the Obstetrical Data section as well as to numerous Protocols. I have separated the monograph in this manner for two reasons. The first is to avoid the boring inclusion of 178 tables and charts into the various discussions, and the second reason is to make the same charts and protocols easier to find and use.

CHAPTER 1

The Fetus as a Person (or the Importance of Maternal Tranquility)

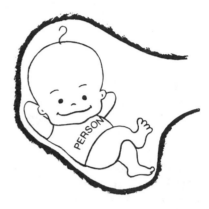

Introduction

FETAL RESPONSES

"For behold, when the voice of your greeting came to my ears, the babe in my womb leaped for joy." Although St. Luke (Luke 1:44) obviously appreciated that the human fetus was capable of responding to external stimuli, like many today, he believed that the sound stimulus was transmitted through its mother's sensory system.

Present available data would suggest that the mature human being *in utero* is neither in a stupor nor in an hypoxic coma[548] and that it will respond to various extrauterine stimuli and to maternal emotions. Even though fetal tympanic membranes are dampened by amniotic fluid, the German research Peiper demonstrated more than 50 years ago that the *in utero* human being responds independently to extrauterine sound as early as the 26th week of pregnancy. Likewise, Smyth[640] showed that a bright light shining on the fetal vertex through the mother's abdominal wall provokes a fetal heart rate (FHR) response. Recent investigators,[344, 621] using the brightly lit fetoscope, have observed that even the second trimester fetus turns its head away from the light source. The human fetus also responds to pain, by movement and FHR changes, as early as 26 weeks when stuck by the needle during amniocentesis[244] or to temperature as when cold saline is flushed through an intrauterine catheter.[277]

Studies of FHR change and fetal movements suggest that a fetus responds to changes in position of its mother, such as tilting. Reynolds[572] has disagreed with the concept of fetal responses to maternal changes, for he concluded that prior to fixation of the fetal presenting part in the maternal pelvis, the *in utero* fetus is like an individual in space, as it is floating free in amniotic fluid and is not subjected to the forces of gravity. (I've tested his hypothesis by swimming underwater in the swimming pool of a ship which was in rough water. It was obvious to me, some 4 ft. below the surface of the pool, that I was very much aware of the ship's motion without touching any fixed wall.) Observations of fetuses maintained in a fetal incubator (Chapter 13) likewise suggest that immature fetuses have active proprioreceptor input as they turn with movement of the immersion fluid, and with real-time ultrasound, even the 10-week *in utero* fetus is seen to respond to shaking of its mother's uterus. The demonstrations by Korner and Colley[412] that the direction of rocking or cuddling of a newborn had influences on whether it is content or irritable suggests that we have a well-developed tactile and spatial sensation at the time of birth. As with all newborn responses, it seems unlikely that these proprioreceptor responses could be developed within the first few minutes of being born without prior activity and practice *in utero*. In all probability, the *in utero* fetus is similarly responding to changes in its (and its mother's) position. Indeed, observant gravida report that their fetuses "like" certain maternal sleeping positions (right or left side) and protest other positions by "protesting" movements.

Sir Liley,[443] as well as Eastman,[178] would have us believe that the human fetus is constantly turning *in utero*, that it is forever seeking a comfortable position, that it is physically active in attempting to seek the best out of its *in utero* life. Sometimes an accident occurs and it is caught in an awkward position, such as a transverse lie, when the membranes rupture or labor begins. But in general, it apparently has enough sense to align itself with the pelvic axis and to protect its umbilical cord. Since it has been demonstrated that the fetus probably is the initiator of labor in most term pregnancies, it would appear that we have an unusual amount of common sense while residing *in utero*.

FETAL SENSORY RECEPTORS

Bradley and Mistretta[65] have reviewed fetal sensory receptors. For hearing, all of the structural components are present by the 24th week of gestation and as noted, the youngest fetus reported to respond was at 26 weeks. The vestibular apparatus has reached morphological maturity by 14 weeks in the human fetus, but no data are available as to whether it functions. Hooker[349] has reported that the earliest a definite human fetal vestibular response has been observed is at 25 weeks.

The human fetus responds to tactile stimulation as early as the seventh week, as demonstrated by Hooker using calibrated von Frey hairs. I noted that the human fetus will respond to cold saline flushed into the amniotic space at 18–20 weeks with FHR changes and movement, but not to saline at 42°C. I concluded that these responses presumably reflect intact temperature receptors in the fetus.

Human fetal taste buds are morphologically mature at 12 weeks. DeSnoo[155] showed that 34–38 week *in utero* fetuses swallowed more amniotic fluid when saccharin was injected into the amniotic fluid, and Liley[443] showed less fetal swallowing with injection of noxious-tasting substances. As discussed in Chapter 8, taste bud receptors apparently induce fetal apnea when materials other than amniotic fluid are present in the fetus' nasopharynx. Bradley has suggested that fetal taste buds are constantly monitoring the composition of the amniotic fluid. Presumably, meconium-stained fluid would induce less swallowing, and perhaps fetal apnea, than does unstained amniotic fluid. It seems reasonable then that fetuses with stained or scanty amniotic fluid might respond with swallowing (and better nourishment) if its fluid were "sweetened."

Human olfactory epithelium and nerve are developed by the 12th week. No information exists on *in utero* function, but by birth, Engen and associates[189] showed at least minimal function.

The human eye continues to develop even after birth, although most photoreceptor development is complete at term.

Fetal Movements

Apparently the first written record of human fetal movements is that reported in Genesis when Rebecca, wife of Isaac, reported "the children struggled within us." Preyer[548] almost single-handedly founded the field of fetal physiology a century ago (1885), but incorrectly concluded that the *in utero* mammalian fetus was normally in a stupor and/or coma. While clinical obstetrics has been greatly influenced by Preyer's concepts, laboratories such as Hamburger's in St. Louis have actively studied fetal movements in laboratory animals.[315] His group has shown that in the rat fetal movements are not necessarily related to uterine contractions, that local complex patterns are built up from less complex units, and that their occurrence seems to be related to the development and organization of the spinal cord.

FETAL MOVEMENTS IN EARLY PREGNANCY

In 1885, Preyer recorded movements of extrauterine human fetuses, apparently from therapeutic abortions. He concluded that spontaneous fetal movements could occur before they are felt by the gravida, that fetal movements continued for considerable time even when the fetus was without oxygen supply, that fetal movements were affected by temperature, that they could be elicited by stimulus (such as touching with a feather), and that these fetal movements were apparently independent of the mother's condition.

In modern times, Minkowsky[474] was one of the first to systematically investigate fetal movements. He used only human fetuses obtained by hysterotomy of mothers who had been "normal and uncomplicated." These fetuses were of 8–20 weeks gestation. Minkowski described early fetal movements which were slow and irregular, had a peculiar wormlike characteristic, and produced minimal locomotor effect. The fetal movements, as observed by Minkowski, included extension, lateral flexion, and rotation of the head, flexion or extension of the trunk, as well as full range of movement of the fetal extremities. Minkowski further noted that tactile stimuli elicited more forceful and rapid movements than occurred spontaneously.

Efforts to mimic the normal *in utero* environment during fetal movement studies were made by the American, Hooker.[349] He studied previable human fetuses immediately placed into an isotonic saline solution at a physiologic temperature. Their movements were recorded with time-lapse photography and included the interval from time of placental separation until the second minute of life, using carefully defined tactile stimulation. He noted that the reflexes first occurred at about 5½ weeks of gestation. When stroked, the fetus responded with a contralateral flexion of the head and trunk. At 7½ weeks of pregnancy, perioral stimulation produced contralateral flexion of the head and trunk. At 8½ weeks of pregnancy, perioral stimulation produced contralateral flexion of the head, neck, trunk, and pelvis. At 10½ weeks, there was extension of the head and trunk, and isolated head movements were also observed. At 13 weeks, the fetus apparently swallowed, and there was frequent movement of the fetal head. At 12½ weeks, tactile stimulation of the palm of the hand or fingers caused flexion of the head. Hooker's investigations were continued by Humphrey[363] who described the fetus at the 18th or 20th week of pregnancy as having total body movements. After this time, there began to appear regular reflexes with obvious sequential changes (Tables D-128–D-133).

Barcroft and Barron[36] had described fetal movements in sheep similar to those noted by Humphrey except that they appeared to be spontaneous. These spontaneous movements ceased once the fetus was removed from the amniotic sac. Barcroft and Barron described a major difference in fetal behavior within the amniotic sac with the umbilical cord attached and those of the fetus when removed from the gestational sac. They reported that as long as conditions were optimal, the previable fetuses continued to make spontaneous movements without any external stimulation. Nearly all observers have agreed that asphyxia markedly reduces fetal movements and those reflexes that are later in appearance are lost first as asphyxia develops (Tables D-130).

Reinold[565] has been the first to use ultrasonic techniques in the systematic study of the normal human fetus *in utero* and has observed that it is not until the 10th or 11th week that fetal movements become prominent and are sufficiently forceful to change the position of the fetal body. He described a series of fetal movements, some of which are strong and brisk, others of which are slow and sluggish movements. Stephens and Birnholz,[663] using ultrasonic equipment with higher resolution than was available to Reinold, found that the normal fetuses have rolling movements as early as 6 weeks of gestation. (The absence of these fetal movements, even with a beating fetal heart, seems to indicate serious fetal illness and impending miscarriage.)

The strong and brisk fetal movements as observed by Reinold in the first trimester fetus are characterized by sudden onset with a forceful motor activity which involves the entire fetal body and shifts the fetal position in the amniotic sac. After the movement has subsided and the fetus returns to the bottom of the gestational sac, it may either go through the same movements again or it may lie still in a new position. [Our studies with the fetal incubator (Chapter 13) showed that human fetuses at fourteen weeks of gestation made constant body "rolling and twisting" movements much like an earthworm as long as they were floating free in the immersion media. Once the fetus was against any sort of surface, these movements generally ceased.] The slow and sluggish fetal movements of the early second trimester fetus are usually isolated and do not appear to be a part of any overall motor activity. These movements occur at the slow rate of only one to four per minute. Reinold, like Stephens and Birnholz,[663] believes that sluggish movements or absence of fetal movements may be a sign of poor fetal health. They have attempted to correlate these early fetal activity patterns of brisk movements, sluggish movements, or absence of movements with clinical outcome. Reinold suggests that there may be some correlation between early fetal movement patterns and subsequent clinical course. He also studied the fetal movements after a "provocative test" (shaking the uterus) and suggested that evaluation after such stimuli may be a useful clinical test.

FETAL MOVEMENTS IN LATE HUMAN PREGNANCY

In 1965, Payne and Bach[529] reviewed the relevant literature on human fetal activity and studied the fetuses of five cooperative prenatal patients. These gravida kept detailed records and apparently had active fetuses. These investigators concluded that the human fetus demonstrated a sleep–awake rhythm as manifested by fetal movements that corresponded to their subsequent immediate noenatal activity patterns. Review of the literature relative to the time of maximal fetal activity is confusing as it is said to occur at anywhere from 1700 to 2400 and from 0100 to 0300. Nearly all reports agree, though, that the fetus is least active in the early forenoon (0800–1200). Our own studies, from analyzing 300 records compiled by normal prenatal term patients, indicate that a majority of gravida appreciate the greatest fetal activity at some time in the late evening and only a minority in the early morning (0100–0200). When we studied five term fetuses of normal gravida with 24-hour continuous fetal heart rate (FHR) monitors, the time of greatest beat-to-beat FHR variability (Chapter 9) was at around 0100. This corresponds to Sterman's[665] studies suggesting that fetal activity is greatest during maternal REM sleep. The differences in our observations with the monitor and those reported by the majority of gravida may reflect the variation in the "deepness" of their sleep in the early morning hours. Sterman concluded after a survey of the literature through 1971 and his own studies[665] that the recurrent periods of motor activity observed in the near-term fetus are intrauterine manifestations of the fetal REM state or basic rest–activity cycle. The earliest that these fetal activity cycles occurred was 21 weeks, and such activity cycles frequently contained a slower cycle not seen in newborns. Regardless of the significance of these circadian cycles of fetal movements, investigators such as Sadovsky and Polishuk[602] consider that "fetal movements are an expression of fetal well-being."

Our own unreported studies also suggested that the hyperactive child is perceived to be hyperactive *in utero* and is often a source of concern to the gravida. We know of four infants who have been documented to be hyperactive children whom their mothers had considered as hyperactive *in utero*. On the other hand, we have records of two fetuses who were hyperactive *in utero* but as children are apprently normal, indicating that there is not a perfect correlation between fetal activity *in utero* and activity as a child. Walters[727] has recorded fetal movements (Fig. 1-1) and demonstrated fetal activity was correlated with childhood neurological and motor development. The value of such studies is uncertain, chiefly because the concept of the newborn being a miniature adult as far as its ultimate intellectual development is concerned has come under severe attack. Lewis[436] has apparenlty shown that there is little correlation (except in extreme cases) between motor and

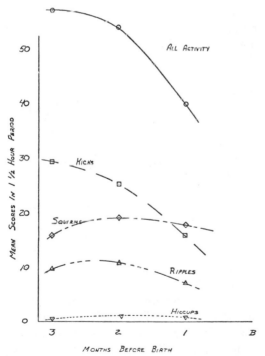

Fig. 1-1. Fetal activity as recorded by gravida during last month of pregnancy. (From Walters, C.B.: *Child Del* **35**: 1249, 1964. Reproduced with permission.)

intellectual test during the first 6 months of life and an individual's subsequent development. However, Sontag[648] reported that hyperkinetic fetuses, as children, exhibited a pattern of apprehension in peer situations.

Fetal movements are apparently necessary for proper development of bones, joints, and limbs. With gravida in whom fetal movements are restricted either by loss of amniotic fluid or by use of maternal tranquilizers, multiple skeletal and soft tissue anomalies occur (Chapter 15).

While maternal anxiety and apprehension (as will be noted) are deleterious to the fetus' development, so is excess sedation and tranquilization. It would appear that there is an optimal amount of fetal activity required for proper development, but there is an absence of studies designed to determine what fetal activity level is optimal for its development. If we knew the ranges of normal fetal movement, then fetologists would be in a position to change the *in utero* activity patterns in order to assure an optimal newborn.

PSYCHOLOGICAL ASPECTS OF *IN UTERO* LIFE

Life *in utero* for the human being has been variously conceived as ranging from living and growing in the quiet contentment of one's mother's womb where all wants are gratified to a more stressful situation in which one can, as a voyeur, spy upon our parents having sexual relations, to sometimes a living hell where the mother's negative emotions and apprehensions can predispose to congenital malformations and abnormal cerebral development. The psychiatric literature would suggest that life in the womb is a time of contentment. (As discussed in Chapter 4, in addition to maternal emotional effects, it should be emphasized that there are sometimes severe limitations of *in utero* nutrients and oxygen which may likewise adversely affect developments within uteri.)

Salk[606] demonstrated in 1960 that human newborns exposed to the sound of a heart beating at 72 bpm (a "calm" mother's heart rate) were more calm than a controlled group. Others had suggested that newborn development is improved with appropriate heart rate sounds, but Palmquisth[523] was unable to substantiate that playbacks of simple audible heart rates at 72 bpm improved the newborn's weight gain. However, Salk's observations have been confirmed; when the heart rate sounds broadcast in the nursery are speeded up to 128 bpm (corresponding to maternal anxiety), the newborn becomes restless and irritable. These newborn observations suggest the following three correlations: (a) that the fetus becomes apprehensive when its mother does, (b) that a fetus learns from its *in utero* environment, and (c) that the maternal anxiety is apparently deleterious for the fetus, as judged by the effects of "anxious sounds" on newborns.

Ellis[187] has reported that more than 10 centuries ago the Chinese had "prenatal clinics," not for our purposes of dispensing iron and vitamins, but rather to ensure tranquility to the mother for its assumed benefit on the unborn child. While no one has seriously recommended anything other than tranquility for pregnant women, yet we in America do little in our prenatal clinics to assure maternal tranquility, other than to attempt to establish "good" patient–physican relationships. There is indirect evidence that tranquility or reassurance to pregnant women is very important, for how else can we explain the obvious benefits of "good" prenatal care. It must be only the assurance and tranquility which comes from being a part of a "study," with its specialized attention, which can possibly explain the various benefits that have been claimed for a wide range of therapeutic modalities (versus controls) for a wide range of maternal–fetal illnesses. These include the use of hormones, vitamins, psychotherapy, and diuretics, for problems such as repeated miscarriage, prevention of toxemia, and prevention of premature labor. Again, regardless of the circumstances, the study group with its added attention invariably does better than the control group. (Perhaps negative results *do not make* the literature, biasing this impression.) In our hospital, as elsewhere, it is the unregistered gravida that has the greatest incidence of eclampsia, premature labor, miscarriage, amnionitis, and so forth. It seems probable that such an underserved population would benefit from efforts to assure tranquility, reassurance, and general well-being (as well as vitamins and iron). The question is whether the affluent of a good social background would similarly benefit from added efforts of prenatal clinics to assure tranquility.

Schuller and Larsen[614] did a retrospective study among our obstetrical patients at the Sacramento Medical Center. They found that the occurrence of maternal dysphoria, depression, anger, and tension were significantly correlated with newborn complications. Likewise, at the University of California, Davis, primate center, a male monkey and his harem are frequently housed in a corn crib type of cage. No privacy is provided and presumably tension exists among the various female members who sit at different levels in the cage. Those females on the lowest point of the cage (and social order) have the highest rate of reproductive loss. Attempts by the primate center's staff and by us at the medical center to improve reproduction by reducing tensions between our two different groups of patients have been equally unsuccessful.

CARDIOVASCULAR RESPONSES AND FETAL MOVEMENT

Hoff and Green[347] demonstrated that the cortical nerve cells associated with motor function and with cardiovascular function (CVF) in cats and monkeys are in close anatomical relationship. As noted in Chapter 8, spillover of activity from the muscular activity cell can activate those cortical cells associated with CVF. Rudolph's laboratory has shown (Williams *et al.*[753]) that, in fetal lambs, stimulation of the hypothalamus produces hypertension and tachycardia (Chapter 8). A bradycardia often follows the tachycardia ("undershoot," Chapter 12). The bradycardia was abolished by vagotomy and the entire hypertensive–tachycardia was abolished by alpha adrenergic blockage.

Human fetal movements are usually associated with a tachycardia and if prolonged, by an undershoot. Such tachycardia (accelerations of FHR) is usually considered a sign of good health, as the fetus is "obviously" moving (Fig. 1-2). These FHR responses have been labeled "FAD" by Lee *et al.*[430] and presumably indicate good fetal health. In the near future, it will be possible to categorize these FHR responses according to fetal maturity and type of movement using real-time ultrasound equipment. Presumably, different FHR patterns will be observed which could be useful in studying fetal psychology and/or maturity.

Aladjem *et al.*[11a] have proposed a classification of apparent random variations of FHR responses to fetal movements. They identified two types of fetal movements (as reported by the gravida), isolated and multiple. FHR patterns were classified according to their configuration into an omega (Ω) (Fig. 1-3), or brief period of tachycardia, and lambda (λ), tachycardia followed by undershoot (Fig. 1-

4). Isolated fetal movements elicited the omega pattern while the lambda was elicited by multiple fetal movements. They believe that gestational age did not influence these FHR patterns.

FETAL AROUSAL LEVELS

There are a number of techniques for determining fetal arousal levels. The simplist is to ask a gravida "how active" her fetus is. After being convinced that her inquiror is serious, gravida in their third trimester seldom have any doubts about the degree of fetal activity, responding, "It is very active," "hardly moves," "is active only at night," and so forth. While each gravida has an impression of her fetus' activity pattern, our problem is that sometimes her impressions fail to correlate with our indicators of fetal arousal. Our indicators of fetal arousal levels include measuring beat-to-beat reactivity and ultrasonic viewing of the fetus, and we have managed to correlate the degree of FHR reactivity (Chapter 9) with arousal levels. The best example is to take the fetus with low FHR

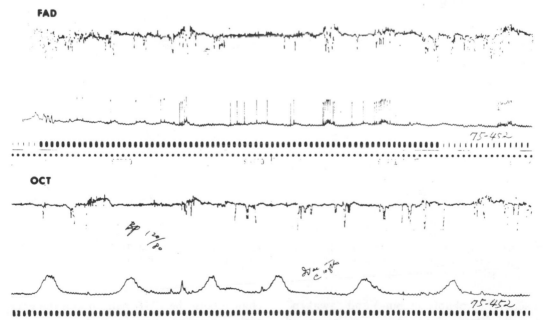

Fig. 1-2. A positive fetal activity acceleration determination (FAD) with a negative oxytocin challenge test. (From Lee, C., *et al.*: *Obstet Gynecol* **48:** 19, 1976. Reproduced with permission.)

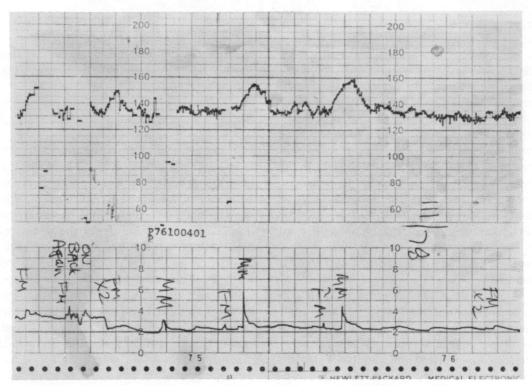

Fig. 1-3. Two omega (Ω) patterns following individual fetal movements (FM) (panel 75). The fetal heart rate (FHR) was obtained by ultrasound. FHR baseline 130 beats per minute. (From Aladjem, S., *et al.*: *Br J Obstet Gynecol* **84**: 487, 1977. Reproduced with permission.)

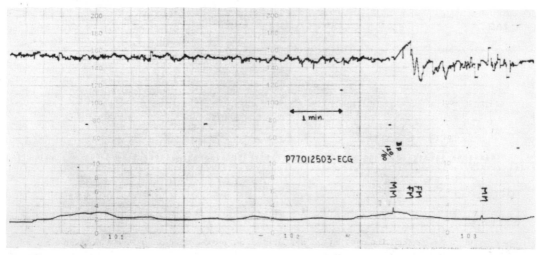

Fig. 1-4. A lambda (λ) pattern (panel 103) following a prolonged fetal rest period. The FHR was obtained by indirect electrocardiogram. FHR baseline 150 beats per minute. (From Aladjem, S., *et al.*: *Br J Obstet Gynecol* **84**: 487, 1977. Reproduced with permission.)

reactivity (probably sleeping) and "awaken" it with extrauterine stimuli such as sound (Fig. 1-5) (or needle stick), and in so doing, change both the FHR pattern and the gravida's impression of fetal activity.

The occasional lack of correlation between

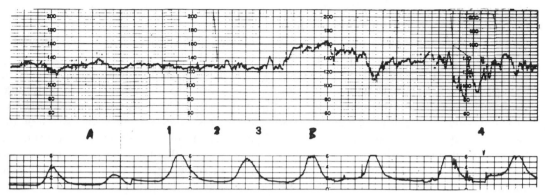

Fig. 1-5.   FHR recording during early labor when the fetus was relatively nonreactive. (A) A 2000-Hz sound stimulus was applied at "1, 2, and 3." At (B), fetus was more aroused.

what the gravida "feels" and what we "see" with either the FHR monitor or real-time scanner may reflect the various "states" of the fetus. The FHR beat-to-beat variability (or reactivity) probably correlates with EEG patterns. In the newborn, the EEG is an important parameter in "state" determinations, being much more definitive than gross movement patterns. The gravida, on the other hand, probably feels fetal limb movement, which may not always be correlated with the fetal EEG pattern or total fetal activity. It is clear that many fetal movements (as seen on the real-time ultrasonic scanner) are not discerned by the gravida. Apparently it is not then possible to precisely correlate the gravida's impression of fetal movements closely with our definition of fetal arousal (FHR reactivity) or with actual fetal movements (real-time ultrasonic scanning). In the assessment of fetal health, these are very much related, as the sickness of the fetus is apparent by all three monitoring techniques. However, insufficient data are available to determine the role of each technique in the monitoring of neurological–psychological fetal development.

CLINICAL APPLICATION

Given that the fetus does respond to extrauterine stimuli, the question arises, "Can such stimuli affect *in utero* development?" Using a rather crude extrauterine graphic recording device, Sontag and Wallace[644]

showed 45 years ago that increased fetal activity occurred during episodes of maternal fear and anxiety, fatigue, and positional changes. More recently, Ferreira[199] demonstrated in a series of controlled studies, the impact of the gravida's emotional attitude upon the fetus. It is apparent from his monograph that his own studies (and those selected references from the literature) have convinced him that maternal emotions have an adverse effect on the fetus. Ferreira explains these adverse maternal effects on the fetus through the various maternal hormones such as ACTH, catecholamines, and the use of drugs such as tranquilizers.

Sontag[644] did record fetal bradycardia during maternal emotional upset. He also noted that during maternal smoking fetal bradycardia occurred, presumably due to the effects of nicotine. However, he subsequently demonstrated the same FHR change when the mother was only shown a cigarette. Clearly, maternal emotions and stress directly affect her fetus.

In 1970, Shaw and associates[626] demonstrated that the more anxiety-prone mother (Taylor Manifest Anxiety Scale) gave birth to infants of lower birth weight. Adamsons and Myers[4] have been able to interpret this sort of old wives' tale about maternal anxiety causing fetal harm on a scientific basis. They have shown that the infusion of catecholamines or nicotine in pregnant rhesus monkeys could reduce the uterine blood flow to the point of producing asphyxia in the fetus. When anxiety was likewise produced in these pregnant primates, the same sort of reduced uterine blood flow occurred. There are two basic methods of maternal anxiety producing fetal distress: one is through reducing uterine blood flow; the other, in the monkey at least, is by inducing strong uterine contractions. Adamsons suggests perhaps phenobarbital for the anxious gravida, but found the most effective therapy to be counseling and psychotherapy.[3] A related study is of Japanese gravida living near a jet airport; when matched with controls, they had lower serum HPL levels and smaller newborns.[18]

Several years ago I saw a gravida at term who had been shot at close range in the arm, with only minimal blood loss, but had fainted in fright. The gravida was in good condition, but her fetus was dead. Since then, I have seen one other such case, and heard of two others—cases in which maternal fright was extreme, but physical damage was nil, and whose fetuses died.

Stott[668] has recommended that society needs to concentrate on assuring women an undisturbed pregnancy. He does not mean "undisturbed" in terms of wealth or physical activity, but rather the avoidance of interpersonal tension. With the cooperation of health officers in Glasgow and Lanarkshire, Scotland, he was able to follow children up to 4 years of age. He found that the great majority of mothers who had suffered from interpersonal tension during their pregnances had "unhealthy" children. Such children had a "handicap score" of 30.3, compared with a score of 16 for those of other parents.

Stott was able to expand his studies in Canada and concluded that the effects of marital discord are expressed in childhood conditions which he terms "congenital." Many of the children he studied were "neurally impaired." The following are some of the infant clinical manifestations he considered indicative of marital discord (the most ominous maternal discord arose when the gravida moved from her mother: "Being jumpy, easily startled, afraid of loud noises as a baby; con-

tinual vomiting, respiratory difficulty at birth; small for age; defective tooth enamel; wandering and hyperactivity; and excessive timidity."

Stott goes so far as to suggest that the excess of central nervous system malformations seen in Germany from the mid-1930s to the 1950s reflected the social stress of the population under Hitler's government. He believes that all animal species that have been studied show similar events. The handicaps produced in the young are caused, in Stott's opinion, by interaction between the mother's and the child's genetic constitution owing to specific types of environments. He suggests that prenatal care should be concerned with normal maternal psychological states. An equally interesting question, however, is whether the nonstressed, normal gravida engages in physical activities, eating patterns, or has changes of mood which are apparently within our accepted normal standards, but which may have an imprint on the fetus' personality and development. It would be undesirable obviously to strive to have all newborns be alike, but it is necessary to determine the optimal psychological *in utero* environment for the developing human so that obstetrical behavioral therapy may be correctly applied. This thought borders on the concept of psychiatric programming of people, which Packard[521] and others consider repugnant. Nevertheless, "directing" normal development may be an area in which fetology can make its greatest contribution, for it may be that even the apparently normal pregnancy does not provide the optimal *in utero* environment.

In 1940 Sontag and Newberry[647] demonstrated that human fetuses "learned" (or habituated) to extrauterine sound stimuli. Their report was largely ignored until 30 years later when, for a 2-year period, we again tested the term fetus' ability to learn (or become adapted) *in utero* (Goodlin and Schmidt[276]). We learned that most human fetuses quickly became adopted to a 2000-Hz sound stimuli when tested in the prenatal clinic. After as few as three tests with such a 100-decibel sound, many fetuses "learned" by ceasing to change heart rates or move. Normal fetuses subjected to repeated sound stimuli at each prenatal visit, as newborns did not respond to a similar stimulus in the newborn nursery. (In one case, we suspected the correct diagnosis, that the fetus was deaf, later shown to be the result of a CMV infection.)

We then attempted to "teach" a fetus to be tranquil, by having near-term gravida listen repeatedly to the same high-pitched music during times they considered to be tranquil for them. The concept was that such high-pitched music would, to the "taught" fetus in the newborn period, act as a pacifier. I had four cases in which the mothers felt that this form of "*in utero* teaching" was successful in that the same music (Debussy) did act as pacifier to their newborns. There were, of course, other cases which did not "learn," but I rationalized my way out of this apparent failure of the technique be believing that some mothers actually were not able to achieve tranquility while they were listening to the music. Another application of the extrauterine sound presumably could be useful for the small-for-dates (SFD) infant (or the large-for-gestational-age infant) to regulate fetal activity so as to increase or decrease fetal swallowing. As Liley[443] observed, fetal swallowing can be a significant part of fetal nutrition and presumable, with the SFD infant, increased swallowing of amniotic fluid nutrients would be a help. The same would probably be true for the macrosomic fetus who presumably is swallowing excessively *in utero*.

Our prediatric colleagues for years preached and practiced noninterference with the newborn, and it was not until they appreciated the importance of active intervention with endotracheal tubes and umbilical catheters that neonatology became a specialty. I believe that the same skepticism surrounding the role of fetologists with human fetuses is likewise preventing the development of fetology (maternal–fetal medicine) as a respected subspecialty. These same colleagues look askance when I speak about active interference in terms of planned fetal stimulation, attempting to alter fetal activity cycles, and use of drugs to assure fetal tranquility. Just as they (neonatologists) are concerned now about nursery noise and stimulation, so should we obstetricians be concerned about the *in utero* environment. There must be more to the perfect life *in utero* than optimal nutrients and oxygen.

The fetal physiologist, G. S. Dawes, has commented on the importance of a normal *in utero* environment and sensory stimulation for subsequent development, also that *in utero* "practice" may be necessary for the development of the various psychologic functions. He cites the observations of Hubel and Wiesel[360] that occlusion of newborn kitten eyelids permanantly reduces the number of neurons of their visual cortex. Thus, while periods of tranquility are apparently important for normal fetal development, so must there be adequate stimulation. Studies of fetal behavior may then be the area in which fetologists can make their greatest contribution.

From a practical standpoint, obstetrics should focus on fetal development. Now that the problems of maternal mortality are largely resolved and cesarean section is employed to solve all the intrapartum problems (real or imagined), the only period of obstetrical care which has promise of significant advance is the antenatal period. In addition to exploring hormonal and enzymatic tests, FHR and ultrasonic patterns, we must also give attention to fetal behavioral patterns. As hopefully demonstrated, these patterns are easily described in terms of fetal movement and response to stimuli (Fig. 1-6).

Case No. 1-1

A 31-year-old anesthesiologist was seen in her 20th week of pregnancy. She related that her first child had been a very active fetus and had severe colic and appeared to be hyperactive. She inquired as to whether efforts to induce fetal tranquility might be of help for future development. My views on the importance of tranquility during pregnancy were discussed, and she was asked to keep a detailed diary. She reported that the fetus

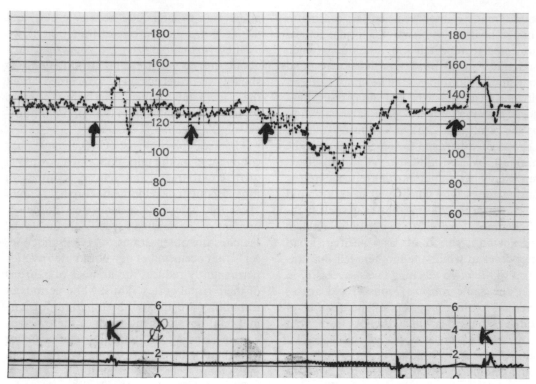

Fig. 1-6. Recording of an antenatal fetus who responded to a sound stimulus (arrows) until its mother developed the hypotensive syndrome. (Note maternal hyperventilation.) After maternal lateral position, fetus again responded to sound.

became hyperactive with frequent kicks and squirms when she was in the operating room for longer than 3 hours. This excessive fetal activity apparently was relieved by resting and lying on her left side. She also reported that the fetus "enjoyed" the maternal left lateral position at night, being much more active when she would lie on her right side or supine. After the 30th week of pregnancy, she regularly lay down for 30-min periods after an evening cocktail and listened to a Debussy recording. During this time, she reported that the fetus became more calm as she did. She also noted that the fetus would awaken her regularly between 1 and 2 AM. Following an uneventful delivery, she reported that the same Debussy recording served as perfect pacifier for his colic although it was some 4 months before the infant slept through his 1 to 2 AM activity. This was no suggestion that this child was hyperactive.

I suggest that this case is an example of "learning" *in utero*.

Case No. 1-2

While working with the fetal monitors in the labor room one evening, I was called to the delivery room because of an "hysterical" patient. She had received a caudal anesthetic and her labor had been uneventful except that the fetus remained in a persistent occiput posterior position. Her obstetrician had turned the vertex by "lifting" it out of the pelvis and rotating it at the level of the pelvic inlet. This, he claimed, had been easily accomplished but as he began to apply traction with the fetus in the occiput anterior position, the obstetrical staff, the patient, and her husband heard an apparent fetal "cry." As the obstetrician began to apply more traction on the forceps, the fetal "cry" become louder and the mother began to cry in an hysterical manner. The anesthesiologist then used a general anesthetic (Pentothal) and the child was delivered without further event. It appeared in good condition, and except for some forcep's marks, had a normal neonatal course. The patient, however, remained most concerned during the postpartum period and accused her obstetrician of brutality and was very hostile toward all those who associated with her delivery. In a subsequent delivery, she delivered under the Lamaze technique and made certain that forceps were not applied to the child's head.

Whether this is an example of "vagitus uterinus" (Ryder[596]) is unknown, but the history would suggest it to be so—and that forceps may be painful for the fetus.

Another Point of View

As noted, the arguments against active interference in the developmental processes of the apparently normal intrauterine human fetus are rather compelling. The first requirement must be the demonstration that such fetuses need some form of therapy and that the therapy, above all, will "do no harm."

Another argument concerns the fate of children born "out of wedlock" and who subsequently are adopted into reasonably stable families. Such individuals should have been subjected to more hostile-than-average *in utero* environments, and yet have often done well after adoption.[339, 743] As argued in the chapter on nutrition (Chapter 2), it may be that a loving and well-supported childhood can overcome most any previous deprivation for the individual *in utero*.

Chamberlain[94] made careful observations of a group of children aged 2 and was unable to document any behaviors that were predictive of these children's adaptation to school at age 6 or 7. Apparently only extreme poverty, poor physical health, and gross psychiatric disturbance consistently indicates high risk factors.

Worse yet, even if these high-risk children could be identified at age 2, Korsch[414] suggests that effective types of intervention are unknown. If behavioral medicine offers so little to the sick child at age 2, one could argue that it would be especially hopeless for sick fetuses *in utero*.

The National Institute of Child Health and Human Development is now engaged in studies of cognitive, social, and personality development in the early years of life. Their studies are extensive, following the same child from birth to 3–5 years, looking at the neonatal period, maternal and paternal influences, intrapartum factors, and so forth. However, in their protocols, there appears to be a complete void of matters related to intrauterine life. Apparently our fetal period of development is considered insignificant as regards subsequent social and personality characteristics.

Anders and Roffwarg[14] studied sleep patterns of three mothers and their newborns, as well as fetal activity in the third trimester. They concluded that the activity cycles of the fetus were independent of the maternal processes, but are dependent on the fetal CNS system.

While it is generally assumed that the development of one's personality begins after birth, Korner[412a] has suggested that statistically significant behavioral differences exist among healthy full-term newborns. Freud stated his conviction that "each individual ego is endowed from the beginning with its own peculiar dispositions and tendencies."[207a] The psychoanalytic literature has continued to stress the importance of pedispositions in the development of neurosis. However, there remains a void in the psychiatric literature as to how to direct a gravida to be an optimal "fetal incubator" for development of her fetus's personality. Helper *et al.* noted psychiatric theories which suggest that life stresses may interfere with the women's psychological affiliation with her newborn.[329a] Two sets of circumstances represent particular threats of a woman's adjustment to pregnancy: rejection of the pregnancy by the fetus's father, and a past experience of having delivered an abnormal child.

CHAPTER 2

Nutrition During Pregnancy

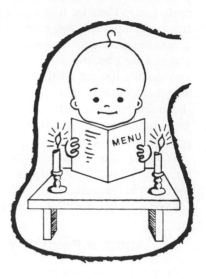

Historical Aspects

During the past 25 years in America, a complete reversal has occurred in the type of nutritional recommendations made to pregnant women. Earlier advice was for near starvation and low-protein diets, while the present advice is for high protein and a diet, or calories, "according to appetite." These radical changes in dietary concepts have not been associated with similar changes in perinatal mortality rates, although there is a suggestion that newborns are bigger now than before. This minimal response to change in diet suggests that nutrition, or at least our technique for giving dietary advice during pregnancy, is not of much importance to the *in utero* human.

In the past, the fetus was considered a perfect parasite, fulfilling its needs by taking from its mother. Among the data to support this concept are higher concentrations of iron, vitamins, and amino acids in the umbilical cord than in the maternal blood stream (Table D-142). However, a lower serum concentration of other substances (such as glucose, oxygen, and fatty acids) in the fetus than in

its mother suggests that while the placenta is programmed to build a fetus, it competes with all other maternal organs for day-to-day nutrients (oxygen, glucose). For example, if the maternal liver is starved for glucose, so too will be the fetus, but the fetus competes better than the liver for amino acids. However, the dreadful experience of the people of Leningrad in World War II, as reported by Antonov,[19] offers grim evidence that there are limits to this restricted concept of the human fetus as a "perfect" parasite. During the Siege, amenorrhea with supposed anovulation was frequent resulting in a tremendous decline in birthrate. (From the teleological viewpoint, anovulation may be a defense against the added stress of pregnancy during starvation.) In those cases in which women did become pregnant, the stillborn rate was 5.6%, and the rate of prematurity was 41.2%. In severe starvation, as with other maternal stresses, the first priority is given to the mother rather than the fetus.

The differences in interpretation of obstetrical data of World War I as compared with World War II probably explain the American reversal in nutritional dogma for pregnancy.

American obstetrics traditionally has been much influenced by the German literature. During World War I, as reported by both Warnekros and Gessner,[732] the incidence of eclampsia decreased significantly in Germany, but rose after the Armistice. Apparently believing that the German data were accurate, that all German gravida were well fed during peace time, and that they had been starved during World War I, the *JAMA* editorialized[180] and concluded in 1917 that restriction of fat and meat during pregnancy reduced the incidence of toxemia.

The American academicians were also influenced by the studies of Prochownick, a 19th-century German obstetrician. In 1889 he studied malnourished pregnant rats and then developed a diet which would assure smaller newborns for women who had suffered a previous perinatal loss because of their contracted pelvis. For these cases of multigravida with contracted pelvis, Prochownick[556] prescribed a fluid-restricted, low-calorie (1800–2000 cal), high-protein (160 g) diet for the third trimester, and reported improved perinatal mortality rates. The women were able to deliver vaginally because their newborns were smaller, but the feature of Prochownick's reports which attracted the Americans' attention was that these smaller newborns developed normally, doing well subsequently as children and adults. Prochownick apparently never intended that such diets be recommended for all pregnant women or that the diets had any other virtue than reducing the size of newborns. The American academicians, however, focused on the fact that the mothers and infants did well with such calorie-restricted diets, and believing that it reduced toxemia, recommended the diet to pregnant women in general.

The Johns Hopkins University's clinical obstetrical experience has had a major influence on American concepts of nutrition (and obstetrics in general) in as much as its professor of obstetrics wrote many editions of an obstetrical text long considered a classic. Their clinic clientele was black and had a high incidence of essential hypertension.

From such a clinical population, the Hopkins group became convinced that many women normally have a "low reserve kidney" and that it was necessary to protect such kidneys during pregnancy. This concept, coupled with the information from Europe that starvation apparently reduced the incidence of pregnancy complications, led to the general recommendation that American pregnant women be given a low-calorie and a low-protein diet. Even the ninth edition of the Williams' obstetrical textbook by Stander,[657] published in 1945, still recommended severe dietary restrictions during pregnancy. It is difficult to understand today, but these older American textbooks treated normal pregnancy as a disease.

For those physicians who had worked with mice colonies, the German experience of decreased incidence of eclampsia in World War I had an obvious explanation. Stated simply, under times of stress only the "proven breeders" (multiparous) reproduce, whether they be mice, pigs, or, presumably, humans. Therefore, the percentages of pregnancies from primigravidas should decrease markedly during times of malnutrition. This has been demonstrated to have occurred in Germany during the periods of World War starvation and is the apparent explanation for the marked reduction in eclampsia; that is, the percentage of primigravidas was reduced markedly. That social circumstances determine, in part, the incidence of eclampsia is further illustrated by comments of Chesley[100] about its height during the siege of Madrid in the Spanish Civil War. The siege apparently brought together many young men and women, and the incidence of primigravida was unusually high, as was the incidence of eclampsia.

Coupled with the low-protein, low-calorie diet, the American authorities compounded their error by recommending a low-salt diet. Ever since the time of Zangemeister's studies[767] in 1903, it had been known that excess salt intake during pregnancy leads to increased fluid accumulation. However, it has since been demonstrated that restriction of salt in pregnant women (who probably are salt-losers) leads to depletion of the renal juxtaglomerular apparatus. While such salt deficiency during pregnancy is apparently fairly benign, this is not true in warm climates. Under circumstances of heat and "glowing," pregnant patients on a low-salt diet can actually go into hypotensive shock because of reduced blood volumes. The present concepts are that pregnant women need salt, and that while excess salt intake may lead to edema and perhaps hypertension, certainly women should be encouraged to take a normal amount of salt throughout their pregnancies.

Recent Studies

Another feature of Prochownick's rat and human studies was that caloric starvation in the third trimester apparently was benign, producing only small but otherwise normal newborns. His studies indicate that protein and not calorie content was important in pregnancy, but Widdowson and Cowen's[748] more recent rat studies indicate that calories are equally as important as protein! Humans and rats can be compared for reduced caloric intake during human pregnancy reduces subsequent birthweight as similar results have been suggested from the Guatemala human studies. These studies of malnourished women in Guatemala (who were given supplemental food at various times in their pregnancy) indicate that increasing caloric intake produces a significant increase in the fetal retention of nitrogen (Mata et al.[465]).

The Americans missed the fact that Prochownick's starvation diet was applied only in the third trimester, presumably beyond the time when the essential fetal organ development has occurred. The effect of maternal diet on pregnancy is brought into focus by the studies of Stein and colleagues[661] in the prenatal exposure of Dutch women during the famine in 1944–1945. The Dutch famine was, from a scientific aspect, remarkable in three respects. (1) Valid data were available concerning the population according to diet, social strata, pregnancy outcome, and newborn development. (2) The famine was sharply circumscribed both in time and place. (3) Follow-up studies were available on subsequent development of the individuals who had been starved in utero. Routinely, Dutch males are medically examined and psychologically tested at age 18 as part of the military induction procedures. These results were available to Stein and colleagues. Amazingly enough, the 18-year-old males who had been starved in utero did slightly better in some tests, and no worse in all of the various examinations, than the controls. (Fig. 2-1). Another unexpected result from these data was that fatness or leanness of the young men was related to the time of their starvation while in utero. Starvation near to or after birth led to leanness, while starvation during early in utero life led to fatness. The authors (Ravelli et al.[562]) suggested that some early in utero effects on the hypothalamus caused fatness, while later starvation reduced the number of the newborn's fat cells. Susser and Stein[674] further noted (as has been shown in rodents) that starvation in the third trimester had the maximal effect on newborn weight and neonatal mortality.

Smith[635] had studied the same Dutch perinatal data to demonstrate the apparent deleterious effects of starvation on fetal and neonatal wastage and suggested that spontaneous miscarriages and fetal deaths were increased. But when Stein and colleagues[661] restudied the total development picture, an entirely different interpretation became apparent. They offered several possible explanations for the apparent "beneficial" effects of starvation in utero (besides the obvious one that pregnancy diet makes no difference): (1) "Selective survival of the fittest" or that the malformed ill and pooly developed fetus dies in utero because of the stress of starvation, leaving only the "more fit" fetuses to survive; (2) that the postnatal learning in the periods from birth to military induction might have represented an overcompensation in care and teaching because it was known that the subjects had had poor fetal existence; (3) the

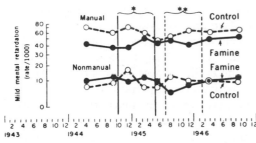
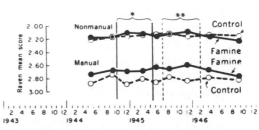

Fig. 2-1. Left: Rates of mild mental retardation in Dutch men examined at age 19, for manual and nonmanual classes according to father's occupation, by cohort of birth in famine and control cities. Solid vertical lines bracket period of famine, and broken vertical lines show the period of births conceived during famine. Right: Mean grouped scores on Raven progressive matrices test of Dutch men examined at age 19, for manual and nonmanual classes according to father's occupation, by cohort of birth in famine cities and control cities. Solid vertical lines bracket period of famine, and broken vertical lines show the period of births conceived during famine. (From Stein, Z., and Sussar, A.: *Science* **178:** 708, 1972. Reproduced with permission.)

possibility that the developing brain has sufficient reserve to overcome early dietary impairment. These unexpected results (Fig. 2-1) should have influenced American nutritional experts, but they have responded mostly by questioning the validity of the Dutch data.

Placental Transport

Robertson and Karp,[576] in a 1976 review of placental transport of nutrients, have concluded that the placental uptake of glucose and its transport to the fetus are primarily determined by maternal oxygen and glucose levels (Fig. 2-2). During maternal hypoxia in sheep, maternal glucose levels rose, but there was no similar rise in the fetus. With our fetal rabbit studies, we demonstrated a rise in blood sugars in hypoxic fetuses.[259] While such data are of interest in discussing fetal hypoxia responses (Chapter 8), it really is not relevant to the nonhypoxic fetuses. For the non-stressed fetus, the fetal blood levels of glucose are lower than but also depend on maternal values (Tables D-134).

Fetal sheep studies by the Battaglia group have challenged the dogma that glucose is the primary fetal fuel[302, 386]; lactate, amino acids, etc., may be equally important. From a clinical view, the fetal effects of maternal hypoglycemia are uncertain. Diabetic experts are convinced that repeated episodes of hypoglycemia in adults are sometimes associated with chronic brain syndrome and likewise view

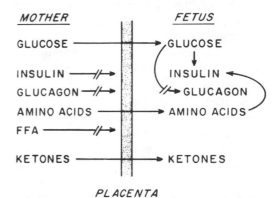

Fig. 2-2. Maternal–fetal fuel and hormone exchange. Glucose, amino acids, and ketones are transferred from mother to fetus while insulin, glucagon, and free fatty acids (FFA) are not. Glucose in the fetal circulation stimulates secretion of insulin and inhibits secretion of glucagon by fetal islet cells. Amino acids are also potent stimuli of fetal insulin secretion. (From *Med Clin North Am*, 1977. Reproduced with permission.)

any episode of maternal hypoglycemia as detrimental to fetal brain development. Meyer[472] reviewed the literature concerning fetal outcome of psychiatric patients treated with insulin shock and concluded that hypoglycemia occurring after 10 weeks gestation had no influence on fetal development, but that such hypoglycemia prior to 10 weeks invariably induced severe malformations and in some cases induced abortions. However, gravida with insulinomas[587] have normal children. In rodents[98] prolonged maternal hypoglycemia is associated with fetal brain damage, but not in fetal lambs.[459] I believe the fear of maternal hypoglycemia is exaggerated, as does White,[746] and that the evidence is overwhelming for close control of blood sugars in the pregnant diabetic, despite an occasional episode of hypoglycemia.

Insulin apparently does not cross the placenta and at the same time, it seemingly is hydrolyzed by placental activity. In the years 1959–1960, while at the University of Minnesota, I cared for five gravida with known anencephalic fetuses. After what was an appropriate explanation, permission, and preparation for those times, labors were induced and the umbilical cord prolapsed. In three cases, radioactive insulin was injected into the umbilical artery and the fetuses remained alive with "good" heart rates. Appropriate sampling from the maternal veins showed that the radioactive marker had been separated from the insulin and that only the marker itself had crossed the placenta. In two other patients, the radioactive insulin was injected into the mother. Again only the marker crossed and, furthermore, the insulin circulating in the maternal blood likewise was separated from its marker. This separation of the insulin and its marker did not occur when radioactive insulin was injected into the maternal vein immediately after the placenta was delivered. This concept of the placenta "destroying" insulin has made sense to me. Pregnancy in diabetics and nondiabetics is associated with increased maternal insulin production, and often even the most severe insulin-dependent diabetics do not require any insulin supplement in the immediate postpartum period, for presumably the increased insulin production lingers into the immediate postpartum period. The concept of placental transfer is shown in Figure 2-1.

Amino acid movement across the placenta is usually an active transport, for the fetal–maternal ratio is above 1.0 for most amino acids. However, the rate of placental transport at term of palmitic and linoleic acids accounts for only about 20% of the fetal fatty acid deposition. In times of stress, the fetus may derive energy from fatty acid catabolism and by oxidation of amino acids.

Ketones readily cross the placenta and 10% of the fetal calorie needs are supplied by ketone bodies. These sources of energy may be particularly important to the fetal brain. This may explain the newborn's (and fetus's) apparent well-being during severe hypoglycemia.

Maternal Blood Volume

As noted elsewhere (Chapter 3), increase in maternal blood volume is one of the most important changes that occurs during pregnancy and can be measured as early as the 10th week of pregnancy. Zangemeister[767] described the significance of reduced blood volume in toxemia. Even in normal pregnancies, Gibson[227] found an inverse relationship between lowest hemoglobin concentration and newborn weight. In our experience, a reduced maternal blood volume is an unfavorable sign for the fetus and its mother, as it indicates a risk of premature labor or of growth retardation for the fetus and toxemia for the mother (Chapter 3). Our experience further suggests that such a fetus of a toxemic gravida with reduced expansion of her blood volume can be salvaged only by delivery or by expanding the mother's blood volume.

Assuming that an expanded blood volume is of such importance, it would seem logical that prophylaxis for increased blood volume should begin early in pregnancy. These include (1) a high-protein diet to assure adequate serum proteins, (2) excess fluid intake—to approximately 3 or 4 liters of fluid per day—and (3) frequent rest in the horizontal lateral position. Like many recommendations concerning diet in human pregnancy, it is difficult to prove the value of these prophylactic procedures, even though both renal and uterine blood flow are improved by the lateral horizontal position. Dieckmann[157] demonstrated more than 50 years ago that excessive fluid intake expanded blood volume in women with EPH gestosis and served as a diuretic. An attempt at proving the value of such a prophylactic plan was that of Atkinson[123] who reported (as have many others with a wide variety of other recommendations) a reduced incidence of EPH gestosis.

Iron Therapy

Associated with the marked increase of blood volume during pregnancy is a fall in the maternal hemoglobin concentration. Despite this decline of the hemoglobin concentration, the hemoglobin oxygen carrying capacity actually increases an average of 18% above the increased oxygen requirements of pregnancy (Hytten and Leitch[367]), because the maternal red cell mass increases but at a slower rate than does the blood volume, as indicated in Figure 2-3. As has been demonstrated again and again, this discrepancy between increase in blood volume and red cell mass is greatest in the early third trimester, but usually is fairly well compensated at term. The "calculated need" of increased iron is clinically inadequate to prevent a fall in the hematocrit at term in most pregnant women. Instead of 6–7 mg/day, 120–240 mg/day of elementary iron are often required in order to maintain a normal hematocrit throughout pregnancy. Hytten and Leitch[367] suggest that such large amounts of iron may actually have a stimulatory effect upon erythropoiesis.

Since iron therapy corrects to a degree the physiologic decrease in hematocrit seen in normal pregnancy, it has been standard procedure in American obstetrics to recommend iron therapy for all pregnant women. No one has really addressed the problem as to whether such iron therapy can be detrimental. Maternal deaths have occurred from the administration of either intramuscular or intravenous iron (Battle and Miller[40]) and the iron pills themselves are well known to cause gastrointestinal upset. A more serious concern, however, is childhood iron poisoning with its associated intestinal scarring and death. Iron is the fifth leading cause of poisoning deaths of children in the United States (Battle and Miller[40]). In my experience, two children have died in the hospital where I was serving because of ingestion of their mothers' prenatal iron supply. I have attempted to find a reported study which demonstrates unequivocally that maternal iron therapy has saved either maternal or fetal lives in apparently normal pregnancies. As was to be expected, I could find no such report, nor were the members of the Committee on Nutrition for the American College of Obstetrics and Gynecology able to supply references for this type of study.[278, 544]

Pritchard has found that 4% of gravida in midpregnancy with normal iron stores had hemoglobin values less than 10 g%.[550] Additional studies by Lawrence[425] and by Liley[442] agreed with Pritchard's findings. The obvious explanation is that such gravida have adequately expanded their red cell volumes to a normal degree, but have expanded their

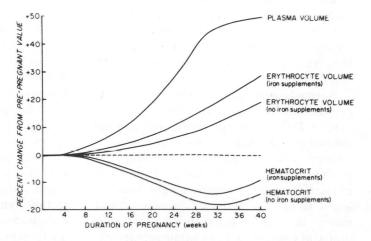

Fig. 2-3. Change in maternal plasma and erythrocyte volume and hematocrit during pregnancy. (From Pitkin, R.M.: *Clin Obstet Gynecol.* Reproduced with permission.)

blood volumes even more markedly. Presumably, those women with the greatest blood volumes would be providing a more optimal *in utero* environment, despite their decreased hemoglobin concentration.

Whether the fall in hematocrit, which is commonly seen in pregnant women between their 28th and 32nd week, requires therapy is argumentative. In America, however (ACOG Committee[1]), reduced hemoglobin concentrations are considered as "anemia" and a disease requiring some form of therapy. Elsewhere, the temporary decrease in hemoglobin concentration in women in their late midtrimester is often accepted as a normal physiologic phenomenon (Hytten and Leitch[367]). Indeed, within limits, we have argued that a gravida who fails to demonstrate a falling hemoglobin concentration is at increased risk of preeclampsia (EPH gestosis) owing to probable failure to increase her blood volume (Chapter 3).

VITAMINS

Specific dietary deficiencies are difficult to study in humans. Pregnant-rat studies indicate that deficiencies of vitamin A cause multiple anomalies,[731] insufficient amounts of folic acid causes throat abnormalities,[341] deficiencies of pantothenic acid causes exencephaly,[452] shortage of riboflavin causes cleft palate,[229] and so forth. But it is zinc deficiency which should frighten us all as it produces severe and multiple fetal anomalies.[365] While such laboratory observations are useful in providing clues as to the etiology of various abnormalities, unless we are concerned about pregnant rats, they probably have limited clinical application.

Normally, in pregnant women, lower levels of vitamins B_6, B_{12}, and folate are found (Tables D-207). As with serum iron and hemoglobin concentration, whether decreased vitamin levels are detrimental to either the mother or the fetus is debatable. Blood levels of vitamins in the newborns are 2–6 times the blood levels of vitamins of the mother, and except in cases of malnutrition, it remains doubtful whether routine vitamin supplementation is indicated during pregnancy. However, American women expect to be given vitamin supplementation during their pregnancy. Unfortunately, sometimes when they are not feeling well, they will double or triple their daily dose of vitamin pills, thinking that "if a little bit of vitamins is helpful, a great deal of vitamins would be truly beneficial." In laboratory animals, excesive vitamin intake has been found to be detrimental. In humans there are specific syndromes suggested in newborns of mothers who have ingested excessive vitamins. Vitamin D may produce "supravalvular syndrome,"[707] and excessive vitamin C intake can cause vitamin C dependency in the infant. However, having dealt with many pregnant women who believed in the megavitamin cult, I can only conclude that the newborn risks of such excessive maternal vitamin therapy must be low, as we have failed to recognize any particular problem with the newborn of such mothers.

There is abundant evidence that maternal folate requirements are increased during pregnancy. The British[342] have had more concern about folic acid deficiency during pregnancy in the past than we Americans, and have ascribed anemias and even abruptio placenta to it. While Americans, with all of their vitamin studies, have been unable to substantiate the need for additional vitamins during pregnancy,[502] there is worldwide agreement that if any vitamin deficiency exists in apparently normal pregnant women, it would most likely be folic acid deficiency.

The newborn of a poorly controlled diabetic often looks not unlike the newborn of the mother with severe vitamin B_6 deficiency (beriberi). For these fetal indications, a few obstetrical clinics began in the 1940s to add extra B_6 supplements to the diets of their pregnant diabetics. However, the appearance of newborn seizures in infants born of mothers with supplemental pyridoxine discouraged this practice. The additional B_6 was of questionable benefit to newborns of diabetic mothers, and the seizure of the newborns of diabetic mothers was an unacceptable risk for the therapy.

Recently, Spellacy,[656] in this country, and Bennink and Schreurs,[43] in England, have again raised the issue of pyridoxine supplementation during the pregnancy of a diabetic woman. Spellacy found that pharmacological doses of pyridoxine (100 mg/day vitamin B_6 for 2 weeks) improved the intravenous glucose tolerance curves of pregnant women with gestational diabetics. During pregnancy, the insulin levels are in excess of nonpregnant states, and a relative pyridoxine deficiency has been offered as an explanation for this "insulin resistance" of pregnancy. Apparently xanthurenic acid (which may increase during the vitamin B_6 deficiency) binds to insulin and reduces its biologic activity. We have delivered three women in whom pyridoxine apparently converted their antenatal abnormal glucose tolerance test to "normal." However, all delivered newborns weighed more than 4500 g.

GENERAL COMMENTS

Present nutritional standards for humans are to a large degree based on studies of nutritional requirements in rodents. Similarly, much of the nutritional information used in clinical obstetrics has come from laboratory study of rodents. Rodents are excellent laboratory subjects for studying such problems as immunogenetics, but I submit that even when pregnant, they are inappropriate for determining the nutritional requirements of human pregnancy. In mice, the rate of fetal growth is tremendous as compared with the human since a litter of fetal mice is a much greater fraction of the pregnant mother's weight than is the human fetus. A few days starvation is disastrous in a mouse and indeed, Cockburn[110] has estimated that 2 days starvation in pregnant mice is equivalent to a month's starvation in pregnant humans. In addition, pregnant mice will resorb their fetuses without apparent cause or even abort them if frightened or placed in strange surroundings.

Differences between mice and humans frequently are ignored in our nutritional literature. By contrast, no one attempts to apply to humans data from the pregnant American brown bear, which as noted by Cahill,[84] hibernates throughout her entire pregnancy and bears healthy, vigorous newborns. Though hibernation is not the same as malnutrition, this difference between the pregnant brown bear and humans is less than those between pregnant rodents and humans. Application of nutritional data from pregnant mice to pregnant women seems inappropriate owing to differences between the two with respect to fetal weight, effects of starvation, and tendencies toward resorption and abortion of fetuses.

Nutritionists in America have also sought to interpolate from populations with poor diets and dreadful socioeconomic surroundings to the American pregnant women. The studies of the poor pregnant women of Guatemala or Eastern Africa are, of course, important, but to compare and interpret the outcome of their children who are subjected to both a deprived *in utero* environment and often a dreadful *extra utero* environment with American gravida who have only poor diets seems especially inappropriate.[183] The circumstances which allowed Stein and her colleagues[661] to study Dutch women and their children in World War II in a controlled manner were unique and hopefully will never occur again. This one of a kind study described the *absence* of the expected harmful effects of poor *in utero* nutrition, and the study should surely be given more attention than it has received to date. It does seem that the deprived human *in utero* can be adequately compensated with optimal childhood care. This comment is not meant to imply that pregnant women should be starved or subjected to any sort of unfavorable conditions, but rather to suggest that improvements of the American pregnant women's diet by itself will not bring about the better newborn outcome that many nutritionists would have us expect.

In pregnant guinea pigs, Crawford and colleagues[126] from the Nuffield Institute demonstrated that the placenta and fetus radically modify the maternal phospholipids. They found a high proportion of C20 and C22 polyunsaturated fatty acids in the lipids of the developing fetal brain. They point out the obvious—that we are ignorant of many things. Since we lack information on the fetal metabolism of what is quantitatively the most important structural group in the brain cell, about which we have much less data than about other fetal nutrients, it is inevitable that discussion of fetal nutrition will remain incomplete.

Whether "bigness" of newborns is "better" is another unanswered question. Churchill's[104] data from twin studies would indicate that there is some virtue in being a large newborn for one's future development. Neel[503] has proposed that the genetic selective advantage of diabetes mellitus is that such women produce larger newborns with greater survival and fitness. While the virtues of bigness at birth remains somewhat theoretical, there are disadvantages to large size which seem rather obvious. On our service, with the abandonment of caloric restrictions during pregnancy, the incidence of shoulder dystocia associated with fetal macrosomia has increased markedly. This is not to be dismissed lightly, for many of these infants bear permanent neurological damage from brachial plexus damage. Another problem of bigness at birth as noted by Pockett and Cole[534] is its positive correlation with future fatness. Considering the advantages of leanness in adult life, a fat newborn may suffer subsequent detrimental effects from his obesity.

Worldwide, supplemental diets are recommended for pregnant women although the evidence to support their use is meager.[395, 519] In clinically malnourished gravidas such as apparently occurs in Guatemala and in our ghettos, added calories and proteins[307, 427] are of obvious advantage to the mother and her fetus. However, in a well-nourished population, there is no evidence to date that increasing maternal caloric and protein intake is of any particular advantage to the fetus.[183, 235] This is particularly true in the otherwise normal gravida who fails to gain weight in her third trimester. To suggest an added caloric intake to such a woman may be analogous to administering estrogen to those gravida with declining serum estriols. How a normal fetus and its placenta "signals" its mother to gain weight, increase her blood volume, seek rest, and so forth, remains unclear. The message for these actions is obviously much more than simply elevated serum estrogen and progesterone. If a gravida has failed to gain weight in the latter portions of her pregnancy, it may be the "pregnancy" itself which is "sick," with the fetus dysmature, and actually suffering some chronic distress. Several times we have instructed our prenatal patients about their need to gain weight and increase rest when actually what we should have been doing was carefully assessing the health of their fetus. With impressive frequency (in about one-fourth of our dysmature fetuses), the only clue we had to the diagnosis of a dysmature fetus was that the gravida failed to gain the expected amount of weight during the third trimester. Likewise, Elder et al.,[185] from London, reported that maternal weight gain was significantly less in gravida delivering dysmature infants than in those of the control group.

Nutrition during pregnancy is obviously important, but pretending that our inadequate knowledge will solve our present problems in obstetrics serves no useful purpose. Rather than present only an iconoclastic view, it should be noted that the Churchill et al.[106] and Stehbens et al.[659] studies of pregnant diabetics suggest that even a brief period of starvation ketosis may have a deleterious effect the fetus's subsequent intellectual development. Presumably, abrupt curtailment of energy supplies to fetuses of all pregnancies, diabetic or not, should always be avoided.

Susser and Stein[675] described a prenatal project in 1000 black women in New York City of supplementing, or complimenting their diets. They found no benefit of added protein, indeed there occurred a higher rate of premature and of growth-retarded fetuses. They suggest that the previously reported benefits of supplementation during pregnancy may be on the affective state and activity of a malnourished mother.

Case No. 2-1

A 21-year-old para 0-0-0-0 gravida was seen at approximately her 20th week of pregnancy. She was one of identical twins, both of whom had a diagnosis of anorexia nervosa and both claimed to have had no menses for approximately 3 years duration. Both she and her sister had weighed as much as 130 lbs., but now weighed approximately 90 lbs., were 5 ft. 6 in. tall, and appeared thin and emaciated. The patient was unable to estimate her length of gestation as she denied the possibility of pregnancy. She continued to do very poorly, refusing therapy and requiring frequent hospitalization for malnutrition. During these times she was given intravenous nutritional support (although the technique was inadequate), tranquilization, sedation, and other psychiatric medications. The patient continued on a downhill course and when thought to be about 36 weeks gestation, was delivered by cesarean section of an 1840-g, apparently growth retarded, male fetus. The patient, at the time of her cesarean section, weighed 81 lbs. She was eventually discharged from the hospital but committed suicide 2 years later. (Her twin sister, by contrast, recovered and subsequently had two normal pregnancies.) Arrangements were made for private adoption of the infant and while its first 6 months of life were somewhat stormy, reports when he was 11 years of age were that he was "an excellent student, and above average athlete." His adoptive parents insisted that his overall performance was above average and that he was the "best" of their three adopted children.

Thus, it may be possible to overcome a very deprived *in utero* environment.

Another Point of View

One of the leading nutritional authorities in America, Roy M. Pitkin of the University of Iowa, has stated the obvious when he notes that increased amounts of all nutrients are required during pregnancy. He further suggests that the underweight gravida faces the risk of delivering the low-birth-weight infant, while the overweight gravida faces the risks of hypertension and diabetes mellitus. Dr. Pitkin believes that birth weight is a crude index of fetal development, though he does not provide limits for the ideal birth weight. Also unclear from his discussion is whether he believes that the macrosomic infant of the uncontrolled diabetic mother is really better ''developed'' than the small newborn of a healthy, highly motivated woman who refuses to let herself gain weight during her pregnancy.

As a member of the Committee on Nutrition of the American College of Obstetricians and Gynecologists, it is not unexpected that Dr. Pitkin quote the committee's recommendations that the average and probably optimal weight gain during pregnancy is 10–12 kg. This weight gain is nearly linear from the beginning of the second trimester to term, and averages approximately 0.4 kg a week. Dr. Pitkin's diagram of the components of this weight gain during pregnancy (Fig. 2–4) indicates that the mother con-

Fig. 2-4. Pattern and components of maternal weight gain during pregnancy. (From Pitkin, R.M.: *Clin Obstet Gynecol.* Reproduced with permission.)

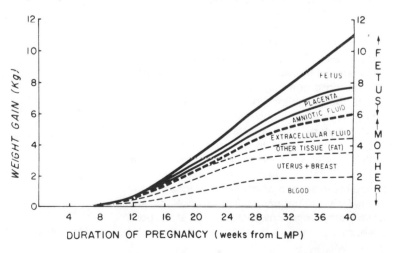

tributes slightly more than half of the gain. It is obvious that in early pregnancy the significant weight gain is maternal, while in the third trimester, the gain is mostly fetal.

A helpful feature of Dr. Pitkin's article is that he presents definitions which allow us to categorize various pregnant patients. The "underweight" has been defined as a prepregnant weight of 10% or more below the ideal weight for height and age, while "overweight" applies to a prepregnant weight of 20% or more above the ideal. "Excessive weight gain" during pregnancy is defined as 3 kg or more per month, while "inadequate weight gain" is defined as 1 kg or less per month. (Again, it is unclear whether inadequate weight gains are the cause, or the result, of a sick pregnancy.)

ENERGY

The total added energy needs of the average pregnancy is, according to Emerson et al.,[188a] approximately 28,000 kcal. As the pregnant woman gains additional weight as term approaches, it is only logical that her energy needs increase. An obvious exception to this would be if pregnant women restricted their physical activity in the third trimester, a possibility which is not usually recommended to the normal American gravida, but is common in other cultures.

PROTEIN

Protein requirements have been variously estimated at 11–15 g/day to as high as 30 g/day. As noted, caloric intake must be adequate or proteins are simply used as a source of energy in the pregnant woman.

Attempts at active intervention with dietary supplements have failed to show benefits except in cases of true malnutrition.[519] However, Aubry[26] of New York believes that the maternal urinary ratio of urea nitrogen to total urea (UN/TN) is useful in evaluating the adequacy of any diet during pregnancy. When this index is low (<60), the pregnancy has a negative nitrogen ratio, providing a technique for logical application of dietary supplementation. In the past, it has been impossible to design an ethical controlled study which would test the effects on gravida of caloric restrictions or excessive caloric diets in women who, prior to pregnancy are normal weight, underweight, or overweight. Aubry's method may now make such a study possible.

CALCIUM

The recommended daily intake of calcium for nonpregnant women is 800 mg, yet the majority of the world receives less than this amount. In calcium-deficient areas, the mothers produce normal babies that have normal skeletons and teeth. (The obvious exception, of course, are those deprived populations with osteomalacia, which fortunately appears to be a disease of the past.) Nevertheless, it is recommended that pregnant women receive an additional 50% increase of calcium, or 1200 mg/day. Pitkin's[533a] extensive review of calcium metabolism during pregnancy should be required reading for all.

We have argued against iron and milk recommendations for all pregnant women, as previously noted—against iron because of the associated risk of poison in children and gastrointestinal upset, and against milk because of the widespread lactose intolerance in most nonwhite women. It is obvious that such arguments are an exaggerated concern and are made only to emphasize the need for individualization of prenatal care. Without exception, every discussion of optimal prenatal care in both medical and lay journals recommends routine iron therapy and extra milk intake.

There are those who write as if they believe that certain diets will solve our perinatal problems. Brewer[73,74] and his associated organization preach that (contrary to the Swedish and Dutch studies) chronic fetal distress, fetal dysmaturity, and so forth are solely the result of poor maternal nutrition. Others, perhaps failing to separate poor maternal environment from cases with both poor maternal and childhood environments, have tended to support his thesis.[158,500,760] If the malnourished fetal brain given adequate infant nutrition is unable to rebound after birth, then our belief in infant compensation for inadequate *in utero* environment is in error. Indeed, the Guatemalean studies have indicated that caloric and protein supplement during pregnancy can perhaps break the dreadful cycle of the underprivileged begetting underprivileged. Naeye et al.,[500] after reviewing abruptio placenta in the collaborative project, suggest that poor maternal nutritional may contribute to the "genesis of the abruptio placenta."

VITAMINS

The views on the need of folic acid supplementation during pregnancy have taken a transatlantic switch. Recent British studies[313] suggest that despite a decrease in serum folate concentration during pregnancy, there is no decrease in total serum folate during normal singleton or in twin pregnancy. The decrease in serum levels apparently reflect the normal blood volume expansion of pregnancy. Repeated British studies[313] also suggest that women with low serum folate concentrations do not suffer more often from such complications as congenital malformations of the fetus or abruptio. Folic acid supplementation is therefore no longer recommended during pregnancy for British women.

In America, however, Kitay[405] apparently now believes that folic acid deficiency is associated with serious reproductive problems, although he concludes his argument by stating that "folic acid deficiency in pregnancy is an easily determined sign of inadequate nutrition rather than the cause of a number of casualties in gestation."

Knutzen and Davey[410] have suggested that female nutrition in childhood is an important determinant of subsequent perinatal mortality rates. Maternal height is the best indicator of childhood nutrition. These South African investigators found that short women had a higher perinatal mortality than those of medium height and double the perinatal mortality of the tall group.

Current concepts in nutrition during pregnancy have been reviewed by Howard Jacobson[371a] of the New Jersey–Rutger's Medical School. He notes that pregnant women synthesize new tissue at a rate greater than at any time during their lives, and their balance studies have shown that the observed nitrogen retention markedly exceeds the amounts predicted, and furthermore, that the efficiency of protein utilization is lower than has been assumed. These findings have resulted in the recommendations for an additional 30 g/day protein for healthy women. Jacobson further discusses the difficulties of any evaluation of supplementary diets during pregnancy but does state that the positive effects of the (WIC) program on prenatal care for low-income women can hardly be overestimated. He fails to delineate what these positive effects are.

And finally, the California Department of Health[88] has instructed physicians that marked caloric restriction in even the obese pregnant woman is potentially harmful for the fetus. They suggest that caloric intake during pregnancy for obese gravida should be adequate to support a progressive weight gain of at least 24 lbs. They do admit that there is a paucity of information in this area and that obese gravida face increased risks.

CHAPTER 3

EPH Gestosis

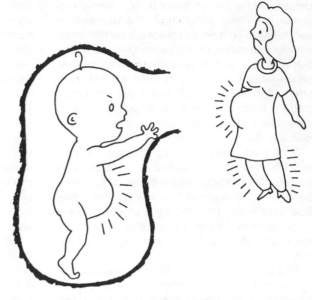

Historical

Many American texts suggest that eclampsia was known to the early civilizations, but Chesley states otherwise. Chesley[101] suggests that the European literature on eclampsia began in the 17th century in France, because it was there that male physicians first began to practice obstetrics. Considering how dramatic is the gravida with eclampsia, it is difficult to understand how the older and ancient writers missed such happenings. (It is tempting to believe that, like syphilis, it was imported into Europe by Columbus' crew from the New World during the 16th century, if its very nature did not render such a concept ridiculous.) The famous French obstetrician Mauriceau (1694) gave considerable attention to eclampsia among his many writings. Mauriceau apparently believed that the fetus was in some way responsible for eclampsia. Bossier De Sauvages, a Frenchman, first introduced the term "eclampsia" in 1793. He stated that the term originated with Hippocrates, although Chesley was unable to confirm his impression. De Sauvages did distinguish between epilepsy and eclampsia, but it is only during the last generation that "eclampsia" has been accepted as having a pure obstetrical etiology.

While the occurrence of eclampsia is dramatic, so is the appearance of massive edema which likewise evoked little mention in the older literature. In what now seems to have been an astute observation, De la Motte (1726) considered edema to be benign unless associated with convulsions. However, Zangemeister[767a] emphasized the association between edema, weight gain, and preeclampsia. This association suggested to many physicians that weight gain should be restricted during pregnancy, and the concept was so convincingly presented that a number of American obstetricians as late as 1933 (Cummings) were recommending antenatal purges with Epsom salts three times weekly. Dieckmann[157] likewise was overly concerned about excess prenatal weight gain and edema and their relationship to the development of EPH gestosis (preeclampsia). He was distressed that only one-third of his pregnant patients followed his request to limit their weight gain during their last 6 months to 200 g/week.

A truly significant contribution in our understanding of EPH gestosis was made by

Hytten and Thomson[368a] when they reported that a substantial proportion of pregnant women without other signs of preeclampsia have edema. They found that infants born to mothers with edema were heavier (and presumably more "healthy") than those without edema (Fig. 3-1). They concluded that minor degrees of generalized edema in healthy and pregnant women was normal, owing in part to increased serum estrogen levels. This excess water is often bound to connective tissue ground substance (skin, breasts, uterus, etc.) and is *not* accessible to the kidney or diuretic agents. (Women with EPH gestosis, of course, often have pathological amounts of edema.) They demonstrated further that most women who gain above the average are not destined to develop preeclampsia.

Lever (1843) is credited with the discovery of proteinuria in eclampsia. He is quoted[698] as saying, "In NO cases have I detected albumen, except in those in which there have been convulsions, or in which symptoms have presented themselves, and which are readily recognized as the precursors of puerperal fits." Simpson (1842) also noted the presence of proteinuria, but one of his fatal cases also had chronic nephritis, leading him to believe that eclampsia was a manifestation of Bright's disease.[101]

The indirect method of measurement of blood pressure did not become available until 1875 and Vaquez and Nobecourt (1897) are generally credited with the description of eclamptic hypertension.[101]

Dieckmann[157] states that prior to 1926, preeclampsia, eclampsia, nephritic toxemia, and chronic nephritis were confused and credits De Snoo, Stieglitz, Corwin, and Herrick with demonstrating that chronic renal disease was rare and that the persistence of hypertension reflected instead the presence of essential hypertension.

Smith (1849), according to Chesley, was the first with the concept of eclampsia as resulting from a toxin. The concept was so widely accepted that Williams, professor of obstetrics at Johns Hopkins University, suggested in 1912 (Williams' *Obstetrics*, 3rd ed.) that investigators should look for toxins specific for each of the many disorders of toxemia (i.e., acute yellow atrophy of the liver, pernicious vomiting, eclampsia, and so forth).

Magnesium sulfate was reported by Blackfan and Hamilton[57] to lower blood pressure and promote urinary output. The Johns Hop-

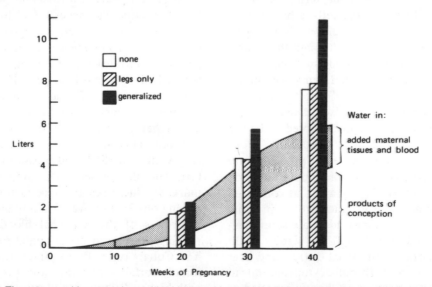

Fig. 3-1. The measured increase in total body water (deuterium space) in three groups shown as vertical bars against the amount of water estimated to be accumulated in the products of conception and added maternal tissue. (From Hytten, F.E.: In *Hypertension in Pregnancy*, M.R. Lindheimer, A. Katz, and F. Zuspan, Eds. Wiley, New York, 1976. Reproduced with permission.)

kins school was then to recommend it in large doses to prevent convulsions, following Lazard[425a] and Dieckmann's[156a] suggestions. Another important paper was by Pritchard and Pritchard[554] who reported 154 cases of eclampsia without a single maternal death, using magnesium sulfate and hydralazine.

The Problem

"Toxemia of pregnancy" is a term and concept which many American academicians find objectionable, for despite much effort on their part, no "toxin" has ever been demonstrated in toxemic gravida. To me, toxemia and preeclampsia continue to be useful terms for several reasons. First of all, I am not embarrassed for having failed to find a "toxin." The toxin concept could still explain the thrombocytopenia which occurs frequently in the white gravida with severe EPH gestosis (in the absence of other disorders of coagulation) and the thrombocytopenia of their newborns.

Second, there are many terms in medicine whose original meaning has changed or actually come to mean the opposite of what its originators intended. For the semantic purist, hematologists still use the term "anemia," although absence of red cells is hardly ever seen in any clinical condition. Pathologists use the term "autopsy," although the examination is hardly a "self-examination."

The third reason that I think we should retain the terms "toxemia" and "preeclampsia" is that the entire malady is one of great confusion and is repeatedly noted to be the "disease of many theories." "Toxemia" probably includes several different processes and in my experience, its manifestations are often very different in white gravida as compared with the black. For instance, we see in white gravida seizures despite adequate serum levels of $MgSO_4$ (of 4 mg% or higher), right upper quadrant abdominal distress and liver dysfunction, and thrombocytopenia all in much greater proportion than is reported to occur in black gravidas. Be that as it may, the terms "toxemia" and "preeclampsia" are now passé, and I have adopted the term "EPH

gestosis" as used in the European literature mainly because I consider the term "pregnancy-induced hypertension," as preferred by some American authorities, to be inadequate and severely limiting.

THE SIGNIFICANCE OF BLOOD PRESSURE

Friedman and Neff[211] have completed an exhaustive analysis of the hypertensive disorders of pregnancy as related to fetal and neonatal outcome, using the data from some 59,000 pregnancies of the "Collaborative Project." The investigators suggest that their study indicates that an entirely new prospective should be taken on those maternal parameters associated with perinatal loss. They found that "toxemia" was a major cause of prematurity, stillborns, neonatal deaths, and leave the reader with the feeling that if we had a cure for "toxemia," much of the fetologist's work would disappear. This belief, of course, is reminiscent of the American obstetricians of the 1920s and 1930s who likewise believed that toxemia was the single greatest problem for obstetricians, and the topic was the center of most obstetrical academicians' pursuits for nearly an entire generation. The etiology and cure for toxemia was never found, a name was never found for the cornerstone of the Chicago Lying-In Hospital (Fig. 3-2), yet its incidence decreased and our perinatal mortality rates have improved spectacularly during that time period.

Friedman and Neff found that any maternal diastolic pressure recording above 85 torr places her fetus at increased risk of being stillborn. This risk factor is increased markedly with diastolic blood pressures above 95 torr, and the presence of proteinuria also markedly increases the risk factor. (A surprising observation was that any proteinuria, regardless of the maternal blood pressure readings, increased the perinatal risk factor.) The Collaborative Project indicates that perinatal mortality rate increases progressively with higher diastolic blood pressures and degrees of proteinuria.

The studies from Friedman and Neff are important for they suggest that we obstetri-

Fig. 3-2. Photograph of the "cornerstone" at the University of Chicago demonstrating the blank stone for the discoverer of the etiology of toxemia. The other stones are named for Palfyn (1650–1730), Van de Venter (1651–1724), Smellie (1697–1763), and Porro (1842–1902).

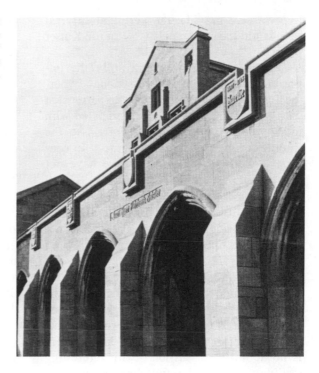

cians should be more concerned about even slight elevations of blood pressures and any protein in the urine when we consider fetal outcome. A problem with having such information is the probability of labeling a large percentage of pregnancies with normal outcomes as "high risk," which appears to defeat the purpose of such a category. Presumably the reasons for establishing categories for high-risk patients is to alert the fetologist (and neonatologist) that various types of interference (including their associated risks) may be necessary in these pregnancies which would otherwise be hazardous in normal gravida. The "high-risk" category has become so meaningless on our service that we instead identify the "low-risk" gravida (Goodwin score of 1 or less), and simply see all "non-low-risk" gravida in a special clinic. The only disadvantage of this type of classification has been in the public relations aspect for we have lost our claim for caring for mostly "high-risk" gravida.

An analysis of pregnancy-related hypertension which appears to me to be much more compatible with clinical experience (than that

of the Collaborative Project) is that of Page and Christianson.[522] These investigators studied the records of approximately 13,000 gravida who were registered with the Kaiser program in Northern California. These authors reasoned that since blood pressure is traditionally lowest in the midtrimester, blood pressure determinations at this time would most accurately reflect the patient's basic values. They found, as did those with the Collaborative Project, an amazingly low maternal blood pressure which appeared to be critical for fetal prognosis. The *mean* blood pressure that Page and Christianson labeled critical was 92 torr, which could correspond to a blood pressure as low as 125/75 torr. However, this low critical level meant that 13% of all white gravida and 18% of all black pregnant patients would be included in this group of "increased fetal risk." Yet the differences in pregnancy outcomes of those gravidas whose pressures were below and above this level were perinatal survival of 98.4% versus 97.3%. Even if we obstetricians had the techniques and the knowledge to give a 100% effective rate of intervention in these hypertensive gravida, the perinatal survival rate would have risen only 0.5% in the Kaiser program.

Page and Christianson did make the important observation that gestational hypertension (pregnancy-induced hypertension with no proteinuria) was not associated with increased perinatal loss, in contrast to the findings of the Collaborative Project. In contrast to both of these studies, we have not considered proteinuria of less than 2+ (100 g or more per 24 hr) to be significant.

One feature of the Collaborative Project that was intriguing was that maternal hypotension (diastolic blood pressures below 65 torr) was also associated with increased perinatal loss. Since elevated blood pressures were found to be related to obesity in the Collaborative Project, one might presume that decreased blood pressures would reflect underweight or malnutrition, although there is no definitive discussion of this interesting finding. The Collaborative Project also suggested that increased weight gain in gravida "at risk because of hypertension" did not improve the fetal outcome regardless of the prior pregnancy weight.

What the practising obstetrician or fetologist needs is a controlled study of women at risk and offered various modalities of treatment. The English experience (Redman et al.[563]) suggests that even the gravida with severe hypertension, if carefully managed with hypotensive agents, bed rest, and so forth, is associated with perinatal mortality rates that are far from hopeless. And in Dallas, the University of Texas group (Hauth et al.[323]) has shown that hospitalization with only restricted physical activity apparently provides excellent treatment for those women with EPH gestosis. The Collaborative Project indicated (in contrast to the British experience) that hypotensive agents, diuretics, and even apparently active intervention in pregnancies did not necessarily improve perinatal rates. Assuming that the Collaborative Project and the Kaiser Project are correct in ascribing to even minor elevations of blood pressure a significant role in perinatal loss,

we need information on which therapeutic modalities, if any, will bring about decreased perinatal mortality rates in these "mildly" hypertensive gravida.

ETIOLOGY

In the English literature alone, there are several recent treatises on the pathophysiology of EPH gestosis (preeclampsia),[99, 211, 448, 652] as well as repeated discussions of the concepts of Brain and associates[67] on the associated microangiopathic disorders and those of McKay on disseminated intravascular coagulation.[497] Given this large body of medical literature, it is easy to derive many concepts for the responsible mechanisms for all of the abnormalities seen in severe preeclampsia. As shown in Figure 3-3, my proposed sequence of development for the symptoms of many cases of severe preeclampsia begins with the failure of the gravida to appropriately increase her blood volume commensurate with the increase in the size of her uterus. Most gravida begin to increase their blood volume by the 10th week of pregnancy, but as was shown by Blekta,[59] women destined to have "preeclampsia" may not appropriately increase their blood volume. I make the analogy of such hypovolemic cases to chronic shock, which then leads to generalized vasoconstriction. This latter case is responsible for the disorders of vital organs such as the kidneys, placenta, and liver. If a significant increase in mean blood pressure occurs in these women, blood flow to these vital organs is at least partially maintained and the patient's symptoms are related chiefly to her hypertension. On the other hand, if the degree of hypertension is inadequate, then the significant organ dysfunction becomes obvious. The gravida with severe EPH gestosis can then present with symptoms which may be attributed to her liver, intestinal tract, placenta, kidneys, or eyes, resulting in my concept of severe EPH gestosis being an imitator of other diseases.

While it is unlikely that after all these years of study and discussion any one parameter is

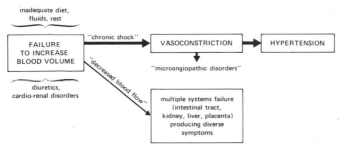

Fig. 3-3. Schematic diagram of proposed mechanisms of EPH gestosis. (From Goodlin, R.C.: Severe pre-eclampsia: Another great limitation. *Am J Obstet Gynecol* **125**: 747–753, 1976. Reproduced with permission.)

the "etiology of EPH gestosis," I believe that the failure to adequately increase blood volume in pregnancy is at least part of the fundamental problem of severe EPH gestosis. The vast majority of American investigators believe that the reduced blood volume is secondary to hypertension resulting from increased vascular reactivity to pressor substances.

Types "A" and "B" EPH Gestosis

There may be an important variant of severe EPH gestosis (severe preeclampsia) that on occasion is especially responsive to blood volume expansion. I refer specifically to the case with inappropriately high hematocrit and BUN, thrombocytopenia, multiple organ dysfunction, and other indicators of reduced blood volume. The following cases illustrate the subclassification (type B) of EPH gestosis, the spectrum of response to volume expansion, and the variety of manifestations of the disease process.

Ten white patients with severe hypertension, proteinuria, and edema were treated during a 14-month period at the Sacramento Medical Center. For the sake of discussion, the patients are divided into two groups (Table 3-I). Group A includes three young gravida who had eclampsia (fits) and were unregistered, while those in group B were referred from other hospitals and had received adequate prenatal care. They had evidence of multiple organ failure and were older than group A and frequently multigravida. The women in group B usually had elevated BUN (12–24 mg%), elevated uric acids (6–9 mg%), reduced creatinine clearance (<100), abnor-

TABLE 3-I. Clinical Profile of Groups A and B Severe EPH Gestosis at Time of Admission to Sacramento Medical Center

	Group "A" N = 3	Group "B" N = 8
Parity > 0	0	5/8
Age < 18 yrs	3/3	0
Gestation < 31 weeks	0	5/8
Hematocrit > 37%	2/3	8/8
Prior UTI	1/3	4/8
Reduced Cr/Cl	0	6/8
RUQ pain	0	7/8
Elevated SGOT	—	7/8
Ascites	0	3/8
Fits	3/3	0
Thrombocytopenia	0	8/8
Infant affected	0	6/8

mal liver function tests (SGOT 240–1000+ units), and thrombocytopenia (22,000–60,000 mm^3). Both groups of patients had elevated hematocrits (36–45%), normal fibrinogen and fibrin-split product studies.

Therapy consisted of intravenous MgSO$_4$ (serum levels 4.8–8 mg%), volume expansion with albumin, plasma or whole blood (to decrease hematocrit by 15%), and phenobarbital (to the point of drowsiness).

Table 3-I lists the differences in clinical profile between groups A and B. Group A includes only those gravida who convulsed despite intravenous MgSO$_4$. The major difference between groups A and B is that group B were older; their disease process began earlier in pregnancy and they were often multigravida. Indeed, one-fourth of group B had had similar disease processes in their first pregnancy. Despite this feature of recurrence, all "B" patients were apparently normal at the time of their 6-week postpartum visits, and therefore represent a form of EPH gestosis.

These cases suggest that there may be at least two separate disease processes within the group of EPH gestosis (severe preeclampsia). Those with eclampsia (group A) were typical of cases described in our textbooks: they had no prenatal care, minimal evidence of hemoconcentration or multiple organ failure, and their infants did well; volume expansion played only a minor role. On the other hand, those in group B had had adequate prenatal care, had evidence of liver dysfunction, renal dysfunction, and thrombocytopenia, and had appeared to especially benefit from blood volume expansion. These disease processes in group B gravida, which were often mirrored by their infants, suggests that there may indeed be a "toxin" which affects both mother and fetus in some types of "toxemia."[288]

We have used volume expansion in more than 150 gravida with both "A" and "B" EPH gestosis and when our protocols were followed, have yet to see a case in which the therapy appeared to have been deleterious. The volume expansion therapy apparently has reversed the disease process, allowing fetal maturity in approximately 10% of the gravida with B-type severe EPH gestosis. In the others, it seemingly improved their condition (blood pressure, thrombocytopenia, renal function) for a short time interval. Case 3-1 illustrates the value of volume expansion, as her disease process was reversed and she was able to carry the pregnancy an additional 7 weeks after being admitted to the hospital with signs of severe EPH gestosis. Our modern textbooks suggest that such therapy is of no value (Williams' *Obstetrics*, 15th ed.; Danforth's *Obstetrics*, 3rd ed.), and may even be hazardous.[82]

PATHOPHYSIOLOGY

Disorders of the coagulation system continue to be a controversial aspect of severe EPH gestosis. Normal pregnancy is characterized by decreased platelet count[730] and Pritchard[554] has recently revised his prior ob-

servations[552] that thrombocytopenia was common in women with the severe variety of this disease process. There are, however, multiple reports which suggest that severe EPH gestosis is associated with a relative thrombocytopenia and that perhaps the degree of the thrombocytopenia can be related to the degree of fetal growth retardation or illness.[623] In our own studies, we have found decreased fibrinogen levels and other evidence of DIC in only 2 out of 43 EPH gestosis cases with platelet counts below 70,000 mm^3. In animal studies, Whitaker *et al.*[747] showed that catecholamine shock produced microangiopathic anemia, which could be prevented by a vasodilator.

The hemoconcentration, thrombocytopenia, and multiple organ dysfunction are perhaps explained by the concept of chronic shock with vasoconstriction in the gravida who has failed to adequately expand her blood volume (Fig. 3-3). Proper therapy then would include volume expansion agents and thus expanding the microcirculation. This therapy appears to be logical for all gravida with severe EPH gestosis. Even those with type A gestosis respond with diuresis and tolerate epidural anesthesia after blood volume expansion.

Those gravida with multiple organ dysfunction and with other signs of EPH gestosis (severe hypertension, edema, and proteinuria) seem to be a different clinical entity than those which manifest hypertension and fits. The literature would suggest that the multiple organ syndrome (group B) has been described primarily in white gravida while hypertension and fits (group A) appears in black gravida. The clinical features of these two groups of patients is so different that perhaps different terms should be used to describe their illness.

Studies in our institution with the Swan–Ganz catheter has shown that in those gravida with type A EPH gestosis, cardiac output is sometimes exceedingly high. In view of their increased blood viscosity and vasoconstriction, this has been an unexpected finding. Such patients may have an increased mean systemic pressure (Guyton) from elevated catecholamine levels with increased venous return. (Smith[637] described reduced cardiac output and Assali et al.[21] reported normal values in toxemic gravida.)

The fluid distribution of severe EPH gestosis has long been appreciated (Fries et al.[207]) and was recently studied in a postpartum toxemic patient by Freund et al.[208] They found a markedly reduced plasma volume and red cell mass. The findings of high pulmonary wedge pressure and low colloid osmotic pressure without pulmonary edema suggest that such gravida may have increased pulmonary lymphatic flow.

The mechanism by which serum albumin is reduced in EPH gestosis is unclear. Many such B-type gravida have liver dysfunction, their renal glomeruli often show ultrastructural damage with capillary endotheliosis and disruption of the basement membrane. The protein content of their edema fluid is high.

While antihypertensive therapy alone may correct the vasospasm, volume replacement will also reduce peripheral resistance and reduce the workload of the heart.

As the incidence of mild cases of EPH gestosis continues to decline, these serious cases are going to become more apparent. Therapy is a problem for, in many cases, we have failed to prevent complications (fits, liver and renal dysfunction) or to send the postpartum patient home with a live infant. Perhaps earlier attempts to expand blood volume will be at least a partial answer.

Severe EPH Gestosis—The Great Imitator

My own views on severe gestosis are obviously somewhat different from those prevailing in America. As indicated before, we found a high incidence of thrombocytopenia and liver dysfunction in white gravida with "severe EPH gestosis, type B." Many of these women came to our attention because of the associated thrombocytopenia or liver dysfunction, although many were complaining of symptoms which were compatible with hepatitis, cholecystitis, renal failure, detached retina, heart failure, and so forth.[288] In other words, we found that severe EPH gestosis could imitate many other diseases (and of course the converse is true—that many other diseases in gravida can imitate preeclampsia). By definition, EPH gestosis type B hardly ever has normal liver functions (SGOT, LDH values), platelet count, and BUN are invariably abnormal (above 10 mg%), in addition to having the standard findings of hypertension and proteinuria. (Pritchard and associates,[553] from a large clinical experience, in contrast to our clinic, found that only 26% of gravida with eclampsia had platelet counts below 150,000.) It was these abnormal laboratory values in sick gravida that enabled us to determine that they truly had EPH gestosis, instead of such illnesses as hepatitis, nephritis, retinal detachment, and so forth.

THERAPEUTIC BENEFITS OF BLOOD VOLUME EXPANSION

The reduced blood volume concept as an etiologic mechanism has several advantages for the fetologist. It offers a definition of which women are at increased risk from fetal death for in our experience of some 200 patients, fetal death occurs when the reduced blood volume is not, or cannot, be corrected (as indicated by hematocrits). On the other hand, when blood volumes were expanded (decreasing hematocrits), fetal survival was good. (See Case 3-1.)

Another advantage of this reduced blood volume concept is that it suggests a logical prophylaxis against the occurrence of all types of EPH gestosis. Gravidas can be instructed to consume sufficient proteins and fluids so that their blood volumes will be adequately expanded. Daytime rest in the horizontal position is also recommended.[23]

The third value of the reduced blood volume concept is that it offers another form of therapy for severe EPH gestosis (in addition to $MgSO_4$, hypotensive agents, sedations, and so forth). Intravenous albumin, plasma, or low-molecular-weight dextran (protocol P-IV) have produced dramatic results in some cases.

Reduced blood volume in severe EPH gestosis has been recognized since the time of Zangemeister in 1903 and was enthusiastically endorsed by Dieckman[157] in the 1930s and 1940s. He believed that the intravenous use of 20% dextrose was the most significant therapeutic agent introduced in the treatment of severe EPH gestosis.

On our own service, we are concerned when the primigravida fails to have a reduced hematocrit at the 27th–30th week of pregnancy. While Pritchard and Stone[552] were unable to confirm a relationship between hematocrits and blood volumes, they have been traditionally used as indicators of relative blood volumes. Dieckman used hemoconcentration as an index of severity of eclampsia and EPH gestosis and recommended routine serial hematocrit measurements as indicators of relative blood volume.

ALBUMIN THERAPY

A recent review of the use of human serum albumin has been presented by Tullis.[708] He notes that its use has increased precipitously in America and that its high cost is placing a major financial burden on the cost of medical care. The safety of albumin is very high. While there is debate whether saline solutions are adequate for treating hypovolemic shock, such solutions have no place in the therapy of severe EPH gestosis.

We limit our use of albumin to two units (protocol P-IV) unless a significant increase in urine output occurs. With diuresis, albumin is repeated to correct their thrombocytopenia, hypertension, etc. Because the only cases I have seen of pulmonary edema during expansion therapy occurred while the CVP was "normal," we do not monitor the patient with a central venous pressure line. Others have used plasma and low-molecular-weight dextran. With albumin therapy, much is lost in the urine and dextran would perhaps be better except in cases of thrombocytopenia. Twenty percent dextrose, as recommended by Dieckman, is no longer used because of its hemolytic effects on red cells.

We also monitor the gravida's colloid osmotic pressure (COP). Because of their low albumin blood levels, all gravida have low COP values. This is particularly striking when they mobilize their excess tissue fluid as when placed at bed rest or in the postpartum period. COP is of course raised by albumin therapy and lowered by salt infusions. However, some gravida with severe EPH gestosis, while increasing urine output markedly during a salt infusion, actually raise their COP and other blood component levels. They must then be contracting their blood volumes, despite the salt infusion and diuresis (a most undesirable effect!).

One thing we now begin to understand from our measurements of pulmonary wedge pressures and colloid osmotic pressure (COP) is these gravida with severe EPH gestosis. With apparently normal central venous pressures (less than 8 cm H_2O) they sometimes develop pulmonary edema. Those that do not develop pulmonary edema (the vast majority) probably have increased pulmonary lymphatic flow.

HYPERPLACENTOSIS

There is one form of EPH gestosis seen in gravida with abnormalities of the fetus, placenta, and sometimes with thecal luteal cysts. When the gravida is hydropic herself, I call it the "maternal" or "mirror" syndrome (Chapter 5). At times, however the gravida appears to have the more usual EPH gestosis. Ballantyne[33] described the triple edema aspects (fetal hydrops, edematous placentae, and maternal edema) and Kaiser[392] has reviewed the more recent literature. Scott[620a] analyzed these cases in three British hospitals. He noted that the toxemia occurs early in the pregnancy, that primigravida are infrequent, and that fits are rare. While these gravida most always have hydramnios, Scott believed that it was the increased placental trophoblastic tissue and activity (hyperplacentosis) which was responsible for the "toxemia."

We continue to see these cases with an initial diagnosis of "hydatidiform mole and live fetus" or those associated with gross fetal anomalies and whose toxemia is secondary.

These cases were associated with gross fetal anomalies[161a] or with a markedly hydropic placenta. The latter patient had two such pregnancies, both terminated in her midtrimester for severe toxemia. The placenta in both instances was markedly hydropic (Fig. 3-4) and there were large thecal luteal cysts.

Scott argues that this type of toxemia seen with fetal hydrops, hydatidiform mole, and perhaps diabetes and plural pregnancies is different than the usual form of EPH gestosis. Chesley[100] suggests that they are the same, as their kidneys have the typical lesions found in the usual EPH gestosis. My own experience suggests that such cases with excessive placental mass are a distinct category of toxemia, because they are repetitive and are infrequently associated with fits or proteinuria. Believing that hyperplacentosis is the etiology, I would consider that a small dose of a folic acid antagonist might be indicated, were the toxemia severe in early midpregnancy and the fetus appeared normal. It would be essential to keep HCG levels in the normal range of pregnancy and to recall that such drugs are especially teratogenic in early pregnancy.

IATROGENIC ECLAMPSIA

There is one form of eclampsia (severe EPH gestosis with fits), which I have seen at least nine times, that appears to be induced by saline infusions (an etiology not accepted by the responsible anesthesiologists). This "iatrogenic eclampsia" occurs in the primigravida in labor, usually demonstrating only mild EPH gestosis but with a relatively high hematocrit. Following anesthesia (usually an epidural) moderate hypotension occurs which is treated with a rapid infusion of a balanced salt solution. Postanesthesia, the patient has a grand mal seizure with only minimal "other" signs and symptoms of EPH gestosis. In Dieckman's[157] 1952 text, there is a description of an intravenous salt load test for distinguishing between pseudo-preeclampsia and preeclampsia. In the latter group of gravida, increases in proteinuria, blood pressure, edema seizures, and even deaths after a salt infusion have occurred. Fortunately, the patients have all done well in my experience. The mechanism of the worsening of symptoms must be related to the rapid rate of the salt infusion, for the total salt load is only 12–24 g.

Case Reports and Discussion

Case No. 3-1

The syndrome of right upper quadrant epigastric pain in a pregnant woman should always suggest the possibility of severe EPH gestosis. Such right upper quadrant pain may

Fig. 3-4. Photograph of 540-g fetus with 1340-g "hydropic" placenta, delivered at 25 weeks because of "severe toxemia." Placenta showed hydropic degeneration. (Photograph courtesy of Dr. R. Niles.)

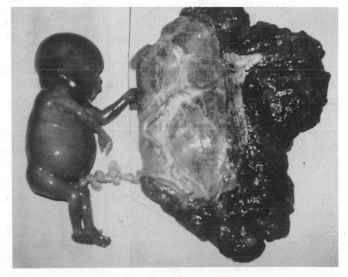

be misdiagnosed as renal stones, choleli-thiasis, or hepatitis. The following case illus-trates the significance of reduced blood vol-ume in the pathophysiology of severe EPH gestosis in the gravida with right upper guad-rant pain, potential dangers of intravenous urography and cholecystography, and the usefulness of expanding the blood volume in fetal therapy.

The patient was a 34-year-old gravida 2, para 0, Ab 1 at 27 weeks gestation. She was referred from another institution because of deteriorating renal function and persistent hypertension. Approximately 6 weeks prior to her admission elsewhere, she had devel-oped mild hypertension and peripheral edema and had been treated with a low-salt diet and bed rest. She subsequently developed right upper quadrant and epigastric pain un-responsive to antacids, local heat, and anal-gesics. At this time, she was started on Diupres (Chlorothiazide + Reserpine) 500 mg/day due to a blood pressure of 170/120. Because of nausea, vomiting, weakness, right upper quadrant pain, and occasional palpi-tations, the patient was hospitalized at the other institution and underwent an intrave-nous pyelogram and an oral cholecystogram a day later. Both tests were within normal limits except to demonstrate twins.

On her admission elsewhere, her labora-tory work showed hemoglobin of 12.7 g%, WBC 10,100/mm^3 with normal differential, amylase 86 units, creatinine 1.1 mg%, BUN 15.2 mg%, SGPT 373 on admission. Two days following the intravenous pyelogram, the patient's serum creatinine was 6.3 and BUN 46 mg%, creatinine clearance 28 cm^3/min and a platelet count of 60,000 per mm. Her hypertension persisted despite hydrala-zine 25 mg p.o., t.i.d. The patient was then transferred to the Medical Center.

The patient's physical exam on admis-sion showed no significant abnormalities ex-cept a blood pressure of 150/100 and 2+ pretibial edema as well as epigastric tender-ness to palpation. The diagnosis of severe EPH gestosis with thrombocytopenia was made and the preeclampsia blood volume

expansion protocol (P-IV) was started and appropriate coagulation studies (subse-quently negative) were drawn. The patient received 25 g of salt-poor albumin and 1 unit of plasminate, phenobarbital 60 mg p.o., q.i.d., and 3 days of MgSO$_4$ intravenously. Her hematocrit fell to 26% and she was then given 2 units of whole blood.

The patient responded to the protocol with an increase in her platelet count and gradual recovery to normal of her creatinine clearance and BUN. She was eventually discharged to outpatient care with the highest blood pres-sure in the clinic being 140–160/100. (Highest blood pressure at home was 130/80 torr.) The only medication was phenobarbital 60 mg p.o., q.i.d. She was followed with biweekly estriols and weekly OCT's. At 34 weeks, the patient developed a painless vaginal bleeding episode with physical examination and ultra-sound showing no evidence of abruption or placenta previa. Amniocentesis was done and an average L/S ratio of 1.6 was obtained. The decision was made to perform a cesarean section and a female infant weighing 2410 g with Apgars of 8 and 9 with a small, infarcted placenta was delivered; the other infant was a slightly macerated stillborn male weighing 986 g. The patient's postpartum course was complicated by blood pressures of 140–150/100, but by her fifth postoperative day, blood pressures were normal and she and her new-born child were discharged home. Follow-up studies were normal.

The danger of acute renal failure following intravenous urography in individuals who have reduced blood volumes and are dehy-drated has been well documented, especially in cases of diabetes and multiple mye-loma.[168, 296] The mechanism of the renal fail-ure in such cases is based on the obser-vations of Sobin et al.[642] who observed aggre-gation of erythrocytes, marked slowing of the microcirculation, variable degrees of vaso-constriction in both minute arterial and ve-nous vessels in human corneal scleral vessels after administration of urographic contrast media. A similar reduction is postulated in renal vessels, resulting in decreased renal blood flow and glomerular filtration rate. It has been noted that urinary mucoprotein, normally produced by the tubules, has an increased secretion rate in renal disease states with proteinuria and that the secretion is increased proportionately to the degree of proteinuria. The resultant ischemia and decreased urine volume production secondary to injection of a hypertonic urographic material in a previously dehydrated individual, such as a gravida with severe EPH gestosis, theoretically precipitates the urographic material with the urinary mucoprotein. This causes blockage of renal tubules and potentiates the vicious cycle of renal failure.[181] The right upper quadrant pain in women with severe EPH gestosis most likely reflects liver dysfunction with hemorrhage or engorgement. It is generally agreed that most cases of severe EPH gestosis do show evidence of liver dysfunction—by abnormal enzymes, pain, or even jaundice. The liver pathology has been explained on the basis of edema and congestion secondary to either reduced blood flow or microembolization. Grossly, the liver is firm with subcapsular hemorrhage. The histology often shows minimal changes or the same central hepatic necrosis as that seen in hepatitis.[326]

This particular case clearly demonstrated the reduced blood volume effects of severe EPH gestosis and the damage that can occur in such women when renographic or cholecystogram studies are done. It also showed what we feel is the appropriate treatment of the reduced blood volume state of EPH gestosis. Colloids such as albumin or plasminate can often reverse the organ dysfunction and coagulopathy manifested by the severe preeclamptic for a period of time. This therapy allowed the fetus to mature *in utero*.

A number of gravida have been hospitalized in our area with severe EPH gestosis in whom the physician focused on their liver pathology because of intense right upper quadrant pain and seemingly forgot the patient's severe EPH gestosis. Some of these women had exploratory surgery for cholelithiasis and others had extensive work-up (as

in this case) for liver or renal disease. The present case then illustrates the possible harmful effects of misinterpreting symptoms of hypovolemia in EPH gestosis, and ordering normally benign studies (such as intravenous pyelogram and cholecystograms). For the patient in which there is severe hemoconcentration manifested by an inappropriately high hematocrit and right upper quadrant pain, these studies obviously carry a considerable risk and are in fact contraindicated. Treatment with colloids will at times reverse the toxemic processes and allow continuation of the pregnancy.

Case No. 3-2

A 28-year-old P0010 was transferred to our hospital at 32 weeks gestation with mild toxemia (3+ edema) and a positive OCT. Her laboratory work at the other hospital showed a Hgb of 11 g%, slightly elevated SGOT, and a BUN of 11 mg%. On admission to our hospital, the Hgb was found to be 8.8%, BUN 18 mg%, a moderate thrombocytopenia (52,000), a markedly elevated SGOT (450 units), and urine demonstrated a 3+ albumin. Her blood pressure was 160/90 to 180/120 torr.

The OCT was positive (Fig. 3-5), which was corrected by whole blood and albumin transfusion, as was the maternal hypertension (150/90 torr). After steroid therapy and because of liver and renal dysfunction, a 1350-g male was delivered by cesarean section. The child had the Pierre–Robin syndrome. The newborn's course was complicated by thrombocytopenia, renal failure, and breathing problems from which he slowly recovered.

At the time of cesarean section, the mother had marked ascites and her postpartum course was complicated by severe liver dysfunction. However, she recovered fully by her sixth postpartum day and was discharged in good health.

This gravida had severe EPH gestosis, type B and a severe anemia. Presumably, with bed rest at the other hospital, she had mobilized part of excess body fluid, reducing her he-

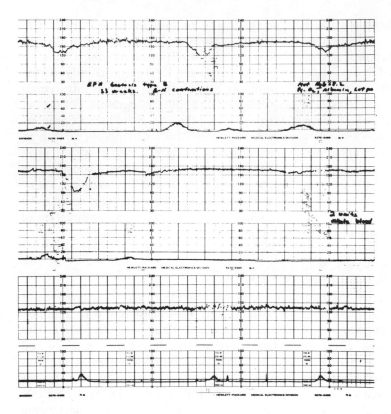

Fig. 3-5. FHR recording of gravida with severe EPH gestosis and anemia. After transfusion the positive OCT (upper tracing) became normal (lower tracing.)

moglobin concentration. (We never found any evidence of hemolysis or of microangiopathic anemia despite repeated laboratory studies.) With further expansion of her red cell mass and blood volume, the signs of fetal distress (positive OCT) abated. As with our other cases, steroid therapy did not correct the maternal or newborn thrombocytopenia. In this case, studies for platelet antibodies were negative.

EPH gestosis, type B, then is a disease process which affects multiple maternal and fetal organs. With a relatively reduced blood volume and red cells mass, apparent fetal distress may occur. Expansion of the maternal blood volume is at least palliative.

Case 3-3: Aspirin in the Treatment of Recurrent Toxemia

A 31-year-old white gravida was first seen at the Sacramento Medical Center in her 29th week of pregnancy in 1976. This pregnancy was characterized by severe hypertension, thrombocytopenia, and she was delivered by cesarean section at her 30th week. The infant weighed 810 g and expired on the fourth day of life with ascites, thrombocytopenia, and renal failure (mirror syndrome). Her first pregnancy, managed elsewhere, had a similar outcome. Between pregnancies her platelet counts were normal, as were all other tests and physical findings.

In the 15th week of pregnancy, she had an elevated hematocrit and a thrombocytopenia. Bone marrow and peripheral blood smear studies suggested peripheral consumption of platelets. All other studies of blood coagulation were normal throughout her pregnancy. She was initially treated with bedrest and forced fluids, and heparin. After a period of 4 weeks time, there was no apparent improvement in her platelet count, and she was therefore begun on aspirin 600 mg t.i.d. This resulted in gradual improvement of her platelet count.

The aspirin was discontinued at her 32nd week because of fear of closing the fetal ductus, following which she began to experience painful uterine contractions and had mild elevations with her blood pressure. After hospitilization and treatment with sedation, her blood pressure and uterine contractions returned to normal. However, by her 32nd week, her blood pressure was 160/100 torr and her platelet count had again decreased to 50,000 with a subsequent rise in her hematocrit. The ultrasonic scan showed apparently normal fetal growth and normal amounts of amniotic fluid until the 32nd week, at which time there appeared to be a cessation of fetal growth and a disappearance of amniotic fluid. The fetus's bladder was observed to fill and empty, however.

She was again given aspirin and her platelet count returned to near normal levels. Since a FHT recording showed apparent severe vagal type decelerations (variable), she was delivered by repeat cesarean section with a 1410-g growth-retarded fetus, with no apparent respiratory distress. Its platelet count was normal, and it did well. Following delivery, the patient's platelet count and blood pressure returned to normal.

This case again demonstrates the thrombocytopenia seen in some cases of recurrent toxemia. It also suggests that there may be a beneficial effect of aspirin therapy as regards both thrombocytopenia and the signs of toxemia.

Dalessio has suggested that aspirin inhibits platelet agglutination in several different ways. It is easy to postulate that platelet agglutination was occurring at the placental site which lead to both platelet consumption and reduced placental perfusion. Aspirin and/or plasma volume expansion may prevent this agglutination.

Another Point of View

From the University of Texas at Dallas, which has provided so much data relative to hypertensive disease of pregnancy from their large clinical experience, an authoritarian viewpoint is often expressed. Gant et al.,[221] speaking about the use of albumin in EPH gestosis, declares "The vascular tree is already filled. If you then place plasma expanders inside the vascular tree, the first place it will come out will be in the lungs. They will begin to bubble, with evidence of pink froth. This has been the case over and over again." It should be noted that the only such patients that I have seen "bubble" numbered two (out of more than 150 cases), each given more than 10 liters (in less than 12 hr) of salt solution because they were oliguric and had "normal" CVP pressures.

From the University of California at Los Angeles, Assali and Vaughn[21] have characterized my concepts of hypovolemia and the analogy to chronic shock (Fig. 3-3) as revealing a misconception of the pathophysiology and a lack of understanding of the most elementary principles of hemodynamics. These California investigators offer data from a small series of anesthetized pregnant sheep to support their view on the importance of systemic vascular resistance and predict dreadful consequences of volume expansion during EPH gestosis. They suggest that a good analogy to the use of volume expansion in EPH gestosis is filling a garden hose, apparently rejecting Guyton's and colleagues' concepts of mean systemic pressure, the importance of pulmonary lymphatic flow, or even the work of Weil's laboratory in Los Angeles (Freund et al.[208]).

Again, from the University of Texas, the rollover test has swept American Obstetrics. Concerning the "rollover" test (an increase in diastolic blood pressure of 20 torr or more after the gravida at 28–32 weeks is "rolled over" on her back after being in the lateral position for 5 or more minutes), Gant and Worley[221] claim that a future preeclamptic patient can be identified 3 months before the appearance of hypertension. This same group of investigators has challenged our current concepts for treatment of EPH gestosis. Their high-risk pregnancy unit at the Parkland Memorial Hospital (Hauth et al.[323]) has markedly reduced perinatal moribidity and mortality by restricting gravida with hypertension to a sendentary life without sodium restriction, antihypertensive medications, or diuretics. This simple clinical approach prevented, in most cases, the development of severe preeclampsia or eclampsia. For definitive therapy, they recommended intravenous $MgSO_4$ to prevent seizures and hydralazine to control hypertension. Using these clinical approaches, the perinatal mortality rate among all preeclamptic primigravidas at Parkland Memorial Hospital in 1974 was an astounding 20/1000 births.

Anderson and Harbert,[15] from the University

of Virginia, promote what they term the conservative management of preeclampsia and eclamptic patients. Their protocol includes stabilizing of the patient's basic cardiovascular status, intravenous $MgSO_4$, diuretics (in 28%!), and antihypertensive therapy when indicated. Like many other southern medical centers, they separate what they term thrombotic thrombocytopenia purpera (TTP) from severe EPH gestosis. (I argue that EPH gestosis probably is all one disease in different degrees and time, including preeclampsia–eclampsia, TTP, and postpartum hemolytic renal failure, and that the nonpregnant state may be represented by immunologic thrombocytopenia purpura.)

In many discussions of EPH gestosis, the role of renin angiotension with sensitized vessels to vasoconstriction is mentioned. As noted, I believe that this is all *secondary* to the gravida's failure to increase blood volume, but the standard American view is that these abnormalities are primary and the decreased blood volume is *secondary*.

A popular project now is to combine both physiologic and immunologic mechanisms for the development of toxemia in pregnancy. This is to assume that the woman destined to have EPH gestosis initially has an enlarged placenta (hyperplacentosis) which, in turn, induces more antibody response to the fetal paternal antigens. The antibodies against placental tissue also react against renal and brain tissue. Against the placenta, they produce some type of destruction which explains the decreased fetal size and abnormalities of placental function. As a defense mechanism, the maternal host mounts production of blocking antibody against the paternal antigens. EPH gestosis is limited to first pregnancies because these blocking antibodies are in more abundance with subsequent gestations.

As a young faculty member, I spend hundreds of hours studying pregnancies of inbred strains of mice and outbred strains of mice and rats. All I proved was that the greater the fetal differences in paternal and maternal histocompatibility antigens, the more the increased fertility and larger newborns. Among humans, there are no data which suggest that inbred cultures versus outbred cultures have any different incidence of "toxemia."

In his 1978 monumental text of EPH gestosis (*Hypertensive Disorders in Pregnancy*), Chesley demonstrates no enthusiasm for blood volume expansion therapy.[102] Indeed, it would appear that type "B" EPH gestosis is an exceedingly rare disease.

Schwartz and Brenner[615a] have suggested that the diagnosis of many cases of thrombotic thrombocytopenia purpura (TTP) in pregnancy may have been inappropriate, with EPH gestosis being the primary problem; others have shown that such TTP may be "cured" with plasma therapy. Thus, there may be more agreement on the use of blood volume expansion in severe EPH gestosis than would appear to the casual observer.

In closing, it should be noted that the patient with severe EPH gestosis has been treated with accouchement force, anesthesia, anticoagulant, bleeding, blistering, dehydration, carbon dioxide, hyperalimentation, hydration, hypotension, lavage, oxygenation, mammectomy, neglect, renal decapsulation, starvation, and tranquilization.[157] (I have always thought that splenectomy should be tested!)

CHAPTER 4

Chronic Fetal Distress

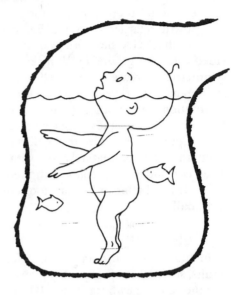

Introduction

As more data become available, it becomes increasingly difficult to define "fetal distress." One concept is that fetal distress includes many types of fetal dysfunction, which have in common an associated small or zero likelihood of complete fetal recovery (or normal development) without some form of intervention. Fetal distress is then very much like an antenatal diagnosis of preeclampsia (EPH gestosis); the diagnosis is suspected, but can only be confirmed in retrospect. The available data and references suggest that most cases of fetal dysfunction are not associated with an acute asphyxial insult, but are chronic or subacute intrauterine problems. Since such events may represent *in utero* metabolic problems, their antenatal diagnosis is difficult.

An example of chronic fetal distress, of course, is the dysmature, small for gestational age (SGA), or the intrauterine growth retarded (IUGR) infant.[92] Some SGA fetuses may represent chromosomal or other genetic anomalies, including multiple defects, and other cases reflect multiple gestation or maternal disease, such as EPH gestosis. Despite appropriate histories and studies, approximately 50% of the SGA newborns deliver unexpectedly unless every effort is made to monitor uterine growth throughout the antenatal period. From the fetus's viewpoint, such monitoring of its growth is probably the most significant aspect of prenatal care, for it is from the SGA group that the stillborns and the infants with subsequent cerebral dysfunction come.[599]

HISTORY

At the Pacific Coast Obstetric and Gynecologic Society meeting in 1946, R.D. McBurney presented "with much trepidation" a paper on "The Undernourished Full-term Infant." He described the problems of these SGA newborns relative to their increased perinatal mortality and morbidity rates and their increased incidence of congenital anomalies. In a 1958 paper that must be a classic, Sjostedt *et al.*[633] described the "dysmature" mature infant (SGA) as observed in Sweden. In 1957, Clifford[107a] had described the "postmature" newborn which probably was a dysmature infant that had been born postmature. Gruenwald[303] and Lubchenco et al.,[454] independently defined the problem of the two types of low-birth-weight newborns, the gestational premature and the intrauterine growth retarded or SGA. Based on rat studies, the SGA newborn was further divided into two groups by Winick[760] (type I, symmetric decrease in total cell numbers of all organs, and type II, asymmetric growth retardation with normal brain cell counts). Neligan and colleagues[503a] in a study at Newcastle upon Tyne studied the performance of children born prematurely or with SGA. They concluded their study with the phrase, "it is clearly better to be born too soon than too small."

ETIOLOGY

Just as there are many reasons for small adults, so are there presumably many reasons for the small newborn. (Fig. 4-1) In other words, not all small newborns are necessarily abnormal or at a disadvantage, and as noted in Chapter 2, from an obstetrical aspect, the small, normal newborn should be at an advantage. One issue which is hopefully resolved is the lack of effect of paternal size on his newborn infant. Many prenatal forms still ask the father's height and weight, the apparent assumption being that these factors somehow influence his newborn's size. This view was perhaps best expressed in Maeck's presidential address reference to Sacagawea and CPD.[457b] Sacagawea was a female Indian interpreter for Lewis and Clark whose difficult labor Maeck ascribed to her mating with a white man. In actuality, the available data are that in neither farm animals nor humans does the paternal size determine newborn size.

Walton and Hammond, a generation ago, mated ponies and standard-size horses and demonstrated the overwhelming importance of maternal effects and lack of paternal effects upon the size of the newborn. These investigators observed that when the mother was a pony and the father a standard-size horse, the newborn was an appropriate size

for ponies. However, when the matings were reversed and the standard-size horse was the mother, the newborn was of a size appropriate for horses.[728] (And, of course, much larger than when the mother was a pony.) These newborns had the same genotype and were of comparable size when adults, yet obviously the in utero environment was all important in determining the size of the newborns. Similar conclusions have been possible (sheep[364] and rabbit data[714]) from analyses of the atomic bomb survivor data of Japan[485] because of the detailed pedigrees which were collected. In comparing human half siblings, the newborn weights were relative to maternal size and to their siblings when they had the same mother. By contrast, when the fathers were the same (but different mothers) there was no relationship between sibling size but only between the mother and her infant's size. As noted in Chapter 2, maternal diet, her body build, glucose metabolism, and the presence of vascular disease are the all important determinate factors of newborn size. As with all rules, there are a few exceptions, such as in certain cases of chromosomal trisomy, newborn weight is not determined by its in utero environment.

MATERNAL HYPERTENSION

Among our patients, maternal cardiovascular disease is responsible for approximately 30% of the cases of SGA. Fortunately, it is usually associated with type-II fetal defect, meaning that the brain is spared. As a rule, the degree of fetal growth retardation is directly proportional to the degree of maternal hypertension. As noted in Chapter 3, fetal prognosis and growth are more adversely affected with superimposed renal disease (proteinuria). In rats and monkeys, type-II IUGR occurs when a portion of the uterine blood flow is ligated. With such chronic hypoxia, fetal blood flow is preferentially diverted to the brain.

MATERNAL MALNUTRITION

As discussed in Chapter 2, the impact of maternal undernutrition on fetal develop-

Fig. 4-1. Fetal growth curves from several different types of fetal populations. (From Gruenwald, P.: Growth of the human fetus. I. Normal growth and its variation. *Am J Obstet Gynecol* **94**: 1112, 1966. Reproduced with permission.)

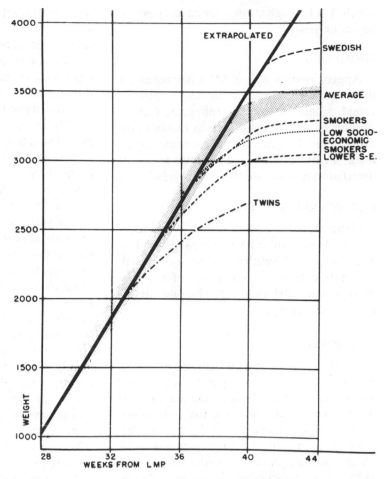

ment is difficult to evaluate, as, unlike animal studies, it is difficult to control psychosocial factors. Niswander *et al.* showed that reduced pregnancy weight gain, when a reflection of undernutrition, adversely affected birth weight.[506] The Guatemala Studies[307] demonstrated about a 400-g increase in birthweight of newborns whose mothers had been malnourished, but when given, in a controlled project, adequate supplementation.

The type-I (all organs retarded to approximately the same extent) growth retardation occurs with maternal cyanotic heart disease and is seen in New York City in pregnancies of underweight women with inadequate caloric and protein intake.[585a] It also occurs with such anomalies as Potter's syndrome (renal agenesis) or chromosome defects. In rats, a mother which herself was stunted *in utero*

may produce small newborns.[130a] If a rapid succession of pregnancies occurs, newborns are smaller and more likely to be impaired.[349a]

TWIN PREGNANCY

Plural pregnancy accounts for about 10% of the SGA newborns. Churchill,[106] using the Collaborative Project data, has shown that there is an increased risk of SGA with mental defects for twins.

INFECTIONS

Maternal infections, such as herpes, rubella, cytomegalovirus, toxoplasmosis, and syphilis, are a cause of SGA. As described by Feldman,[196] their action may be through placentites (herpes, vaccinia, CMV) or fetal cellular affects (syphilis, herpes, vaccinia, CMV, rubella) or through chromosomal injuries (rubeola, herpes).

ANOMALIES

Approximately 20% of SGA newborns are the result of anomalies, including chromosomal, single gene, or morphogenic factors. Besides chromosomal defects as Down's syndrome, renal agenesis, osteogenesis imperfecta, heart lesions, and various forms of dwarfism are associated with SGA newborns.

METABOLIC DISORDERS

General metabolic disorders working at various fetal cellular levels were suggested by Sabel et al.[599] of Sweden as a cause of growth retardation from their findings of the dysmature and SGA newborn who later developed CNS damage.

DIAGNOSIS

A 1976 study by Whetham and colleagues[745] of Toronto suggests that certain antenatal clues can lead to the diagnosis of SGA. Their study indicated the various suspect antenatal categories for SGA as the following: a past history of a previous SGA child (present in 37%); maternal illnesses (17%); the obstetrician's impression that *in utero* growth was inadequate (was relatively inaccurate in the absence of other clues, but still contributed to 15% of their cases). The discouraging feature of these investigators' report is that even when the gravida was referred for ultrasonic examination with a diagnosis of suspected SGA, these examinations were actually able to discern only 60% of the SGA cases. In Toronto, as elsewhere, there is a trend to accept ultrasound as the final arbitrator. (Our experience is similar and we have "watched" as two supposedly 27-week gestation fetuses died *in utero*, only to discover that they were actually more mature SGA fetuses. In both of our cases, inaccurate menstrual histories and repeated ultrasonic scans had been the basis of our error.)

These Canadian authors recommend that the scans begin somewhere in the 20th–24th

week and that there be follow-up scans at 2–4 weeks. The obvious problem for the obstetrician is that unless there are some clues, such as past history of chromosomal disease, viral infections, or maternal cardiovascular renal disease, it is most unusual to suspect fetal dysmaturity at the midpoint of pregnancy. It is only in the third trimester in the unsuspected case that the obstetrician finds reliable signs that the fetus is failing to grow, at which point serial ultrasonic diagnosis has less to offer, because the rate of growth for even the normal fetus is relatively small.

The various endocrine assays for the SGA fetus are almost legendary; they include such tests as the clearance of radioactive salts from the myometrium, the use of serum HPL, diamine oxydase, oxytocinase, estriols, and so forth (Protocol P-20, Tables D-6–D-21). Nearly every one of these tests has such a wide standard deviation of values that it is virtually impossible to discern the specific case based simply on a single abnormal laboratory value. We have been impressed by Spellacy's reports[654,655] in the United States and the many reports from the United Kingdom on the value of HPL in the problems relative to placental insufficiency and the SGA fetus.

A survey of the SGA infants delivered on our service suggests that almost any informed medical student should be able to make the correct antenatal diagnosis in 90% of the cases (yet with our combined efforts of faculty, residents, and students, we missed 50%). In all of our cases, the newborns were delivered of mothers with either (a) severe EPH gestosis or (b) plural pregnancies or (c) who were drug addicts or (d) who had failed to gain weight accurately. These maternal diagnoses were so obvious that it is a puzzle as to why we missed one-half of the cases.

Actually, we have a "type-III" SGA—the case in which repeated and expensive examinations suggest SGA, but the fetus is "normal." When we have made the diagnosis of SGA, we have been accurate only 30% of the time. Such a dismal record suggests that only the obvious case is diagnosed *in utero* with precision at the Sacramento Medical Center, yet Dr. Robert Creasy (University of California, San Francisco) states that his obstetrical service has not missed a single SGA case. Drillien[164] of Dundee has likewise suggested that we should be able to make the diagnosis in the second trimester. I like to believe that our poor record reflects our patient population with their inaccurate menstrual histories. Despite the cost and effort and sometimes unnecessary interference, it probably is acceptable to have a relatively high ratio of "type-III" SGA, as compared with types I and II.

Therapy

OXYGEN

Most fetal physiologists now seem to discount the rather logical beliefs of Sir Joseph Barcroft, as expressed in his "Mount Everest *In Utero*" concept that the normal term fetus escapes the constant danger of hypoxia only when being born. The modern viewpoint seems to be that even though fetal oxygen tension is low, the increased fetal hematocrit provides an adequate oxygen supply. However, it may be that Barcroft was correct in part and that even under normal *in utero* conditions, oxygen supply to the fetus is not optimal and that increasing fetal P_{O_2} could be of benefit to the ill fetus and perhaps even to the normal fetus.

A number of years ago, I was working with an inbred mice colony in an attempt to determine what, if any, maternal environmental factors might be teratogenic or deleterious to the fetuses. Among the many factors I studied was a maternal environment of increased oxygen tension. Based on my prior concepts, I assumed that such an environment would be detrimental because of maternal accumulations of carbon dioxide (reduced ventilation), possible uterine artery constriction induced by hyperoxia, effects of oxygen poisoning on sulfydryl enzymes, and so forth. Much to my surprise, the litters of mice exposed to increased oxygen were larger than the controls. My hopes for a research grant at that time

were to find environmental detrimental factors for fetal health and not for those which may increase fetal size or health! Furthermore, I was unable to demonstrate that oxygen tension was elevated in these mice exposed to high oxygen, but this may have been an artifact of collection. At any rate, I was unable to pursue the matter further but did continue to puzzle over the reasons for the statistically significant increases in fetal size that occurred to these mothers in high oxygen.

It has long been known that pregnant women with cyanotic heart disease have smaller fetuses, but there has been an absence of data which suggest that increasing the oxygen environment of normal women with normal fetuses will increase the fetal size. The effects of oxygen therapy await technical advances which will allow presentation of a continuously rich oxygen environment to the ambulatory gravida.

WORK

Metcalfe[471] and associates at the University of Oregon had been reinvestigating the effects of maternal exercise on pregnancy outcome, and their preliminary investigations suggest that maternal exercise may indeed be detrimental. Longo and colleagues[425a] have observed, in both pregnant sheep and guinea pigs, that maternal exercise reduces placental exchange and/or uterine blood flow. It does seem that an exercising muscle mass does rob the uterus of oxygen[484] and, indeed, such exercise tests have long been used clinically as evaluators of *in utero* health in the form of abnormal FHR recording after maternal exercise.

Beltram-Paz and Driscoll[41a] compared the placentas of SGA fetuses with normal fetuses and found that 90% of the normals had normal placentas and that 95% of the SGA's had abnormal placentas, a most remarkable observation. Nevertheless, it seems almost axiomatic that the placenta is abnormal when there is SGA and repeatedly, one wonders which is the cause and which is the effect. If placental transfer is the culprit in these cases, it seems apparent that our proposed therapy of maximum physical rest is logical. On the other hand, if the intrinsic defect lies within the fetus as with chromosome abnormalities and the fetus controls the size of its placenta, then such therapy really has little to recommend it.

The effects of hard physical maternal work was demonstrated in a clear manner more than a hundred years ago in Bavaria (Ploss, 1886)[153] where maternity leave became compulsory for working pregnant women. The perinatal mortality rate decreased spectacularly after the instigation of this rule. I believe that one of the most foolish recommendations that American obstetricians have given to their patients is the recommendation for increased physical activity during their pregnancy. As best as I can determine, this recommendation apparently stems from our concern over constipation, as it has been reasoned that physical activity would keep "one's bowels moving." (Constipation is more likely related to the pregnant woman's failure to consume adequate fluids.) At any rate, maternal physical work probably never is of benefit to the fetus.

Common sense and the experience of working gravida tells us that most women have a uteroplacental transport mechanism which is adequate and has sufficient reserve to allow for physical exercising without exposing the fetus to any significant stress or risk.[484] However, in those borderline placental transfer situations such as occur in SGA, it may be that restricted physical activity and forced physical rest for the mother should be the rule. Bed rest in the lateral position offers increased uterine and renal blood flow and increased maternal blood volume. Whether in addition to recommending absence from as much physical activity as possible, one should also propose brief periods of oxygen therapy are argumentative indeed. These other measures will be difficult to prove by anything short of a huge collaborative study.

GENERAL THERAPY FOR SGA

Since becoming aware of Sontag's studies of the 1930s (Chapter 1), I have thought it logical that in any sort of stressful situation, in addition to providing emotional support, one should prescribe tranquilizers to reduce maternal catecholamines and increase prolactin levels, bed rest to assure maximum uterine blood flow, and forced fluids to assure maximum blood volume. (Oxygen therapy, as with a modified space suit, is unproven and impractical.)

Whether therapy in the form of complete maternal rest in the lateral position is sufficient to prevent most cases of SGA seems unlikely. Whether additional fetal nutrition in the form of intraamniotic feedings is unsolved and probably hazardous and efforts to increase fetal swallowing (Chapter 2) are untried. Nutritional effects have already been overemphasized, but the effects of malnutrition on placental size should be mentioned again. Laga and colleagues[419a] found a 19% reduction in placental parenchyma in mothers who were malnourished.

Drillien[164] has suggested that the growth-retarded fetus (or SGA) may suffer adversely *in utero* from its hostile environment and may benefit from early delivery and modern neonatal care. American neonatologists, on the other hand, speak of the need of allowing fetal maturity so that the newborn will have a neurological system providing for temperature control and so forth. As noted repeatedly in this dissertation, it is from these SGA (dysmature, small-for-dates) infants that come the cases of cerebral palsy, minimal brain damage, and other causes of cerebral dysfunction. We may be approaching the time when obstetricians will be able to diagnose these fetuses early and terminate the pregnancies so that they will have an optimal opportunity for development.

One issue that needs to be addressed in America concerns the relative rights of the fetus for the "best of all possible *in utero* life" and its mother's right to "do as she wishes with her own body." A pregnant diabetic in America can purposefully mismanage her diabetic control and the heroin addict can refuse adequate care, both knowing that such action is probably detrimental to their fetus' welfare without fear of criminal charges. The issue concerns gravida of all social classes. I have known gravida to exercise their work maternity benefits by taking leaves in the third trimester, only to go skiing at 10,000 ft. The concept that such maternity benefits are for their fetus' welfare and not their own pleasure never occurred to them.

In concluding, it now appears that from an obstetrical viewpoint, the significant problems of the growth-retarded fetus are, first, diagnosis, perhaps therapy, and, most important, determining when the fetus is "better out than in."

Another Point of View

McCullough et al.[496] have demonstrated that maternal environment can be a factor in the growth-retarded fetus. They found a progressive decline in birth weight as altitude increases. Intrauterine growth retardation began earlier (placenta reached its maximum growth sooner)

and newborn respiratory deaths were more frequent. If there is a correlation between low oxygen environment and IUGR, then perhaps oxygen therapy might aid the IUGR fetus whose mother is at sea level.

Bjerre and Bjerre[56] reported an incidence of only 4.9% of low birth weights in Malmo, Sweden, or about one-third to one-half of the rates usually reported in America. In these Swedish studies about half of the cases had no recognizable etiology, 15% were associated with twin births, and only 15% with toxemia. Such figures suggest rates of LBW which we can achieve and also the limitations of our present clinical techniques in its prevention.

Contrary to Longo's studies,[452a] Curet et al.,[133] in their studies of exercise effects on pregnant sheep, demonstrated no change in stroke volume or total uterine blood flow. Interestingly, blood flow distribution during exercise in these pregnant animals changed in favor of the placenta. Therefore, those who argue that exercise is desirable during pregnancy have some laboratory data to support their claim.

CHAPTER 5

Mirror Syndromes

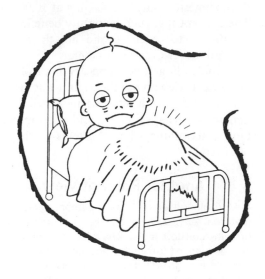

Introduction

There are a number of illnesses which seem to affect both mother and fetus, so that one "mirrors" the other. The human placenta is selectively permeable to IgG. Any maternal disease process dependent on the serum IgG fraction may also affect the fetus. Sometimes such IgG fractions are apparently harmless (as the C_3 nephrotic factors) to the fetus, other times they are detrimental (myasthenia gravis, Graves disease, immunologic thrombocytopenia purpura).[137a] Fetal disease may likewise affect its mother (maternal syndrome with hydrops fetalis, fetal neuroblastoma), presumably by transplacental mechanism. Scott consider the affected infant of the diabetic mother to represent a transplacental factor, although this is less clear.[620a] The fetus may also be affected by maternal malignancies, such as malignant melanoma, leukemia, carcinoma of the breast, and so forth.

MATERNAL SYNDROME

The mirror syndrome about which much has been written is the "maternal syndrome," seen frequently in cases of fetal hydrops (also

Chapter 21). The fetus and its placenta are hydropic, and the gravida mirrors the condition of her fetus with marked edema, sometimes hypertension, and often pruritus.[238] Kaiser[392] believes that the common denominator of the hydropic fetus, placenta, and mother are the placental factors. Many of these gravida have elevated serum HCG levels and thecal luteal cysts. Some of these cases are apparently unrelated to problems of isoimmunization, for I have seen two in which the fetus and placenta were hydropic and the mother edematous on the basis of fetal heart disease. Priscoll[166], MacAfee et al.[457a] described cases related to tumors of the umbilical cord, placenta, fetal heart, EPH gestosis, maternal anemia, and so forth (Table 5-I). Kaiser[392] suggested that the occurrence of a hydropic fetus, placenta, and gravida by termed "Ballantyne triple edema syndrome," after the British physician who described four cases in 1892.

On our service, we see one to three such "maternal syndrome" cases a year and, unless related to isoimmunization or fetal anomalies, have been unable to determine the etiology of the syndrome. The syndrome may sometimes be related to the fetus' inability to swallow because of lesions or illness with resulting hydramnios and placental hydrops. In my experience, regardless of the etiology, the appearance of this interesting "maternal syndrome" in a gravida means that the fetus has a disease process from which it cannot be salvaged.

MYASTHENIA GRAVIS

Myasthenia gravis is a disease process that affects both the gravida and her newborn. Dunn[171] suggested that there is a specific serum factor which blocks cholinergic receptors at the neuromuscular junction which can cross the placenta. As with many of the other "mirror" diseases, this factor may be an immune complex which could theoretically be removed from the newborn by exchange transfusions. While only approximately 10% of the newborns are affected in mothers with myasthenia gravis, in my experience, the sicker newborns are often born of mothers that have minimal disease. This is especially so when a mother has had removal of her thymus. The newborn paralysis is apparently easily treated, responding nicely to edrophonium (Tensilon) 0.1 ml subcutaneously.

NEWBORN HYPERTHYROIDISM

Newborn hyperthyroidism sometimes occurs when their mothers are hyperthyroid or have been treated for hyperthyroidism (Protocol P-45). Newborn hyperthyroidism is especially common if the mother has ophthalmopathy or pretibial edema. Most such cases of newborn hyperthyroidism are associated with elevated levels of "long-acting thyroid-stimulator" (LATS) or "LATS protector" or some immunological factor which stimulates the thyroid. In the only case that I have treated, it was easy to make a diagnosis of *in utero* hyperthyroidism. The gravida had a high LATS titer and the fetus had a persistent tachycardia. The newborn responded very nicely to Lugol's solution and was perfectly well at the age of 5 weeks.

TABLE 5-I. Etiology of Hydrops Fetalis (188 Cases, Caucasian)

Rh-blood-group incompatibility	81%
Non-Rh-blood-group incompatibility	1%
Congenital malformations (major) (heart abnormalities, hamartoma of lung, tracheoesophageal fistula)	4%
Congenital malformations (minor) (Talipes, ectopic kidney, double ureter, dislocated hip, hepatitis, chorioangioma)	4%
Twin pregnancies	3%
Severe EPH gestosis (toxemia)	2%
Maternal anemia	1%
Idiopathic	4%

Modified from Ref. 457a.

IMMUNOLOGIC THROMBOCYTOPENIA

Approximately 50% of newborns of mothers with ITP (immunologic thrombocytopenia purpura) demonstrate thrombocytopenia at birth or in the newborn period. This may occur even when the mother is in remission, apparently because of her platelet antibodies. The argument continues as to whether such fetuses should be delivered by cesarean section. Territo and colleagues[693] recommended that delivery be accomplished by cesarean section as a prophylactic measure against the development of newborn intraventricular hemorrhage. While the recommendation has a certain logic because so many of the fetuses have thrombocytopenia, and whose brains presumably should be protected from intraventricular hemorrhage, it is impossible to support such a plan from the literature.[422] My own series includes 10 infants whose mothers had ITP with platelet counts varying between 4000 and 70,000 mm^3 at the time of delivery. All the infants were delivered vaginally and none of them showed any evidence of CNS or other trauma. Several of these infants required steroid therapy, as they developed profound thrombocytopenia at age 3 to 10 days. For therapy of both the maternal and newborn thrombocytopenia, a steroid should be used which will cross the placenta (hydrocortisone or beta methasone) in hopes of preventing the newborn thrombocytopenia. Our one such case, in which the mother was treated with beta

methasone (and apparently responded herself), was an apparent failure, as her 3-day-
old child developed a severe thrombocytopenia. While the recommendation to perform
routine cesarean section in these patients is
unproven, it is important that the newborn be
followed very carefully for at least 1 week, as
thrombocytopenia may occur as late as the
fifth or sixth day of life.

EPH GESTOSIS

A newborn "mirror" syndrome is seen occasionally in mothers who have severe EPH
gestosis and is often lethal to the newborn.
The occurrence of parallel symptoms in
mothers and fetus of pregnancies complicated
by EPH gestosis suggests that there may be a
transplacental factor which is responsible
both for the maternal and fetal illnesses. In
our experience, approximately one-third of
the newborns of gravida with "severe EPH
gestosis marked by thrombocytopenia and
multiple organ failure" will themselves have

a similar disease of renal and liver failure and
thrombocytopenia. These infants are usually
premature (less than 1500 g) and, in our
experience, have not done well. Therapy in
this situation seems rather hopeless as their
pregnancies have invariably been terminated
because of the severe maternal disease. This
newborn outcome is in contrast to the severe
EPH gestosis marked either by fits or only
severe hypertension (and no thrombocytopenia) whose newborns usually do very well
(Chapter 3).

Other maternal immunes diseases often affect the fetus, but the newborn shows little or
no "mirror" effects. These include maternal
diseases such as lupus erythematosus (abortion rate is high apparently as a result of
reduced uterine blood flow and antibodies),
herpes gestationis, and cholestasis of pregnancy.

Fetal endocrine-producing tumors, such as
neuroblastoma, can cause maternal sweating,
headache, and so forth.

CHAPTER 6

Orgasm and Its Possible Deleterious Effects on the Fetus

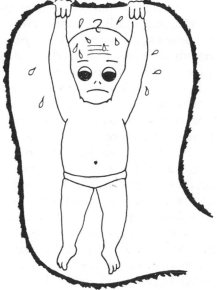

Few subjects in obstetrics have engendered such diversity of opinion as has the issue of whether "sex" during pregnancy is detrimental to the fetus. Most obstetrical opinions (often drawn from personal experience) suggest that coitus is not (detrimental). The adage that "if intercourse harmed pregnancies, there would be no newborns" apparently holds as true today as ever. I disagree with these views, which, unfortunately, aligns me with those in our specialty who still support certain prudish positions.

A stance similar to mine is taken by Roman Rechnitz Limner,[449] author of the popular paperback *Sex and the Unborn Child.* In this work—subtitled "Damage to the Fetus Resulting from Sexual Intercourse During Pregnancy"—Limner concludes that the original sin was violation of the natural sex taboos appreciated by all other pregnant animals; he believes that Adam had coitus with a pregnant Eve. Limner quotes Masters and Johnson frequently, particularly as regards hyperventilation during coitus and uterine contractions during orgasm. He associates the latter with fetal asphyxia and probable brain damage. I agree, at least in part, that maternal

orgasm may be detrimental in terms of initiating labor. However, the relationship between maternal orgasm and newborn cerebral palsy is completely unsubstantiated, and would be most indirect under any circumstances.

I believe maternal "orgasm" may be detrimental to the fetus for the following reasons: It is associated with increased maternal levels of oxytocin, prolactin, catecholamines, and probably prostaglandins; it is also associated with uterine contractions and probably decreased uterine blood flow.[269] I have sought to measure relative uterine blood flow with a pulse sensor (photoelectric plethysmographic probe) placed in the lateral vaginal fornix of two women in the third trimester. When these women achieved orgasm (by self-manipulation), there was a marked decrease in the blood volume pulse of the lateral fornix of the vagina. Presumably, a decrease in flow occurred in the uterus as well. (My assumption has always been that the vaginal fornix and the uterus have the same functional arterial supply.)

Most pregnant women who believe that they achieve orgasm in the third trimester report that they do experience strong uterine contractions, which often continue up to 30 min following the termination of the coitus. Unlike Braxton–Hicks contractions, the orgasm-related uterine contractions are often painful, and usually are followed by a sense of fullness and discomfort in the pelvis. Some gravida have reported that the fetus is hyperactive in the postorgasmic phase.

In one gravida in whom we externally monitored fetal heart rate, significant bradycardia occurred during the orgasm-induced uterine contraction (Figs. 6-1 and 6-2). In ignorance, we interpreted this FHR bradycardia as evidence of fetal distress. A more educated appraisal, which we would make now, would be that the fetus was undergoing some form of stress during these contractions. For many years, in interviewing women who have lost a fetus in the third trimester, I have inquired about the possible relationship between the death and orgasm. However, I have never definitely been able to establish a connection (and actually have been happy not to do so).

Orgasm and breast massage have long been considered effective means of inducing labor by people of various cultures and among gravidas of different economic backgrounds.[475] Indeed, both orgasm and breast massage are associated with increased levels of serum prostaglandins and oxytocin.[475] When the cervix is ripe, particularly in the multigravida, uterine contractions achieved through orgasm are often sufficient to initiate labor. When a patient at term has a ripe cervix, I continue to recommend either breast massage or orgasm for elective induction. I find that if strong uterine contractions occur, the success rate for inducing labor is approximately 60%.

What then are the specific detrimental effects of maternal orgasm in pregnancy? I believe that in late pregnancy there may be two: one is induction of premature labor; the other is initiation of abruptio placentae. While at Stanford University, I studied 200 pregnant or immediately postpartum women in regard to frequency of orgasm during pregnancy and the possible association with premature labor. After most of the factors reputedly associated with premature labor were

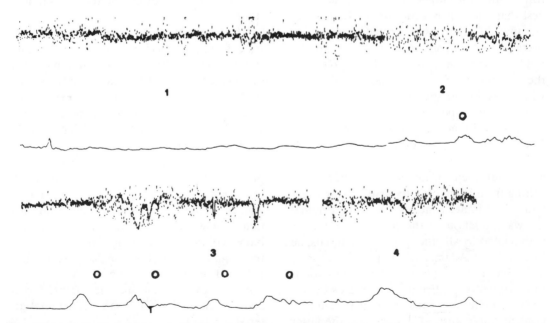

Fig. 6-1. Recordings from a Smith–Kline fetal monitor with fetal heart rate recorded in upper tracing and uterine tension in lower. "O" refers to maternal orgasm. Basal fetal heart rate is approximately 155 beats/min and dips to 96 beats/min. (From Goodlin, R.C.: *Obstet Gynecol* **39:** 125, 1972. Reproduced with permission.)

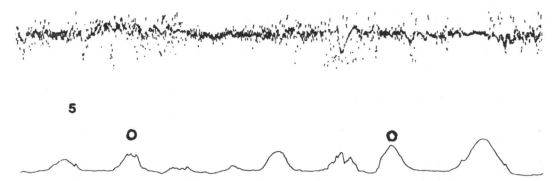

Fig. 6-2. Terminal orgasmic episode (O). Note bradycardia (vagal type). (From Goodlin, R.C.: *Obstet Gynecol* **39:** 125, 1972. Reproduced with permission.)

matched, a significant correlation remained between orgasm in the third trimester and premature delivery. However, these findings have not been substantiated by Solberg *et al.*[643] or by Wagner *et al.*[721] There are some possible explanations for these discrepancies.

Without being critical of anyone's personal behavior, I think it is accurate to say that, in retrospect, the study group at Stanford University Hospital in 1970 represented a wave of the future. They were using illicit drugs, often had multiple sex partners, and experienced frequent and prolonged coitus during pregnancy. Many also had gonorrhea.

These apparent factors were brought into focus when I later moved to another hospital, only 18 miles down the freeway from the Stanford University Hospital, which had a relatively large Chicano population. As best I could determine among gravidas in the second hospital, coitus during pregnancy was brief, orgasm was rare, and fewer of the women were "promiscuous." The incidence of premature labor and/or cystitis was markedly lower than among women in the Stanford Hospital study group.

My explanation for these observations then is that vaginitis and cervicitis are more frequent with promiscuity and that orgasm and its associated uterine contractions, with cervicitis, are related to deciduitis. The arguments over the role of uterine infection in premature labor are extensive, but I continue to believe that infection (deciduitis and chorioamnionitis) and breakdown of the decidua with its relase of prostaglandins is a common

cause of premature labor (Chapter 19). These same sexual factors are also responsible for the increased incidence of urinary tract infection, which I believe accounts for the relationship reported between asymptomatic urinary tract infections and premature labor.[396]

I continue to obtain histories of premature labor following orgasm. Therefore, it seems to me that women who have no orgasm or coitus during pregnancy have a lower incidence of premature labor than do women who have prolonged orgasmic experiences and coitus (particularly if they have multiple sex partners).

Throughout this discussion, I have emphasized orgasm over coitus. While vaginal coitus can introduce both prostaglandins and infectious agents into the vagina, our matched studies at Stanford would suggest that maternal orgasm is the most important factor in "sex" inducing premature labor. I became especially convinced of this after obtaining histories of induction of premature labor either through maternal masturbation (where uterine contractions are stated to be stronger) or when gravidas would "dream" of orgasm.

My studies of uterine contractions and FHR monitoring during maternal orgasm were terminated for two reasons: one was the difficulties I encountered in data collection and its possible adverse effect upon physician–patient relationship. I found it necessary to spend at least twice as much time with patients during their prenatal visits when I asked about orgasm as when I did not, and I sometimes created patient anxiety upon broaching the matter. To my surprise, I found that many gravidas were quite concerned about being nonorgasmic during pregnancy, and they wished instantaneous improvement. I had no easy answer for this need and could tell them only that it would be "better" after they had delivered. Women who experienced orgasm were often interested in a prolonged discussion because of uterine contractions and their possible deleterious effects. A third group of patients resented such questioning. Thus, the overall effect of my "study" on patients was negative in that I alienated some women and was unable to help others.

The second reason for terminating the studies was a probable abruptio placentae induced by orgasm. A 19-year-old gravida 2, para 1, Ab 1, in her 28th week of pregnancy told one of our house officers that she was unable to tolerate coitus and orgasm because of associated severe, painful uterine contractions. Since the patient had a soft, relatively ripe cervix, she was cautioned about orgasm and advised to abstain until the 34th week of pregnancy—when she was to participate in our "pregnancy–orgasm" studies.

Upon reaching the 34th week, she appeared as instructed and was monitored for 30 min before inducing uterine contractions through masturbation. During the preorgasmic period, she had only one obvious uterine contraction. But following orgasm, uterine contractions became more frequent and painful. Within 1 hr after orgasm, she began to have heavy vaginal bleeding and her uterus was tense. A diagnosis of abruptio placentae was made. The membranes were ruptured, and 50 min later she was delivered of a 1806-g male infant who required 3 weeks of care in the newborn nursery. The placenta showed an area of separation over approximately 30% of the maternal surface.

I kept insisting to the patient that it was probably only a "coincidence" that the abruptio occurred after the painful uterine contractions during the course of our study. But I have lingering doubts, and, therefore, have never again encouraged a woman to undergo such studies. Since this case, I have learned of other gravidas whose abruptios apparently began immediately after orgasm.

One of the risks of having sex when pregnant is that during foreplay air is sometimes blown into the vagina (aerocolpos). The California Maternal Mortality Studies have documented several cases of maternal death from air embolism during sex play. While I have never found a comfortable or easy way to warn patients about this hazard, considering present sex practices, I do think that the risk should definitely be brought to their attention.

My view on sex in pregnancy is to attempt to adjust to whatever are the current cultural practices. There can be no doubt that a significant number of gravidas in early labor have vaginal coitus immediately prior to leaving for the hospital. (Such "lay" therapy for prolonged latent periods appears even more common with our home style deliveries.) (Protocol P-XVI.)

Given such circumstances, I try to explain to my patients the relative risks of coitus, including venereal disease (especially herpes and gonorrhea), premature labor, and prolonged annoying pelvic discomfort (round ligament pain?). I also mention that forced abstinence causes many otherwise-faithful husbands or lovers to establish sexual contacts elsewhere—sometimes for the first time.

It is my hope that the gravida and her mate will evaluate her orgasmic response, the importance of orgasm to both individuals, and weigh the relative risks. If the gravida has strong orgasmic responses with painful uterine contractions or a history of premature labor, placenta previa, or miscarriages, perhaps she and her mate can agree on abstinence from at least maternal orgasm. On the other hand, if she is without obstetric complications and wishes to continue her coital relationship with her mate, or if orgasm is important to her, she should obviously ignore my advice (which I think 100% of gravida do in this context).

In the event that a gravida has a poor obstetric history and a strong orgasmic response but continues to have vaginal coitus,

I recommend use of vaginal antibacterial suppositories precoitus for I am convinced that premature labor is rare in the absence of deciduitis,[166] especially when related to orgasm (Chapter 19). With tongue in cheek, I also suggest to patients that they try to achieve nonorgasmic sexual responses only during their pregnancies.

Case No. 6-1

A 33-year-old gravida had one premature infant who survived, three early spontaneous miscarriages, and then four midtrimester abortions of whom none survived. A hysterogram was normal and the last two pregnancies had been treated unsuccessfully with cervical cerclage. During all of these pregnancies, the gravida experienced frequent postcoital orgasm after her obstetrician's assurance that "sex" was not harmful. During the current pregnancy, we prescribed a high protein and caloric diet, forced fluids, abstinence from orgasm, and frequent periods of physical rest in the left lateral supine position. The gravida was able to avoid orgasm from the 18th to the 32nd week, at which time she claimed to have "dreamed" an orgasm which was followed by coitus associated with further

orgasm. Within 30 min, the patient began painful uterine contractions which continued 2 days despite bed rest, intravenous alcohol, and forced fluids. She delivered spontaneously a 1620-g male infant who survived.

Other Points of View

Papers have appeared, mostly in our free journals, stating that "sex" is safe throughout pregnancy. Pion and Reich[542] suggest that avoidance of sex during pregnancy is necessary only in the presence of "some" complication. They quote S. Leon Israel, "In my 36 years of practice, I have never observed harm to anyone resulting from the average loving act of intercourse between husband and wife." In Dr. Israel's obstetric practice, it is entirely possible the length of coitus was brief, and that the various venereal diseases (herpes, CMV, gonorrhea, etc.) were absent.

While Wagner and associates[721] were unable to demonstrate any relationship in 19 cases of prematurity with coitus per se during pregnancy, they do suggest further study. In a personal communication, Limner has indicated that he has important new information which demonstrates the deleterious effects of coitus during pregnancy. (Adapted from: Goodlin, R. C.: Can sex in pregnancy harm the fetus? *Contemp Obstet Gynecol* **8**:21, 1976.)

CHAPTER 7

Antenatal Care—Or How to Have a Normal Baby

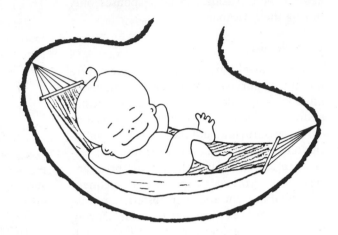

Historical

In 1902 Ballantyne, a Scottish physician, postulated that routine prenatal care might safeguard the life of the gravida and her fetus. He suggested that comprehensive antenatal care could delineate the many maternal and fetal factors that cause fetal disease and mortality. In America, the first organization, in 1902, to bring antenatal care to all expectant women was the Instructive Nursing Association of Boston, under Mrs. William Putnam. However, American physicians maintained a general apathy toward perinatal loss, as many apparently believed that such was the work of nature and to do otherwise would only preserve the defective and weaken subsequent generations. Mrs. Putnam finally went to Baltimore to see J. Whitridge Williams, professor of obstetrics at Johns Hopkins University. After a brief period of trial with routine prenatal care, Williams presented a landmark paper in 1915, "The Limitations and Possibilities of Prenatal Care," to the American Association for the Study and Prevention of Infant Mortality. This same organization in 1909 had suggested a model law for the registration of births and infant deaths which allowed some understanding of the problem as it existed in America. However, the emphasis in prenatal care remained, in America at least, with protection of maternal health and the prevention of toxemia. In 1974 the American Board of Obstetrics and Gynecology certified the first specialists in Maternal–Fetal Medicine. For reasons that are not clear, American perinatal mortality figures have failed to improve at rates comparable to those in Europe and Japan.

To Have a Normal, Healthy Baby

No question is more frequently asked by gravida and is more difficult to answer in scientific terms than, "How do I have a normal, healthy newborn?" Fortunately, for our specialty, western countries have experienced improving perinatal mortality rates over the past decade, even without any new knowledge or specific therapy.

THE FRENCH EXPERIENCE

France has enjoyed the greatest improvement of perinatal mortality rates of any developed nation, which at first glance appears to be the result of a previously well-organized and federally financed program. In 1968, a French committee headed by Sureau studied the national problem and determined that there was a lack of proper equipment in public hospitals, an excess of small, private institutions, a lack of organization among the various obstetric professions, a general lack of organized interest among most pediatricians and anesthesiologists in perinatal problems, a deficiency in the recruitment of new obstetricians, and an overall lack of financial support for perinatal research and programs. Much as in America, despite a feeling among certain obstetricians, most French people were apparently convinced, in 1968, that all obstetric problems had been solved and that pregnancy was a "natural" phenomenon, and that the only problem to be seriously considered was the psychological aspects of pregnancy and delivery. This view is now expressed in California for more humanistic births by "lay" midwives.

However, there subsequently occurred a consensus of feeling among French pediatricians and obstetricians that there was a national "perinatal" problem and a study was undertaken which concluded that a national effort should be made in the field of perinatology, not only for obvious ethical reasons, but also on economic grounds. The study concluded that the cost of perinatal problems to the French community was equal to approximately 2.5% of their gross national product.

The French perinatal program, as undertaken in 1971, included seven points. The first was teaching and training of students, anesthesiologists, obstetricians, and hospital staff about perinatal problems. This apparently was the part of the program which met with the most difficulties because of problems with university appointments, the problems of residency training, and the general lack of interest in obstetrics among French medical students. The second portion of the program included obtaining an accurate definition of the French problems in perinatal care and securing support for relevant research. The third feature was routine vaccination against rubella and the fourth was improvement of prenatal care. At that time in France, the official number of prenatal visits was 4; but in practice, the number was found to be only 3.5. Part of the new program was to increase the number of prenatal visits to perhaps 7 for all gravida and 10 for those judged to be high risk. The fifth part of the prenatal program, directed toward both private and public institutions, was improvement of the conditions surrounding delivery. For the public hospitals, an effort was made to purchase monitoring equipment, particularly in the high-risk centers. Sixth, direct efforts were made to ascertain that all institutions had adequate instruction and equipment for resuscitation of the newborn. Those institutions which could not meet these standards were to be closed. In the seventh step, neonatal intensive care units were established.

At the same time, nongovernmental efforts were made by the French medical profession in reorganization and enlarging some private institutions and the establishment of a society of perinatal medicine. There were also planned organizations of perinatal multidisciplinary research teams.

Five years after undertaking and funding the national effort, the French perinatal rate had decreased from 23.3 in 1971 to 16.9 per thousand in 1976. These results were considered outstanding, but in retrospect, the decrease in perinatal rates had actually started before the inauguration of the national perinatal program in 1971. The projected decrease in perinatal mortality for 1980 had actually been reached (without planning) by 1971.

After cost analysis, the "resuscitation of the newborn" was the most successful of the French programs and the "rubella vaccination" the least. Fetal monitoring was difficult to evaluate, but was one of the most costly parts of the program.

THE AMERICAN EXPERIENCE

While no such official program has been undertaken in America, the results in perinatal rates have been similar to those achieved in France.[735] Now that the American perinatal rates are decreasing, many disciplines are taking credit, such as the abortionists, birth control centers, nutritionists, neonatal intensive care centers, and the organizers of regionalization.

The decline seen in France and America in perinatal rates has also occurred worldwide. As shown in Figure 7-1, the perinatal mortality rates improved steadily in England and Wales over the past 20 years and in California over the past 10 years (Figs. 7-2–7-4). No sudden change occurred in these perinatal rates, but rather a gradual improvement appeared, suggesting no particular medical event or technique was responsible for this gratifying happening.

Our patients, their lawyers, and neonatologists now take seriously our claims that by monitoring of fetal health and development, we are able to achieve a "better" newborn. The only aspect of our present malpractice dilemma which is perhaps beneficial is that it has forced the obstetrician to realistically inform the gravida of the likelihood of her newborn having a serious birth defect, and at the same time indicated our relative inability to prevent or ameliorate the occurrence of such tragedies. My experience in court has taught me that the same physician who modestly implies in his office of being omnipotent, in court confesses his inability (as well as that of the medical profession) to modify the course of events that produce such abnormal newborns.

THERAPEUTIC ABORTION

A concept that seemingly appeals to layman and physician alike is a program designed to diagnose *in utero* fetal anomalies. In the event that an anomaly is diagnosed which prevents the fetus from functioning as a normal human being (such as Down's syndrome, severe meningiomyelocele, hydocephalus, and so forth), the gravida is presumably offered a therapeutic abortion. I have argued in a letter to the editor of the *American Journal of Human Genetics* against this widely held concept, proposing somewhat facetiously that we instead practice infanticide. The midtrimester human fetus, which is the period of fetal life when such therapeutic abortions are done, is, from a developmental standpoint, the same as the newborn. Only 20 weeks of life separate the two. The truth of these similarities is illustrated by how frequently physicians and hospital staffs are disturbed by the performances of midtrimester therapeutic abortions.

I was one of the originators of the midtrimester abortion techniques in America[256] and therefore cannot base my arguments against the procedure on either moral or religious grounds, but simply argue from the standpoint of efficiency of diagnosis and maternal safety. In my letter, written in 1969, protesting a series of articles which pleaded that more money should be expended in developing techniques for *in utero* diagnosis of congenital anomalies, I argued that the number of anomalies which could be diagnosed *in utero* was small (pp. D-68–D-75), that the *in utero* diagnostic techniques were subject to error, and that the risks to the gravida of therapeutic abortion in midtrimester were greater than the risks of delivering at term. Given a newborn with suspected anomalies, the diagnosis could be more accurately confirmed than is possible *in utero*, and presumably death would be no more painful to such

Fig. 7-1. Perinatal mortality rates; stillbirths and first 28-day neonatal deaths. Similarity between perinatal mortality rates (all weights) is even more pronounced when single-year figures for Sheffield are plotted against national figures. (From Gordon, R.: *Br Med J* 2: 1202, 1977. Reproduced with permission.)

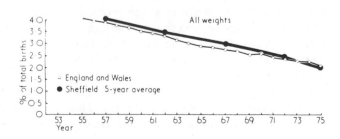

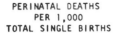

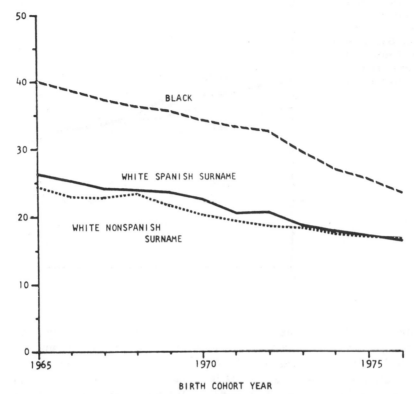

Fig. 7-2. Direct method of adjustment to 1960 California single total births by age of mother. Source: State of California, Department of Health, Maternal and Child Health, Birth Cohort Records.

a newborn in the nursery than while a mid-trimester fetus. Given the wide range of severe anomalies which can be diagnosed at birth as compared with those detectable *in utero*, and the difference in cost of detecting anomalies at these two time periods, the cost benefits of infanticide are much greater to society than are those of therapeutic abortion.

The editor's response to my letter was prompt. While acknowledging the basic correctness of my concept, he rejected outright publication of such a letter (the only rejection I have had in some 50 letters to the editor). His argument was that the field of human genetics was not prepared to accept the burden of a doctrine of infanticide, for such a concept evoked (in him, at least) the horrors of Nazi Germany's genocide program.

I continue to believe that a society which applauds therapeutic abortion at 20 weeks gestation (and even pretends that it is "good" for the fetus) while at the same time rejecting the concept of infanticide for severe anomalies as dreadful and inhumane, is indeed schizophrenic. As an example of this viewpoint, on some occasions it is necessary to make certain an anencephalic is stillborn, because of the neonatologist's inclination to "preserve life" and to maintain such an individual with considerable anguish in the nursery until it dies. The preceding discussion has not been pleasant or tranquil, but it does concern the problem of preserving the fetal right to be heard (precise tests) and of assuring the gravida that she will take home from the hospital a normal child. I hope that the argument will not be taken out of context.

PRENATAL TECHNIQUE

Given the constraints of our society and

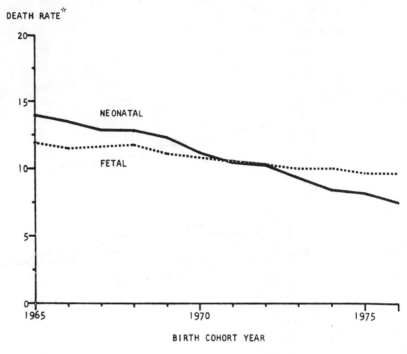

Fig. 7-3. Direct method of adjustment to 1960 California total births by age of mother. Fetal death rate per 1000 total births, neonatal death rate per 1000 live births. Source: State of California, Department of Health, Maternal and Child Health, Birth Cohort Records.

the limitations of our knowledge, our techniques for helping couples obtain a normal child are as follows (protocols P-1–P-49): First, we determine whether the gravida is low risk (protocol P-48), which really requires minimal time and effort. Past obstetrical history is the most important item of our evaluation, for clearly those women who are proven reproducers will likely remain "low risk" for subsequent pregnancies while those women with prior reproductive loss have a reduced chance of having a subsequent normal child. For example, there is a familial spectrum of repeated reproductive defects from spontaneous miscarriages to delivery of children at term with CNS defects. Gravida with unexplained prior premature births are more likely to have a subsequent premature birth. The risk factors are also obviously increased if the gravida has previously delivered a child with anomalies. Maternal age, general health, socioeconomic status, drug addiction, and so forth (protocol P-48), are all factors which remove a gravida from the low-risk category. If, after thorough exploration of all these possible factors, a patient still is in a low-risk category, we assure her that

the probability of having a normal pregnancy and newborn are very high. Indeed, we offer these patients the "homestyle delivery" in our hospital, or delivery by the midwife (protocol P-XVI). I believe that the obstetrician has little to offer such low-risk gravida other than reassurance and perhaps the added benefits of tranquility. Those associated with the homestyle delivery program or the midwife can seemingly do this as well, if not better, than most obstetricians are able to.

Second, the gravida's personal habits should be thoroughly, but quickly, explored. An adequate high protein diet is probably desirable (Chapter 2) as is increased rest (Chapter 4).

For the sake of optimal fetal outcome, any women in the reproductive age group (and perhaps males, too) should refrain from drug ingestion when contemplating or attempting pregnancy. Following implantation of the embryo, and during organogenesis, the fetus is more sensitive to detrimental effects, including not only drugs, but pyrexia, viremia, and perhaps even excessive physical activity (Table D-51) (Fig. 7-5). While there appears to be only four drugs (thalidomide, andro-

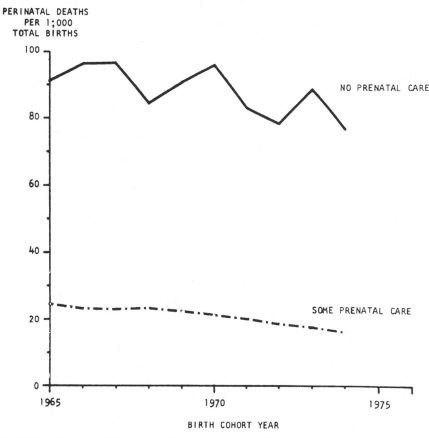

Fig. 7-4. Perinatal deaths per 1000 births. Source: State of California, Department of Health, Maternal and Child Health, Birth Cohort Records.

genic hormones, folate antagonists, methyl mercury) that have been definitely proven to be teratogenic in humans (Tables D-51 and D-91–D-97), there is a suggestion that many drugs may lower the threshold to expression of detrimental fetal abnormalities, especially in this critical time period. The data for this latter statement are soft, but it is best substantiated by comparing the incidence of cerebral palsy and congenital anomalies in infants born in Scotland with those in America. When this is compared with a history of drug ingestion, in both instances, the rates of drugs and anomalies is about one-third of that in the United States. Confirmation of this impression awaits the equalization of drug ingestion by pregnant women in America with Scotland. It is hoped that the rates in America will decrease to that of Scotland.[343a]

The use of drugs in the third trimester seems to be more acceptable than at other times during pregnancy. The presumed deleterious effects of drugs are less marked during this period and presumably both the patient and her physician are aware of her condition and will use caution. At the same time, many gravida are most uncomfortable during this time period and since I regard the achievement of tranquility as so important, I am willing to prescribe tranquilizers and mild analgesics during the third trimester. Admittedly, there are limitations to this viewpoint, as aspirin, for instance, does cause abnormalities of platelet agglutination in newborns and tranquilizers cause the floppy newborn syndrome.

ITCHING DURING PREGNANCY

Pruritus during pregnancy can sometimes indicate an ominous situation for the fetus. It

Fig. 7-5. The critical stages of development of the main structures of the human embryo. (From Tuchmann-Duplessis, H.: *Drug Effects on the Fetus.* Seaforth, Addis, 1975. Reproduced with permission.)

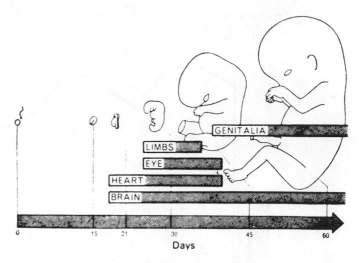

can represent the "maternal syndrome" (Chapters 5 and 22) or cholestasis of pregnancy. The latter is much more common in Scandinavian countries and Chile.[190a] The perinatal mortality in cholestasis of pregnancy can be devastating, with perinatal mortality rates reported as high as 9% and frequent occurrences of unexplained fetal acidosis during labor. Pruritus itself, without obvious cause, is sometimes equally ominous for the fetus. With all itching during pregnancy, Ylostalo and Ylikorkala[766a] of Finland reported associated maternal toxemia to occur in 24–33% in the various series and urinary tract infections in 24%. Obviously, itching with these complications could represent side effects of the various maternal therapies. The management of itching in pregnancy is outlined in Protocol P-33.

CHORIONIC FLUID

One of the difficult areas to treat or offer prophylaxis is "premature rupture of the membranes" (Chapter 22). Many cases that we see in midpregnancy are, in my view, rupture of the chorionic sac. These fluids are more yellow, limited in amount, and the pregnancy usually suffers no ill effects from loss of the fluid. Like with so many problems in obstetrics, the diagnosis only becomes obvious in retrospect. I do believe in the reality of the chorionic sac, however. For, as noted (Chapter 14) occasional amniocenteses done

at 16–18 weeks show a bloody brown fluid. This fluid represents, in my opinion, the chorionic fluid which is usually reabsorbed by this time.

HEPARINIZATION

A gravida with thromboembolism must be anticoagulated or the mortality rates are approximately 15%. However, almost all other indications for anticoagulation are uncertain. These include deep vein thrombosis, HbS trait, or history of past embolism. If the anticoagulation is carried on through delivery, the risk of signifiant postpartum bleeding is 15–20%, even with only 5,000 units of heparin t.i.d. And then, too, such heparin schedules apparently are, at times, associated with a thrombocytopenia. We continue to use prophylactic heparin in these gravida.

PREVENTION OF FETAL INFECTION

The prevention of fetal infection (see Tables D-107–D-113) would seemingly be the one area in which physicians could provide their patients with useful information. Unfortunately, the most common chronic infections of neonates are generally the results of relatively asymptomatic infections in their mothers.

CMV

Cytomegalovirus (CMV) may be totally

asymptomatic in the affected gravida or may present as a flu or as the infectious mononucleosis syndrome. Among pregnant women, ranges of 3–28% have been reported to have positive cervical cultures for CMV and the virus may apparently be venereally transmitted. Approximately 4% of all pregnant women excrete the virus in their urine, but fortunately only a small minority of their infants demonstrate any problems. Asymptomatic mothers have been reported to deliver repeatedly infected children, and it is known that the virus may affect only the placenta and not the fetus or that it may only affect one of twin fetuses. While CMV is perhaps the most common serious infection of newborns, and may be a significant cause of cerebral dysfunction (Chapter 23), it has no known effective prophylaxis or therapy. At the moment, about all obstetricians can recommend to their patients regarding prophylaxis is that they not work in newborn nurseries. Unfortunately, not even this very limited recommendation can be proven to be valid, as adult or neonatal infection has not been demonstrated to occur from newborns.[319]

TOXOPLASMOSIS

All gravida should probably have toxoplasmosis titers determined early or prior to their pregnancy. If serologically negative, they should be advised not to eat uncooked meat and avoid direct contact with cat feces, as it is assumed that these are the two major sources of infections for the human. In my experience, so many women have positive toxoplasmosis titers that the routine use of the test becomes almost useless. Even if toxoplasmosis can be diagnosed during pregnancy, as evidenced by a marked rise in titers associated with flu-like symptoms or lymphadenopathy, chemotherapy is probably unacceptable in view of the unknown toxic effects of the recommended drugs on the fetus. This is especially so since the direct correlation between maternal acute toxoplasmosis and subsequent fetal infection is not clear. In the few cases that I have dealt with apparent

acute maternal toxoplasmosis, the gravidas have elected to have a therapeutic abortion (and in none was the fetus infected).

RUBELLA

All women should be immunized against rubella and rubella titers should be determined on all pregnant women. The use of higher titer immune globulin following maternal exposure is questionable, although I did recommend this prophylaxis in the past. (My view may change for we recently had a gravida who was given the live rubella vaccine in error when the physicians and nurses involved intended to give the "high rubella titer immune globulin.") The need of therapeutic abortion after apparent rubella later than the 15th week of pregnancy is likewise uncertain.

HERPES

Recommendations concerning herpes type II infections in pregnant women are also confusing. Whether the appearance of herpes type II maternal antibodies might protect the fetus of an affected woman is debatable and whether placental transmission is a significant mode of infection for the seriously ill newborn is also unanswered. However, we have recently had a case in which twins were delivered, the first one having the classical TORCH syndrome with cerebral calcifications and hydrocephalus and the second twin being essentially normal. The latter twin had a mild neonatal case of herpes and recovered, and the first twin fortunately expired. The mother was totally asymptomatic, but demonstrated positive herpes viral cultures from the cervix and vagina. Presumably the first twin represented transplacental infection and the second represented infection by contact.

It has been my experience that women with chronic herpes are not the ones who deliver the seriously affected neonates, but rather these sick neonates are delivered from essentially asymptomatic women. Nevertheless, our present protocol (p. P-22) is to test the amniotic fluid for herpes virus in any woman who appears to have active genital herpes in the last 2 months of her pregnancy. If the amniotic fluid culture is negative, she is offered a cesarean section after we explain our understanding of the risks. Virtually all women have elected cesarean sections when told the dreadful consequences of congenital herpes, but I am unconvinced that this is the proper management. A series of brief papers in the *New England Journal of Medicine* by Chang and O'Keefe[97] have raised the question again of whether maternal herpes antibodies may protect the fetus and whether the woman with such protective antibodies is at risk of delivering an affected infant. It is hoped that this question will soon be resolved.

Hepatitis B virus may also be a venereally transmitted disease, as the virus has been identified in the vagina. Such vaginal infections, at least theoretically, pose risks to the fetus during delivery, as well as to the gravida's sexual partner. The evidence for fetal hepatitis B transplacental infection is also confusing. It is probably accurate that transplacental hepatitis B infection can occur, as HAA positive umbilical blood has been described, but most neonatal infections occur during the birth process. In gravida with hepatitis B infection, there are no present data which would indicate that cesarean section is indicated for nonobstetric reasons. Such gravida should have the same care as nonpregnant women with recommendations for rest, adequate diet (of undocumented benefit), and probably gamma globulin injections of their unaffected close contacts. Other gastrointestinal pathogens (*Escherichia coli, Shigella,* etc.) are also now transmitted venereally.

SYPHILIS

Failure to check a woman's VDRL after treatment for gonorrhea is perhaps the reason for the sharp increase in syphilis that is now occurring. This devastating disease, for whose control so many Nobel prizes were awarded, is now appearing in our unregistered neonates. Fetal syphilis is apparently rare prior to the 18th week of pregnancy, although Harter *et al.*[322] have suggested that the spiro-

chetes may be found in the placenta of midtrimester fetuses. Given the promiscuous nature of our society, it is wise to repeat the serological test for syphilis late in pregnancy and again at the time of admission to the hospital.

URINARY TRACT INFECTIONS

During the past 15 years, we have alternated between routine cultures and urinary sediment analysis for bacteria in asymptomatic gravida. Despite glowing reports from Boston[396] and Dallas,[726] we have failed to demonstrate the benefit of routine urine cultures in preventing either future maternal symptoms or premature labor in the truly asymptomatic gravida. Nevertheless, we periodically feel obligated to undertake the expense of such cultures after reading of other institutions' experience. Although it is only an impression, I believe that the reported correlation between cystitis and pregnancy complication both reflect the frequency and duration of coitus during pregnancy (Chapter 6).

NORMAL VAGINAL FLORA INFECTIONS

The vaginal bacterial infections are ones that are readily diagnosed, but therapy again is uncertain. The group B streptococcus is now a cause of neonatal deaths in approximately one out of every thousand newborns.[32] The recorded incidence of group B streptococcus in the cervix and vagina of pregnant women varies from 5 to 25% and the bacteria is probably venereally transmitted.[564] Our own experience is that neonatologists are undecided about the proper course of management when informed that the mother harbors such bacteria in her vagina. Therefore, we have ceased doing routine cultures for B strep as it is expensive to identify and is difficult to eradicate from the women's vagina and above all, apparently leads to no useful information for the neonatologist. Listeria monocytogenes has been held by those in Israel as the cause of miscarriage and sometimes neonatal infections, and it may be a cause of premature labor (with intact membranes),[12] but its presence in the maternal vagina likewise evokes no special care or therapy from the neonatologist.

GONOCOCCUS

The *Neisseria gonococcus*, of course, should be screened for in both early and late pregnancy and should be treated. Chlamydia is now recognized as a common venereal disease.[744a]

ACTIVITY

As discussed in Chapter 6, I recommend to women that coitus should be enjoyed in pregnancy as at other times, except if they have postcoital bleeding, pain, a history of prior premature birth, reproductive loss, or if their mate may have been exposed to one of the many venereal diseases.

I recommend to gravida that they seek maximum physical rest. This is a difficult concept to sell, both to the medical profession and to lay persons alike, as it has been a standard American recommendation that physical exercise prevents constipation, develops muscles appropriate for labor and delivery, controls weight gain, and is generally healthy. But, if a gravida is judged to be high risk for reasons of heart disease, cardiovascular disease, fetal growth retardation, prior premature labor, and so forth, the standard American recommendation is for limited physical activity. If such recommendations are appropriate for the high-risk gravida, then they are likewise appropriate for the low risk.

The recommendation that is the least accepted and perhaps the most difficult to defend is that pregnant women should avoid crowds. The likelihood of viral infection increases with exposure. The data relative to Coxsackie virus concerning congenital heart lesions, influenza associated with increased fetal anomalies, rubella, and so forth (and indeed most every known viral infection apparently an increase in miscarriages and general anomalies) is sufficient to caution our patients to avoid possible exposure.

When gravida are found not to be low risk, then we recommend frequent prenatal visits with techniques toward maternal and fetal surveillance appropriate to whatever their problem may be. As best we can, we attempt to preserve the patient's tranquility in this "non-low-risk" group and still increase our monitoring techniques so that they will benefit from whatever knowledge we may have about the prevention of fetal loss and congenital anomalies.

PRENATAL CARE

In addition to defining the low-risk gravida (protocol P-48), we have attempted to list some of the abnormalities which indicate that the pregnant woman may be high risk (Protocols P-1–P-47). Our recommended diagnostic procedures and care of these high-risk gravida is outlined in the various protocols with their appropriate references and, when appropriate, cross-indexed with this monograph. Defining the low- and high-risk gravida leaves an undefined group which we simply term "undefined risk." In the women delivering at the private obstetrical services in Northern California, approximately 40% of them are low risk and 15% high risk with the remaining 45% being undefined risk. Other clinics have used a much broader definition of the high-risk patient, and using the index as recommended by the California State Board of Health, such an affluent county as Santa Clara in Northern California appears to have 65% of its gravida high risk. This is an absurdity and is the reason for our more rigid definitions. The undefined group are, for all practical purposes, treated as "normal" as concerns their prenatal care, differing only from the low risk in that they are not offered a "homestyle delivery" or delivery by the midwife service. As with all of these definitions, a gravida can change her risk factor during pregnancy.

What then do we recommend to our pregnant patients? Our instructions are listed in protocol P-37, but in brief, it is to be "tranquil," eat a high-protein diet, lie down every 4 hr, drink three quarts of liquid per day, avoid promiscuity, and be aware of certain danger signs. If the gravida requests, we prescribe prenatal vitamins; for others, oral iron, with precautions.

It is important that gravida be informed about our concerns regarding fetal development and the occurrence of rare but serious maternal complications. While such teaching could perhaps best be done by the maternal–fetal medicine specialists, from a practical standpoint, trained nonphysician personnel do a better job. Public health nurses, midwives, nurses, or social workers, through both individual and group teaching, can adequately inform gravida as well as achieve the tranquility which is so important. (I argue, for instance, that only three antenatal physician visits are necessary for optimal results for low-risk gravida.) Since physician time is reduced, such a program has definite cost benefits. It is important that a program such as warning all gravida of the signs of premature labor or of chronic fetal distress be consistently and thoroughly applied.

Case No. 7-1

A 43-year-old P0-0-0-0 Mexican-American female had an amniocentesis for determination of fetal karyotype. Despite having had the purpose of the amniocentesis fully explained to her, when the fetal karyotype was found to be 47XX (trisomy 21) she refused a therapeutic abortion (even after having visited a home for children with Down's syndrome). Her labor at 42 weeks of gestation was terminated by cesarean section for "failure to progress." The newborn was a typical Down's syndrome with multiple minor anomalies, and required prolonged hospitalization.

Case No. 7-2

A 22-year-old P 3-0-1-3 white female was found at the 33rd week of her pregnancy to carry a hydrocephalic fetus. Repeated ultrasonic and computerized tomography (CT) scans indicated that the fetal cerebral mantle (cortex) was very thin (4–5 mm) and would not be functional. The patient and her family were told by our neurosurgeon that the fetus had a 1% chance or less of having normal intelligence. Nevertheless, they all elected to have the fetus delivered by cesarean section instead of fetal decompression and vaginal delivery.

These two patients represent 25% of all cases of intrauterine diagnosis of "fetal anomalies incompatible with normal life" made by our service over a period of 1 year. It is possible that a similar percentage of all gravida undergoing intrauterine diagnosis with negative tests would likewise have refused therapeutic abortion if the tests had been positive. Thus, much of my discussion about therapeutic abortion or infanticide may be in vain, because the gravida has the final decision in such matters.

Other Points of View

INFANTICIDE

The problems relative to infanticide have recently been discussed in *Perinatology-Neonatology* (Vol. 1, No. 2, 1977). In an editorial, David Abramson of Georgetown University states that, first, all jurisdictions have specific laws against homicide. Second, the infant–patient is further protected by the doctrine of an informed consent. Furthermore, Abramson is strongly opposed to all decisions to "not treat" any hospitalized infants. In the paper itself, entitled, "Care of the Newborns: The Decision not to Treat," by M. J. Garland, three categories of babies in intensive care are listed according to their need for treatment. These categories are (1) those who must be treated; (2) those who, at the parent's discretion, may either be treated or allowed to die; and (3) those who should be allowed to die. Garland refers to an extensive bibliography and notes that the very discussion of these matters (infanticide) inevitably raises the spector of Nazi Germany where "merciful" euthanasia policies lead to the horrors of genocide. Garland states that active euthanasia (in America) is not exempt from criminal laws prohibiting homicide. He believes that the exclusion of active euthanasia is necessary as it serves as a check against abuse. Garland defines the problem as he is emphatic that any such discussion (of infanticide) should only apply to infants in need of medical intervention to prolong their lives. Indeed, throughout the paper, there is no consideration of a case in which a child would have to be actively killed. Dr. Garland is coordinator of the Bioethics Program, University of California, San Francisco, and believes that this restriction is important to society as a symbol of the value of life and a safeguard for security. Nontreatment of the deformed newborn does not always ensure that death will follow and quoting Lorber, Garland suggests that a case in which the infant survives nonintervention should be treated as if the decision had initially been to treat the child. Garland believes that the three categories offer some conceptual tools for analyzing and discussing situations which "inhibit a gray landscape." In their monograph, *Ethics of Newborn Intensive Care,* by Jonsen and Garland, they explore in detail some of these issues. It seems clear that they and most other authorities have completely separated the right to life of the fetus of the therapeutic abortion in the 20-week pregnancy and infanticide after it is delivered.[700a]

ANTENATAL CARE

As a medical student I was taught that "good prenatal care accomplished more than the use of antibiotics, blood transfusions, and anesthesia." The California State Board of Health has recently declared that all pregnant women should be seen after their first missed menstrual period and that the minimal number of prenatal visits should be 12 (once every month through the seventh month, every 2 weeks during the eight month, and every week during the ninth month). The same organization also declared that adequate nutrition is critical for the delivery of a healthy child. Similar thoughts and phrases are repeatedly proclaimed by our various national organizations and governmental agencies. There is no doubt that the gravida who follows these directions has a better outcome of her pregnancy than does the unregistered gravidas seen first in early labor. Whether prenatal care and all of its various dogma is responsible for these correlations is the question.

During visits to obstetric hospitals in Western Europe, Japan, and Hong Kong, I have been impressed with the large facilities they have for hospitalization of the antenatal patient. I have always assumed that such facilities are in part responsible for their low perinatal mortality rate.

In America, the Dallas group[726] has similarly found that simple antenatal facilities are able to dramatically improve perinatal mortality rates, even in the high-risk patient, and even when the facilities are of the minimal care variety. However, studies have recently appeared from Britain in which randomized controlled trials of bedrest were compared with ambulation in cases of hypertension of late pregnancy and also with women with twin pregnancies.[463, 734] Much to my surprise, bed rest offered no better outcome than did normal activity at home without sedation. If bed rest is subsequently demonstrated in other studies to be without benefit in these high-risk patients, then I shall have virtually nothing to offer in terms of prenatal care.

ELECTIVE TERMINATION OF PREGNANCY

Neonatologists would have us do amniocentesis before every elective cesarean section or induction of labor.[121, 232] Years ago we reevaluated our policy at Stanford University of doing repeated cesarean sections only after the gravida was in labor, in order to avoid the problem of prematurity. This policy was compared with more than 600 repeat cesarean sections done prior to the onset of labor. To my surprise, *none* of the infants born prior to onset of labor died, even those showing respiratory distress, and all weighed more than 2800 g. There was obviously a bit of luck in obtaining such a good result, as many of these gravida had had the time of their repeat section selected at their first prenatal visit. However, we abandoned our policy of awaiting the onset of labor for timing repeat sections as we were often doing the cases when the woman was already dilated and in the middle of the night when conditions were less than optimal. Indeed, the cesarean section experience at Stanford was baffling. In addition to this superb result with repeat sections, we noted that most cesarean sections done for "cephalopelvic disproportion" occurred at specific times of the day. None were done between the hours of 0250 and 0550, whereas peak occurrence was between 1700 and 1800 (after office hours) or 2200 and 2300 (before the change of shift). While it is always possible that certain circadian rhythms were responsible for such a time distribution ("failure to progress"), staff convenience appeared to be the more logical explanation.

Cowett and Oh,[121] neonatologists, would have us believe that routine amniocentesis with its risks and costs is better than clinical dating of pregnancies for elective termination of pregnancy. But, as Harris and Mead have pointed out,[320] routine amniocentesis is not without its risks. I personally have had three fetal deaths from routine amniocentesis in near-term fetuses and we have done several stat cesarean sections for apparent fetal hemorrhage (in more than 2000 amniocenteses). With more use of ultrasound, dating may become more accurate and amniocentesis more safe, but then we may find that ultrasound is not without its risks.

Harrison et al.[321] have evaluated eight methods for assessing fetal development from amniotic fluid (AF). They found that the L/S ratios, late ultrasound cephalometry, and AF creatinine values were much better tests than the nile blue sulfate stain, the hematoxylin and eosin stain, AF urea or uric acid levels. The mean gestational age as determined from combining the first three reliable tests was more accurate than any single test. (See Table D-44.)

PERINATAL MORTALITY RATES

The entire problem of comparing perinatal mortality rates has been reviewed in a series of letters in *Lancet* (June 1977 through August 1977). It is apparent that perinatal rates are markedly influenced by local ground rules, such as including 500-g fetuses as liveborn infants. In our own hospital, we average about two transfers per month of patients at 26–28 weeks of pregnancy in late labor. Out of the last 15 newborns weighing 500–800 g, only one lived (with hydrocephalus), which of course adversely affects our perinatal mortality rate. At the same time, other maternity hospitals in our area are announcing through the local news media that their perinatal rates have decreased to 6–9 per 1000 births.

An interesting turn in arguments over perinatal rates is that made by Tew[694] from the United Kingdom. Using national statistics, she shows that stillborn rates among patients delivering in hospitals are higher than those delivering at home. These stillborn rate differentials are uniform even when high-risk and low-risk groups are compared and she concluded that trends toward increasing hospital confinements are dangerous and wasteful. One explanation is that gravida originally booked for home delivery but transferred to a hospital have high perinatal mortality rates with the fetus often dead at the time of the transfer.

Naeye, in a 1977 review of perinatal deaths from the collaborative study,[501] states that excluding those cases with "no known diagnosis," 73% of the deaths were due to disorders in which the pathogenesis is so poorly understood that it is not clear how they can be prevented! These disorders include the amniotic fluid infection syndrome, abruptio placentae, premature rupture of the membranes, congenital anomalies, large placental infarcts, thrombosis of the placental vessels, extensive fibrosis of placental villi, intervillous thrombi, hydramnios, and growth retardation of the placenta (Table D-21).

AMNIONITIS

An important argument against the significance of amnionitis in the etiology of prematurity is made by Ledger[428] who states that neonatal mortality is not influenced by the presence or absence of prenatal amnionitis. However, in a more recent publication, Bobitt and Ledger[62] suggest that in cases of premature labor, the role of unrecognized amnionitis should be re-evaluated.

ULTRASOUND

Most obstetricians using ultrasound consider it a precise diagnostic tool as regards placental localization. As noted, this has not been our experience, but King[402] and Kurjak and Barsic[418] explain errors in diagnosis by "placental migration." In 63 out of 67 cases in the latter study in whom the lower margin of placenta was initially found to reach the internal os of the uterus, placental migration occurred, involving a movement of 3–9 cm toward the uterine fundus. The apparent "migration" is perhaps best explained by formation of the lower segment. It appears that only the placenta of a total placenta previa remains fixed and that repeated ultrasonic examinations are required near term to confirm the diagnosis of a previously diagnosed low-lying placenta.

RADIATION RISKS TO THE FETUS

Bross and Natarajan[79] analyzing data from a Tri-State leukemia survey have concluded that there is a 50-fold increase in leukemia of children in 1% of the individuals previously exposed to diagnostic radiation. Uchida had showed in 1960 that diagnostic radiation prior to conception similarly produces chromosome abnormalities.

The American College of Radiology and The American College of Obstetricians and Gynecologists have similarly suggested that diagnostic radiation prior to ovulation is harmful to future progeny. That such diagnostic radiation is no more harmful to the human embryo than to the nonfertilized ovum. Thus, there is no measurable advantage to scheduling diagnostic x-ray examinations at any particular time during a normal menstrual cycle.

ACTIVITY

The role of exercise in pregnancy is unresolved. The ACOG pamphlets for pregnant women recommend exercise for a "healthy" pregnancy and Curet[133] and associates found that in pregnant sheep, uterine blood flow was not "changed" following exercise. As a matter of fact, the distribution of uterine blood flow was altered in favor of the placenta. Curet's study was done (in contrast to that of Longo et al.[4526]) with microspheres injected into the maternal aorta.

The ACOG, in one of its medical guidelines, has declared, "normal women with uncomplicated pregnancies and normal fetuses in a job presenting no greater potential hazards than those encountered in normal daily life in the community, may continue to work without interruption until the onset of labor and may resume working several weeks after an uncomplicated delivery." Thus, ACOG (Dale Dunnihoo, Jan Schneider, and Louise Tyrer) does not accept the concept that rest is beneficial for all pregnancies. ACOG, of course, covers itself, stating that when fetal growth retardation is diagnosed or women have hypertension, plural pregnancies, or work in an unhealthy environment, obviously, work is unacceptable. It is interesting that ACOG reached its conclusions without the benefit of controlled studies.

In a 1978 review of physical training during pregnancy, Dressendorfer[167] concluded that hard physical training had no disturbing effect. In one gravida studied through two pregnancies, he noted that physical training can improve maximal oxygen uptake and endurance performance. Erkkola et al.[190] studied the physical fitness of 120 healthy primigravida 2 weeks prior to term. They subsequently demonstrated a negative correlation between physical fitness

and intrapartum maternal lactic acid levels/umbilical lactic acid levels. Since umbilical lactic acid levels sometimes reflect fetal hypoxia, the assumption is made that maternal physical fitness is desirable in avoiding fetal hypoxia. As indicated, I believe this assumption is nonsense.

EFFECTS OF PERINATAL CARE

There are data which suggest that the introduction of certain perinatal measures specifically improved perinatal outcome. An obvious event was the widespread use of Rh immune globulin in Rh negative women.

Bjorn Westin has shown that in his hospital in Danderyd, Sweden (Fig. 7-6), perinatal rates improved with the use of the "partogram" and when the availability of fulltime pediatric coverage was introduced at 1 (at 2 of Fig. 7-6), with the gravidogram project (graphic comparison between changes in symphysis–fundus distance, girth, weight, and blood pressure and HPL) (3 of Fig. 7-6), and when the high-risk ward was in full use. It is interesting that compared to American hospitals, the incidence of stillborns among post-term pregnancies was only 1 per 10,000 births in this Swedish hospital and that less than one intrapartum death occurred per 1000 deliveries in the Danderyd Hospital. This remarkable Swedish record occurred despite inadequate resources for electronic fetal monitoring!

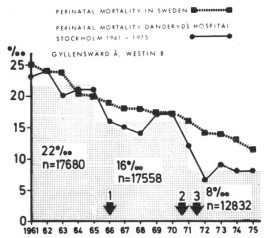

Fig. 7-6. Perinatal mortality in Sweden and the Danderyd Hospital, Sweden. Significant decreases in perinatal rates ascribed to improvements in perinatal care. See text for details. (From Westin, B.: Gravidogram and fetal growth. *Acta Obstet Gynecol Scand* **56:** 273, 1977. Reproduced with permission.)

CHAPTER 8

Fetal Cardiovascular Responses to Stress

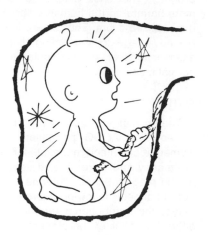

Introduction

This review is undertaken because of what I consider are two prevailing, but inaccurate, obstetrical concepts. The first is that the fetal heart rate is somehow a precise indicator of fetal health (in contrast to the recognized inadequacy of heart rate responses for health screening in adults) and that electronic fetal monitoring will prevent all intrapartum fetal deaths or cases of cerebral palsy. The second is that the fetus is always acting in its own best interest with its various intrauterine cardiovascular responses to stress.

Alexander Pope admonished that "The proper study of mankind is man," but hopefully, the clinician will not reject this review because of its emphasis on laboratory animals. Admittedly, there are large areas of obstetrics in which sheep data are not applicable, but, on the other hand, it is possible to carry out many of the required fetal physiologic investigations only in the laboratory. The sheep or goat fetus has been the standard fetal research preparation since the 1884 animal studies of Cohnstein and Zuntz[115] and this review will also concentrate on sheep data. However, reference will also be made

to fetal primate and adult diving studies.

The "fetal hypoxemic–asphyxial response" (FHAR) (cardiovascular response) is repeatedly mentioned and is considered to include vasoconstriction, hypertension, bradycardia, and in its most ominous form, reduce cardiac performance and output.

The Chronic Fetal Preparation

A point to be emphasized in discussing fetal research from different laboratories is the circumstances surrounding the fetal preparation. While Assali and associates[21] disagree many investigators believe that seemingly benign surgical and anesthetic procedures alter fetal physiologic functions.[143, 403, 589–594] For instance, in chronic fetal preparations umbilical vein pressure decreases and umbilical flow increases during the postoperative period[589] and the basal heart rate slows,[403] which are important changes if fetal cardiovascular function is being studied. The clinical usefulness of data obtained from acute or even exteriorized fetal sheep preparations is not meant to be denied as the obstetrician sometimes attempts to interpret responses of human fetuses that have been stressed or drugged with similarly decreased precision. However, in order to identify the various mechanisms responsible for fetal cardiovascular responses, it is necessary to study fetuses in good health, free of drug influences or elevated catecholamine levels. Unless otherwise noted, quoted fetal sheep data will be that obtained from fetuses of chronic preparations, at least 2 days postsurgery and apparently in good health. Friedman and associates[210] apparently believe that chronic preparations should be studied only after the 10th to 13th postoperative day, a view which would essentially limit this review to their publications. Longo and associates[452b] have further defined the nonstressed preparing by showing that prior "training" of the pregnant sheep results in higher P_{CO_2} values during their studies, even in the chronic preparation.

The Diving Reflex

The FHAR is much like the adult diving response and because it has been extensively studied, this adult response is briefly discussed. More than a century ago, the French physiologist, Paul Bert, described the cardio

vascular events associated with diving, and this has remained a popular topic for scientific inquiry. The ability of mammals to remain submerged for long periods of time was unexplained until Irving[370] proposed the "heart–brain" preparation. Briefly, he reasoned that during anoxia, through a process of selective vasoconstriction, blood would be diverted from nonessential organs (skin, muscle, gut) to essential ones (heart, brain). (The adrenal is now included in the essential group.[16]) (Fig. 8-1).

The adult diving reflex includes apnea, bradycardia, systolic hypertension, selective vasoconstriction, and peripheral lactic acid accumulation.[16,373] Features of the adult diving reflex which are presumed to be analogous to the FHAR are that ventilation abolishes the responses,[385] that hypocarbia reduces its selective vasoconstriction, that cardiac output decreases in proportion to the bradycardia, that atropine abolishes the bradycardia, and that the entire diving reflex is inhibited by general anesthesia.[373] Face or nasopharyngeal immersion has been considered to be the initiating event of the diving reflex, but since the fetus is constantly im-

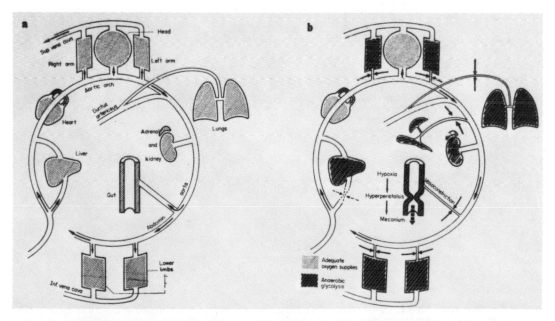

Fig. 8-1. Schematic diagram of fetal cardiovascular response to stress. With selective vasoconstriction (b), blood flow is maintained to fetal adrenal, brain, heart, and placenta. (Modified with permission of Saling.)

mersed in warm amniotic fluid, it has been difficult to understand why these immersion reflexes are not evoked during *in utero* life. An answer may be Johnson and colleagues[385] demonstration that a variety of physiologic fluids such as amniotic fluid or sheep's milk do not produce apnea when instilled into the newborn sheep's nasopharynx. The inhibition of the immersion reflex is apparently through the superior laryngeal nerve from the taste receptors. Thus, the same reflexes which are initiated by immersion in the adult are evoked by hypoxia in the immersed fetus.

As discussed below, the umbilical circulation is very insensitive to vasoactive drugs.[143] However, the fetal body tissues are sensitive to vasoactive drugs. With propranolol, a beta-blocker,[114] the fetal hypoxic response is compromised because total cardiac output is further diminished and because blood flow to the placenta is significantly reduced due to lack of fetal body vasoconstriction.

Apnea obviously is crucial for diving in mammals and apparently plays an important reflex role in maintaining selective vasoconstriction and bradycardia, since rapid lung ventilation alone initiates reflexes which override both the vasoconstriction and bradycardia of either dry or wet apneic asphyxia.[373, 385, 413] However, in Rudolph's laboratory, when a fetus of a chronic preparation in good condition and with normal heart rate was hyperventilated through a large bore catheter with either warm saline or gas mixtures, there was no consistent FHR or blood pressure change other than that due to intrathoracic pressure changes (Fig. 8-2). Unfortunately, these studies were not done during a period of fetal bradycardia, which presumably would have shown changes in FHR with ventilation. Dawes[144] has reported an arrest of fetal breathing in fetal sheep during hypoxemia, but again, studies in Rudolph's laboratory suggest an inconsistent breathing response, as sheep fetuses dying an asphyxial death did not show consistent agonal breathing patterns.

Scholander[612, 613] subsequently proved Irving's hypothesis of the "heart–brain preparation" and furthermore, demonstrated in seals a lactic acid accumulation in muscle during diving. When the diving animal sur-

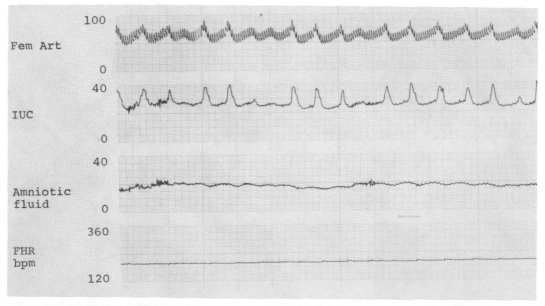

Fig. 8-2. Recording from a 120-day fetus of a chronic sheep preparation ventilated *in utero* through a tracheal catheter (Rudolph's laboratory). Each abrupt rise in fetal inferior vena caval pressure (IVC) represents lung expansion. Note absence in change of FHR.

faced and the selective vasoconstriction was relieved, lactic acid was washed out, producing a brief acidemia. The immediate newborn has been shown to have a similar lactic acid washout at birth, presumably as a result of a degree of fetal selective vasoconstriction during terminal labor. An obvious comparison has been made between the immediate newborn and the adult diving reflex,[188, 374] although it is unclear as to what "releases" the vasoconstriction in the newborn. The "release" could be initiated by lung ventilation, or temperature and blood gas changes, or almost anything that the newborn experiences in the immediate period after birth.

The fetus appears to readily evoke the selective vasoconstriction response to hypoxia and other stress[604] (Fig. 8-1), but the value of such a reflex in fetal hypoxic survival is difficult to assess. For instance, those drugs which diminish or abolish the diving reflex, such as atropine or barbiturates, are in proper dosage protective of the fetus against asphyxia.[246, 259] This "drug hypoxia protective" effect is thought to operate through reduced metabolism and inhibition of vagal reflexes. In contrast, these same drugs reduce the time an adult mammal can stay submerged[17] by altering the heart rate and the selective vasoconstriction, and presumably have the same effect on the FHAR.

Dawes[141] has objected to comparing the fetal asphyxial response to the diving reflex because the associated biochemical protective mechanisms are so different, i.e., fetal stores of liver and cardiac glycogen and diving mammal's stores of myoglobin. Nevertheless, the aspects of the FHAR of bradycardia and selective vasoconstriction seem best understood (for purposes of discussion) in terms of the fetus employing at least a modification of the adult diving reflex.

The baroreflex, an essential feature of both the fetal hypoxic response and the adult diving response (Fig. 8-3), was first described in dogs by Etienne Marey (Marey's law of the heart) in 1859 and was studied in sheep fetuses 85 years later by Sir Joseph Barcroft.[37] It is one of the oldest reflexes, being present in primitive fish. The reflex also appears early in fetal life and its development has been carefully studied by Rudolph's group.[629] Rudolph and Heymann[590] have pointed out the possible detrimental effects of the reflex on fetal cardiac output and has suggested that its appearance may not be to the fetus' advantage. It includes changes in heart rate, arterial and venous dilatation, and cardiac performance, all in response to blood pressure alterations. The baroreflex effect on FHR is mediated by the vagus nerve. Vagal nerve stimulation has an especially negative inotropic (decreased cardiac function) effect as the fetal heart has diminished sympathetic innervation.[210]

The baroreflex is modified by P_{O_2} and P_{CO_2} levels, and its pressure set points are continuously modified.[628] While chemoreceptor responses to hypoxia and hypocarbia have been shown repeatedly to arise both centrally and in aortic and carotid centers, the opposite effects of low fetal oxygen (in-

Fig. 8-3. Fetal lamb, 138 days gestation, 3.8 kg. At each small arrow 0.8 mg of a sodium cyanide solution (0.2 ml) was injected into the ascending aorta before and after section of the cervical vagi and carotid nerves, demonstrating the selective vasoconstriction with the baroreflex [decreased femoral flow and the importance of the afferent (vagus) and efferent (carotid) loops]. (From Dawes, G.S., *et al.: J Physiol* **195**: 55, 1968. Reproduced with permission.)

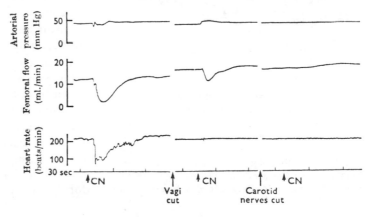

creases) and carbon dioxide tension (decreases) on fetal peripheral resistance has more or less been ignored.

Cardiac Output

Rudolph and Heymann[590-593] have shown that in fetal sheep, the combined ventricular output is about 490 ml/kg/min. The right ventricle accounts for two-thirds of the cardiac output despite the fact that right and left ventricular pressures are essentially equal as are those in the aortic and pulmonary trunk (Fig. 8-4). One explanation for the marked fetal variations in ventricular output is the different resistance against which the two ventricles must pump. About 60% of right ventricular output goes to the umbilical circulation, which is relatively nonreactive to

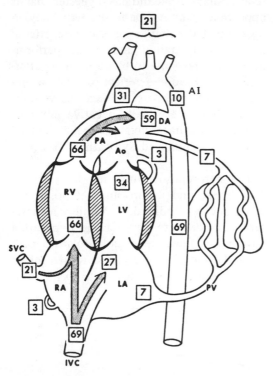

Fig. 8-4. The percentages of the combined ventricular output that return to the fetal heart, that are ejected by each ventricle and that flow through the main vascular channels. Figures are those obtained from late gestation lambs. Note that right ventricle output is twice that of left. AI = aortic isthmus. (From Rudolph, A.M.: *Congenital Diseases of the Heart.* Year Book, Chicago, 1974. Reproduced with permission.)

drugs and stress and has a low resistance. In contrast, the left ventricle faces a relatively high resistance at the aortic isthmus. These relationships are, of course, modified by changes in flow which occur across the foramen ovale. Such changes in flow apparently occur when left atrial pacing is used in the laboratory or during atropinization.[210] When generalized vasoconstriction and increased peripheral resistance occur, as during the fetal hypoxia response, it is the left ventricle which should be primarily affected and its output falls. However, with increased umbilical cord resistance, the major effect is on right ventricular output. These observations of Rudolph and Heymann[594] suggest that the two ventricles function independently of one another largely because of the differences in afterloads they serve. Barcroft proposed in 1937, based on this fetal injection and oxygen saturation studies, that there may in effect be two fetal circulations, an upper served by the left ventricle and a lower served by the right ventricle. Assuming that these concepts are in general correct, it is apparent that the output of each ventricle is largely dependent on the afterload it faces, as well as the relative flow across the foramen ovale.[403, 594]

Stroke Volume

Another important observation from Rudolph's laboratory is that both fetal ventricles are restricted in their ability to increase stroke volume when compared to adult hearts. During the adult diving response and probably during most fetal periods of brief and abrupt bradycardia,[17, 594] the Frank–Starling law of the heart seems to fail, probably because they are operating at the apex of their ventricular function curves.[292] This means that stroke volume does not increase and cardiac output is not maintained during the bradycardia. Rudolph and Heymann[590] found that sheep fetal cardiac output increased only 15–20% when end diastolic pressure was increased by saline infusion from 8–10 to 25–30 torr (in contrast to an adult increase of 300–400% during similar circumstances). With its decreased cardiac performance, the fetus is (at least initially) unable to increase stroke volume during bradycardia associated with a major increase in peripheral resistance.

Human intrapartum heart tone recordings from either Doppler or microphone pickups indicate that the intervals between opening and closing of ventricular valves (ejection time), or between the first (S_1) and second (S_2) heart sounds (the systolic time) (Fig. 8-5), are likewise relatively fixed during bradycardia just as in the sheep fetus.[162, 318, 487] With acute decreases of FHR below normal ranges, these intervals remain relatively constant, suggesting that stroke volume does not significantly increase and often that cardiac output falls (except that within 6–10 heartbeats, human fetal recording suggests that systolic times often begin to increase).[282] This cardiac response to time may be an effect of catecholamines secretion to stress as described by Comline and Silver.[118]

The relatively constant fetal $S_1 - S_2$ interval has been appreciated,[265, 318] but its significance in terms of reduced cardiac output has not had much attention. Furthermore, the bradycardia (and reduced cardiac output),

considered to be of benefit during adult diving (because it conserves work), appears to be of no advantage in fetal hypoxemia. For, except in circumstances like maternal hypoxia or abruptio, the placenta during fetal hypoxia should be a source of additional oxygen supply and CO_2 excretion, if the umbilical flow could be increased. This seemingly illogical fetal cardiovascular response of bradycardia during hypoxia which reduces cardiac output is why the baroreflex is considered an "inappropriate" reaction. For instance, in the diving seal, constant stroke volume, bradycardia, and reduced output probably reflect reduced effective circulating blood volume and the need to conserve oxygen.[17, 188] But when the fetus reduces cardiac output during many cases of hypoxia, it may be similar to an adult decreasing his cardiac output and pulmonary blood flow when suddenly moved to high altitude. As noted, one reason a fetus can tolerate these abrupt (vagal) type bradycardias is that the systemic vasoconstriction diverts more of the cardiac output to the umbilical circulation. As a corollary, anything (sedatives, hypocarbia, anesthetics) that reduces the systemic vasocon-

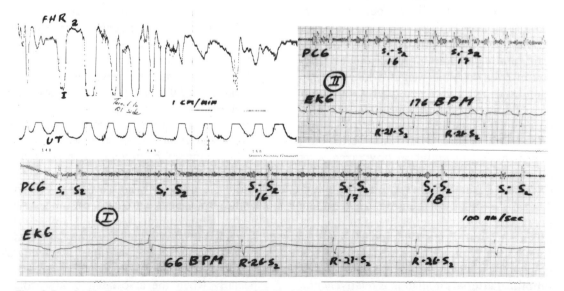

Fig. 8-5. A simultaneous recording of FHR and UT, fetal heart sounds and EKG during periods of bradycardia (I) and tachycardia (II). ($S_1 - S_2$) is unchanged when FHR is 176 bpm (II) and when 66 bpm (I). (From Goodlin, R.C., and Lowe, E.W.: Unexplained hydramnios associated with a thanatophoric dwart. *Am J Obstet Gynecol* **118**: 873–875, 1974. Reproduced with permission.)

striction could remove blood flow diversion and reduce umbilical and brain blood flow.

Umbilical Circulation

The umbilical circulation has always been recognized by both layman and physiologist as of uppermost importance to the fetus. Rudolph's laboratory has studied its control in detail and their work has made it possible to better understand the mechanisms controlling its flow.[47] The amount of any given material transported by the umbilical circulation is dependent on (a) the rate of umbilical flow and (b) the differences in concentrations between the umbilical venous and arterial bloods. For instance, in a desperately ill fetus with reduced cardiac output, the umbilical venous blood (which represents "arterial blood") oxygen content may be high. This is because umbilical placental flow is markedly reduced allowing the fetal red cells to come into complete oxygen equilibrium with the maternal red cells, unlike the normal situation. Therefore, measuring umbilical venous blood gases (and finding a high O_2 content) would give an entirely erroneous impression of the fetus' health under such circumstances, as the amount of oxygen delivered to the fetus is low because of the reduced umbilical flow.

The term sheep fetus has an almost constant umbilical flow at approximately 180–200 ml/min/kg fetal weight, while its corresponding combined ventricular output is 450–500 ml/kg/min. Except under the influence of drugs, an acute sustained rise in umbilical flow apparently does not occur, but a persistent fall in umbilical flow, even when all other parameters apparently are normal, often means fetal demise within 1 or 2 days. There is a direct relationship between fetal heart rate and/or arterial pressure and umbilical arterial flow. Rudolph's laboratory found that to physiologic doses of vasoconstrictors, and in a chronic preparation, the umbilical arterial circulation is relatively nonreactive *in utero* as even systemic norepinephrine constricts only the systemic circulation (Fig. 8-6). Under circumstances in which fetal

blood norepinephrine levels might be high, placental perfusion is elevated, providing the fetus with an important mechanism for maintaining umbilical blood flow during stress.

Novy *et al.*'s[510] studies in a relatively acute fetal preparation suggest that the sheep's umbilical circulation does respond to catecholamines, indicating that repeated stress may negate the funis' ability to maintain flow. But in less stressful studies (from Rudolph's laboratory) it has been shown that during asphyxia in fetal sheep, the umbilical circulation receives an increased proportion of the combined ventricular output. Because fetal cardiac output decreases during acute bradycardia, this asphyxial defending mechanism is not all that beneficial, as bradycardia is most always present during the usual FHAR. It is because of this detrimental effect of decreased cardiac output that atropine has been recommended to prevent acute bradycardia (Chap. 22). However, more detailed studies are required, as Parer[525] found that atropine did not increase oxygen tension in the hypoxic sheep fetuses of mothers who were themselves hypoxic. It was uterine oxygen supply that was limited in his studies and increasing umbilical flow under these circumstances could not be helpful to the fetus. As noted in Chapter 10 though, many events causing fetal bradycardias with hypoxia originate within the uterus.

Rudolph and associates have demonstrated that cardiovascular drugs could be divided into three groups as regards their effect upon umbilical flow.[47] These groups of drugs' actions depended on whether they are injected into the umbilical circulation or in the fetal IVC, whether they produced systemic (fetal) hypertension, and/or whether they increased umbilical–placental vascular resistance. As noted, norepinephrine and acetylcholine increased fetal systemic blood pressure and had no effect on umbilical resistance. As would be expected, umbilical flow was increased, especially when the associated bradycardia (or the baroreflex) was prevented by atropine. On the other hand, the prostaglandins E, E_2, and F_2, as well as angiotensin II, bradykinin

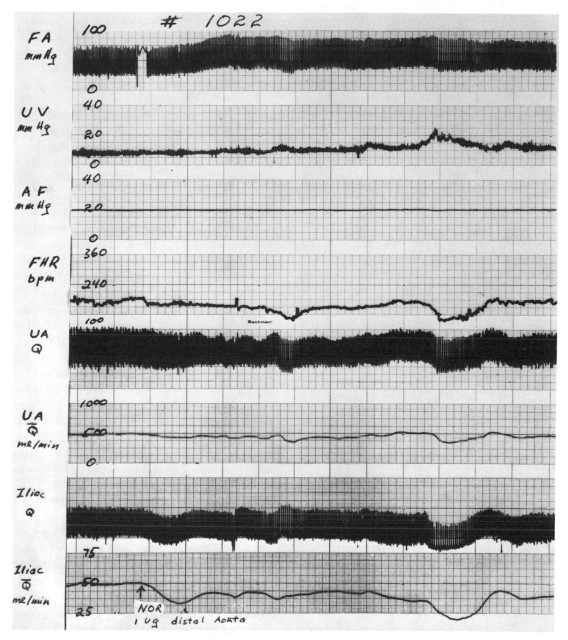

Fig. 8-6. Recording from a 127-day chronic fetal sheep preparation. FA = fetal aorta, UV = umbilical artery flow, Iliac Q = iliac artery flow. When norepinephrine (NOR) is injected into fetal aorta, the baroreflex occurs with fetal hypertension and bradycardia and peripheral resistance is increased (iliac flow diminished) but umbilical flow is maintained.

and 5-hydroxytryptamine, increased umbilical resistance and therefore decreased umbilical flow. When used in small doses, histamine, tolazoline, dopamine, and isoproterenol had no effect as they produced neither hypertension nor increased umbilical resistance.

Power and Longo[541] had proposed that in the sheep, the maternal circulation generated a placental tissue pressure which controlled the fetal umbilical circulation. Thus, under such a concept, any significant increase in uterine venous pressure would reduce umbilical flow, as might be expected in the maternal supine hypotensive syndrome or during a uterine contraction. However, Rudolph's laboratory, using an elegant chronic fetal preparation, demonstrated that such a "sluice" or "waterfall" relationship between the maternal circulation and umbilical blood flow does not exist.[47] These later studies suggest that fetal cardiovascular dynamics and baroreceptor and chemoreceptor mediated reflexes, rather than uterine vascular pressures, are the critical determinants of umbilical blood flow in the fetal lamb. In a way, Rudolph's groups' demonstration that the "sluice" theory was not applicable is unfortunate, for the theory offered a convenient explanation for the bradycardia associated with uterine aorto-caval compression (see Chapter 10).

The Central Mechanisms

As in the adult, fetal cardiovascular functions are presumably influenced by medullary, hypothalamic, and cerebral cortical activity. Dawes and associates[144] have stressed the importance of the fetal arousal level and circadian CNS activity patterns, noting that bradycardia and respiratory activity frequently accompany fetal sheep EEG patterns characteristic of rapid eye movements.

While the medullary centers appear to influence cardiovascular responses in a variable manner, higher cortical–hypothalamic activity associated with fetal movements or increased arousal levels seems to evoke a specific pattern of fetal tachycardia and hypertension. Rudolph's group made the observation that when the fetal sheep hypothalamus was stimulated, the most frequent fetal cardiovascular response was a brief pressor-tachycardia.[754] The importance of their observation is that hypertension in these fetal studies is associated with tachycardia, quite the opposite of the baroreflex. (The baroreflex is, of course, a peripheral response of the barore-

ceptors to hypertension which itself is secondary to increased peripheral resistance.) This pressor-tachycardia is perhaps a more common event and is commonly seen in a healthy fetus with any sort of movement.

A chronic fetal sheep preparation (in Rudolph's laboratory), when decerebrated by a supracollicular cautery incision, showed a reversal of vagal activity (Fig. 8-7). Besides a loss of beat-to-beat variability and breathing activity, acceleration of FHR activity was observed during uterine compression (Fig. 8-8). Katzin and Rubinstein,[400] in adult cats, have shown essentially this same reversal of vagal activity. They reported that a tachycardia response to hypoxia is obtained after midcollicular decerebration, which is mediated by the vagus. There was no bradycardia response to hypoxia as observed in the intact animal. They demonstrated that the tachycardia response is integrated in the pontomedullary region. In the past, such tachycardia was ascribed to sympathetic effects or to respiratory changes in hypoxia, but it now appears that such tachycardia responses are at least in part vagal. Katzin and Rubinstein further demonstrated that halothane anesthesia is quantitatively indistinguishable from midcollicular decerebration. Similarly, we noted that tranquilizers functioned like supracollicular decerebration in fetal sheep, converting the usual bradycardia response to tachycardia. Thus, the use of various anesthetic and tranquilizing agents renders any fetal preparation useless for study of heart rate responses. These studies also may demonstrate why fetal tachycardia occurs unexpectedly in parturients after various drugs. Also, atropinization can abolish tachycardia ("shoulders" of Figs. 12-3) since such accelerations of FHR represent vagal accelerator activity.

The use of drugs with a significant cortical effect (anesthetics, tranquilizers, opiates) may then be associated with sheep fetal (vagal) responses of heart rate acceleration or brief spurts of tachycardia. Persistent tachycardia also may reflect elevated catecholamine levels, fetal fever, or loss of vagal tone in the

Fig. 8-7. Recording of twin sheep fetus from Rudolph's laboratory. "A" has been decerebrated at supracollicular level. "B" is dead. With uterine contraction, the decerebrated fetus (B) with loss of BBV, shows tachycardia. (The usual response with uterine contractions is a moderate hypertension and bradycardia.) After atropine, the associated tachycardia was abolished, the blood pressure decreased, and the fetus expired.

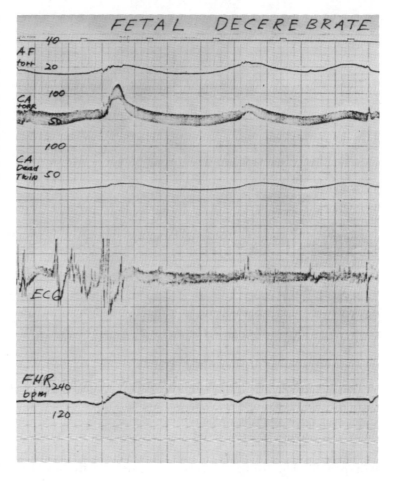

otherwise intact fetus. All of this is in contrast to the response of the fetus free of drugs, prior stress or fever who responds to hypertension with the baroreflex (or bradycardia).

In 1865, Traube postulated that activity from the respiratory center in the brain stem crossed over into cardiac autonomic centers, giving rise to rhythmic variations in heart rate correlated with breathing. In addition to this "spillover" activity in the brain stem, other reflex mechanisms relating changes in heart rate to breathing include those reflexes arising in the chest from increased venous return during inspiration (Bainbridge reflex) and those arising from respiratory changes in blood pressure (baroreflex).[413] There are both reflexes from lung movements which affect heart rate and also local cardiac factors such as blood pressure fluctuations in the sinoatrial

(SA) node blood supply that relate breathing to heart rate alterations.[433, 706]

As we demonstrated several years ago,[265] recordings of the human fetal scalp pulse during labor demonstrates changes in vasomotor tone (α waves) and heart rate presumably related to *in utero* fetal breathing (Fig. 14-3). These oscillations of arterial pressure at a presumed breathing frequency of approximately 40–60 Hz are probably Traube–Herring waves. In fetal sheep, Dawes[145] has described a similar cyclic variation in FHR and blood pressure related to breathing. Thus, several adult mechanisms are known which may relate fetal heart rate fluctuations to fetal breathing. Such effects of breathing would be expected to have a frequency of that reported for fetal chest wall movements, or 30–60 Hz.

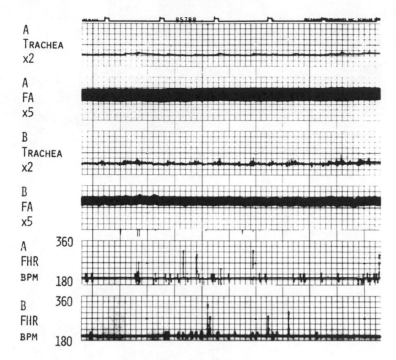

Fig. 8-8. Recording of twin pregnancy with A fetus decerebrated at level of supracolliculus. In contrast to B, A shows no BBV, no breathing, and no fluctuations in blood pressure.

Beat-to-Beat Variability (BBV)

The degree of fetal heart rate irregularity (arrhythmia index, beat-to-beat variability, baseline FHR variability, reactivity, or rapid heart rate change) has received clinical recognition as an indicator of fetal well-being (Chapter 9). Unfortunately, this heart rate irregularity is influenced by several factors (arousal levels, gestational age, heart rate, and drugs) not necessarily pertinent to the acute state of fetal health. As noted in Chapter 9, the quantification of beat-to-beat variability (BBV) is complex. This present discussion will only be concerned with FHR variability on a beat-to-beat basis (short-term variability) which has a different clinical significance and mechanism than does long-term beat-to-beat variability.

It is stated traditionally that fetal heart rate is controlled by the sympathetic and parasympathetic nervous systems under the influence of the cardioaccelerator and cardioinhibitor centers in the medulla. While this concept may be correct as regards other than acute heart rate changes, only the parasympathetic (vagal) system's reactive time is fast enough to effect beat-to-beat heart rate changes.[230, 231, 398] Warner and Russell[733] have calculated that equally brief and simultaneous vagal and sympathetic stimulation of the SA node would be expected to produce a brief bradycardia and overshoot heart rate pattern. In adults, reflex vagal stimulation or withdrawal has been shown to play the primary role in regulating rapid heart rate changes.[413] Catecholamines may also increase BBV, for after complete atropinization, both human and sheep fetuses maintain a small degree of BBV.[144] A β blocker such as propanolol removes this residual BBV (Goodlin, unpublished). The assumption is that this effect reflects changing sensitivity to the cardiac pacemaker system. The vagal concept of control of BBV is complicated by the fact that as noted, the vagus contains significant accelerator fibers.

In the past, BBV was considered a physiologic "hunting" for the optimal heart rate, much as a driver constantly adjusts the steering of a car on a straight roadway.[328, 495, 765a] But the phasic changes of respiratory function, arterial pressure, and especially the input from higher centers, with spillover from other active systems are sufficient to account for BBV.[160] This distinction is important as there is a tendency to equate BBV to a specific input, such as fetal breathing movements. The available evidence is that the vagal centers are affected in a multiplicative manner with these outside impulses having their greatest effect when the interval between beats is the longest (or heart rate the slowest).[230, 733] As the fetus matures and its vagal tone correspondingly increases, basal heart rate slows and BBV increases.[87] Actually, instead of "vagal tone," Dong and Reitz[160] have proposed the concept of "phasic sensitivity" as vagal outflow occurs in bursts synchronous with arterial pulse. The effects of vagal bursts depend on the cardiac cycle phase in which they are delivered to the pacemaker tissue (SA node). Figure 8-9 is modified from a report of Glaze and Dong showing the main control loops of the cardiovascular system postulated to regulate the medullary centers. As an example, when efferent impulses increase vasomotor tone, afferent impulses are increased by the baroreflex. Of all the various inputs to the vagal centers, those from CNS seem the most important.

If BBV is an indicator of total CNS activity, it is logical that loss of this variability can be a sign of almost any fetal condition, from impending death to normal sleep. Drugs with a central depressive and/or atropine effect can be expected to reduce this variability. Also, bursts of catecholamines can increase BBV, even in terminal events before death. Separate from the effects of vagal tone, drugs, or asphyxia on BBV is the effect of tachycardia itself, as variability of heart rate on a beat-to-beat basis is mechanically reduced at rapid heart rates.

Fetal Tachycardia

Brief periods of fetal tachycardia or FHR accelerations have been considered a cardiac response to the distress of hypoxia both in sheep and human fetuses.[113, 592, 604] As noted previously, in both human and sheep fetuses, brief periods of tachycardia are associated with fetal movement. In sheep fetuses, tachycardia responses to hypoxia generally are rare unless either general anesthesia has been used or the fetal preparation is exteriorized

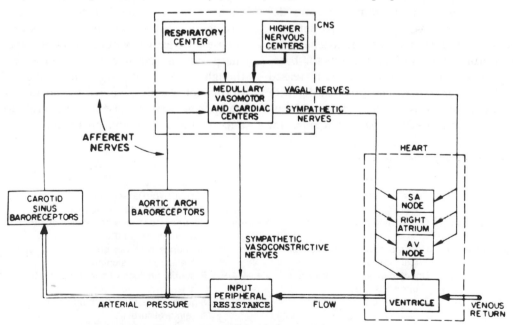

Fig. 8-9. Control loop for heart rate as modified from Glaze and Dong. The double lines represent hydraulic events and the single lines neural links. The vagal centers are affected in a multiplicative manner with the higher centers being the major source. (From *Obstet Gynecol* **49:** 371, 1977. Reproduced with permission.)

or even if it is acute. Brief periods of increased heart rate (acceleration) also occur along with prolonged periods of tachycardia during times of increased catecholamine levels[379, 571] which is part of the FHAR. All types of tachycardia are more likely to occur in the younger fetus when vagal tone is less. In sheep, as well as human fetuses, partial umbilical cord occlusion may be associated with brief episodes of tachycardia (accelerations)[280, 376] (Fig. 8-9). But as the funis occlusion becomes more complete, the heart rate response includes bradycardia (deceleration). Brief or prolonged periods of tachycardia are not consistently associated with any particular blood gas determination. In the healthy, nonstressed sheep fetus, spurts of simultaneous tachycardia and hypertension occur in association with fetal movement or when it is aroused.[594] Just as in adults, brief periods of tachycardia (accelerations) can represent a wide spectrum of fetal physiologic states, from severely stressed and drugged, to healthy and highly aroused fetuses.

Bradycardia

Two types of brief bradycardia are described in detail because they apparently reflect two different and specific mechanisms. The abrupt bradycardia represents the baroreflex which in turn is a response to increased peripheral resistance. The bradycardia with a more gradual onset reflects decreased cardiac performance. Obviously, FHR slows for other reasons (Chapter 10) unrelated to vagal activity.

Since this discussion mostly reflects sheep studies, no attempt will be made to use clinical terms as "type I or II dips" or "early or late decelerations" since their definition depends upon the relationship of heart rate changes to uterine contractions. Sheep uterine contractions, although they accomplish their mission as well as the human does, are much less intense than those of the human uterus and probably effect fetal cardiovascular function less than in the human. This is admittedly another one of the serious limitations when attempting to extrapolate from sheep to humans, but still the characteristics of the sheep uterus (which allows intrauterine manipulation) are of tremendous advantage to the investigator.

Abrupt Bradycardia (Table 8-I)

HYPOXIA

In fetal sheep preparations, small quantities of sodium cyanide have been traditionally used to mimic hypoxia stimulation of the chemoreceptor. When injected into the fetal circulation, cyanide elicits among other responses, selective vasoconstriction and a sharp rise in peripheral resistance.[141] Although the relatively large umbilical circulation is not usually involved by vasoconstriction, the general increase in peripheral resistance in the fetal body, plus a high cardiac

Table 8-I. Abrupt, Brief Bradycardias

Stimulus	Mechanism	Usual Severity	Comment
Hypoxia	Chemoreceptor → vasoconstriction	2+, 3+	Abrupt hypoxia and no hypocardia or sedatives required for response
Funis (cord) occlusion	Obstruction of umbilical cord	1+ → 4+	Response depends on relative obstruction of both arteries and vein
Uterine contraction	Uncompensated rise of umbilical pressure	1+	Response requires greater rise in umbilical pressure than amniotic
ad compression	Uncompensated pressure upon fetal head	1+ → 4+	Probable etiology of second stage bradycardia
Grunting	Fetal valsalva?	4+	Significant rise in intrathoracic and umbilical vein pressure
Seizures	Drugs, toxins, asphyxia?	4+	Severe acidemia, duration depends on seizure activity

output, is still sufficient to produce fetal systemic hypertension.[138] With hypertension, the baroreflex then produces an abrupt bradycardia proportional to the mean blood pressure increase.

Dawes and co-workers[141] in England documented these pressor effects of fetal hypoxia (and sodium cyanide) in sheep and also observed that with hypocarbia, the selective vasoconstriction response to hypoxia either was blunted or did not occur.[29] The response was further studied in Rudolph's laboratory with documentation of the reduced blood flow to the nonvital organs (Table 8-II).[113] The generalized vasoconstriction has been subsequently shown to be diminished by general anesthetics, opiates, and barbiturates (Goodlin, unpublished). Since hypoxic bradycardia occurs in part because of selective vasoconstriction, anything modifying the latter will affect the former; or, in other words, if fetal P_{CO_2} is reduced by maternal hyperventilation, so should the incidence of fetal hypoxic bradycardia.[690] While preventing bradycardia and decreased cardiac output may be of advantage to the hypoxic fetus, we observed that umbilical flow was maintained less well in hypoxic fetal sheep with low P_{CO_2} than when P_{CO_2} was normal or elevated during hypoxia. One explanation may be that with normal or high P_{CO_2}, the increased lower body peripheral resistance and associated hy-

Table 8-II. Effects of Hypoxemia and Asphyxia on Fetal Lambs[a]

	Hypoxemia	Asphyxia
Cardiac output	−5%	−25%
Stroke volume	+30%	+8%
Umbilical flow	+9%	+8%
Total body blood flow	−20%	−48%
Organ blood flow		
gut	−20%	−50%
spleen	−65%	−82%
kidneys	−20%	−50%
carcass	−35%	−60%
lungs	−65%	−60%
heart	+205%	+240%
brain	+186%	+150%
adrenals	+405%	+280%

[a] Modified from Cohn et al.[113]

pertension diverts a greater percentage of the decreased cardiac output towards the passive umbilical circulation, thus maintaining umbilical flow.[113]

It is possible that the baroreflex is not always involved in the FHAR. In Rudolph's laboratory, with fetuses sedated in an acute preparation and after injection with NaCN, no hypertension occurred, but still an abrupt bradycardia did occur. Since atropinization did not prevent the bradycardia, the implication is that there are active chemoreceptors within the heart. Green et al.[299] observed that mild hypoxia itself is seemingly able to invoke a direct bradycardia response even in the chronic preparation. Thus, as more studies are done, it is apparent that there are variations to the FHAR which are incompletely understood and that the response is indeed complex. In general, in the absence of hyperventilation, sedatives, or illness, the fetus evokes the baroreflex at the slightest excuse.

UTERINE CONTRACTIONS

In sheep with either spontaneous or induced uterine contractions, umbilical blood flow sometimes decreases a few seconds before any discernible rise in amniotic pressure is noted. During the subsequent uterine contraction, relative fetal hypertension (to increased amniotic fluid pressure) and bradycardia are present. One possible explanation is that umbilical circulation may be effected by uneven distribution of myometrial tension, giving rise to increased vascular resistance. Also, when a catheter is wedged into a sheep maternal uterine vein, occasional rises in its pressure are seen which are associated with fetal hypertension and bradycardia, all without any apparent changes in amniotic fluid pressure levels, (Figs. 8-10 and 8-11). While such localized or uneven uterine contractions appear infrequently in sheep, these observations offer an explanation for the laboratory observation of fetal hypertension and bradycardia seen sometimes during uterine contractions or even the abrupt episodes of fetal hypertension and bradycardia observed dur-

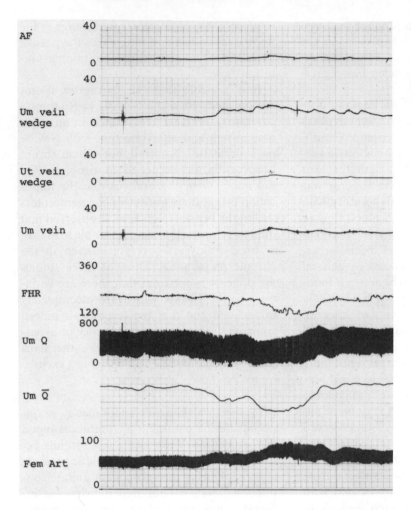

Fig. 8-10. Recording of a 126-day chronic fetal sheep preparation from Rudolph's laboratory. Catheters have been "wedged" into umbilical vein toward placenta and maternal uterine vein toward myometrium. An unexplained resistance occurs in placenta with resulting baroreflex (hypertension and bradycardia) in fetus. (From *Am J Obstet Gynecol* **129:** 618, 1977. Reproduced with permission.)

ing uterine diastole. These rises in fetal blood pressure, unrelated to at least the degree of uterine tension, may also explain fetal bradycardia associated with uterine contractions, the so-called "head compression" FHR pattern. When these episodes of decreases in umbilical flow occur prior to either a localized or generalized contraction, the flow quickly recovers during the subsequent period of reactive fetal hypertension.

FUNIS OCCLUSION

Barcroft and Barron[37] demonstrated in exteriorized and anesthetized fetal sheep that acute occlusion of their umbilical cord produced an immediate fetal hypertension and abrupt bradycardia (Fig. 8-12). Hon,[354] noting the FHR pattern similarity between observations of Barcroft in fetal sheep and his own FHR recordings of human fetuses, proposed that similarly abrupt human FHR patterns indicated umbilical cord compression. He confirmed his impression by occluding the umbilical cord of term human fetuses delivered by cesarean section and produced an abrupt bradycardia, but apparently also concluded to reverse, that all abrupt bradycardia (variable decelerations) represented funis occlusion. Barcroft further noted that vagotomy abolished the abrupt onset of cord compression FHR patterns with the resulting pattern being a more gradual heart rate deceleration. Presumably the original FHR pattern reflected the baroreflex response, but after vagotomy the less abrupt bradycardia represented asphyxia-induced decreased car-

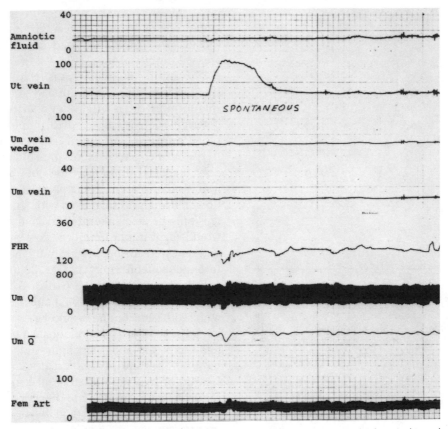

Fig. 8-11. Same preparation as Fig. 8-10. This time, an unexplained increase in the uterine vein occurred, associated with fetal baroreflex and decreased umbilical flow.

diac performance in the presence of increased peripheral (funis and systemic) resistance.

In 1955, Reynolds[569] reported that umbilical vein occlusion alone produced a severe bradycardia apparently due to decreased venous return, but we found in both humans and sheep fetuses that such occlusion was associated with a tachycardia (Fig. 8-13). Perhaps the differences between Reynolds' and our observations reflected the degree of obstruction of venous return. In humans, many funis compressions are seemingly first suggested by tachycardia (accelerations) during uterine contractions. We[280] have interpreted this observation to mean that early funis compression may involve only the umbilical vein, sometimes to a minimal degree, or that minimal vagal stumulation accelerates FHR. Yeh *et al.*[766] has reported cardiac conduction defects (in fetal baboons) during cord compression, which were abolished by atropine and has noted similar "heart blocks" during severe bradycardia in human fetuses.[765b] Compression of the funis obviously represents both artery and vein compression, with both hypertension and decreased venous return being produced. The exact FHR response depends upon the degree of these two components, as well as the degree of vagal stimulation.

HEAD COMPRESSION

Head compression may be a fetal bradycardia response to hypertension. If in the chronic sheep preparation the fetal head is slowly compressed through the intact uterus, bradycardia does occur. The more abrupt the increase in head pressure, the more severe the bradycardia and reduced cardiac output. Fetal hypertension is not always present.

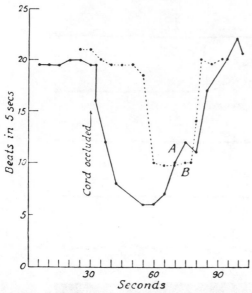

Fig. 8-12. Barcroft's FHR recording of funis occlusion of an exteriorized fetal goat. A = first gasp when vagus was intact. B = first gasp when both vagi had been cut. (From Barcroft, J.: *Researches on Prenatal Life.* Blackwell, Oxford, 1946. Reproduced with permission.)

In humans, the more severe forms of head compression may occur during late labor when the vertex is subjected to pressures greater than the amniotic fluid pressure as it negotiates the maternal pelvis.[446, 617] It seems likely that abrupt head compression is the usual explanation for the severe and abrupt fetal bradycardia in humans as commonly seen in terminal labor. Atropinization will often abolish or blunt this heart rate response.

GRUNTING

Another cause of abrupt bradycardia is that associated with what we have termed fetal grunting. As observed in sheep, fetal gasping or sighing appears frequently and their occurrence suggests good fetal health since apnea may indicate hypoxia. By fetal grunting, we mean breathing activity associated with a rise in tracheal and intrapleural pressure and its occurrence may have the opposite implication of fetal sighing.[275] Fetal grunting includes a rise in mean blood pressure and intraperitoneal pressure and, most importantly, a significant rise in umbilical vein pressure. Prolonged fetal grunting is associated with prolonged bradycardia and decreased umbilical flow. (Fig. 8-14).

The umbilical circulation is relatively passive,[141, 143] meaning it is normally unresponsive to most drugs or stimuli and its flow is determined by fetal cardiac output, mean blood pressure, and umbilical vein pressure. A rise in mean fetal blood pressure appreciably increases umbilical flow, but a rise in umbilical or placental vein pressure decreases flow. During grunting, even with fetal hypertension, the rise in umbilical vein pressure would suggest that umbilical flow is reduced and repeated episodes of grunting may therefore induce fetal asphyxia (Fig. 22-5).

Fetal grunting may be part of (Figs. 8-14 and 8-15) the fetal valsalva maneuver during which time meconium would be expected to be passed. Thus, the relationship between fetal hypoxia and meconium-stained fluid may be opposite of that usually conceived. Instead of hypoxia initiating meconium passage, the act of grunting and passing meconium itself may induce fetal hypoxia. Fetal grunting then may be another example of the fetus inappropriately using a response designed for extrauterine life. Grunting in the immediate newborn increases pulmonary vein oxygenation, but *in utero* it probably decreases umbilical flow and therefore decreases fetal oxygen consumption.

The stimulus for *in utero* grunting in sheep is unknown. Stimulatory drugs or vagal stimulation may initiate grunting, but the umbilical flow decreases are less than with spontaneous grunting. Atropine usually abolishes grunting.

SUCKLING

In human fetuses with face presentation, with suckling (the examiner's finger), bradycardia occurs. Similar FHR changes are sometimes seen in sheep fetuses with dips in esophageal pressures. Such FHR responses are diminished with fetal sedation.

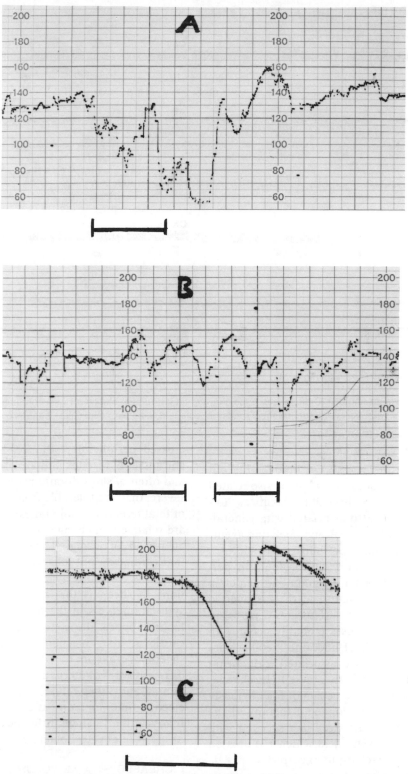

Fig. 8-13. Recording from a 682-g human fetus with prolapsed umbilical cord. In A, entire umbilical cord clamped for 85 sec. In B, only the umbilical vein is clamped and in C, after atropine, the entire cord is clamped for 2 min. With umbilical vein clamping, only tachycardia occurs. Note overshoot, especially after atropine. (From Goodlin, R.C., and Lowe, E.W.: Multiphasic fetal monitoring. A preliminary evaluation. *Am J Obstet Gynecol* **119:** 341, 1974. Reproduced with permission.)

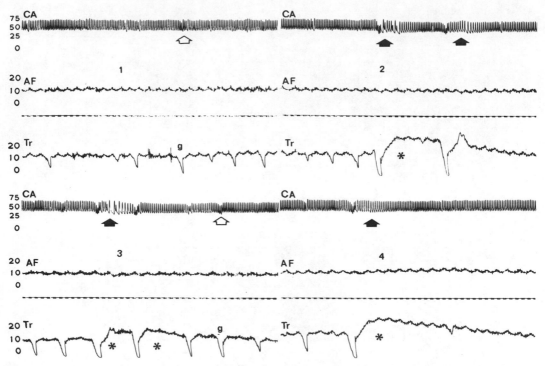

Fig. 8-14. Recording of 128-day sheep fetus showing fetal grunting (closed arrows) contrasted with gasping (open arrows). With increased fetal tracheal pressure (asterisk), fetal cardiovascular changes occur.

SEIZURES

One type of fetal abrupt bradycardia observed in the laboratory, which is also related to hypertension, is difficult to classify as "tolerable" as it is also associated with generalized seizures. When calcium chelating agents were injected into the fourth ventricle of a fetal sheep,[275] seizures with profound hypertension, bradycardia, gasping, and acidemia occurred and the fetus' death was averted only with the use of barbiturates (Fig. 8-16). Similar fetal responses probably occur with toxic serum levels of lidocaine. Fetal seizure activity apparently is associated with abrupt bradycardia and whether these FHR changes should be considered benign or not obviously depends on the etiology and therapy of the seizure. The seizure itself is associated with high levels of lactic acid which requires an adequate cardiac output to correct.

COMMON MECHANISM OF THE VARIOUS ACUTE AND ABRUPT FETAL BRADYCARDIAS

The preceding fetal bradycardias have in-creased peripheral resistance, hypertension, and intact baroreflex and are of abrupt onset and often of short duration (Fig. 8-17). If not severe, they are tolerable from the standpoint of fetal reserves. In all of these, ejection times are relatively unchanged during the immediate periods of decreased heart rates suggesting that cardiac output falls with these bradycardias. The clinical relevance of these observations in sheep is that the measurement of systolic intervals in the human fetus during labor supports the concept that these same cardiovascular mechanisms (observed in sheep) operate in the human despite their different types of uterus and placenta. In both human and sheep fetuses, stroke volume (or ejection time) increases after 10–70 sec of the bradycardia.[282] These differences may reflect drugs or fetal catecholamine levels.

INCREASED STROKE VOLUME

The previous bradycardias are characterized by increased peripheral resistance and hypertension causing vagal-type bradycardia

Fig. 8-15. Recording at variable paper speeds from Rudolph's laboratory of 119 fetal sheep (chronic) preparation. When fetus grunted (arrow) there was decrease in right ventricle output, hypertension, bradycardia, and decrease in pulmonary trunk flow.

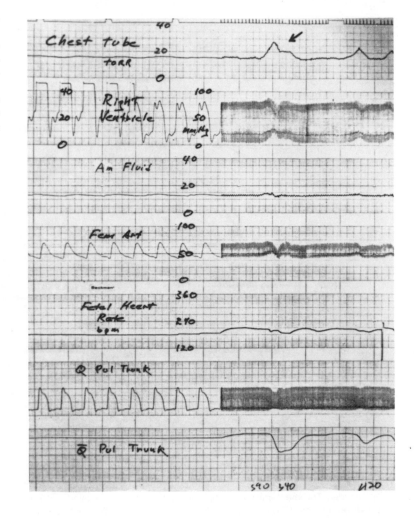

Fig. 8-16. Recording from a 2.8 K intrauterine fetus with a catheter in the second cerebral ventricle. NaHCO$_2$, 1 mEq, was injected, and 75 sec later marked hypertension, bradycardia, and rhythmic frequent breathing occurred, apparently all associated with a fetal seizure.

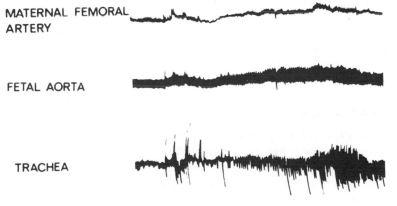

in both sheep and human fetuses. When marked decreases in rate occur *without* increased peripheral resistance, stroke volume (ejection times) *does* increase. An example is during marked beat-to-beat variability where peripheral resistance is unchanged (Fig. 8-18). Stroke volume changes proportionally to instantaneous heart rate change, suggesting fetal operation of the Frank–Starling law of the heart when afterload or resistance is not

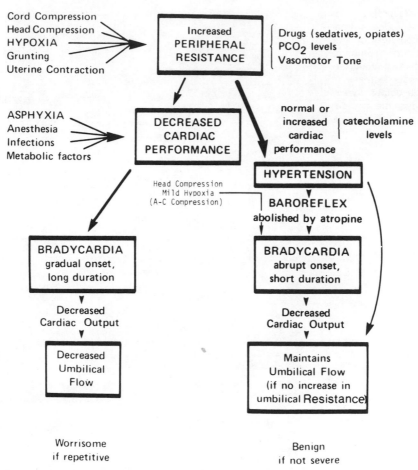

Fig. 8-17. Proposed mechanisms of fetal reactive bradycardia. Head compression may directly produce vagal bradycardia. The mechanisms of the right and left side may overlap so that atropine or inotropic agents may abolish both types. (From Goodin, R.C., and Haesslein, H.G.: Fetal reacting bradycardia. *Am J Obstet Gynecol* **129:** 845–856, 1977. Reproduced with permission.)

altered. The same is true when fetal heart rate changes gradually. Similar findings are also seen with sytolic time interval determinations in the late antenatal period.

GRADUAL BRADYCARDIAS

In 1958, Reynolds and Paul[571] noted the heart rate alone was not a reliable indicator of fetal hypoxia in fetal sheep, but that heart rate and blood pressure taken together appeared to be useful indicators of fetal well-being. The following bradycardias illustrate this concept for they differ from those previously discussed in that their occurrence may be ominous, they are gradual in onset and of long duration, and they are *not* associated with hypertension.

Decreased Cardiac Function

VENOUS OBSTRUCTION

In the laboratory, obstruction of the fetal inferior vena cava above the liver or complete obstruction of the umbilical veins in the absence of arterial obstruction produces a profound fetal bradycardia, hypotension, and fall in cardiac output. Fortunately, a comparable pure umbilical cord vein obstruction is apparently rare in clinical situations.

ACUTE BLOOD LOSS

The immediate fetal response to significant blood loss is a bradycardia.[279, 701a] Its mechanism is not understood although it probably is similar to venous obstruction. With time or

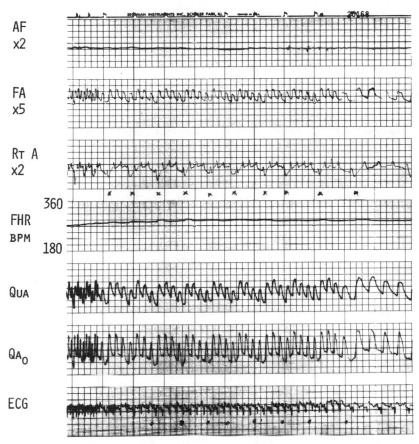

AF
x2

FA
x5

Rᴛ A
x2

FHR
BPM

360

180

Qᴜᴀ

Qᴀₒ

ECG

Fig. 8-18.   Recording from Rudolph's laboratory of a chronic fetal sheep preparation. Rt. A = right auricle, QUA and QA₀ refer to flow of umbilical artery and distal aorta. ×2 or ×5 refer to gain of recorder, asterisk = fetal gasping. Associated with fetal breathing are changes in BBV (·) and aortal flow. Note α waves in FA, and increased flow (stroke volume) with respiratory bradycardia.

anesthesia, the fetal heart rate response may change to tachycardia.

IMPAIRED OR DECREASED CARDIAC PERFORMANCE

The final fetal bradycardia to be discussed and the type which should be of greatest concern to the obstetrician is that which represents impaired cardiac performance. While its etiology is most often fetal asphyxia, it may also be the result of drugs such as lidocaine or halothane, or infections, metabolic disorders, and so forth. Under these circumstances of reduced myocardial performance and even with peripheral vasoconstriction and increased resistance, hypertension does not occur and the bradycardia reflects inadequate cardiac function. It seems logical that a time delay would occur between the in-

crease in peripheral resistance and the manifestations of poor cardiac function (decreased heart rate) with this clinical situation, and that the bradycardia would be much less abrupt and slower in onset than in those related to the baroreflex. Such bradycardias in clinical terms are often termed late decelerations, delayed recovery, type-II dips, etc.

Brinkman and associates[75, 76] have demonstrated an increase in placental and ductus venous resistance during hypoxia. Therefore, in cases of bradycardia without hypertension, but with decreased cardiac output (CO) and a rise in placental resistance, it would seem reasonable that umbilical flow would not be maintained. Such bradycardias would aggravate the fetal asphyxia and cardiac recovery would be expected to extend beyond the time of the asphyxial event or when peripheral resistance is again normal. In acute fetal monkey preparations, Myers and colleagues[491] and James et al.[375] observed that bradycardia in the absence of hypertension is associated with asphyxia and is a "late deceleration." Myers further suggested that decreased cardiac performance was probably the basis of the deceleration and poor fetal health as catecholamines improved the clinical situation.

BRADYCARDIAS IN GENERAL

Studies in chronic fetal sheep suggest that only a minority of fetal heart rate decreases are secondary either to the baroreflex, or to decreased cardiac performance. Perhaps some of the more common bradycardias reflect decreased arousal levels or changing metabolic rates. Bradycardia (and apnea) is associated with REM sleep in prematures,[220] and it seems logical to assume the same is true of the fetus in utero. Urbach et al.[711] showed accelerations of FHR with crying in the newborn and deceleration with hiccough, valsalva maneuver, and so forth. Some of these bradycardias would clearly include increased stroke volume. Regardless, without the underlying mechanisms of increased resistance or decreased performance in these nonspecific bradycardias, stroke volume should increase at lower heart rates and cardiac output be maintained.

Fetal Osmotic and Colloid Pressure During Stress

In 1946, Barcroft wrote of his surprise in learning that the fetus required even more water than oxygen. Water exchange between fetus and mother is determined by placental gradients of both hydrostatic and osmotic pressure. It seems obvious that maternal blood pressure and osmotic pressure change appreciably during any normal day of activity, rest, and fluid intake and that likewise, fetal blood pressure changes in relationship to alterations in its activity and arousal level. It is indeed a wonder that fetuses are not regularly alternating between being either hydropic or dehydrated. Faber[191] believes that one of the main determinants of water exchange across the placenta is fetal placental capillary blood pressure. This is in turn related to umbilical flow, which should be markedly altered during times of fetal distress. Presumably, the many "variables" work to produce a new, steady state across the placenta under all these changing conditions so that proper water transfer rates to the fetus are maintained.

The factors controlling fetal colloid osmotic and placental hydrostatic pressures and therefore its water balance are an unknown. As noted, it cannot be entirely passive and under maternal control. In our interest in EPH gestosis, we began measurements of COP in gravidas under varying conditions. We noted (as have Heitten and others) that there are sometimes tremendous shifts in maternal body fluids during a 24-hr period. Extracellular fluid collects in the gravida's lower extremities during the upright position. When changing to the horizontal lateral position, fluid is moved by reduction in hydrostatic pressures into her vascular compartment. This movement of fluid results in marked decrease in COP. Indeed, we found changes as great as 25% in blood COP in some edematous gravida, on being put to bed. Such women obviously had a profound diuresis. The question, of course, is how does the fetus maintain its own water supply in face of such changes (which probably would be even greater with diuretic agents) in maternal COP pressure?

Clinical experience teaches us that the fetus is not entirely independent of its mother's COP. Prochownick[555] found that when gravida were restricted in their fluid intake, their newborns were dehydrated. Likewise, with "hydropic" gravida, newborns also have excessive body fluids (mirror syndrome). Newborns with renal or pulmonary agenesis demonstrate no striking abnormalities of fluid balance except perhaps a tendency toward hemoconcentration. (Ever since I studied tracheal excretion in fetal rabbits, described in Chapter 13, I have sought to find a function for fetal lung alveolar electrolyte excretion and believe that it may be in osmoregulation.) Even in the mature fetus, renal function is known to be immature and amniotic fluid COP seems correlated with maternal and not fetal serum COP. Thus, there are no clinical clues as to fetal organs involved in osmoregulation.

In Rudolph's laboratory,[431] Levin, he and Dr. Hymen were producing fetal hypertension in sheep by constricting a fetal renal artery (Goldblat kidney). In addition to all of the fascinating implications relative to the fetal mechanism of hypertension, I found the preparation interesting, because fetal blood COP did not change with its associated hypertension.

It seems probable that the placenta maintains the proper COP and osmotic gradients despite the major changes in maternal–fetal hydrostatic and osmotic pressures. Since hypertonicity is lethal, this placental function may be especially important in times of fetal distress. Perhaps prolactin, the ancient hormone controlling fish gill regulations of osmotic pressure, plays a part.

On the other hand, it is possible that none of the above mechanisms are determinants of water transport across the placenta. Curran has proposed that water transport in the intestine is a passive process resulting from active solute transport.[133a] The proposed mechanism is based on the marked differences in the permeability properties of two membranes arranged in series and separated by a closed compartment, such as occurs in the placenta.

Other Points of View

It has been long presumed that beat-to-beat variability (BBV) increases with vagal tone, and therefore is increased during slower heart rates, reflecting vagal activity. The younger fetus has a lesser beat-to-beat variability and a higher heart rate than does the term fetus. This association presumably reflects the reduced level of vagal activity and indicates that tachycardia on a mechanical basis reduces the short-term BBV. However, workers from Dawes' laboratory[135, 136] challenged this viewpoint. In chronic sheep preparations, they found poor correlation between heart rate and the degree of BBV. Instead, they observed that BBV was increased at certain times of the day, unrelated to heart rate, and that often when heart rate was increased, BBV was likewise increased. Furthermore, they emphasized the common observation that many times BBV increased or decreases without apparent change in FHR.

The definition of BBV is an unresolved problem. Interpretations will differ significantly if brief periods of tachycardia (accelerations) are termed increased BBV, rather than if BBV is strictly defined in terms of the amount of change of any successive R wave to R wave interval. The latter has been our definition and probably explains some of the differences in views found in our recent literature. Differences between the English and American schools may revolve around the attention given to the mechanisms of heart rate changes when considering changes in BBV. If the rate change reflects increase in vagal tone, then our repeated observations have demonstrated the reverse relationship between heart rate and degree of BBV. If decreases in FHR are unrelated to increased vagal tone, then there is no reason for a relationship to exist between heart rate and degree of BBV. When discussing the question of whether BBV is related to heart rate, one should likewise discuss the degree of apparent vagal tone. Gradual changes in FHR are not likely to be due to increases in vagal activity.

Dawes' group also reports that fetal respiratory paralysis with gallamine is associated with a loss of BBV. We did not find this relationship to be so when respiratory paralysis was achieved with succinyl choline. This apparent disassociation between BBV and breathing was the basic observation for our conclusion that BBV was not necessarily reflective of fetal breathing activity. We believe the differences between Dawes' group and ourselves is simply related to the fact that gallamine inhibits the cardiac vagus and succinyl choline does not. This difference in views reinforces the impression that vagal activity is usually necessary for increased BBV, and that its inhibition (with atropine, gallamine, etc.) is usually associated with loss of BBV.

Reacting fetal bradycardias have been presented in this discussion in a simplistic fashion; i.e., when hypertension is present, the bradycardia is tolerable, but when hypertension is absent, the bradycardia is worrisome. Like many other simplistic explanations of physiologic responses, there are many obvious exceptions to this classification.

In the chronic fetal sheep preparation, it is possible to achieve acute bradycardia by head compression without an associated hypertension. Since this bradycardia is inhibited by atropine, it must reflect direct vagal stimulation initiated by increased intracranial pressure with no relationship to the baroreflex. On the other hand, systolic time determination shows a relatively constant ejection time during head compression of the human fetus, strongly suggestive of an associated hypertension. Thus, the precise role of the baroreflex in "head compression" fetal bradycardia has not been completely defined. (See Chapter 10 for further discussion.)

In the acute FHAR response, there may be no hypertensive event and many[21, 113, 299] have rejected our concepts.

In our own acute fetal sheep studies with a "delay loop" separating the aortic from the carotid chemoreceptors, we occasionally observed a hypoxic response (bolus of sodium cyanide) consisting of bradycardia and *Hypotension* (Figs. 8-19 and 8-20). However, the subsequent carotid response was almost always that of hypertension and tachycardia. I had assumed that the combined response of the aortic

and carotid chemoreceptors was hypertension and bradycardia and Dawes' group,[141] in more elegant studies, showed that the hypoxic response was indeed hypertension and bradycardia mediated by the carotid and vagal nerves.

In an acute fetal sheep preparation, Siassi[630] and colleagues showed that the cardiac chemoreceptors may elect bradycardia without hypertension to a hypoxic response. This is certainly true when a bolus of sodium cyanide is injected into the heart of almost any animal. The point is that in our studies of the carotid and aortic chemoreceptor nerve loop, the fetal cardiac chemoreceptors were unresponsive to all but severe hypoxia (or asphyxia). Thus, there are many complex reflexes to hypoxia (including vagal tachycardia) which may be expressed under varying circumstances.

As noted, the available data suggest that the fetal myocardium is unable to perform as well as does the adult's heart. Friedman and colleagues, in a series of studies,[210] have demonstrated that the resting tension of the fetal cardiac muscle is higher and that the active tension is lower than in adults at all points along the length–tension relationship curves. Furthermore, it also appears that even under normal circumstances, fetuses are close to the apex of their ventricular function curves and that the Frank–Starling relationship may therefore be

Fig. 8-19. Schematic diagram of carotid delay loop in intrauterine fetal sheep. The small black masses represent chemoreceptor bodies. The tourniquet prevents collateral circulation between aorta and carotid bodies.

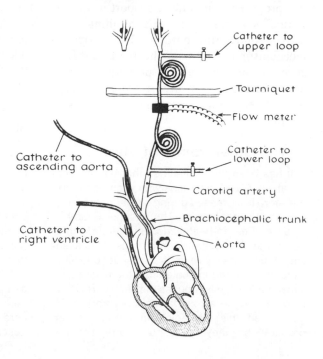

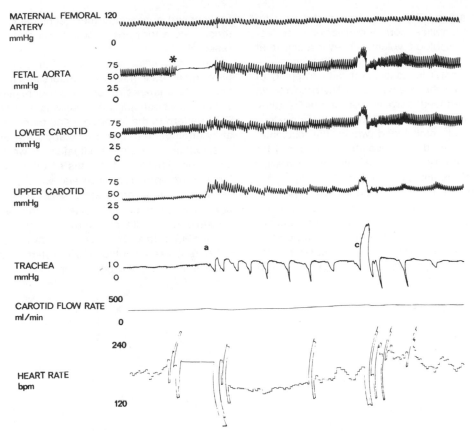

Fig. 8-20. Recording from a 4.1 K intrauterine fetus with a carotid delay loop. Nicotine 100 μg injected into ascending aorta at (*). The aortic response "a" consists of gasping (with moderate grunting), bradycardia (rate meter driven by aorta BP), and at carotid response "c", significant grunt, hypertension, and tachycardia. This "c" type of "grunting" has opposite cardiovascular effect as that initiated by hypoxia with tracheal pressure. The carotid flow rate was 210 ml/min; the volume of delay tubing was 41 ml and time between a and c was 13 sec.

limited to a small portion of this curve. In addition, vagal stimulation compounds the apparent fetal myocardial deficiency as its activity independently decreases cardiac performance. But, fetal myocardial performance is not always inadequate, for when the heart rate changes for reasons other than increases in peripheral resistance or decreased cardiac performance, stroke volume does increase as heart rate slows. This is seen clearly in beat-to-beat changes in both sheep (Fig. 8-17) and human fetuses (Fig. 8-20). As noted, the antenatal fetus does increase ejection times during periods of bradycardia. Presumably, these unexplained fetal bradycardias have different etiologies from those which often occur in labor.

Friedman's group has recently attacked Rudolph and Heymann's conclusion concerning decreased cardiac output during acute bradycardia. They base their conclusions on studies of fetuses' changing heart rates under no apparent stress, while Rudolph's laboratory findings were from fetuses under atrial pacing or vagal stimulation. Even if one accepts Friedman's objections, it still appears that Rudolph's studies more closely approach human fetal conditions found during labor.

Strang and associates have reported in nonacidotic, exteriorized term sheep fetus of chloralose anesthetized animals, that the variability of the FHR was inversely proportional to fetal P_{O_2} within the range of 10–26 torr. It is unclear from their discussion, how the investigators related such a study preparation to any clinical situation, but apparently do not consider a loss of BBV to indicate hypoxia.

Pecorari and Trovati[531] argue that the brady-cardia of umbilical cord compression is protective of fetal blood volume. They assume that partial cord compression (umbilical vein obstruction only) is associated with trapping of fetal blood within the placenta. The bradycardia and its reduced cardiac output results (they believe) in less umbilical flow, and therefore less trapping of fetal blood within the placenta. These authors do not mention the tendency for umbilical artery spasm with even minor manipulation of the umbilical cord.

There are, then, many conflicting reports in the literature concerning fetal cardiovascular responses to distress, which, in my opinion, are often due to differences in the fetal preparation and techniques. While we all resist regimentation, it almost appears that investigators should be licensed concerning their technical competence before they are allowed to report on fetal research.

Fetal cardiovascular responses are very complex and at least in terms of understanding fetal heart rate changes, often remain unexplained. We all have been guilty of observing a particular FHR pattern in the laboratory and then immediately attempting to incorrectly apply the limited observation to a clinical situation. If we could just understand why the fetus so often evokes the baroreceptor response and what changes vagal stimulation bring about, FHR interpretation could be much more scientific than is now possible. About all that is known is that a normal vagal FHR relfex (bradycardia with increased BBV) requires an intact CNS system and the relative absence of drugs.

CHAPTER 9

Fetal Heart Rate Monitoring

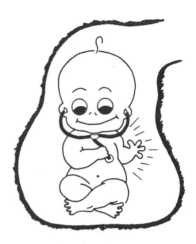

Introduction

HISTORICAL ASPECTS

In Western medical literature, Mayor of Geneva (in 1818) is credited with being the first to report the presence of fetal heart tones (FHT). Its presence was extensively publicized by Kergaradec in 1821. Legends would have us believe that the former discovered the FHT while with his girlfriend, and the latter by attempting to hear the fetus splash in the amniotic fluid of one of his patients. At any rate, Kergaradec quickly appreciated the clinical implications of his own finding and within a decade, physicians everywhere were listening for the fetal heart.

In 1833, Evory Kennedy[401] of Dublin published a monograph concerning auscultation of the human fetal heart (Fig. 9-1). He was attempting to convince his fellow accoucheurs of the value of the fetoscope, which had been introduced only 12 years previously by Kergaradec. Several copies of Kennedy's various books are still in circulation at the Lane Library (Stanford Medical Center) and their file suggests that they were popular with the 19th-century San Francisco physicians.

Although some of his views on the significance of fetal distress have not stood the test of time (such as those relative to uterine "flatus"), most of his clinical impressions regarding FHR auscultation appear remarkably up to date.

In his 1833 book, Kennedy commented upon Merat's experiments with newborn rabbits. These suggested that since newborn's hearts beat longer when excised, they were more resistant to anoxia than were adult hearts. Kennedy also mentioned Bodson's descriptions of fetal distress ("sufferance of the fetus") which stated that the most ominous fetal heart rate pattern was "slowness of its return when a contraction is passing on"—probably the first description of a late deceleration FHR pattern. Kennedy also noted the importance of fetal head compression on fetal heart rate and the effects of funis compression. He finished this discussion with accurate reflections on the significance of meconium-stained fluid. Despite what was an accurate and widely disseminated clinical description of intrapartum fetal distress by Kennedy, von Winkle is usually cited in American textbooks as the pioneer in relating FHR

OBSERVATIONS

ON

OBSTETRIC AUSCULTATION,

WITH

AN ANALYSIS

OF THE

EVIDENCES OF PREGNANCY,

AND

AN INQUIRY INTO THE PROOFS OF THE LIFE AND
DEATH OF THE FŒTUS IN UTERO.

By EVORY KENNEDY, M.D.,

LICENTIATE OF THE KING AND QUEEN'S COLLEGE OF PHYSICIANS
IN IRELAND, LECTURER ON MIDWIFERY,
AND THE DISEASES OF WOMEN AND CHILDREN, AT THE
RICHMOND HOSPITAL SCHOOL,
AND LATE ASSISTANT TO THE DUBLIN LYING-IN HOSPITAL.

Fig. 9-1. Frontpiece of Kennedy's monograph (courtesy of Dr. L. Longo.)

WITH

AN APPENDIX CONTAINING LEGAL NOTES,

By JOHN SMITH, Esq.,

BARRISTER AT LAW.

DUBLIN:

PRINTED FOR HODGES AND SMITH,
21, COLLEGE-GREEN;
LONGMAN, REES, AND CO., SIMPKIN AND MARSHALL,
LONDON; MACLACHLAN AND STEWART, EDINBURGH;
SMITH AND SON, GLASGOW.

1833.

patterns to fetal distress. This has occurred even though von Winkle's 1903 paper was published some 70 years after Kennedy's book.[717]

It is interesting to speculate as to why Kennedy's concepts were essentially lost to the 20th-century American obstetrical text. In part it may have been due to the respect that American authors had for the German writer or to our predecessors' overwhelming interest in maternal welfare or perhaps their fear of advocating more obstetrical interference. At any rate, 125 years later, with the problem of maternal deaths largely resolved, American obstetricians are turning again to Kennedy's concerns for the welfare of the fetus and the significance of its heart rate patterns.

Prior to the advent of fetal scalp sampling, electronic, and ultrasonic monitoring, the intrapartum clinical criteria of fetal distress were (a) tachycardia (a FHR of more than 160 bpm), (b) bradycardia (a FHR of less than 100 bpm), (c) "irregularity" of FHR (never precisely defined), (d) passage of meconium in vertex presentation, and (e) gross alterations of fetal movements (never defined). Controlled studies suggested that these criteria were of little predictive value, but undaunted, many obstetricians attempted to develop various scoring indexes for determining when apparent fetal distress was "real" (a problem that is still with us).

The experience of Cox[121a] in the 1950s in Australia is representative of studies reported during that time period. Mainly, there was a minimal increase in newborn morbidity and perinatal mortality when only one of these clinical signs of fetal distress was observed on only one occasion. However, when these clinical signs were observed in combination or repetitively, the morbidity and perinatal mortality rates were much higher. Except for Walker's[723] study in South Africa, there appear to have been few efforts in that era to objectively evaluate the clinical signs of fetal distress. Then, as now, most obstetricians responded to apparent fetal signs of distress and concluded that the resulting newborn morbidity or perinatal mortality were related to the intrapartum stress and not to the operative interference. However, Walker demonstrated in a relatively large series that operative interference in cases of suspected fetal distress (according to criteria available at that time) did not improve the newborn's condition. For the present, these clinical criteria of fetal distress (without the use of the electronic monitor) have been largely discarded in most American academic centers. The recent study of Haverkamp and associates[325] in Denver, comparing clinical monitoring with electronic monitoring, is one clear-cut exception.

ABDOMINAL FETAL ECG

In discussions of the development of methods for recording of the fetal ECG, the story is often retold of Cremer's 1906 *in utero* human fetal ECG recording.[129] In some reports, his subject is described as his pregnant wife and in others, as a volunteer from von Winkle's hospital ward. At any rate, in 1906, some 3 years after Einthoven published his original description of the adult ECG, Cremer placed an abdominal electrode over the uterine fun-

dus and inserted a vaginal electrode into a pregnant woman. The recordings showed distinct fetal ECG complexes (Fig. 9-2). The intervening literature on abdominal fetal ECG's (FECG) has been voluminous and confusing. The abdominal FECG tracing has been used for the diagnosis of the fetal position, twins, congenital heart defects, the presence of fetal life, and the general state of fetal health. The most enthusiastic supporter for the FECG was Larks,[421] who reported a discernible abdominal FECG as early as 11 weeks after conception, and suggested that the FECG complex itself was (as in the adult) useful for determining the fetus's health.

Ward and Kennedy[729] reported a success rate in abdominal FECG recordings varying from 70% at 20 weeks to 100% at term. However, others were seldom able to achieve such success.[134] In practical terms, often nothing more than a slight interruption of maternal abdominal ECG (which supposedly occurred

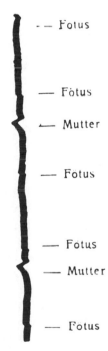

Fig. 9-2. Initial fetal electrocardiogram recorded by Cremer in 1906. The fetal complexes are indicated by the disruption in the baseline. (From Larks, S.D.: The fetal electrocardiogram in multiple pregnancy. *Am J Obstet Gynecol* **77:** 1109, 1959. Reproduced with permission.)

at the fetal heart rate) was taken as a positive finding. Under circumstances of such poor recordings, it is easily understood how a high incidence of false positive tests of FHR recordings occurred and how the impression developed that sometimes the dying fetal heart discharged at 300–400 bpm. Some of these technical difficulties, such as losing the fetal ECG at 28–34 weeks, were ascribed to vernix, and at other times to the position of the placenta. There has been no agreement on the reasons for failure to pick up the abdominal FECG, and the literature remained undecided about its clinical usefulness.

Various fetal arythmias were diagnosed from the abdominal FECG. While arythmias do occur, it would appear that many such recordings were actually artifact. Since the overwhelming percentage of such fetuses turned out to be normal newborns, the impression developed that fetal cardiac arythmias were benign. This question has not been resolved as even our modern techniques for abdominal FECG are often inadequate in the prenatal period.[466]

Borrowing techniques used in *extra utero* humans, several early investigators attempted to describe the changes of hypoxia and asphyxia in the fetal ECG (FECG) complex. Larks[421] described "notching" of the FECG complex with depression of the ST segments during fetal hypoxia. But the abdominal FECG tracings he used were so poor under most circumstances that his interpretations are probably another example of over diagnosis from inadequate data collection.

Several years ago, Hon[352] analyzed the fetal ECG's of nine dying human fetuses and challenged the concepts put forward by Larks and others that the form of the FECG's (no matter how obtained) was somehow useful in determination of fetal health. Hon noted that bursts of normal FECG complexes occurred right up to the time of fetal death. The concepts of Southern[653] (who believed that diagnosable ST depressions occurred) and Bernstein[50] (who diagnosed fetal PR changes) have been reactivated and once more we are

hearing of the necessity for analyzing the FECG complex itself. Recording of FECG is now recommended as a necessary technique in the analysis of fetal cardiac arrythmias, and with worrisome FHR patterns. Adamsons and Myers[4] noted in the monkey, and Organ et al.[517] noted similarly in the human, that fetal postural changes have much more impact in the configuration of FECG than does myocardial function or oxygen level.

In summary, the abdominal FECG is useful only as a technique for determining fetal heart rate (FHR). While enthusiasm for using this modality of FHR determination was waxed and waned over the last 70 years, the technique is once again a matter of great interest. Complications with the direct scalp monitoring techniques are now more obvious, and in many obstetricians' views there is a need for a safer method of FHR monitoring than internal techniques.

To count the FHR from abdominal leads requires a technique for removing the maternal ECG (MECG) complex from the tracing as well as exclusion of myometrial and maternal muscular activity. The MECG complex is of greater voltage and its R wave of greater slope than that of the FECG complex. Older techniques attempted to subtract the MECG complex from the recording, either by filtering or by cancellation with special placement of the abdominal and chest wall electrodes. The simultaneous cancellation techniques had to be precise, or else artifacts are created in the recordings which may erroneously be counted as FHR. More recent techniques have sought to exclude the MECG. These techniques are based on difference in voltage and demand that the MECG be larger than the FECG by a ratio specified by each manufacturer.

Even if all of these systems perform without error, there remains the problem of simultaneous beating of the maternal and fetal hearts. This latter problem occurs in 10–40% of the fetal ECG complexes. Several fetal monitor manufacturers now "fake" a FECG complex whenever the two hearts beat nearly or actually simultaneously. Such "faked" fetal heartbeats destroy the concept of accurate fetal beat-to-beat determination. An improved system designed by Widrow and colleagues[749] employs up to 18 electrodes placed on the maternal chest and abdomen and a computerized "noise cancellation" system. This technique is actually able to pick out the FECG from an abdominal wall tracing which to the eye contains only the MECG and noise (Fig. 9-3). Unfortunately, the system demands a great deal of computer ability, and to date is expensive and cumbersome.

FETAL ECG DETERMINED BY THE INTERNAL METHOD

The concept of obtaining the FECG directly from the *in utero* fetus apparently originated independently in both South America and Europe. Caledryo-Barcia and colleagues[86] in Uruguay inserted needles directly through the maternal abdominal wall into the fetal buttock and transcervically into the fetal scalp. Smyth[638] in England, Sureau[671] in France, and Kaplan and Toyama,[393] in America, all inserted various electrodes into the amniotic space, coming to rest against the fetus. Ross,[585] in Australia, employed a suction electrode attached to the fetal scalp. In America, however, it was Hon and Lee's[351] modification of a Michelle skin clip in the mid-1960s which made possible the widespread use of direct pickup of the scalp FECG.

LaCroix[419] developed a fish hook scalp electrode which was easy to use, but its manufacture never actively entered the commercial market (Fig. 9-4). Kitahama and Sasaoka[404] of Japan originally described the "screw" fetal scalp electrode in 1967. Ruttgers and Kubli[595] designed a device for applying such an electrode, but it has never been as popular as that described by Hon *et al.*[356] in 1972. The popularity of the disposable screw scalp electrode has resulted in a number of lawsuits for infringement upon various patents. The screw electrode has recently come under reevaluation for a scalp abscess rate of approximately 5% and reports of newborn deaths from sepsis.[194, 516, 762]

Concern over possible scalp trauma from

Fig. 9-3. Result of wide-band fetal ECG experiment (bandwidth, 0.3–75 Hz; sampling rate, 512 Hz). (a) Reference input (chest lead); (b) primary input (abdominal lead); (c) noise canceller output. (From Widrow, B., *et al.*: *Proc I.E.E.E.* **63:** 1692, 1975. Reproduced with permission.)

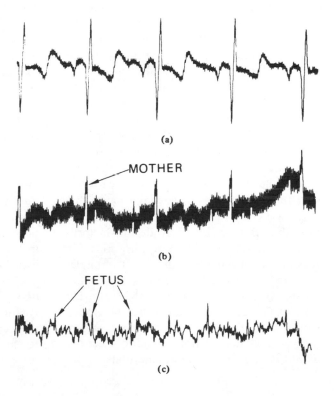

(a)

MOTHER

(b)

FETUS

(c)

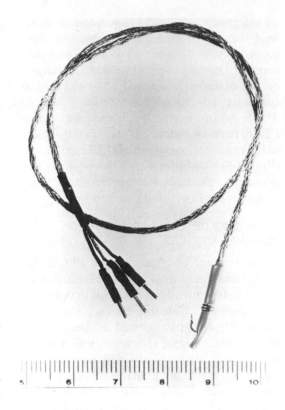

Fig. 9-4. The fish-hook scalp electrode designed by L. A. Croix which was easy to apply and worked well.

the "Hon" clip electrode prompted us to develop an "atraumatic" suction scalp electrode.[267] In its final form, the suction electrode contained an ECG terminal, a heat thermister to monitor fetal scalp temperature, and an infrared pulse sensor to determine fetal scalp pulse and fetal oxygen saturation. Unfortunately, in three infants (out of approximately 250) in which it was applied, scalp hemangiomas (the size of the suction electrode) appeared at the site of electrode placement. It was therefore necessary to redesign the electrode as a flat, nonsuction disk (Fig. 9-5). Although at one time commercially available, this "disk" electrode satisfactorily recorded in only 60% of its applications. For reasons that are unclear, the FECG complex obtained from the fetal buttock is of much greater voltage than that from the scalp. The disk ECG electrode (as any other electrodes) works well, therefore, with a breech presentation and such a nontraumatic electrode would be useful in face presentations.

THE ACCEPTANCE OF ROUTINE FETAL MONITORING

In order to understand the wide acceptance in America of electronic fetal monitoring to the point where it is considered "intrinsic to routine obstetrics care" (Aladjem and Brown[11b]), it is necessary to briefly trace (without judgmental views) the development of the corporation Corometrics and its relationship to E. Hon. For Corometrics was to conduct extensive educational and advertising programs after its inception, concerning the "need" for electronic fetal monitoring. Professor Hon was largely responsible for the prestigious role of electronic fetal monitoring in America, and was recognized by the American College of Obstetricians and Gynecologists with a special award for his contributions.

Hon's laboratory at Yale University was the center of clinical obstetrical biometrics research in America in the mid-1960s, and his extensive studies have stood the test of

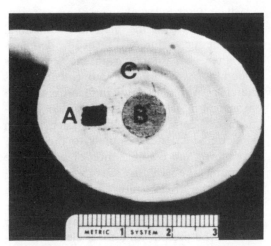

Fig. 9-5. The combination nontraumatic fetal probe (which was held against fetal tissues by uterine or vaginal pressure). A—solid state photoelectric emitter and sensor (for scalp pulse and oxygen saturation); B—ECG terminal; C—thermistor (for fetal temperature and pulse).

time very well. In 1966, Corometrics Corporation was organized among Dr. Hon's laboratory staff to render certain engineering and consultation services to Yale University. In 1967, when I visited Dr. Hon's laboratory at Yale, he was most generous in demonstrating to me his techniques for maternal and fetal monitoring. His staff's enthusiasm was contagious. I also noted that his engineers had completely disassembled a prototype fetal monitor designed by Hammacher (manufactured by Hewlett-Packard) based on fetal heart sound recording, and they were discussing the design of a similar apparatus based on fetal ECG for the American market. (My 1968 updated Hewlett-Packard monitor is still functioning 10 years later.) By 1969, Ed Hon had become Professor of Obstetrics and Gynecology at the University of Southern California. According to 1968 and 1971 prospectus filed at Securities and Exchange Commission, Professor Hon conducted research for Corometrics while at the University of California, and was supplied with a full-time engineer by the company. He was likewise hired by Corometrics as its Medical Director.

One feature of the Corometrics monitor was that it functioned well and was given the greatest of all flattery by a competitor (Berkeley Bio-Engineering) who essentially "copied" their machine. Professor Hon subsequently authored and coauthored many widely read papers using the Corometric apparatus, which acknowledged his position as Professor of Obstetrics at USC, but none have apparently acknowledged his relationship with Corometrics. An amazing aspect of American obstetrics was that Corometrics' viewpoint on the importance of fetal monitoring were accepted (myself included) without controlled studies. (Their original statement that electronic monitoring appeared to reduce the incidence of cesarean section has been dropped.) Professor Hon's generous support from governmental agencies never corrected this obvious deficiency. Today's Federal Drug Administration regulations would probably have prevented the widespread use of fetal monitors.

In 1976, a controlled study in Denver on the use of fetal monitoring was published[325] comparing electropic monitoring in high-risk pregnancies with expert nursing care. This study suggested that monitoring by electronic means only increased rates of cesarean section. A comparable situation with medical apparatus had occurred in American medicine, when Waganstein had introduced gastric freezing for treatment of duodenal ulcers. When the gastric freezing apparatus was found to be ineffective by controlled studies (1972) it was quickly abandoned, despite its introduction by a distinguished group and the manufacture of hundreds of units. The freezing apparatus was uncomfortable for the patient and not much fun for the physician.

On the other hand, we have not scrapped the fetal monitor since the publication of the Denver study. The difference may be that the fetal monitor brings into the labor room a certain degree of "scientific apparatus." I know that I enjoy using fetal monitors, pondering the significance of the fetal heart rate tracings, and attempting to devise better monitoring techniques. I suspect that other obstetricians have found the monitor to be equally satisfying from an intellectual standpoint and it is perhaps for this reason that we continue to pursue our studies despite the difficulties of demonstrating their therapeutic value. Papers from fetal intensive care services have appeared, modestly claiming that their improvements in perinatal care are due specifically to the introduction of electronic fetal monitoring. This introduction (of electronic fetal monitoring) occurred in America at approximately the same time that abortion on demand became available, that neonatal intensive care was developed, that pregnancy diets were changed, that family size decreased, and probably most importantly, that medical interest in the welfare of the fetus became as widespread as interest in maternal welfare (Chapter 2).

Electronic fetal monitoring has been my major academic interest for the past decade and I am unwilling to believe that it (and everyone else's efforts) has all been for nothing in terms of fetal welfare. For the non-low-risk gravida, the unregistered, or for those wishing the latest in scientific care, it still is indicated. My original assumption that it would reduce nursing requirements in the labor ward were soon proved to be very much in error, but its application does bring to the bedside additional obstetrical staff, which must be of fetal benefit. Until otherwise disproven, in the average labor ward, electronic monitoring, plus the added required staff probably does, for the high-risk gravida, improve perinatal rates (as has been so frequently claimed by its supporters). Professor Hon's and Corometrics' message has so impressed the obstetrical world that even the Swedes, with their fantastically low perinatal rates, are exploring the use of fetal electronic monitoring.

PHONOCARDIOGRAPH RECORDINGS

Fetal phonocardiograph (PCG) recordings were apparently first made by Rockwood and Falls in 1923.[578] Using microphones with low-frequency response (between 75 and 105 Hz),

excellent fetal heart phonocardiographs can be obtained from the maternal abdominal wall. The successful PCG recording demands that there be a relative absence of excess abdominal wall noise or movement and is therefore of limited value in recording for an intrapartum FHR monitoring system. Hammacher[317] employed a logic system which converted fetal heart sounds to the square wave form and counted three signals before accepting the sounds as representing the FHR. Thus, a heart rate "accepted" by such an apparatus can be considered to be reliable. The fetal PCG technique has much to offer even in the present time for it clearly distinguishes the fetal systolic from the diastolic intervals. These are (as noted in Chapter 11) of interest for determining fetal cardiovascular function. The fetal PCG also provides a reasonable noninvasive technique for measuring FHR beat-to-beat variability as there is no confusion over whether the systolic or diastolic pulse is being recorded, such as occurs with the use of Doppler transducer.

In utero fetal sounds are often a form of energy developed within the uterus in relationship to either the fetal heart or the pulsations of the placental bed. Both can be a potential source of monitoring. Braxton-Hicks, nearly one hundred years ago, reported on the various sounds that occur from the placental soufflé and their possible interpretation.[573] There is no doubt that these placental sounds give a relative indication of flow or that such flow is a useful indicator of perfusion of the placenta. Various techniques to convert these forms of energy into some sort of reliable diagnostic criteria have failed,[280] (Fig. 9-6) although the adult ballistocardiogram at times will demonstrate fetal complexes.

ULTRASOUND MONITORING

Doppler ultrasound owes its development to underwater detection developed in World Wars I and II. Its widespread use for fetal monitoring awaited the demonstration of its apparent safety. Despite repeated reports describing detrimental effects of the energy

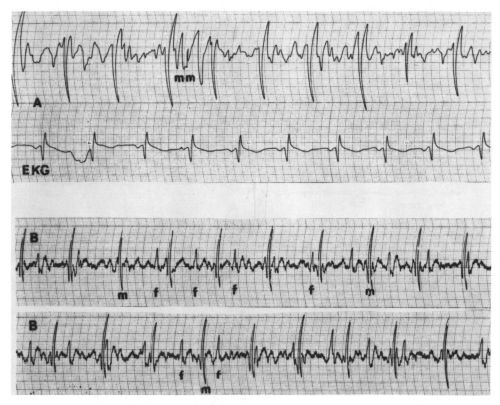

Fig. 9-6. Fetal "ballistocardiogram" recorded with intrauterine microphone. (A) Fetal ballistocardiogram and simultaneous EKG. (B) *In utero* ballistocardiogram showing both maternal and fetal complexes. (From Goodlin, R.C., and Lowe, E.W.: Multiphasic fetal monitoring. A preliminary evaluation. *Am J Obstet Gynecol* **119**: 341–357, 1974. Reproduced with permission.)

from ultrasound on animals and bacteria, Doppler transducers continue to be extensively used for fetal monitoring. Hellman and colleagues[333] concluded in 1970 that at the Doppler level of 1 W/cm, there were no demonstrable deleterious cellular effects, and concluded that "there will be no evidence of genetic safety for generations to come."

At present, the Doppler ultrasonic device is the most useful instrument available for detecting the antenatal FHR during the second trimester. One interesting feature of Doppler transducers is that the beating auricles may give as strong a pulse as do the ventricles or valves[274] (Fig. 9-7). Thus, if there is a fetal heart block, the Doppler fetal heart pulse often suggests the "acceptable" FHR while the FECG (R wave) recording will give one-half or one-third of the value, depending on the degree of heart block. While this is ad-

vantageous in diagnosing the rate cases of fetal heart block, the ability of the auricles to provide a strong Doppler pulse is also one of the severe limitations of the Doppler fetal heart rate monitor. Unless the beam is perfectly focused on the fetus's small beating heart, the reflected Doppler pulse may easily wander between signals generated from either the diastolic or systolic intervals. For FHR determination, this feature is insignificant, but it can be very misleading in the measurement of beat-to-beat variability. The Doppler signal can give a false impression of fetal well-being by suggesting a normal degree of FHR beat-to-beat variability when there is none.

The Doppler beam is reflected from the moving surface, and to a degree, can be quantitated according to the amount of moving surface or blood flow. In other words, an idea

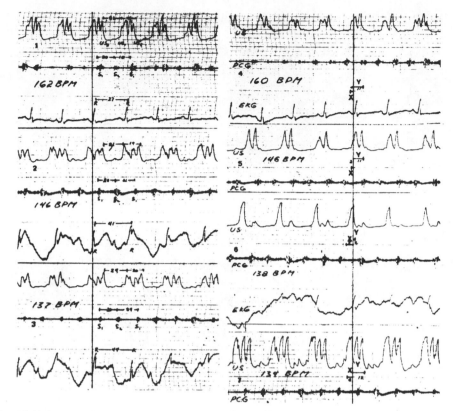

Fig. 9-7. Multiple recordings of simultaneous Doppler pulse, fetal heart sounds, and ECG. Vertical line is drawn through Q-wave, showing varying intervals of Doppler pulse in diastolic time (X) and systolic time (Y). (From *Obstet Gynecol* **38:** 916, 1971. Reproduced with permission.)

of the relative fetal blood flow at the monitored site can be obtained from the volume of the signal. This is one of the exciting future uses of the Doppler device, as presently we have no satisfactory techniques for measuring umbilical or uterine blood flow. Assuming that one could perfectly focus the artery with the Doppler, it should be possible to measure from week to week the relative changes in umbilical or uterine blood flows.

THE FETAL PHOTOELECTRIC PLETHYSMOGRAPHIC PULSE

In 1969, I became interested in determining fetal oxygen saturation with a photoelectric cell applied to the fetal scalp. It soon became apparent that the fetal pulse (blood volume pulse) could be measured with such an apparatus (Fig. 9-8). There is an extensive literature about the blood volume pulse, with demonstrations that it reflects aortic flow and

cardiac output.[265] It became apparent that with a double beam probe placed against the fetal scalp it would record both the fetal scalp BVP and the uterine (or vaginal) BVP. In addition, a probe was also placed on the maternal big toe. I was able to demonstrate that during a uterine contraction, there (often) occurs a decrease in uterine blood flow, a relative fetal hypertension immediately prior to a contraction, and a marked decrease of maternal aortic blood flow (if she were supine). I rushed to get the report into print, only at the last moment to discover that Poseiro *et al.*[539] had previously described the effects in supine parturients of uterine contractions on aortal flow (Fig. 9-9). This latter concept seems to be the most important idea that monitoring has contributed to the routine care in the labor ward. (Avoid the maternal supine position!)

My attempts to find either commercial or

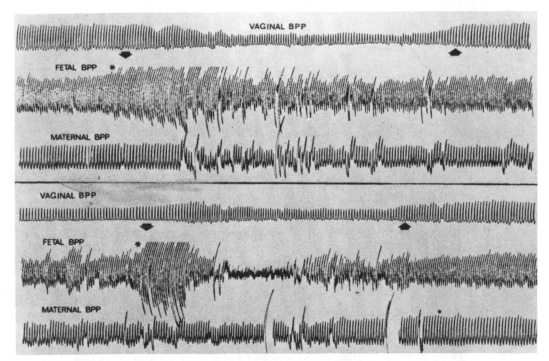

Fig. 9-8. Simultaneous blood-volume pulse recording of upper vagina (vaginal BPP), fetal scalp BVP (fetal BPP), and maternal big toe BPP (maternal BPP). With onset of uterine contraction (downward arrow), vaginal pulse height decreases (decreased flow), fetal hypertension (asterisk) preceding contraction (and movement artifact) and a decrease in maternal big toe pulse (Poseiro effect). During contraction, both maternal and fetal bradycardia occurred.

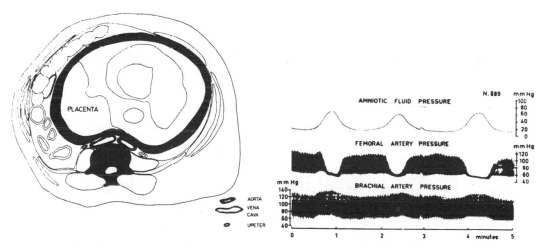

Fig. 9-9. Pregnant uterus obstructing aorta and vena cava at level of LIV vertebrae. On right is recording of femoral and brachial artery pressure, demonstrating a marked decrease in femoral flow and an increase in bracheal pressure during a uterine contraction. (From Poseiro, J., *et al.*: WHO # 185 Washington, D.C., 1969. Reproduced with permission.)

foundation support for the fetal BVP probe have failed, but I persist in the belief that when the importance of fetal oxygen saturation is recognized, the infrared photoelectric cell applied to the fetus will come into its own. (The fetus operates in a low P_{O_2} range which means that changes in oxygen content are on the straight part of its oxygen saturation curve. Besides, saturation is markedly affected by pH, suggesting that oxygen saturation would be a better indicator of fetal health than pH.[456a] The use of the fetal plethysmographic pulse is less clear, as there are better transducers for use in systolic time intervals. The maternal big toe pulse is still useful, particularly when delivering by cesarean section, as it easily indicates the presence of aortal compression by the pregnant uterus (Fig. 9-10).

BEAT-TO-BEAT VARIABILITY (BBV)

The normal FHR pattern shows some 5–10 oscillations per minute on a short-term basis and 10–40 beats per minute on a long-term basis (Fig. 9-11). The earliest studies with fetal FHR variability in the human apparently were those of Sontag and associates[644-648] of Yellow Springs in the 1950s. These pioneer investigators of fetal movement and heart rate changes were begun in 1938 (Sontag and Richards) when they stud-

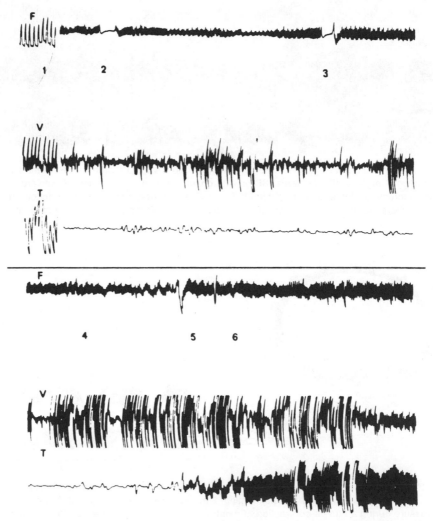

Fig. 9-10. BVP pulse recording during a cesarean section under caudal anesthesia. F—finger; V—vaginal pulse; and T—big toe. 1—control period, 2—maternal hypotension treated by saline infusion (3); 4—uterine incision with vaginal movement (5) delivery of fetal head; 6—delivery of infant with 1 min Apgar score of 2. Note loss of toe and vaginal pulses as the c-section proceeded (varying paper speeds). (From *Obstet Gynecol* **37:** 702, 1971. Reproduced with permission.)

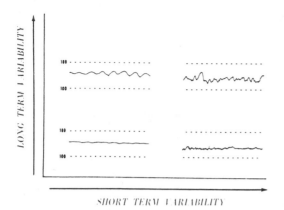

Fig. 9-11. Schematic diagram of LTV and STV showing minimal degree of both in lower left and maximum of both in upper right. (From Schifrin, B.S.: *Workshop in Fetal Heart Rate Monitoring*, 1976. Reproduced with permission.)

ied the effects on the fetus of sound stimuli applied directly to the maternal abdomen. They were able to demonstrate correlations between the emotional state of the mother and her fetus's heart rate pattern. In 1967, they showed that there were distinct differences in the FHR variation patterns between different fetuses. The patterns of FHR variation for a given fetus, however, were consistent from recording to recording (made twice a week). Sontag's group also noted that FHR variability was influenced by playing pleasurable music and by the mother's moods. Other early papers on BBV were by Hammacher in 1967,[317] describing the loss of BBV in the sick fetus, by Caldeyro-Barcia *et al.,*[86] 1966, and by Hon,[354] 1968, in the United States, noting the loss of BBV with atropine.

In 1972, I wrote a letter[272] to the editor of the *JAMA* protesting a paper by Schrifrin and Dame[611] which had presented Hon's FHR interpretation. Hon himself soon recommended the use of BBV (or baseline variability) and Schrifrin's group has since become a leader in its interpretation and understanding. While I modestly consider myself the first in America to suggest the importance of BBV (FHR reactivity) as a parameter of FHR recording interpretation,[267] I would also like to be the first to suggest that its impor-

tance has been greatly exaggerated. Even Schrifrin has been moved to declare that "all that wiggles is not variability."[328a] However, important aspects of BBV have been shown by Martin and associates[461] of Los Angeles, who convincingly demonstrated that loss of BBV in the premature is an ominous sign for its subsequent course in the nursery. But for the term fetus, the unpredictable effects of maternal drugs and fetal arousal levels on BBV is a serious limitation of its use as a sole indicator of its health (Chapter 1).

Caldeyro-Barcia *et al.*[86] in 1966 reported that there were at least two types of FHR variability, short term (STV) and long term (LTV). In 1968, Hon described a visual index related to the amplitude of the FHR. Several investigators have described indexes to detect STV and LTV. The best known are those of de Haan and associates[148] and Yeh and associates.[765a] Schrifrin has shown that there are multiple indices possible from any given FHR recording (Table 9-I) depending on which formula is used. I have argued[288a] that "pure" STV exists only in the eyes of a computer, for when I manually measured changes in time between the peak of two R waves, I found that the changes in STV occurred over four or five heart beats. Short-term variability then has a "long-term" or gradual component which is invariably ignored by a computer. The trend to continue to devise new computer indices for FHR variability reminds me of the ancient argument over how many angels could dance on the head of a pin. The questions tax the ingenuity, but have little practical value. For BBV is like beauty, in my opinion, we can all appreciate its presence, but no computer can accurately define it.

Fetal Heart Rate Reactivity

In 1971, I spoke about baseline "reactivity" of the fetal heart rate. Urbach *et al.*[711] had previously discussed newborn heart rate irregularity and related it to neonatal outcome. As discussed, Caldeyro-Barcia, Hon, and others had recorded the various degrees of irreg-

Table 9-I. Possible Techniques for Quantifying Variability[a]

Number	Description	Formula or Presentation
1	INTERVAL OR RATE HISTOGRAM	HISTOGRAM
2	INTERVAL OR RATE DIFFERENCE HISTOGRAM	HISTOGRAM
3	PEAK TO PEAK RATE DIFFERENCE	MAXIMUM VALVE – MINIMUM VALVE (DURING STUDY PERIOD)
4	AVERAGE INTERVAL OR RATE DIFFERENCE	$\frac{1}{N}\sum_{i}^{N}\mid x_i - x_{i-1}\mid$
5	AVERAGE PERCENTAGE INTERVAL OR RATE DIFFERENCE	$\frac{1}{N}\sum_{i}^{N}\frac{\mid x_i - x_{i-1}\mid}{x_{i-1}}$
6	STANDARD DEVIATION OF INTERVAL OR RATE DIFFERENCE	$\sqrt{\frac{1}{N-1}\left[\sum \Delta x_i{}^2 - N\left(\frac{\sum \Delta x_i}{N}\right)^2\right]}$
7	INTERVAL OR RATE DIFFERENCE SUMMATION	$\underset{\text{Time}=0}{\overset{T \text{ SECONDS}}{\sum}}\mid x_i - x_{i-1}\mid$
8	TRANSFORMATION TO POLAR COORDINATES	$\text{ARGUMENT} = \text{ARCTAN}\left(\frac{x_i}{x_{i-1}}\right)$ $\text{MODULUS} = \sqrt{x_i{}^2 + x_{i-1}^2}$

[a] Notes: x_i are data elements, either interval or rate. Δx_i is the difference between two successive data elements. N is 255 in this study. T is 60 sec in this study.

ularity of fetal heart rate. It was Hammacher,[317] I believe, who first described the ominous significance of the lack of variability of fetal heart rate—the so-called "silent" fetus. My concept was in 1970, and still is today, that the fetus' overall CNS activity was reflected in the irregularity of its instantaneous heart rate. By "fetal heart rate reactivity," I meant the amount of variability of heart rate values above and below the baseline. Hon and others were to use the term "beat-to-beat variability." Initially this appeared to be a better term than "reactivity," but with more experience, I have returned to the original concept of reactivity.

It has been exceedingly difficult to define beat-to-beat variability. Unless it is expressed as a percentage of change of R-R intervals, the values will be related to baseline heart rate (short-term variability) or on an arbitrary length of time. The variability index defined on the basis of succeeding heart rates (STV) will be greater at slower heart rates than at higher heart rates. As noted in Chapter 8, this simply reflects the longer interval between heart beats and the buildup of sensitivity of

the SA node so that it reacts to less stimulus. It also reflects the fact that with a very short interval between beats (tachycardia) there is simply less opportunity for variability of heart rate. On the other hand, when beat-to-beat variability is defined over many heart beats (LTV), accelerations can occur at all baseline rates.

If it is accepted that the reactivity of the fetal heart rate is a valid concept, then there are several techniques for its description. A simplified technique for beat-to-beat variability is that employed in the Berkeley 900R machine which simply shows the baseline FHR changes on an expanded scale and one can inspect the record and have an excellent but subjective value for fetal reactivity. Mondanlou and associates[479] have described a technique of continuous integration of the variability of heart rate values and display on a scale of 0 to 4. They modified the Berkeley 900R so as to continuously display on a recorder the actual integration over a time period of 1 min. I cling to the concept that visual inspection of the recording is the only satisfactory way of determining fetal heart reactivity. We have continued to use the rough guideline that when the range around the baseline is less than 5 beats per minute, the reactivity is absent, when between 5 and 10 beats per minute, it is moderate, and in excess of 10 beats per minute is excessive.

In any determination of beat-to-beat interval, variability, or reactivity, care should be taken in accepting the readout of a recorder. Nearly every commercially manufactured monitor uses a peak detector of the R wave, which is converted into a pulse. When the basline is clean and there are few artifacts, this can be a precise technique. However, given uterine contractions or any other feature which causes a noisy baseline and varying R-wave voltage, often this peak detection method is imprecise and creates an artificial increased BBV. This artifact is seen particularly during bradycardias associated with strong uterine contractions. The only way to circumvent this problem is to use a strip recording or oscilloscope which simultaneously shows the R wave and its derived pulse. Such is seldom available with commercial models.

In summary, fetal reactivity determination from FHR recordings assumes that one has a perfect "peak" detector; when this is not present, one should be very cautious about the interpretation of increased reactivity displayed from any recording. Sleep, drugs, arousal levels, maturity, infection, and probably many other factors affect fetal heart rate activity in addition to asphyxia. In my view, loss of BBV without other worrisome signs in a FHR recording is without clinical significance. Drugs which decrease BBV include atropine, tranquilizers, narcotics, $MgSO_4$, propranolol, and β-adrenergic agents (isoxsuprine, terbutaline).

SIGNS OF FETAL DISTRESS

In 1833, Kennedy[401] suggested that certain FHR had an ominous connotation for the well-being of the fetus. Ever since, obstetricians have been attempting to define and to refine the definitions of patterns which are truly indicative of fetal distress. One of the problems is that fetal distress is often a retrospective diagnosis. Little attention, however, has been given toward maternal reports of "decreased fetal movements" or toward "increased maternal concern about her fetus."[291] In certain fetal illnesses, such as erythroblastosis fetalis,[238] efforts were made to quantitate these maternal impressions. With few exceptions, though (Chapter 1), obstetricians were reluctant to consider such factors in evaluating possible fetal disease. The general belief has been that maternal impressions about fetal health and fetal movements are too subjective to provide any data base on which to act or to evaluate fetal health. My own studies suggest that fetal surveillance should concentrate on fetal movements in the antenatal period, with efforts directed toward finding the silent (sick) fetus prior to the onset of the stresses of labor.

I question the prevailing American view that intrapartum electronic fetal monitoring will adequately identify the fetus in trouble, and that its application will reduce the incidence of stillborns or subsequent cerebral palsy. The history of our speciality has been that all intrapartum fetal monitoring techniques, when actually subjected to studies where controls are offered the same sort of intrapartum intensive care as the monitored subjects, the controls invariably do as well if not better than the monitored fetuses. The basis for this impression is apparent in the comparison of the monitor with the stethoscope,[325] the stethoscope with indirect observation,[723] and so forth. Regardless of whether monitoring with simple auscultation versus no auscultation or electronic monitoring versus auscultation is considered, the only difference between the control and "monitored" groups has been that the controls endured less operative interference.

I have interpreted our own data and those studies reported by others to indicate that the healthy, term human fetus tolerates labor. Although it is prone to certain intrapartum accidents, such a healthy *in utero* human being is not unduly at risk of imminent death or permanent injury. When the rare fetal accidents of prolapsed cord and abruptic placenta have occurred on our service, they have been diagnosed not by the attached FHR electronic monitor, but by the standard techniques of intrapartum surveillance and good nursing care.

Only one intrapartum death of human fetuses weighing more than 2 kg has occurred on my service during an 8-year period. Fetuses weighing less than 2 kg are excluded from this statement due to our inexcusable tendency to underestimate fetal weights. Assuming that the fetus weighed less than 1 kg, we have literally allowed it to die *in utero* despite very ominous signs of fetal distress. Much to our horror, we have found that the subsequent stillborn weighed as much as 1.5–1.8 kg. If we can ignore this deplorable, but fortunately rare, underestimation of fetal weights, we have had an outstanding record during this time of electronic FHR monitoring. In reexamining records from the monitors, however, it becomes obvious that literally scores of supposedly ominous FHR recordings were ignored, and on the other hand, even more relatively benign FHR recordings spurred us onto operative interference. Compounding interpretation of these excellent results even further were hundreds of very brief or technically unsatisfactory FHR recordings.

This clinical experience appears unusually good in terms of fetal outcome, yet actually was based on poor data collection and interpretation. This phenomenon can be interpreted as our and our patients good fortune (while perhaps other institutions who made a similar effort suffered what should have been our misfortune).[107] Other explanations of our good results include possible direct fetal benefits from the increased bedside personnel which are required for electronic FHR monitoring. I like to believe that we now avoid the common iatrogenic causes of intrapartum fetal distress which were associated with maternal supine position, maternal hypotension, and excessive oxytocin stimulation.

I am convinced that the improvement in perinatal mortality rates (Chapter 2) in this country reflects the easy availability of contraception and abortion "on demand," smaller families, neonatal intensive care nurseries, etc. This improvement perhaps occurs in the same way that homicide improves cancer mortality rates. The basis for this last belief is that the most favorable prognostic sign for fetal welfare that I have found in any obstetrical patient is a strong desire for another child.

To my surprise, our experiences now suggest that with adequate perinatal screening, the occurrence of perinatal death among normal term size fetuses is virtually eliminated. When we began intrapartum monitoring in 1968, we secured funds for the purchase of monitors with the conviction that such instruments would prevent approximately three intrapartum fetal deaths per one thousand deliveries, and that we would probably be able to avoid one-half (or 5 out of 1000) of all cases of cerebral palsy. Perhaps this noble concept has not endured the test of time, as it now appears on reflection that intrapartum monitoring accomplishes neither of our expectations.

On the other hand, the important part of fetal monitoring probably takes place in the prepartum period. An inexpensive and good antenatal technique of monitoring fetal well-being is to accept the mother's own impression of her fetus's health (Chapter 1). We use a very simple technique of asking mothers to record fetal movements on a scale of 0 to 4+, over 4–6 hr intervals throughout the day (Fig. 9-12). (Anything more complicated has not worked.) During most pregnancies, the human fetus goes through periods of activity and periods of sleep or inactivity recognized by its mother as increased or decreased fetal movements. As has been noted by pregnant women since the beginning of time, their fetuses slow down as term approaches (Fig. 1-1). The fetuses nevertheless maintain the same circadian patterns of activity and rest.

Pearson and Weaver[530] have evolved a technique of asking gravida (who were apparently very dedicated and had nothing else to do) to count their fetuses movements be-

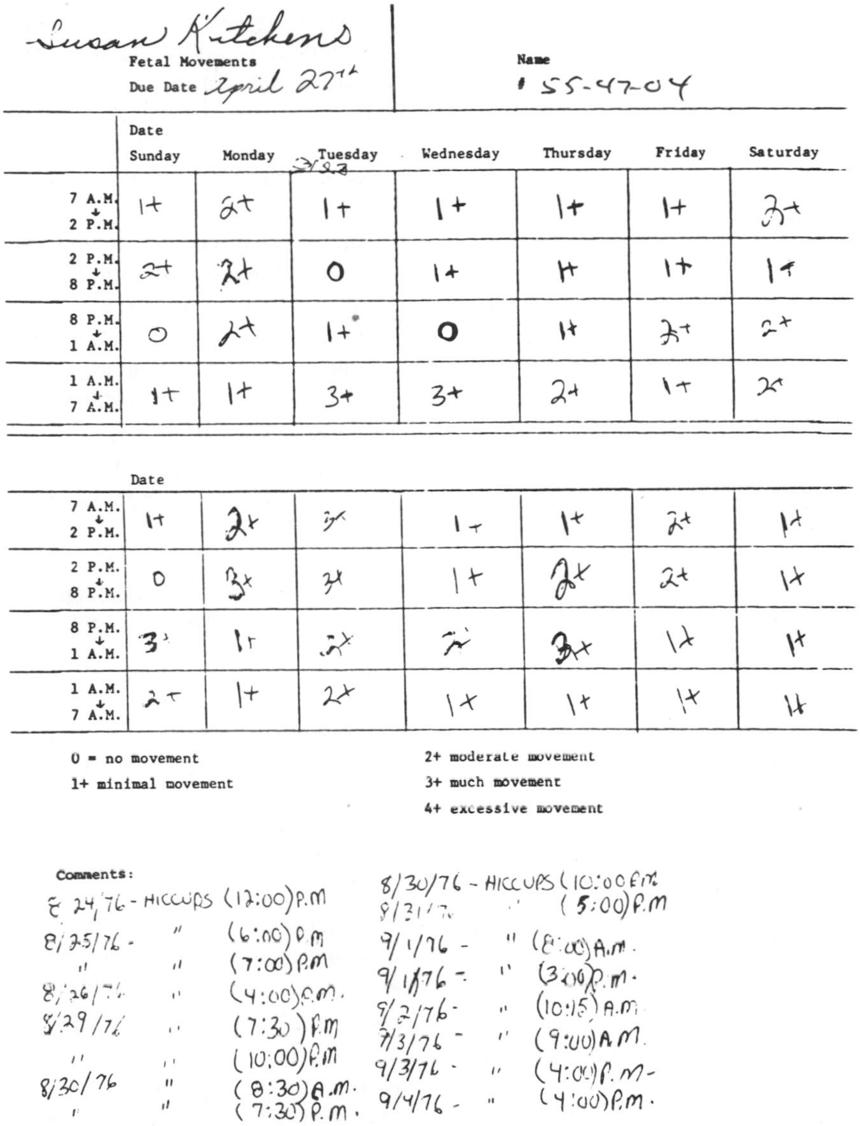

Susan Kitchens
Fetal Movements
Due Date *April 27th*

Name *↑55-4704*

Date	Sunday	Monday	Tuesday	Wednesday	Thursday	Friday	Saturday
7 A.M. ↓ 2 P.M.	1+	2+	1+	1+	1+	1+	3+
2 P.M. ↓ 8 P.M.	2+	2+	0	1+	1+	1+	1+
8 P.M. ↓ 1 A.M.	0	2+	1+	0	1+	3+	2+
1 A.M. ↓ 7 A.M.	1+	1+	3+	3+	2+	1+	2+

Date							
7 A.M. ↓ 2 P.M.	1+	2+	2+	1+	1+	2+	1+
2 P.M. ↓ 8 P.M.	0	3+	2+	1+	2+	2+	1+
8 P.M. ↓ 1 A.M.	3	1+	2+	2+	3+	1+	1+
1 A.M. ↓ 7 A.M.	2+	1+	2+	1+	1+	1+	1+

0 = no movement
1+ minimal movement

2+ moderate movement
3+ much movement
4+ excessive movement

Comments:

8/24/76 - HICCUPS (12:00) P.M
8/25/76 - " (6:00) P.M
   "   " (7:00) P.M
8/26/76 " (4:00) P.M.
8/29/76 " (7:30) P.M
   "   " (10:00) P.M
8/30/76 " (8:30) A.M.
   "   " (7:30) P.M.

8/30/76 - HICCUPS (10:00 P.M.
8/31/76 " (5:00) P.M
9/1/76 - " (8:00) A.M.
9/1/76 - " (3:00) P.m.
9/2/76 - " (10:15) A.m.
9/3/76 - " (9:00) A.M.
9/3/76 - " (4:00) P.M-
9/4/76 - " (4:00) P.M.

Fig. 9-12. Photograph of a fetal movement record of a normal fetus as recorded by its mother.

tween 9AM and 9 PM from the 32nd week of pregnancy onward. They found that only 2.5% of the fetuses moved less than 10 times in 12 hr (Fig. 9-13). Sontag[649] had suggested that each fetus has its own pattern and frequency of movements, unique unto itself. Strict comparison of movement patterns for different fetuses is thus probably of limited value. Once the pattern for a given fetus is established, however, it can be used as a reference for its well-being. Pearson and

Weaver applied modern techniques and found that there was a good correlation between decreased fetal movement, poor outcome, and low estriol values.

Comparison of maternal diaries of fetal activity with fetal outcome suggest that the fetus is healthy as long as it demonstrates circadian patterns of activity. Although we are ignorant of the physiological meaning of these circadian patterns (i.e., what determines the time of peak activity, why some fetuses

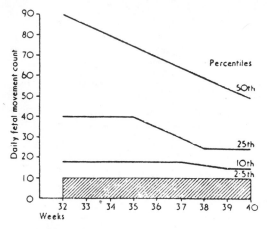

Fig. 9-13. Fetal movements as recorded by patients of Pearson and Weaver. (From *Br Med J* **1**: 1305, 1976. Reproduced with permission.)

have several peaks and others only one) the lack of circadian activity and decreased movements is clearly ominous.

In a limited study, we found that approximately 5% of the gravida keeping records reported decreased fetal movement or activity. Of this 5%, approximately one-sixth showed further signs of fetal compromise, such as a positive oxytocin challenge test, nonstress FHR recording, amniocentesis or amnioscopy, and decreasing maternal serum estriols or HPL. Among those with additional signs of fetal dysfunction, approximately 85% of the newborns were acidotic.

Our plan for antenatal monitoring then is to ask mothers to keep diaries of fetal movements, and when these appear abnormal, to study the fetuses further in the hospital. When a history of decreased fetal movements and at least one other ominous "fetal" test is found, in our experience, one-sixth of the fetuses will have demonstrable dysfunction. On the other hand, in the "normal" group that has been screened by such techniques, when followed in labor with intrapartum electronic monitoring, the yield of finding acidotic fetuses has been embarrassingly low (approximately 0.6%, of which 50% of the fetuses had anomalies incompatible with life).

When a term human fetus is viewed with a real-time ultrasonic scanner, it appears to be moving its limbs much more than is appreciated by its mother. However, ultrasonic scanners may stimulate a fetus, giving the viewer a false impression of great and constant activity. Using both a microphone and Doppler transducer, I became convinced that a fetus with low arousal levels had increased FHR variability occur when the Doppler crystal was activated. Others have disagreed, simply believing that mothers are unable to perceive the fetal movements seen with ultrasound. In order to correlate what is seen with ultrasound and the gravidas' perceptions of fetal movements, I consider fetal movements to be positive only when the fetus moves its body (arches its back). Movement of only the fetus's extremities is not considered positive movement.

The Role of Electronic Fetal Monitoring

In our 1968 thinking, we were following the then current obstetrical opinions that parturition contributed significantly to the incidence of crebral palsy as best espoused by Eastman of Johns Hopkins Medical School. In his famous 1954 paper,[177] "Mount Everest in Utero," he proposed that "while intrauterine anoxia actually kills fetuses, it was logical to believe that sometimes a degree of anoxia was not sufficient to kill the fetus, but large enough to inflict irreparable damage to the cerebrum." As noted in Chapter 8, it would appear that the "all or nothing" doctrine probably operates in cases of fetal distress, and that all we should ask of intrapartum fetal care is that the newborn be delivered alive and undamaged. (Such a statement should not be overinterpreted, for we should always seek to conduct labor with as little fetal stress as is possible.) I simply argue that despite all the platitudes to the contrary, intrapartum electronic fetal monitoring has not been demonstrated to reduce the incidence of cerebral palsy. I do not make this statement as a "devil's advocate," for I was the first to attempt to electronically monitor all parturients[265] (and was on call 24 hr a day), but base it on our own subsequent experience as well as how other societies have achieved a low incidence of cerebral dysfunction.

Since having proclaimed that antenatal monitoring is sufficient to detect the fetus at risk,[290] I have been challenged by a number of case histories which seem to refute my belief. One series of three cases of significant fetal–maternal transfusion (presented by Wertz of Sutter Hospital, Sacramento) have given me pause. In these three cases, there was shown to be approximately 150–250 ml of fetal blood in the maternal circulation following delivery. The gravidas had no symptoms of the fetal blood transfusion (chills, lethargy, or urticaria) and fetal movements were stated to be normal during the antenatal period (but two of the three had complained of decreased fetal movement upon entry to the hospital). In all, abnormal FHR patterns were observed during labor and the fetuses were delivered by cesarean section for fetal distress. At birth, they all demonstrated acidemia and severe anemia (Hgb 6–9 g%). With such blood loss, the fetuses were unable to tolerate the stresses of labor. Thus, routine intrapartum electronic monitoring of seemingly low-risk gravida (whose complaints of decrease FM were ignored) was apparently of value in these rare cases of significant fetal–maternal transfusions.

Fetal Heart Rate Pattern Interpretation

The clinical significance of various types of apparently abnormal FHR patterns encountered remains controversial despite 130 years of study. The following is my present scheme and interpretation of FHR patterns. It is assumed throughout that many FHR unclassified patterns have no pathological significance; that our present understanding of fetal physiology forces us to assume that some FHR changes are capricious. To do otherwise is to subject the *in utero* human to the dangers of overdiagnosis and overtreatment.

BASELINE CHANGES

Severe Bradycardia (100 bpm)

I collected 15 cases in which there were at least 30 min of a baseline FHR below 100

bpm. In the absence of other problems, the newborns—all delivered vaginally—did as well as those whose baseline heart rates were in the normal range. The "study" in which this information was collected was not accepted for publication, correctly (in retrospect), as such negative findings should be confirmed by many more cases.

In the last 3 years, we have refrained from responding to such bradycardias (except do scalp pH's and to give them atropine) and have yet to see an asphyxiated newborn. Nevertheless, the worldwide impression is that these severe and prolonged bradycardias are ominous fetal heart rate patterns. Our own impression could be reversed by delivery of just one asphyxiated newborn which had such abnormal heart rate patterns. I therefore try not to be too cavalier about the occurrence of such baseline FHR below 100 bpm.

Congenital heartblock is a rare cause of fetal bradycardia. Two cases that I have studied intrapartum were reported as having normal FHR until 4–5 weeks prior to term. This indicates that the possibility of a congenital lesion as the etiology of a low FHR in labor should not be rejected just because the bradycardia was missed in (or changed from) the prenatal examinations.

Moderate Bradycardia

Young and Weinstein[766b] have reported on those intrapartum fetal bradycardias in the range of 100–119 bpm. These authors considered such moderate bradycardias to represent a relative cephalopelvic disproportion (CPD). They based this conclusion on finding that neither oxygen administration nor change in maternal position improved the fetal bradycardia, but when the fetal vertex rotated, the bradycardia was relieved. The infants did well, which would suggest that such ranges of FHR are without clinical significance. That fetal bradycardia may represent CPD has not been our experience from reviewing 52 FHR tracings of labor terminated by cesarean section for CPD. We have considered such mild bradycardias as within the normal range and we have lowered the range of significant bradycardia to below 100 bpm.

Tachycardia (above 160 bpm)

Baseline FHR decreases as pregnancy advances, although I have not been impressed that the premature fetus in labor consistently has a relative tachycardia. Tachycardia on our service is most frequently associated with maternal pyrexia. Indeed, one of the benefits of routine electronic fetal monitoring in labor has been the demonstration that many parturients have a brief episode of unexplained pyrexia which is often missed when temperatures are recorded only at 4-hr intervals. The first rule in evaluating any fetal tachycardia, then, is to take the mother's temperature.

The second rule for the evaluation of fetal tachycardia is to record the mother's pulse. Sometimes the FHR seems to mirror its mother's tachycardia without any obvious explanation other than maternal anxiety (Fig. 9-14). Other times maternal drugs such as those with an epinephrine-like action may give both the fetus and the mother a tachycardia. This is especially notable after caudal anesthesia in which epinephrine is mixed with the conduction anesthetic. Figure 9-15 is from a case where the gravida was regularly using Neo-Synephrine nasal drops for a stuffy nose. Only the chance observation of the medication in her purse avoided an emergency cesarean section for "toxemia and fetal distress." Other known etiologies of tachycardia include fetal asphyxia, infection, fetal arrhythmia, and fetal LATS syndrome.

Fetal Heart Rate Accelerations

Brief periods of fetal tachycardia appear to be more common than brief periods of fetal bradycardia. As described in Chapter 8, such periods of brief tachycardia (accelerations of FHR) are frequently associated with fetal movements. (In sheep, such accelerations often occur as a pressor-tachycardia response.)

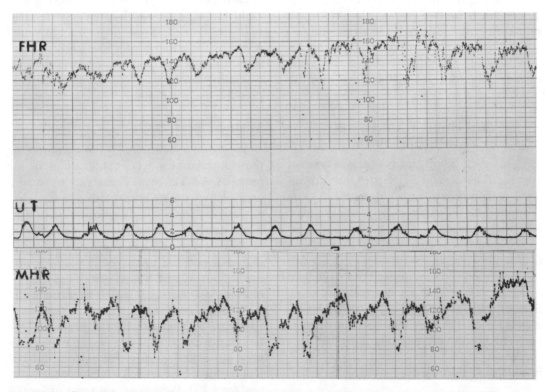

Fig. 9-14. Recording of simultaneous fetal (FHR) and maternal (MHR) heart rates during labor. (UT—uterine tension.) Both mother and fetus demonstrated several vagal-type bradycardias (although fetal was delayed) with uterine contraction. Fetal scalp pH was 7.31 and it was born in good condition.

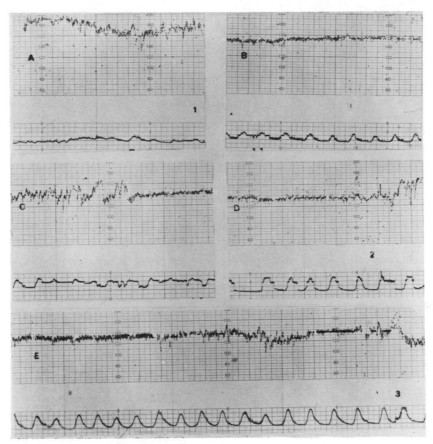

Fig. 9-15. FHR recording of gravida seen for hypertension who was self-administering a Neo-Synephrine nasal spray. A—after nasal spray; B—30 min after spray; C—again after nasal spray; and D—again 30 min later. E—2 weeks later when gravida was in spontaneous labor showing normal FHR patterns.

The more prolonged and more vigorous the fetal movements, presumably the longer sustained the fetal tachycardia and the more common a subsequent terminal bradycardia. The "post-tachycardia" deceleration (undershoot) probably reflects the baroreflex response to the initial pressor-tachycardia response (Chap. 8). Workers in Rudolph's laboratory[754] showed that in the chronic fetal sheep preparation, stimulation of the hypothalamus produced both fetal tachycardia and hypertension. The responses were blocked by an alpha adrenergic blocking agent. These same workers demonstrated that the integrity of the vagus nerve is essential for the undershoot which follows the fetal brief tachycardia.

As described in Chapter 8, the vagus carries accelerations of FHR stimulus as well as decelerations. The deceleration is the predominant response carried, but under special circumstances, atropine will block both the deceleration and acceleration of FHR carried, by the vagus nerve (Fig. 9-16). On the other hand the vast majority of FHR accelerations are abolished by alpha adrenergic blocking agents, implying a predominant sympathetic pathway for tachycardia. Schifrin[611a] has termed accelerations associated with vagal activity as "shoulder" accelerations. They must not be confused with "overshoot" (Figs. 9-17 and 9-18). I originally termed the shoulder variety of acceleration "false" overshoot[280] and believed that they represented minimal funis compression (umbilical vein compression alone). It is also

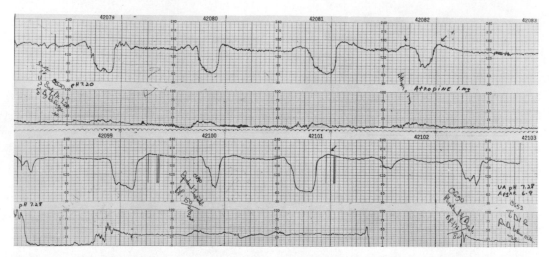

Fig. 9-16. FHR recording demonstrating "shoulder" (FHR accelerations *before* and *after* the bradycardia). After atropine (42082), the shoulders were converted to "overshoot" (42099–42101). In 42103, the atropine was "wearing off," with return of BBV and shoulders.

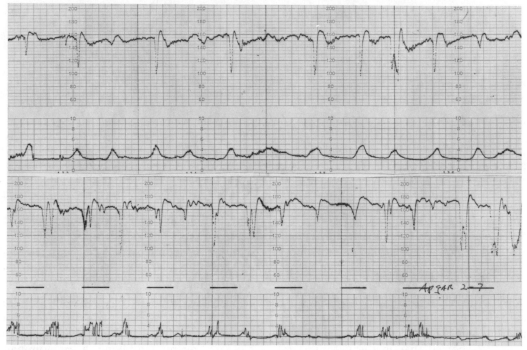

Fig. 9-17. FHR tracing demonstrating overshoot (acceleration after bradycardia). Newborn was depressed and VA pH was 7.12. (Paper speed is 1 cm/min.)

possible that "shoulder" accelerations represent the accelerator fraction of vagal stimulation for atropinization sometimes clears both the vagal deceleration and its associated shoulders.

The occurrence of FHR accelerations is considered to represent an aroused, healthy fetus. Arousal by itself indicates that the fetal health is at least not poor. These indications are particularly true in the antenatal period, but probably should be qualified during the intrapartum period. Intrapartum FHR accelerations may represent excessive fetal stress, reaction to pain, partially obstructed umbili-

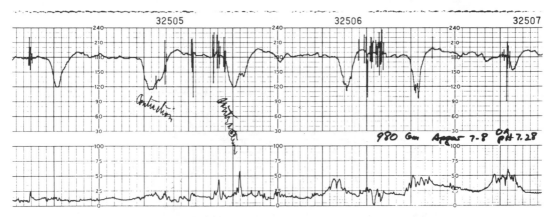

Fig. 9-18. FHR tracing of premature (980) fetus demonstrating "overshoot". Overshoot appears to be less ominous sign in the premature. (Paper speed is 3 cm/min.)

cal cord, excess vagal activity, or a highly stimulated fetus. As noted in Chapter 18, such a highly aroused and overstimulated fetus may perhaps benefit from tranquilization (or atropinization). Such a fetus' metabolic rates must be increased, its oxygen needs raised, and probably its metabolic reserves reduced.

The brief acceleration of FHR is often included in any long-term description of beat-to-beat variability (BBV). Such BBV has an entirely different connotation than has the short-term variability which includes only the changes in rate between individual heart beats (Fig. 9-19). The latter is increased with vagal tone while the former may imply increased sympathetic tone and increased arousal level.

In summary, many clinical conditions associated with highly aroused fetuses such as maternal fever, stress, and anxiety are reflected in the FHR by either brief or prolonged periods of tachycardia. Persistent fetal tachycardia can also represent a partial recovery from a prior episode of severe stress of asphyxia. Though a rare occurrence on our service, if we have no other explanation for fetal tachycardia, a scalp pH is performed.

Decelerations (Brief Bradycardia) of Heart Rate

As noted in Chapter 10, reactive FHR decelerations are proposed to have two dif-ferent etiologic mechanisms: bradycardias reflecting vagal activity, usually tolerated by the fetus, and bradycardias reflecting cardiovascular dysfunction, which can aggravate a compromised fetal situation. There are then at least two types of decelerations of FHR. Based on qualitative visual observation, vagal bradycardia is relatively abrupt in its beginning and end, although this may not be obvious if the deceleration of FHR is minimal. By contrast, bradycardias reflecting cardiac dysfunction are gradual in onset and termination. Also, the greater the area of deceleration of FHR, the more likely it is to have a vagal component.

Second, the two reacting FHR patterns are distinguished by studying the timing of their beginning and end. Vagal effects on fetal SA node are almost instantaneous. Therefore, the onset and finish of the bradycardia, and even the degree of deceleration reflect the event initiating the fetal–vagal activity (e.g., head or funis compression, hypoxia, fetal grunting). The cardiac dysfunction type of deceleration requires time after the initiating event for the "cardiac inadequacy" to become obvious. Hence, both initiation of the bradycardia (deceleration) and its recovery have a lag time in the cardiac dysfunction type. Sureau's laboratory and others have (for the sake of the computer) developed the concept of "simultaneous area" and "residual area" (Fig. 9-20).

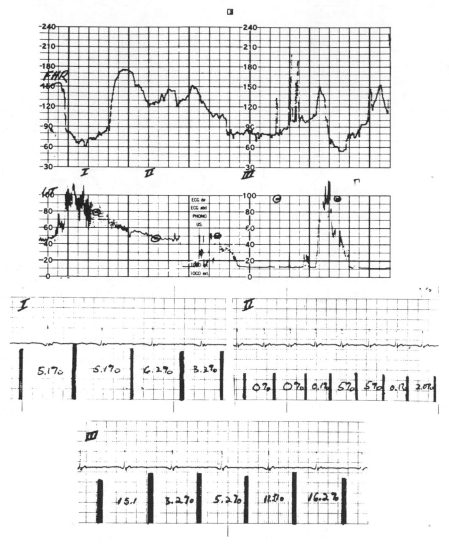

Fig. 9-19. Simultaneous FHR recording, ECG, and R − R intervals. During bradycardia (I and III), the BBV is increased as compared with increased rate II. The bars represent R − R intervals and the numbers (5.1% or 0.1%) reflect percent change in length of succeeding R − R intervals.

In summary then, when inspecting any FHR recording of a deceleration (brief bradycardia), one should attempt to relate it first to the initiating event (usually a uterine contraction) and second, to its form. Decelerations representing cardiac dysfunction recover late and are usually gradual in form. The much more common vagal-type bradycardia is a more severe deceleration. They are modified by drugs with an atropine effect (e.g., meperidine), or with central effects (general anesthesia, especially Ketamine or tranquilizers). By contrast, the cardiac dys-

functional-type bradycardia is modified by ionotropic drugs such as catecholamines or beta mimetics.

Techniques for Fetal Monitoring

My method of interpretation of FHR patterns is to first acknowledge that, in my hands at least, they are an imprecise indicator of fetal health. Whenever in doubt, I obtain a scalp pH or sometimes determine a fetal systolic time interval. If these are normal, then I feel confident that however ominous I thought the fetal heart rate pattern the fetus

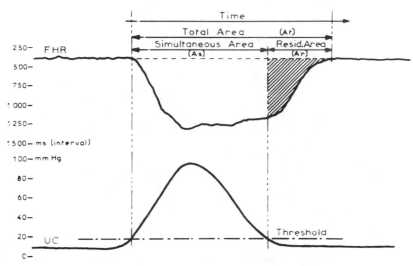

Fig. 9-20. Three different kinds of areas of FHR bradycardia as determined by Sureau's laboratory. (From Sturboid, R., *et al.*: *J Perinat Med* **1**: 235, 1973. Reproduced with permission.)

is at that moment tolerating its stress. However, as discussed in Chapter 8, any FHR bradycardia (deceleration) during labor is probably not beneficial to the fetus, and may have no logical etiology, even though it be very common. Our goal then should be to conduct labor in such a fashion that significant alteration of FHR are kept to a minimum.

My views on electronic fetal monitoring are apparently confusing. House officers often do not understand my displeasure when certain parturients are not "monitored" or when ominous FHR tracings are ignored, for I have publicly stated that I do not "believe" in electronic fetal monitoring.[291] Actually, what I have tried to state is that the low-risk gravida (Goodwin score <2) (protocol P-48) with an apparently healthy fetus (normal fetal movements) is ill-served by intrapartum electronic monitoring. All other parturients, especially the post date, the unregistered, or those judged to be high risk, *must* have electronic monitoring during labor. And we *must* respond to ominous FHR tracings. My view that the majority of ominous FHR tracings are "red herrings" is precisely why I believe that low-risk gravida should not be routinely monitored. The occurrence of such FHR patterns in the low-risk gravida sets in motion certain procedures (scalp pH, preparations

for cesarean section, etc.) which usually bring about some form of unnecessary interference. If we have selected carefully these low-risk patients, fetal monitoring, in my view, only increases the cesarean section of forcep rate and increases the incidence of newborn scalp infections without appreciably improving the health of the newborn. My iconoclastic views on fetal monitoring certainly do not apply to any parturients who are not low risk.

The California Medical Association has sought to require that all hospitals with obstetrical facilities (no matter how small) have available electronic fetal monitors. I have argued that these small hospitals mostly have low cesarean section rates (below 5%) and excellent perinatal mortality rates (below 18 per 1000) and will be forced by the presence of fetal monitors into high rates of delivery by the abdominal route. In addition, I am convinced that any hospital using electronic fetal monitoring should have some other method (i.e., scalp pH, systolic time intervals, etc.) besides cesarean section to confirm their interpretation of abnormal fetal heart rate recordings.

THE ULTIMATE IN INTRAPARTUM MONITORING

Figure 9-21 is a schematic diagram of our complete monitoring, using blood volume

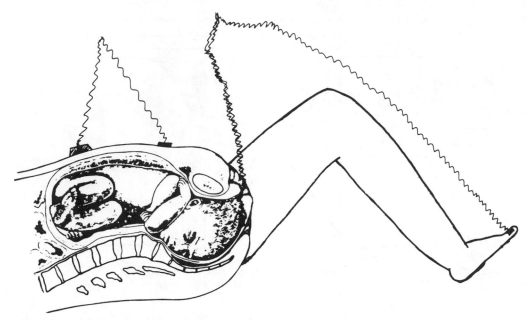

Fig. 9-21. ''Complete intrapartum monitoring'' with microphone and Doppler transducers on maternal abdomen, BVD pulse monitor on maternal big toe, uterus and fetal scalp, plus fetal scalp electrode and intrauterine catheter.

pulse, heart sounds, Doppler, ECG and intrauterine pressure recordings. Figures 9-22 and 9-23 are a result of such effort.

Definitions (As Commonly Used in the American Obstetrical Literature)

Acidemia (as used in fetal monitoring)—Fetal capillary or arterial pH below 7.20 (with normal maternal pH). Scalp pH is usually above 7.30 in early labor and declines to 7.25 in normal late labor.

Asphyxia—Acidemia plus hypoxemia.

Baseline FHR—The fetal heart rate between uterine contractions, observed in the absence of periodic FHR changes. Assessment of baseline FHR consists of the determination of the FHR level in beats per minute (bpm) and FHR variability (± beats).

Bradycardia—Abnormally slow heart rate (<120 bpm).

Fetal electronic monitoring—The continuous simultaneous acquisition and recording of data on fetal heart rate (FHR) and uterine contractions for diagnostic inspection.

Fetal heart rate (FHR) classification—

Marked tachycardia   180 or more bpm

Mild tachycardia	161–180 bpm
Normal heart rate	120–160 bpm
Mild bradycardia	100–119 bpm
Marked bradycardia	99 or less bpm

Hypoxemia—Depressed oxygen pressures in arterial blood for whatever cause, associated with diminished O_2 saturation of arterial blood.

Hypoxia—Interruption of respiratory gas exchange with depression of oxygen tension in body tissues below normal values.

Long-term FHR variability—Fluctuations described in terms of frequency (2–6 cycles/min) and amplitude of change in bpm (normally 6–10).

Periodic FHR variations—Fetal heart rate variations related to uterine contractions (UC). Response to uterine contractions may be categorized as follows:

Acceleration—Temporary FHR increase from baseline in response to uterine contractions, fetal activity or stimulus.

Deceleration—Temporary decrease in FHR in response to uterine contractions, fetal activity of stimulus. Decelerations may be divided into three categories.

1. *Uniform patterns*: Reflect the waveform

FETAL HEART RATE RESPONSE PATTERNS

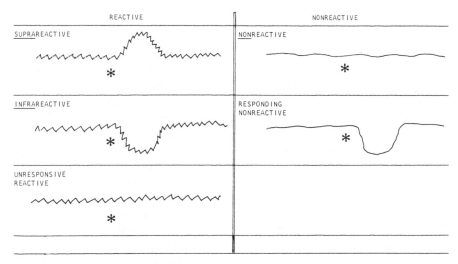

Fig. 9-22. FHR patterns according to fetal arousal level. The most ominous pattern is the responding nonreactive. Asterisks indicate a fetal stimulus, such as sound, uterine contraction, etc.

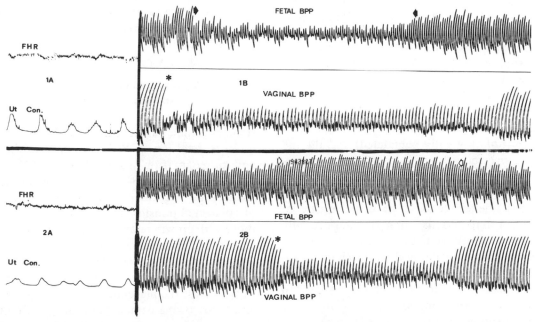

Fig. 9-23. Simultaneous FHR and fetal pulse and maternal vaginal pulse recording as obtained in Fig. 9–21. Uterine contractions between arrows.

of the uterine contraction and occur repetitively, with onset at, or beyond, the apex of the contraction.

a. *Early deceleration pattern* usually has an onset, maximal fall, and recovery coincident with the contraction wave.

b. *Late deceleration pattern* has an on-set, maximal decrease, and recovery which is delayed in time in relation to the contraction wave (due to fetal hypoxia) and is symmetrical.

2. *Variable deceleration pattern*: A non-uniform periodic change in the fetal heart rate, bearing no constant time re-

lationship to the uterine contractions. Has a variable time of onset, a variable waveform, and may be nonrepetitive. The difference from early deceleration (1a) is often only a matter of degree.

3. *Combined or mixed deceleration pattern*: May exhibit characteristics of one or more of the above patterns.

Short-term FHR variability (beat-to-beat-changes)—These changes reflect R wave (R − R) interval differences measured from successive fetal ECG's (normal 1–4%).

Tachycardia—Abnormally fast heart rate (>160).

An Alternate Concept of FHR Definitions

The preceding definitions are used throughout the American obstetrical literature and have become part of our dogma. An entirely different scheme of defining FHR patterns is based on the concept of fetal arousal levels. We believe that we have data to support the concept that the human fetus, like an adult, has varying states of arousal. At the two opposite extremes in arousal levels are the nonreactive fetus which lies motionless *in utero* and maintains a constant heart rate (unless greatly stimulated) and the *hyperactive* fetus which even when not stimulated, exhibits frequent body movements and a constantly changing heart rate. These fetal arousal levels tend to be characteristic of certain time periods, but may change rapidly and markedly, sometimes without apparent cause. Of the available clinical techniques for estimating the levels of human fetal arousal, instantaneous heart rate recordings appear to have the widest application. Presented here are examples of various fetal heart rate patterns presumably associated with different arousal levels.

For the purpose of discussion, fetal heart rate patterns are classified according to their highest level of activity. The patterns are termed *reactive* if changes in baseline heart rate of more than 8 beats per minute occur on a random basis. A reactive fetus demonstrating mostly accelerations of rate in response to stimuli is considered in the highest level of arousal and is called *suprareactive* (I), while a fetus with a reactive pattern demonstrating mostly decelerations is classified *moderately reactive* (II). If stimuli do not evoke a change of heart rate, the fetal arousal level is termed *unresponsive reactive* (III).

When the FHR baseline is constant (flat, smooth, and silent), the arousal level is classified *nonreactive* (IV), and when nonreactive but with decelerations after stimuli, *responding nonreactive* (V). Figure 9-22 is a schematic diagram of our classification of FHR patterns indicative of fetal arousal levels. With ultrasound pickup, it is not possible to determine degrees of FHR reactivity but only gross changes in FHR such as accelerations or decelerations.

De Haan *et al.*[149] have shown in the human newborn different patterns of BBV associated with active sleep and quiet sleep. They speculate that these same BBV changes may be seen in the FHR patterns of the *in utero* human fetus.

PLACENTAL TRANSFER INDEX

As has been suggested by Hellman *et al.*[333] and Hon,[354] BBV should provide a tool to measure placental transfer of drugs and fetal state. Atropine transfer time, (from maternal effect to fetal loss of BBV and tachycardia) and diazepam (from maternal loss of BBV to time of fetal loss of BBV) are the commonly used drugs. We found no consistent pattern of "placental transfer" in toxemia gravida or those with growth retarded fetuses. While the smaller placentas tended to have the shortest "transfer times," there were several exceptions. We tested drugs which normally are slow to cross the placental, atropine bromide and hydroxyzine pamoate (Vistaril), without evidence of abnormal transfer. One drug which appears to affect fetal BBV in abnormal pregnancies (and not normal) is Alphaprodine (Nisentil). Studies should continue for a drug which will distinguish the abnormal placenta.

Other Points of View

It probably is illogical to attack the concept of intrapartum electronic fetal monitoring as I have, for the technique has brought American obstetrics a certain degree of scientific respectability and stimulus to undertake serious laboratory and clinical investigation. While Urbach et al.,[711] Sontag,[649] and others had suggested the significance of beat-to-beat variability, it has really been obstetricians who have contributed the most in this area. However, so much of the research in obstetrics has been dominated by FHR tracings with often unfounded implications to pathophysiology, that our efforts have often been circular, instead of forward. Nevertheless, the new subspecialty of Maternal–Fetal Medicine is largely based on the "science" of intrapartum electromic fetal monitoring and fetal intensive care.

In an international symposium (San Diego, 1976) on intrauterine asphyxia, its organizer, Louis Gluck declared that "the FHR is our most sensitive clinical tool to detect and follow intrauterine asphyxia." He correctly credits Hon and Caldeyro-Garcia with the development of the techniques to quantify FHR patterns. As one who has attempted to read all of Professor Hon and his associates' hundreds of papers, I have learned a great deal about fetal physiology from their pages. The associated group, which has been assembled at the University of Southern California, has been one of the most distinguished and productive in American obstetrics. The group has produced much of our current obstetrical dogma. It may even be accurate that this dedicated staff is indeed responsible for the remarkable decrease in perinatal mortality rates which has occurred at the huge Los Angeles County Hospital.

Others besides Hon, such as LaCroix (Patent No. 3,580,242) and Ruttgers (Patent No. 3,750,650) have patented their fetal scalp electrodes for use in fetal monitoring. That this is accepted practice for physicians is shown by Stanford University, which is proud of how many of its faculty have secured patents on medical devices.[184a]

To argue that electronic fetal monitoring was uncritically accepted by American obstetricians is to ignore the fact that most of our current practices (prenatal care, the "Pap" smear, outlet forceps, value of routine exams, vitamins, and so forth) have been similarly accepted without controlled studies. There is probably no reason to expect our specialty to suddenly become a science rather than an art.

The present state of our confusion over the value of fetal monitoring is perhaps best illustrated by the editorial comments in the journal,

Obstetrics and Gynecology Survey. Despite the fact that a controlled study in the editor's own institution has suggested that fetal electronic monitoring does not improve the perinatal rate, but only increases the cesarean section rate, the journal's editorial comments continue to wonder if monitoring would not have improved the unfavorable outcome of cases which are reviewed. Dr. David Rubsamen, as editor of the *Professional Liability Newsletter*[688] has declared that the courts may dictate the use of the FHR monitor and arguments such as mine may all be in vain. And finally, it is always possible that the vast majority of academic obstetrics will be proven correct and that I will be shown to be wrong about the value of routine intrapartum electronic fetal monitoring.

In the meantime, beat-to-beat variability is of course a useful index when evaluating FHR records. Numerous papers have appeared attesting to its value. As Paul and associates of Hon's group have shown, late decelerations plus loss of BBV is probably the most ominous of all FHR recordings. But out of approximately 8000 FHR recordings, I have seen such a dreadful combination of FHR patterns on five occasions. Only twice, however, was the fetus acidotic. Sureau, who has contributed so much to our understanding of FHR interpretation, has decided recently that BBV was of little importance for the interpreting of the intrapartum FHR record. (He continues to believe that BBV is a useful parameter in the antenatal FHR record.) Sureau has gone so far as to suggest the much less costly averaging type of FHR monitor may be sufficient for labor.

Whereas, as I have noted, most institutions have found an increase in cesarean section rates with the introduction of fetal monitoring, Hughey and associates[361] found this not to be true at Northwestern University. As with most series, fetal distress is one of the less frequent indications for cesarean section. They believe that the increases in cesarean section rate (from 2.6% to 6.9% over a 6-year period) in their institution and others, reflects the changes which have occurred in obstetric philosophy. The present policy for "breech presentation," the "premature," and the "failure to progress" account for most of the increase in cesarean section rate. As with almost all other such series, theirs was not a controlled one.

In leaving the subject of intrapartum fetal monitoring, it should be noted the confusion over terminology exists. "Fetal intensive care" means more to me than electronic fetal monitoring. Such care includes an experienced staff at the bed side with avoidance of iatrogenic problems and close observations for the fetus' welfare, in addition to that provided by the fetal monitor. Renou published an abstract[567] stating that in a controlled study, electronic fetal monitoring was not of benefit to high-risk fetuses. The same group then later published an extended paper which showed that "fetal intensive care" was of benefit to the high-risk patient.[567a] Although the authors state that "it is possible that this improvement results from the use of fetal diagnostic tests of some other factor associated with intensive care," this paper has been used by the advocates of electronic fetal monitoring[559] as evidence of its value. A subsequent publication from that same group by Wood seems to support this view, stating that "statistical methods have shown that fetal monitoring more than any clinical factor, determine the biochemical acid base and gaseous status of the fetus at birth." In a personal communication (1978), Professor Wood suggests that with "good" labor room nursing staffs it may be impossible to prove that electronic fetal monitoring is of benefit even in high-risk pregnancies. (As my colleagues in statistics once told me, when I was looking for a "test" that would show my data to be significant, "the hardest hypotheses to prove are those which are not true.")

It should be noted that my concept of FHR response as determined by the fetal "state" has not been confirmed by others. Schulman, for instance, after studying human newborn heart rate response to auditory stimuli, concluded that there was no effect of "state" on the FHR responses. She did note a significant percentage of FHR decelerations (as we did in the fetus) to sound stimuli. She ascribes these deceleration responses (rather than acceleration) to a relative lack of cardiac sympathetic innervation in the newborn. Schulman also reported that lack of temporal cortex produced only acceleration FHR responses to sound stimuli. It seems apparent (as we have noted) that a functioning temporal cortex is not required for a fetal auditory FHR response and that a functioning cortex is necessary for the usual FHR brief bradycardia (Chapter 8). At the same time, the reports of Cruikshank[131] and ours (Chapter 12), that cerebral dysfunction (squashed brains) are associated with typical FHR patterns suggests a

definite neurophysiologic relationship between cerebral function and FHR patterns.

If it is possible, Sadovsky and Weinstein[601] view fetal movements recording of even more importance than do I. They ask all of their patients to keep written records of fetal movements during the last trimester of pregnancy. These investigators suggest that abnormal fetal movements are such a precise indicator of fetal health that in the third trimester they sometimes reflect the ill-defined entity of gradual funis compression. Furthermore, when fetal movements become rapid and then markedly reduced, these investigators believe that the fetus may be severely threatened.

Other studies suggest (contrary to my findings) that it is impossible to predict antenatally which intrapartum fetus may suffer asphyxia, and that a low-risk pregnancy may turn into a high-risk pregnancy during labor and thus all parturients should be monitored.[345] If this is true, it apparently is a phenomenon of the "scientific" hospital labor ward, for the midwife or home services do better than the hospitals,[694] with low-risk pregnancies.

Hajeri and Papiernik have described the FHR patterns associated with meconium aspiration.[312a] These changes are characterized by transitory decelerations followed by supervening persistent tachycardia, or an increase in the amplitude of rapid oscillations of the baseline. I have reviewed our records of meconium aspiration and find that about one-half fit this description. However, such events are probably more accurately reflective of fetal grunting and the resulting hypoxia.

Cibils[107] proposed that the premature's FHR response is different than that of the mature fetus'. Repeatedly the FHR changes considered ominous have been shown to have more significance in the premature than the term infant. This finding can be interpreted many ways, however, one being that the premature is less tolerant of stress. Another is that the premature's CVR responses are different than the mature. To me, this seems more likely, for in the laboratory the more immature and smaller the mammalian fetus, the more resistant it is to asphyxia.[248]

Oldenburg and Machlin[515] have reviewed the problem of obtaining satisfactory abdominal fetal ECG (FECG). They concluded that different abdominal electrode placements are required for different periods of gestation.

CHAPTER 10

Reacting Fetal Bradycardia

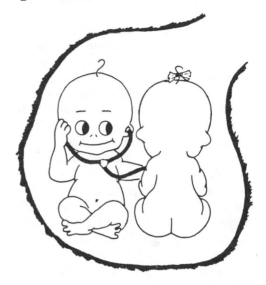

Historical

The first descriptions of human fetal bradycardias were those in which the FHR was responding to a specific stimulus, such as funis or head compression. Evory Kennedy noted in his 1833 monograph[401] that fetal head or funis compression caused fetal bradycardia without providing any specific details. (He also claimed that fetal "thorax compression" caused a "bradycardia.") Schatz (1885) provided more detailed description of umbilical cord compression as did Frey (1925), Hamilton (1947), and Biskind (1958). These studies were all done without the benefit of recorders and reflected only manual FHR determinations. In 1870, Schwartz described fetal bradycardia with compression of the fetal head against the sacrum. Fischer (1976) notes that Kehrer (1867) likewise described head compression FHR patterns. Barcroft's work[38] with fetal sheep umbilical cord compression that demonstrated a functioning baroreflex and vagal transmission had a tremendous impact on our understanding of these bradycardias.

In 1961, Bradfield described human vagal bradycardias occurring from both head and funis compression. Bradfield suggested that excess vagal activity could be one mechanism of unexplained fetal death, as he noted fetal cardiac arrest with fetal head compression (external abdominal pressure).[64a] However, it was the publication of *An Atlas of FHR Patterns* by Hon[354] that categorized such reacting fetal bradycardias into head compression (early decelerations) or funis compression (variable decelerations), which had a major impact on our understanding of reacting bradycardia.

Fetal Reacting Bradycardia

THE PROBLEM

There are many etiologies of acute bradycardia. Even the deinnerated heart responds to the various degrees of asphyxia. I consider *acute reacting* fetal bradycardias to be evoked by two different mechanisms (Chapter 8). The most common mechanism of these bradycardias is usually innocuous and vagal in origin, while the rare mechanism reflects cardiovascular dysfunction and is worrisome (Fig. 8–17). The subject of this chapter is the vagal fetal bradycardias which are characterized by abrupt beginnings and endings and are abolished by atropinization. According to current concepts, vagal bradycardias have only two different etiologies—fetal head compression or funis compression. The latter initially produces a vagal type of bradycardia which may change to the cardiovascular dysfunctional type if the funis compression is not relieved. In the laboratory, it is possible to demonstrate that many acute fetal responses can lead to vagal activity such as fetal seizures, fetal grunting, or any condition (e.g., hypoxia) giving rise to abrupt rises in fetal vascular resistance and the baroreflex (Chapter 8).

I have reviewed for this chapter selected types of fetal heart rate responses from approximately 3000 deliveries, with supplemental information obtained by fetal scalp pH, systolic time intervals, and maternal blood volume pulse recordings. I have also included two recordings of a chronic fetal sheep preparation from Rudolph's laboratory, as they seem to imply important mechanisms for intrapartum fetal bradycardia. These data to be presented suggest that fetal vagal bradycardias often have multiple and complex etiologies, that the simplistic view of considering them to be either the result of either funis or head compression is incomplete. I conclude by suggesting that an alternate interpretation of such FHR patterns, originally recommended by an international committee, be used, and again recommend the prophylactic use of atropine. In other words, I am taking up the battle against the simplistic "FHR interpretation equals fetal health status" concept, one more time. I am interested in determining in this chapter the etiologies of many of the fetal bradycardias which do not seem to fit any specific pattern. Such fetal bradycardias occur frequently, particularly in the high-risk fetus. Then too, the fetal bradycardia of terminal labor is likewise of interest as it appears to have no clear-cut etiology.

On our service, FHR recordings are obtained with a variety of commercial fetal heart rate monitors, including Corometrics, Hewlett-Packard, and Berkeley, as well as the Beckman Research Unit and the Berkeley RSR (systolic time) recorder. (In my opinion, one should not become attached to any one recorder with its particular shortcomings and

recorder scale.) Systolic time intervals were determined with simultaneous recordings of fetal ECG, Doppler, or microphone heart sounds, and Doppler placental pulse (Chapter 11). The maternal pulse (photoelectric plethysmographic pulse or blood volume pulse) was obtained with a Beckman pulse monitor (Chapter 11). Unless otherwise noted, the parturients labored in the lateral recumbent position and were delivered in the dorsal lithotomy position.

For study of the newborn's expulsion bradycardia, immediate newborns' heart rates were recorded after vaginal delivery using a combination of scalp electrodes and a second needle electrode applied either to a newborn extremity or its funis. During nonelective cesarean section deliveries, a scalp electrode was used until the fetal head was disengaged from the pelvis. A Doppler transducer was then applied to the newborn's chest as soon as possible. Initially, the funis was clamped in a random fashion before or after the newborn's first breath, but so many newborns made early breathing efforts that a randomized study could not be completed. The effects of cold and warm delivery environments were studied by recording the newborn's heart rate when delivered into an environment of 40–41°C (supplied by an infrared heater), or when the delivery room temperature fell below 18°C.

The chronic fetal sheep preparation was as previously described by Rudolph and associates and the work was done in his laboratory. In addition to catheters in the amniotic space, fetal aorta, and umbilical vein, and a Clark electromagnetic flow transducer around the common umbilical artery, a catheter was also "wedged" in an umbilical vein towards the cotyledon and in a maternal vein towards the endometrium.

HUMAN INTRAPARTUM FETAL BRADYCARDIAS OF UNCERTAIN ETIOLOGIES

We observed fetal bradycardia in many situations, related apparently to many different causes. Some of these are described below. Unless otherwise noted, all of the newborns described had cord artery pH values above 7.20.

MATERNAL SEIZURE BRADYCARDIA

The fetal bradycardia began simultaneously with the start of the maternal convulsion of eclampsia or drug toxicity, and often continues into the maternal post-ictal state (Fig. 10-1). Such fetal bradycardias are at least partially relieved by atropine. In newborns delivered within 15 min after the end of the maternal drug seizure, the umbilical artery pH has been above 7.25 and none of the anesthetic toxic agents have been found in the umbilical blood.

Fetal bradycardia associated with maternal seizures (either those related to epidural drugs or to eclampsia) begin with the onset of the maternal convulsion, but often last much longer than does the fit. These bradycardias are found in the absence of (1) anesthetic drugs in the fetal blood, (2) a latent period after the maternal seizure, or (3) fetal acidemia. It therefore must be the rise in intrauterine pressure associated with the maternal fit which evokes the fetal bradycardia. Why the bradycardia has such a delayed recovery is unknown. A similar fetal bradycardia pattern sometimes occurs with maternal vomiting, but in our experience, it is not associated with such a prolonged delayed recovery as that which occurs which maternal seizures.

MATERNAL VOIDING BRADYCARDIA

Parturients whose FHR recordings demonstrated profound fetal bradycardias during maternal voiding (Fig. 10-2) were studied for possible correlating factors. Measurements of intravesicle pressure did not correlate with the FHR changes, nor did the fetuses demonstrate acidemia. In many cases, the parturients had just been turned to the supine position; in some there was an increase in uterine tension (as recorded with the external tocograph) and in others, a decrease in uterine tension. With repeated voidings, only 62% demonstrated a similar episode of fetal bradycardia. Membranes had usually been ruptured and in most cases the vertex was engaged. In other words, voiding fetal bradycardia could not be absolutely correlated with either rupture of membranes, station of the fetal head, rise in intrauterine tension, or intravesicle pressure, nor was it always reproducible.

The voiding bradycardia or "bed pan" bradycardia is impossible to explain. It occurs repeatedly with some fetuses and not at all with others and is not necessarily associated with fetal acidemia. It seemingly occurs with or without a rising intrauterine pressure and with or without the Poseiro effect. Similar "bed pan" effects have been described by Hendricks to occur on the patterns of uterine contractions.

INDEPENDENT FETAL BRADYCARDIA

Fetal vagal bradycardia, independent of uterine contraction, is assumed to frequently reflect "grunting" and the fetal valsalva maneuver, Fig. 10-3, which presumably includes the passage of meconium.[258,275] I diagnose

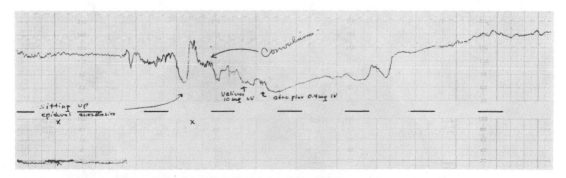

Fig. 10-1. FHR recording demonstrating fetal bradycardia occurring during a maternal seizure secondary to an intravascular injection of bupivacaine for an epidural anesthetic.

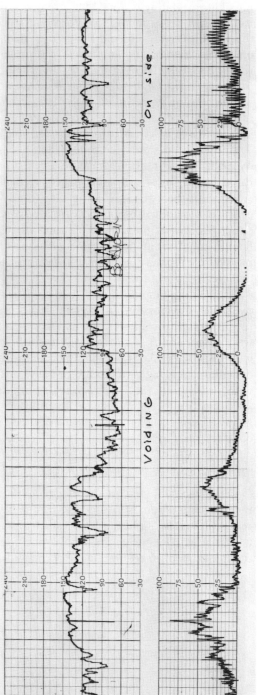

Fig. 10-2. FHR recording showing bradycardia during maternal voiding.

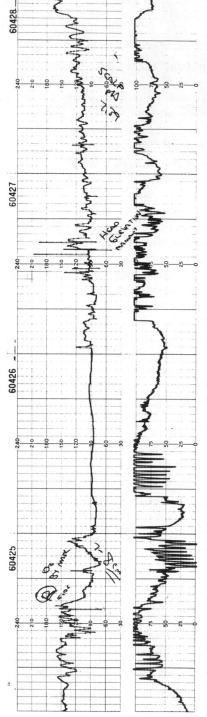

Fig. 10-3. FHR recording demonstrating independent or "grunting" type of fetal bradycardia. The bradycardia apparently began with a "vigorous" vaginal examination and was associated with passage of meconium.

"grunting" fetal bradycardia when the decrease of heart rate is severe (rule of 60, 60 & 60, Chap. 9) and the amniotic fluid appears to become secondarily stained by meconium. This type of fetal bradycardia is also relieved by atropine, and in two of the four cases monitored with scalp pH, there were values below 7.15. The subsequently delivered newborns appeared to have marked vagal activity with frequent bradycardia.

Independent fetal vagal activity (grunting) may also be the source of unexplained increases in fetal-peripheral resistance, hypertension, and bradycardia. I believe its occurrence is well documented in fetal sheep[275] but have been unable to do the same in human fetuses. Certainly in a human newborn, grunting as part of the valsalva maneuver has an associated profound bradycardia.[27] We suggest that these cases described in this report of fetal bradycardia followed by fresh meconium staining represents similar fetal grunting *in utero*. Such fetal grunting may be deleterious because of the associated decreased cardiac output (Chapter 8). Excessive vagal activity is apparently characteristic of

some individuals and is expressed in the newborn and fetus by "valsalving" and profound bradycardia. It may even be related to "cot" deaths in the older infant.

FETAL SUCKING

In face presentation, when the fetus sucks the examining finger, a severe vagal-type bradycardia occurs.

POSEIRO EFFECT BRADYCARDIA

Intrapartum fetal bradycardia associated with aortal–caval compression (Poseiro effect) during uterine contractions in supine parturients (Fig. 10-4) is common during epidural anesthesia, and is characterized by loss of the maternal toe pulse which is relieved by turning the parturient on her side (Chapter 7). Maternal toe pulses were recorded with a standard pulse monitor oscilloscope in more than 300 parturients and the Poseiro effect was presumed to have occurred when the height of the toe pulse is reduced by one-third during the uterine contraction. In supine parturients, the Poseiro effect was present in

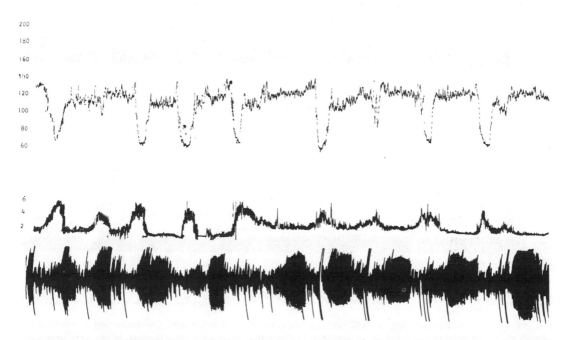

Fig. 10-4. Combined FHR recording and pulse monitoring of maternal big toe showing the Poseiro effect. With loss of maternal toe pulse (aortal compression), there was an associated vagal-type fetal bradycardia.

32% of all cases having effective epidural anesthesia, but in only 21% of women in labor without such anesthesia. Consistent abrupt and brief fetal bradycardia occurred in 56% of all parturients showing the Poseiro effect. The remainder frequently had inconsistent contraction-related bradycardia. Turning the parturient to the lateral position (the rule on our service) relieved 86% of the loss of toe pulse with uterine contractions. Ninety-one percent of the abrupt fetal bradycardias were similarly relieved by turning the parturient to the lateral position.

It is the Poseiro effect (aortal compression during uterine contraction) which appears to be common and is perhaps the most baffling to understand. These bradycardias are correlated directly with uterine contractions which implies a pressure relationship, but instead the effect, as judged by the "measurement" of maternal aortic flow, is apparently one of reduced uterine blood flow. Further confusion occurs since uterine contractions are uniformly associated with reduced uterine blood flow[80] and yet most uterine contractions are not associated with fetal bradycardia. Both Rudolph's group, using a chronic fetal sheep preparation,[47] and Kunzel et al.,[417] using an acute preparation, have noted a fetal vagal-type bradycardia following reduction of uterine blood flow (achieved by occlusion of the maternal vena cava). However, both described a significant latent interval between the decline of uterine blood flow and the occurrence of fetal bradycardia, which both investigators attributed to time required for development of fetal hypoxia. Walker and associates[722] likewise found a significant lag time for lower maternal oxygen tension to be expressed in the human fetus.

In one parturient whose fetus demonstrated severe acute vagal-type bradycardia and she demonstrated the Poseiro effect, with complete atropinization (2 mg) both phenomena abated (Fig. 10-5). With loss of the atropinization, both the fetal vagal-type brady-

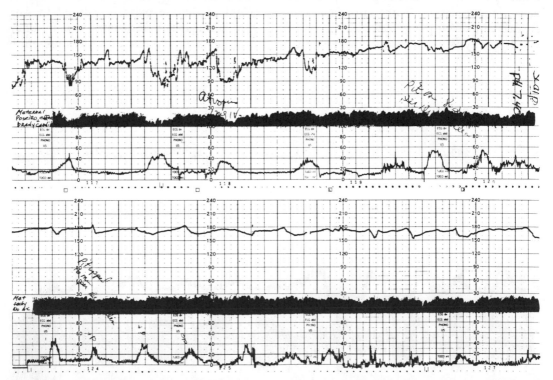

Fig. 10-5. Combined recording of FHR rate and maternal toe pulse (sketched in according to oscillograph recording). After atropine, both the vagal type fetal bradycardia and the maternal Poseiro effect were abolished. When the atropine effect on FHR disappeared, the Poseiro effect and fetal bradycardia returned.

cardia and the Poseiro effect recurred. While the effects of atropine on the fetal bradycardia are certainly understandable, the relationship with aortal compression is not. They may be unrelated, with maternal cardiac output increased by atropine to the point where aortic compression is overcome. On the other hand, the apparent association between the Poseiro effect (fetal bradycardia) and rupture of the membranes, occiput-posterior positions, intensity of uterine contractions, maternal hypotension, and epidural anesthesia suggests that there may be a common denominator for all vagal fetal bradycardias which could be reduced uterine blood flow.

Brotanek et al.[80] in an extensive review of initiation of labor observe that (1) oxytocin reduces the UBF independently from its effect on uterine activity, (2) that amniotomy causes the UBF to decrease, and (3) that contractions are preceded by a decrease in UBF. As noted by Vasicka,[712] there is a delay between the decrease in uterine blood flow and the onset of fetal bradycardia (Fig. 10-6).

Before the sluice theory was disproven,[46] it offered concepts relative to rise in uterine pressure which could explain the immediate onset of fetal bradycardia with the beginning of the contraction, by uterine vein pressure affecting the umbilical vein pressure. Until more data become available, it appears prudent to observe that through unknown mechanisms, an acute decrease in uterine blood flow is able to evoke an equally acute fetal bradycardia.

TERMINAL AND EXPULSIVE BRADYCARDIA

All fetuses demonstrate a pronounced "terminal" bradycardia (Figs. 10-7 and 10-8) of varying duration at the time of vaginal delivery and expulsion. This low heart rate continues post-delivery (expulsion bradycardia) until the newborn ventilates, after which time the newborn's heart rate usually rises abruptly to 160 bpm or higher (Fig. 10-9). When fetal membranes remained intact until the time of delivery, there sometimes is no bradycardia until the time of membrane rupture, but in other cases, fetal bradycardia occurs prior to their rupture. However, with relatively sparse forewaters, bradycardias occur like those of deliveries with early rupture of membranes. Immediate newborns with prior intact membranes until the last possible moment still have expulsion bradycardia until they have ventilated.

In vaginally delivered immediate newborns

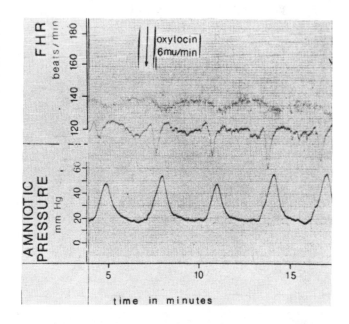

Fig. 10-6. Combined recording of maternal uterine blood flow and FHR recording. The fetal bradycardia and the decreased uterine blood flow are correlated with the uterine contraction. (From Vasicka, A.: *Am J Obstet Gynecol* **88:** 530, 1964. Reproduced with permission.)

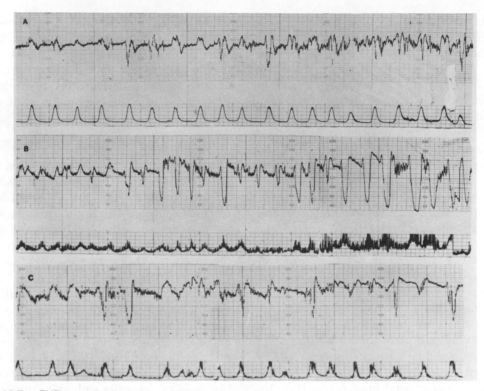

Fig. 10-7. FHR recordings of three different fetuses demonstrating varying degrees of vagal bradycardia occurring during the second stage of labor. All newborns were in good condition. Note "shoulders" in middle tracing.

whose mothers have not received either a general anesthetic or an "atropine-like drug," their heart rates were either below 110 bpm or over 140 bpm. This latter group has ventilated. Eight newborns that failed to have heart rates above 140 bpm at 2 min of age were uniformly depressed, apneic, and required resuscitation. The immediate newborn's heart rate is, then, a very reliable indicator of its condition (Fig. 10-10).

In newborns delivered by nonelective cesarean section, the same "expulsive" heart rate pattern with rates below 110 bpm occurred prior to ventilation in 16 cases. Only with special care of head and funis handling has it been possible to deliver the newborn under gentle conditions and, under these circumstances, no bradycardia occurred.

Terminal fetal bradycardias are more severe in primigravidas or in multigravidas having a "tighter" perineum in relationship to the newborn's head size, and in the pre-mature with a mobile skull. Such bradycardias lasting longer than 20 min are associated with a decreased umbilical arterial pH. Atropine (0.4 mg) administered to the mother 10–20 min prior to delivery was only completely successful in 37% of the cases in relieving this type of bradycardia. General anesthesia (especially ketamine) at times markedly alters the expulsive fetal bradycardia and instead the newborn manifests a tachycardia.

"Terminal" fetal bradycardias also occur when the cervix is incompletely dilated, if the mother is bearing down, or if uterine contractions are particularly severe. The bradycardia is sometimes reduced when the mother is rolled on her side or is delivered in the lateral Sim's position, but the FHR does not necessarily return to baseline when the maternal toe pulse returns to its precontraction level. Many times the maternal toe pulse diminishes when the vertex is deeply engaged without

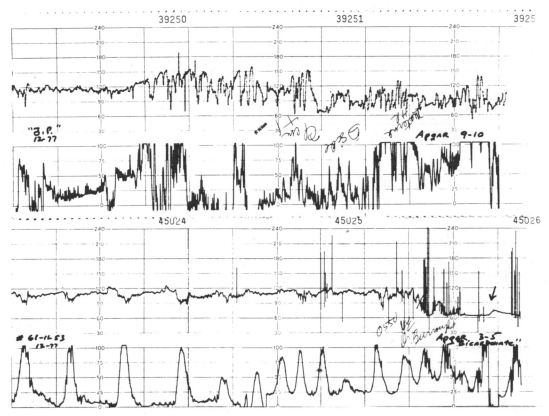

Fig. 10-8. Two FHR recordings of terminal labor bradycardia. Although the degrees of terminal bradycardia are essentially equal, the lower recording is ominous (loss BBV) at arrow and the newborn required active resuscitation. In neither case was the bradycardia explained.

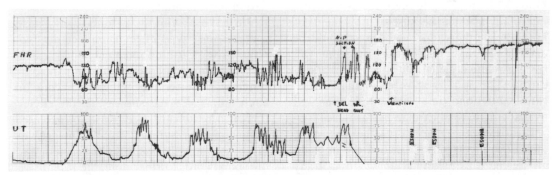

Fig. 10-9. Terminal labor fetal bradycardia demonstrating partial relief of the bradycardia with nasal pharyngeal suction. With esophageal suction, the bradycardia temporarily reoccurred.

apparent effect upon the FHR. Thus, the terminal FHR pattern then seems to represent a variety of mechanisms, including fetal head compression, the Poseiro effect, and possibly funis compression.

Nothing short of ventilation relieves the immediate newborn's bradycardia. When the immediate newborn was warmed with an infrared heater, exposed to a cold environment, exposed to a stream of O_2, when varying lengths of time were taken to clamp the umbilical cord, or when delivered in a

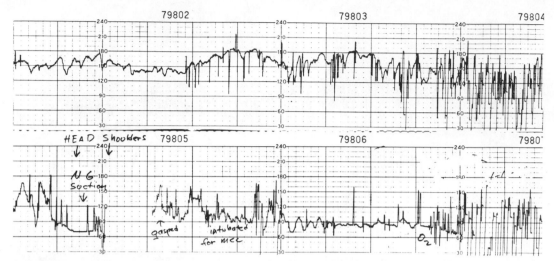

Fig. 10-10. FHR recording showing prolonged (8 min) expulsive bradycardia associated with attempts at tracheal lavage (performed for meconium staining of amniotic fluid). Newborn required intensive care for 2 days for "unknown" reasons.

darkened room, all had no appreciable effect on its bradycardia. In some cases, however, gentle suction of the nasopharynx prior to delivery of the infant's shoulders gave a brief episode of the FHR returning to baseline. (The analogy to the diving reflex with the involvement of the nasopharynx reflexes is obvious.)

The fetal systolic time intervals were determined during the terminal and the expulsive bradycardia and while these recordings contain many artifacts because of movements of both the mother and newborn, it could be determined that the ejection time intervals remain relatively constant during the bradycardia. This is suggestive of increased fetal cardiac afterload (fetal hypertension) as well as inadequate fetal cardiac performance,

Bustos et al.,[83] like many other investigators, have incorrectly described the immediate newborn as having a tachycardia. Brady and James[66] noted the newborn bradycardia, but ascribed it to clamping of the umbilical cord. Just as we have observed, Zilianti and colleagues[768] reported that the immediate newborn's bradycardia was relieved by the newborn's first respiratory movement. These South American observers ascribed the expulsion bradycardia to the reduction in placental vascular bed and subsequent increase

in umbilical vascular resistance and hypertension. Our systolic time interval measurements likewise suggest fetal hypertension at this time. But like ourselves, Zilianti and coworkers found that cord clamping made no difference in the bradycardia, which it should aggravate if hypertension were the etiology. In addition, we found no less expulsive bradycardias in fetuses whose mothers had an atonic uterus, and therefore have no explanation for this bradycardia.

We have previously assumed that "head compression" type of fetal bradycardia represents the "Cushing phenomenon," i.e., increased intracranial pressure accompanied by systemic hypertension. However, work in adult animals[184a] has shown that the elicitation of a bradycardia response to increased intracranial pressure requires the integrity of the connections between the brain stem and the spinal cord. Furthermore, the response is not completely blocked by atropine or by beta adrenergic agents, but it is abolished by alpha adrenergic agents. Unlike clinical "head compression" bradycardia, the vagal reflex is not a critical factor in the bradycardia of the Cushing phenomenon. The mechanism of head compression bradycardia is further confused for in chronic fetal sheep preparations, fetal head compression can elicit a severe acute bradycardia *without* a preceding fetal hypertension or the baroreflex. Such fetal bradycardias are prevented and abolished by atropine. In intrapartum hydrocephalic human fetuses, Mocsary and Gaal[476] showed that head compression bradycardia is evoked only after a threshold intracranial pressure of 55 torr is achieved (Fig. 10-11). Such pressures are reached well after the start of the uterine contraction and abates before the end of the contraction (Fig. 10-9). The deceleration is then unlike the usual clinical "head compression pattern" FHR which often starts and ends with the increase in amniotic fluid pressure (contraction).

Human fetal systolic time interval determinations during terminal bradycardia usually demonstrate unchanging ejection times, an observation which strongly suggests an associated fetal hypertension. Since head compression is considered an important component of terminal bradycardias, it may be that there are at least two types of "head compression bradycardia," one with and one without fetal hypertension.

NUCHAL CORD BRADYCARDIA

In 62% of the cases, the prior FHR recordings of newborns with nuchal cords at the time of delivery show abrupt and moderately severe (variable) bradycardias on more than four occasions. Twenty-four percent showed an initial FHR acceleration with uterine contractions in early labor which changes to decelerations in late labor. A similar fetal bradycardia occurred before terminal labor in only 38% of fetuses without a nuchal cord. The duration of terminal and expulsive bradycardias are seemingly unrelated to the presence or absence of nuchal cord.

As Sureau has noted,[673] there is often a lack of correlation with the occurrence of Hon's definition of an umbilical cord compression FHR pattern and actual funis compression. Unfortunately, we have not clarified the problem. Even when the placental Doppler pulse diminished during the uterine contraction, we did not at the time of delivery consistently find the funis in a position of possible compression. Such false positive "placental pulse" tests may indicate that umbilical flow is diminished in all types of vagal bradycardia and may occur more often than is suggested by Figure 10-1.

Our own analysis suggests that in fetuses with a typical severe funis-type FHR deceleration, in only approximately 65% of the cases is the cord found in a position of possible compression. As discussed below, this false positive rate of 35% for funis compression pattern is markedly increased if the parturient is supine and has an epidural anesthesia (the Poseiro effect). On the other hand, only about 60% of the fetuses with nuchal cords have even occasional "cord-like" bradycardias.

It appears easy to understand the mechanisms of the vagal-type bradycardia with acute and complete funis compression. There

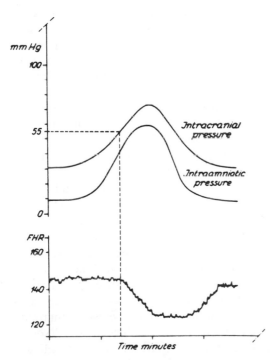

Fig. 10-11. Relationship between fetal intracranial pressure, intra-amniotic pressure, and FHR during uterine contraction. (From Mocsary, P., *et al.*: Relationship between fetal intracranial pressure and fetal heart rate during labor. *Am J Obstet Gynecol* **106**: 407–411, 1970. Reproduced with permission.)

presumably occurs a marked increase in peripheral vascular resistance, since 40% of the fetal cardiac output has been obstructed, followed by an equally abrupt and severe hypertension, which in turn initiates the baroreflex. However, the clinical FHR patterns of umbilical cord compression include many other responses such as accelerations, intermittent recovery, and marked increases in beat-to-beat variability. Based on studies in both exteriorized sheep fetuses and in human with prolapse of the umbilical cord, we[277] have previously suggested that the early acceleration of FHR reflects partial umbilical vein compression. As discussed in Chapter 8, the vagus also carries accelerator fibers and thus it is possible to explain most funis FHR responses as vagally mediated. This is especially so, since atropine abolishes most funis FHR responses, except those related to decreased cardiac performance.

The increase in beat-to-beat variability during funis compression probably reflects the excessive vagal activity and fetal catecholamine levels (Chapter 8).

Despite the American literature, internationally there is no uniformity of opinion over what constitutes a funis compression FHR pattern. Tipton and Chang[700] noted that in depressed newborns born with tight nuchal cords, the prior FHR deceleration patterns were of all types ("early, late and also variable"). Only the area of FHR deceleration correlated with the newborn's condition in Tipton and Chang's experience and not the relationship of the fetal bradycardia to uterine contraction. By contrast, O'Gureck and colleagues[514] found that when the incidence of variable decelerations was greater than 50% with contractions, all of the fetuses had either a short or nuchal cord.

FETAL SHEEP STUDIES

Figure 8-11 is of a chronic sheep preparation of 130 days gestation and 2 days postoperative, from Rudolph's laboratory. Catheters have been placed in the amniotic fluid and fetal aorta (Fem Art) and "wedged" in maternal uterine vein toward the myometrium (Ut vein) and umbilical vein toward uterus (Um vein wedge). The umbilical flow was determined from a Clark electromagnetic flow transducer with pulsatile flow (Um Q) and mean umbilical flow (Um Q̄) recorded. FHR is beats/minute, pressure in torr, and flow in ml/min. A spontaneous rise in maternal uterine vein wedge pressure occurs, which is assumed to represent a localized uterine contraction as no pressure rise is noted in the amniotic fluid. This "localized uterine contraction" is associated with fetal bradycardia and decreased umbilical flow, which is unrelated to a rise in amniotic fluid pressure.

Figure 8-10 is from the same preparation obtained on the fourth postoperative day. On this occasion, prolonged rise occurs in umbilical vein wedge pressure, which is associated with fetal bradycardia, fetal hypertension, and decreased umbilical flow. The clinical implications of these recordings is that the fetal baroreceptor reflex may be initiated by increase of umbilical cord resistance which is not reflected by a similar rise in amniotic fluid pressure or due to cord compression (but placental compression). Thus, they offer an explanation for unexplained fetal bradycardia, or even those "understood" bradycardias (head compression deceleration) beginning and ending with uterine contraction.

The recordings (Figs. 8-10 and 8-11) of the sheep fetus suggest that local areas of uterine tension insufficient to elevate amniotic fluid pressure can be associated with fetal bradycardia perhaps secondary to the fetal baroreflex. Whether such cardiovascular relationships occur in human fetuses is unknown, but similar episodes of unexplained (without apparent contractions) bradycardia do occur. Laboratory recordings of sheep preparations during uterine contractions often suggest a greater rise in fetal blood pressure than amniotic fluid pressure, which would likewise initiate the fetal baroreceptor. The clinical implications of these fetal sheep studies are that fetal hypertension responses related to increased umbilical vascular resistance and the baroreflex which may explain many of the so-called "head compression" or "independent" fetal bradycardias.

GENERAL DISCUSSION

The *in utero* human obviously changes its heart rate for many reasons, some due to changes of fetal arousal or levels of metabolitics and some associated with movement and breathing or in response to stress. This chapter is concerned only with those abrupt intrapartum fetal bradycardias which appear to be mediated by the vagus nerve, sometimes associated with stress, whose mechanisms are, at best, only superficially understood.

Manipulation of the fetal vertex can evoke either fetal tachycardia or bradycardia. We previously described the different fetal responses to the various fetal arousal levels.[276] Others have suggested that minimal fetal manipulation could result in increased uterine tension.[528] As shown in Figure 10-12 with scalp blood volume measurements, there is a suggestion that fetal hypertension occurs with even normal uterine contractions.

This chapter has been an anecdotal account of many different apparent etiologies of fetal bradycardias. The common theme has been that the information at hand is insufficient to explain their occurrences. As described in Chapter 8, it is doubtful that any acute fetal bradycardia is ever "physiologic" in the sense that it is completely innocuous. Furthermore, I believe that it serves no useful purpose to label fetal bradycardias according to their theoretical mechanisms, particuarly when we have been unable to document their occurrence in humans. Others disagree, believing that certain FHR patterns are diagnostic of umbilical cord compression and have recommended immediate cesarean section, even when failing to find the prolapsed umbilical cord.[114] Still others[617] suggest that head compression is the basis of nearly all fetal bradycardia and that the amniotic membrane should be protected. We ourselves have suggested that the maternal supine position should always be avoided.[267] Given this apparent lack of knowledge and disagreement over etiology, I proposed that all abrupt fetal bradycardias simply be referred to as vagal

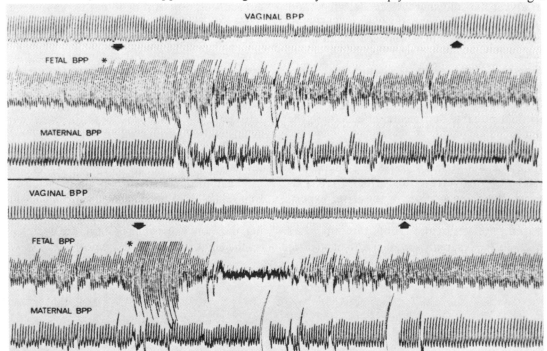

Fig. 10-12. Blood volume pulse recordings from maternal vagina, fetal scalp and maternal big toe. In upper three recordings, a relative increase in pulse pressure occurs prior to the uterine contraction. In lower three recordings, associated with maternal decreased pulse heights in vagina and big toe, are fetal hypertension. (During height of uterine contraction, fetal scalp pulse is lost.)

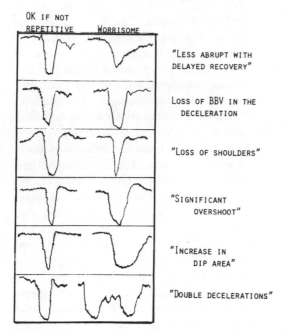

OK IF NOT
REPETITIVE   WORRISOME

"LESS ABRUPT WITH
DELAYED RECOVERY"

LOSS OF BBV IN THE
DECELERATION

"LOSS OF SHOULDERS"

"SIGNIFICANT
OVERSHOOT"

"INCREASE IN
DIP AREA"

"DOUBLE DECELERATIONS"

Fig. 10-13. Interpretation of severe vagal abrupt bradycardia. (After *Kardiotokographie, Lehrbuch und Atlas,* W. M. Fischer, 1976.)

bradycardias and that they be described and treated according to their severity. This concept is not unlike that proposed by an international meeting in 1972. Prolapse of the funis and fetal asphyxia should, of course, always be ruled out but otherwise, the bradycardia treatment should be considered for its own possible detrimental effects upon the fetus.

When we assume greater knowledge than we have about FHR responses, there is a tendency to overreact to various FHR patterns. It has been nearly a universal experience that when FHR monitors are introduced, the cesarean section rate increases markedly. Cesarean section rates of greater than 20% are now being accomplished in some of our private obstetrical services with patient populations that are largely low risk. Although such trends are decried, especially by the group at the University of Southern California, the trend continues. Indeed, even the USC group reports a 16% cesarean section rate in electronic monitored cases, while only a 3% rate in the unmonitored parturients.[528a]

Rudolph and associates have demonstrated in fetal sheep that fetal cardiac output is often heart rate dependent (Chapter 8). Our own systolic interval measurements in human fetuses also suggest that ejection times do not uniformly increase during fetal bradycardia, indicating that during severe and prolonged vagal bradycardia, the fetus cardiac output decreases. Under these circumstances, it is logical to seek to prevent fetal bradycardia whenever possible, even to the extent of using atropine. Parer[525] has failed to find a beneficial effect of atropine in hypoxic sheep fetuses (by inducing maternal hypoxia) and I have never recommended its use under these circumstances. But throughout this chapter, I have attempted to suggest that fetal vagal FHR are not reproducible nor consistent after given event (Poseiro effect, nuchal cord, maternal voiding, etc.), a physiologic independence which is probably of advantage to the fetus. The use of atropine would make the fetus even more independent of these *in utero* events whose detrimental effects on the fetus are often only their associated vagal bradycardia.

Vagal abrupt bradycardias are depicted in Figure 10-13. While no bradycardia should ever be considered to be completely reassuring, the more worrisome patterns are depicted on the right side of the diagram.

CHAPTER 11
Recording Fetal Cardiac Intervals

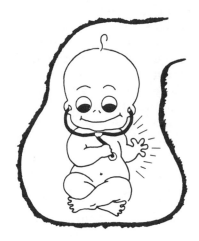

Introduction

The standard electronic fetal heart rate (FHR) monitoring techniques are imprecise indicators of fetal health. They often give the labor room staff nothing more than an idea of whether or not to be "reassured" about the health of the fetus. When abnormal FHR patterns occur, in the majority of cases, more convincing information is clearly required before responding with definitive therapy.

In 1970, in an effort to evolve more precise indices of fetal well-being, we began[274] to apply the concept of adult systolic time intervals to the intrapartum fetus. Following our own and other investigators' efforts, the use of fetal cardiac interval determinations now makes it possible to think in terms of fetal cardiac performance whether an HR recording appears "nonreassuring."

The measurement of systolic time interval, or the time required for the heart ventricle to eject, was introduced more than a century ago by Garrod[222] as an indicator of cardiac function. These measurements are obtained by indirect, noninvasive techniques that give relatively precise determination of myocardial function in adults. While direct invasive

techniques (catheterization) or ultrasound are still considered to be superior for determining cardiac performance, they cannot be used in the human fetus in the usual clinical situation.

Cardiac interval measurements in the human fetus by combining the fetal ECG and heart sounds was reported as early as 1941, and there were sporadic reports from Europe during the 1950s.[277] However, only with the renewed interest in systolic time interval analysis in adults has serious interest been shown in similar measurements in the fetus. Current investigations are based on classic cardiac cycle studies in dogs by Wiggers[750] and on human studies by Katz and Feil,[399] by Blumberger,[60] and by Weissler and colleagues in the 1960s.[741]

Cardiac Performance

Cardiac performance is basically affected by three conditions: preload, afterload, and inotropic state of the myocardium. Preload refers to the degree of stretch of the ventricle just before the systolic phase. Frank, working with the frog's heart in 1895, showed that increasing diastolic volume and pressure in turn increased the output of the heart. Starling, in 1914, concluded that the amount of mechanical energy released was determined by the ventricle's fibers length in diastole. These concepts became known as the Frank–Starling mechanism. As shown by Braundwald et al.[69] in 1958, afterload for the heart is very much determined by mean aortic pressure.

Before discussing the various types of systolic time interval determinations in the fetus, it seems appropriate to review briefly some of the cardiovascular responses of the fetus to stress and to distress. The fetus presumably changes its heart rates for many reasons, such as changing arousal levels, metabolic needs, overall activity, as well as response to stress and distress (Chapter 8). In acute reacting fetal bradycardias, we consider there to be only two basic underlying etiologies (Fig. 11-1). One mechanism (on the left of Fig. 11-1) is cardiovascular dysfunction which is of course worrisome, and the other is through vagal stimulation (on the right of Fig. 11-1) which is usually considered to be tolerable.

Vagal stimulation produces an abrupt bradycardia and the available data seem to indicate that there are, in turn, primary (head compression) and secondary (baroreflex) mechanisms leading to its stimulation in the fetus. A primary vagal stimulation can occur during fetal head compression or mild hypoxia. The baroreflex (Fig. 11-2) is usually evoked by increased peripheral resistance and the resulting hypertension which I postulate results from such in utero events such as severe hypoxia, umbilical cord compression, unequal myometrial contractions, and grunting (Fig. 11-2).

Workers in Rudolph's laboratory, using the chronic in utero fetal sheep preparation, have demonstrated that during fetal bradycardia, cardiac stroke volume remains relatively constant which results in a decreased cardiac output (Fig. 11-3). Determinations of human fetal systolic time intervals also suggest that "stroke ejection time" (S_1S_2) remains constant during many acute bradycardias (Figs. 11-4 and 11-5), suggesting that cardiac output like-

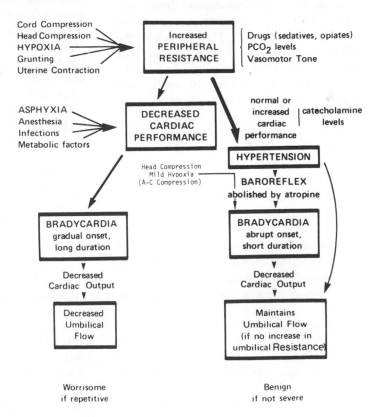

Fig. 11-1. Reacting fetal bradycardias. The right side is mediated by the vagus. The left side reflects decreased cardiac performance. (Same as Fig. 8-17.)

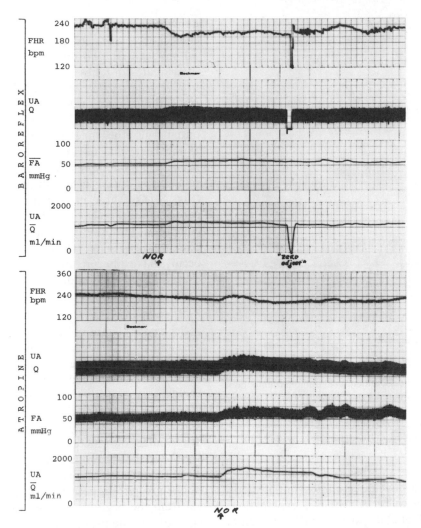

Fig. 11-2. Recording of 0.8 gestation sheep preparation from Rudolph's laboratory with catheters in umbilical artery (UA) and fetal aorta (FA). In upper recording, with injection of norepinephrine, an immediate rise of blood pressure (FA) and bradycardia (FHR) or baroreflex occurs. After atropine, the baroreflex is blocked with norepinephrine injection and umbilical flow (UA) is increased. (From *Obstet Gynecol* **48:** 117, 1976. Reproduced with permission.)

Fig. 11-3. The effects of increasing and decreasing heart rate from the normal resting level on right ventricular output of a fetal lamb at 0.8 gestation are shown. (From Rudolph, A.M.: *Congenital Diseases of the Heart.* Year Book, Chicago, 1974. Reproduced with permission.)

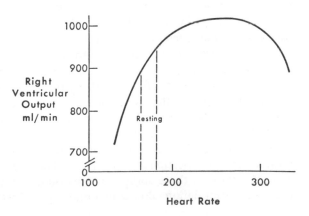

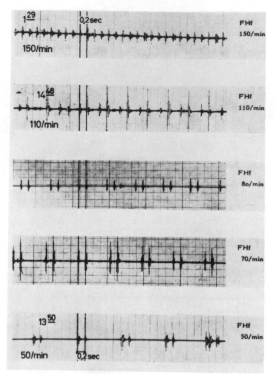

Fig. 11-4. Phonocardiograms demonstrating constant $S_1 - S_2$ intervals over varying heart rates from five different fetuses. (From Hammacher, K.: In *Perinatal Medicine*, H. Bossart *et al.*, Eds. Huber, Vienna, 1968. Reproduced with permission.)

wise decreases and that Rudolph's fetal sheep observations have direct clinical implications. There seem to be at least two explanations for this lack of ability of the fetal myocardium to follow the Frank–Starling law.

Friedman and colleagues,[403] in a series of studies, have demonstrated that the resulting tension of fetal cardiac muscle is higher and the active tension is lower than in adults at all points along the length–tension relationship curves. Thus, fetal myocardial performance is decreased when compared with adults in that the extent of cardiac muscle shortening at any load is relatively reduced. Furthermore, it also appears that even under normal circumstances, fetuses are close to the apex of their ventricular function curves and that the Frank–Starling relationship may therefore be limited to a small portion of this curve.[292] The other reason is in those abrupt bradycardias, the vagal stimulation also compounds the

deficiency, as its activity independently results in decreased cardiac performance.[147] Fetal myocardial performance is not always inadequate, for it has been demonstrated that bradycardia *unassociated* with increased peripheral resistance or decreased cardiac function is not correlated with a fallen cardiac output but rather the stroke volume increases as the heart rate falls (Chap. 8). This is especially notable when wide range of heart rate occurs during beat-to-beat variability[403] (Fig. 8-18). Thus, the relative decrease in cardiac performance of the fetal myocardium compared with the adult and the varying circumstances under which fetal bradycardia occur, make interpretation of its electromechanical time interval difficult.

SYSTOLIC TIMES

Schematic diagrams of the various electromechanical or cardiac time intervals (Figs. 11-6–11-8) and the methods of determining them in the human fetus are presented (Fig. 11-9). In general, the shorter these intervals, the greater the cardiac performance or cardiac "contractility." Asphyxia, depressive drugs, infections, increased peripheral resistance, and bradycardia usually increase the duration of these intervals.

The preejection period (PEP) is that interval from the beginning of ventricular depolarization to the beginning of left ventricular ejection; its duration reflects myocardial performance. The shorter this interval, the less time is required for intraventricular pressure to open the aortic valve and, therefore, the greater the cardiac performance. (Throughout this discussion, the term performance will be used in the absence of a more precise definition for the traditional term cardiac contractility.) The PEP and ventricular ejection time are of proven value in evaluating cardiac function in adults. (Clinical factors affecting cardiac intervals are shown in Table 11-I). However, nearly every institution applying the systolic interval technique to the human fetus described different alterations in the various intervals during times of apparent fetal stress or distress.[274, 282, 487, 518] The impli-

Fig. 11-5. Human simultaneous fetal EKG and heart sounds showing that $S_1 - S_2$ intervals remain constant during heart rates from 142 bpm to 64 bpm (1–5). As a newborn, it showed changing $S_1 - S_2$ intervals with changing heart rate (6–10).

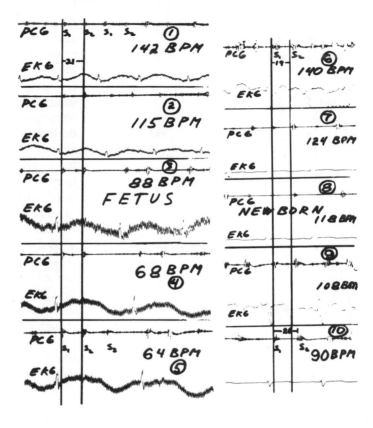

Fig. 11-6. Method of calculating systolic time intervals in adults using carotid pulse. In fetuses, scalp pulse lags R wave by 0.03–0.04 sec.

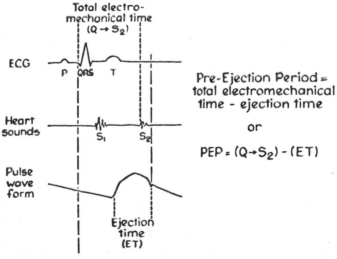

cation was that either systolic interval technique was imprecise or that the physiologic alterations of fetal cardiovascular function during fetal dysfunction are unlike those of the *extra utero* human.

In an attempt to resolve such discrepancies, I arranged to spend time in the laboratory of Dr. A.M. Rudolph of the Cardiovascular Research Institute, San Francisco, I considered this facility to be without peer in the area of fetal cardiovascular research, and it had detailed records of cardiovascular functions

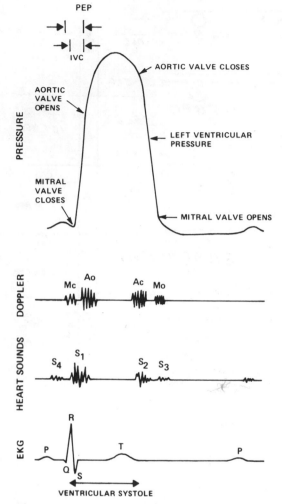

Fig. 11-7. Schematic diagram of electromechanical events of ventricular contraction. PEP—preejection interval; IVC—isovolumetric contraction; Mc—mitral valve closure; Ao—aortic valve opening; Mo—mitral valve opening.

from scores of chronic *in utero* fetal sheep studies just begging for the type of analysis I had in mind. I was interested in studying what I regard as an intriguing finding from systolic time recordings of intrapartum human fetuses. The time intervals between the first fetal heart sound (S_1) and the second heart sound (S_2) did not change during the initial period of acute and severe fetal bradycardia. This seemed to be true for the fetus only during labor. At other times, the $S_1 - S_2$ time intervals change in relationship to heart rate. (With fetal tachycardia, even during

labor, $S_1 - S_2$ has to shorten in order to accommodate the entire cardiac cycle.) The reason for my interest is that the $S_1 - S_2$ interval approximates the ejection time; this, assuming that mean blood pressure is constant, approximates the stroke volume. These observations suggested that when the FHR declines during labor due to increased vagal activity, cardiac output decreases. Others have not agreed with these interpretations[21, 765b] and have even argued that fetal bradycardia may be beneficial during times of stress.

I believe that my interpretations were not accepted by physiologists for the following reasons: first, the groups working with exteriorized, anesthetized sheep fetuses, stroke volume increases with declining heart rate or, in other words, cardiac output is maintained (Chap. 8). Second, since the time of Frank's observations of the frog heart, stroke volume always has been assumed to increase when heart rate slowed. The third reason concerns the one exception in adults to the Frank–Starling rule that occurs during the diving response.[17] Since bradycardia and decreased cardiac output are probably beneficial to the diving seal, others have reasoned that the same is true for the fetus.

However, work in Dr. Rudolph's laboratory showed that during bradycardia in the *in utero* fetal sheep, the cardiac stroke volumes remain relatively constant and that cardiac output falls. This confirmed my clinical impressions and gave me confidence in human systolic time determination. Reviewing many fetal sheep recordings convinced me that this is because many of the acute bradycardias are often the result of abrupt fetal hypertension and the baroreceptor reflex. Fetal hypertension, in turn, occurs because of increased fetal peripheral resistance.

In order to understand why changes in fetal cardiac interval measurements appear to be different than those seen in adults, it is necessary to briefly outline fetal cardiovascular responses already discussed in Chapters 8 and 10.

With central stimulation, or that unrelated to the baroreflex, hypertension and tachycar-

Fig. 11-8. Schematic diagram of methods for determining cardiac time intervals in human fetus at term. Unlike the adult techniques, PEP interval is measured from the R wave to opening of the ventricular valve (which actually corresponds more to the IVC interval). Tx refers to artery transmission time. (From *Obstet Gynecol* **44**: 119, 1974. Reproduced with permission.)

PEP DETERMINATION

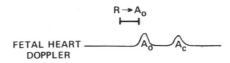

$$PEP = R \rightarrow A_o$$
$$PEP = R \rightarrow S_2 - ET_c$$
$$PEP = R \rightarrow Pl - Txp$$
$$PEP = R \rightarrow Sc - Txs$$

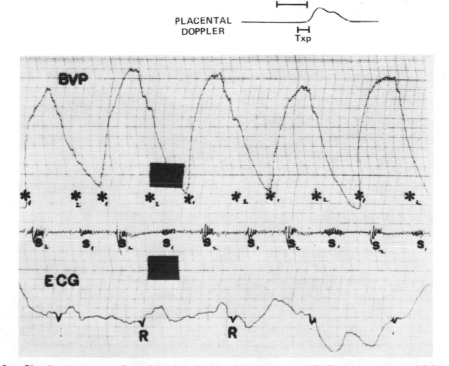

Fig. 11-9. Simultaneous recording of fetal scalp blood volume pulse (BVP), heart sounds (PCG), and EKG. PEP—R $-$ S_2 interval minus ejection time.

TABLE 11-I. Immediate Changes in Systolic Time Intervals during Fetal Bradycardia

Parameters	Conditions		
Etiology of bradycardia	Antenatal arousal change	Intrapartum, benign	Intrapartum, ominous
Myocardial performance	0	0*	↓*
Peripheral resistance	0	↑	↑
Blood pressure	0	↑	0 or ↓
Stroke volume	↑	0	↓
Intervals			
PEP	0	0 or ↑⁺	↑
R–S₁	0	0 or ↑⁻	↑
S₁–S₂	↑	0	↑
R–S₂	↑	0 or ↑⁺	↑ ↑
R–PI	0	0	↑

0 = no change
↑ = increase
↓ = decrease
*With ↑ catecholamine production, myocardial performance may be improved
⁺Changes depend upon degree of blood pressure rise

dia (and not bradycardia) occur. This type of pressor-hypertensive response is seen with fetal movement, with increase in fetal arousal levels, or any other stimulation of the higher CNS. While fetal hypertension can then occur simultaneously during bouts of "spontaneous" tachycardia, the appearance of initial hypertension in a fetus with an intact vagus nerve means abrupt bradycardia.

Factors affecting fetal peripheral resistance, hypertension, and the baroreceptor response are described in Chapter 8. Increased peripheral resistance is part of the adult diving response, and it also plays a role in the fetal hypoxemic response, head compression, uterine contractions. The degree of increased peripheral resistance is influenced by oxygen and carbon dioxide tensions, catecholamine levels, and drugs such as sedatives and narcotics.

In addition to increased peripheral resistance, another reason for the sheep fetus' inability to maintain cardiac output during acute bradycardia was also explained by the concept of reduced fetal myocardial performance. The fetal heart is, therefore, often unable to increase stroke volume during bradycardia secondary to the baroreflex in the face of the associated increased cardiac afterload (increased peripheral resistance).

Since anesthesia, sedatives, or hypocarbia will partially prevent increased peripheral resistance, and catecholamines will increase cardiac performance, bradycardia occurring under these conditions may be associated with increased stroke volume and fetal cardiac output will be maintained. This probably explains the difference between those laboratories using stressed and anesthetized preparations and those using chronic stable preparations.

With this information in hand, it appears possible to explain the changes associated with bradycardia that occur in the various fetal cardiac intervals. In the antepartum period, most FHR alterations probably reflect changes in fetal arousal levels, position, or metabolic levels. These antepartum FHR responses are, in all probability, unlike most intrapartum fetal heart rate alterations that occur secondary to increased fetal hypertension (peripheral resistance). (In the newborn period, fetal cardiac performance increases.) Therefore, in the antenatal period, fetal stroke volume would be expected to increase during bradycardia, and PEP would not lengthen because (for one reason or another) myocardial performance equals the demands of the occasion. It seems important to emphasize this point that we made a number of years ago,[265] that the etiology of FHR changes and demands on fetal cardiac performance are probably different in the antenatal versus the intrapartum periods.

Years ago, work in Reynolds'[511] laboratory suggested what is now even more apparent. In order to understand FHR responses (or systolic times) to stress, knowledge of the fetus' blood pressure changes is essential, and this sort of data are not available in the usual clinical setting. One can, however, clinically estimate relative fetal blood pressure from cardiac interval readings, assuming that cardiac performance remains unchanged.

PEP (PREEJECTION INTERVAL)

While numerous intervals have been described and various indices used in adults, the PEP and ventricular "ejection time" ($S_1 - S_2$ or Ao − Ac) of Figures 11-7 and 11-8 have best stood the test of time in clinical cardiac function evaluation.

The preejection period (PEP) (interval from the beginning of the ventricular depolarization to the beginning of the left ventricular ejection) and its duration is considered to reflect myocardial performance. Reitan and others[566] have shown that $1/(PEP)^2$ is directly proportional to the rate of acceleration of flow of blood through the ascending aorta (or cardiac performance). From a practical standpoint, it is acceptable to consider the better the cardiac performance, the shorter the time (PEP interval) it takes for interventricular pressure to open the aortic valve.[741] In addition to cardiac performance, the PEP interval is also influenced by preload (end-diastolic pressure) and afterload (aortic pressure).

In the fetus, so many of the acute and severe bradycardias represent both hypertension (increased afterload) and vagal stimulation (decreased cardiac performance), that a lengthened PEP interval in the fetus can mean other things (in contrast to adults) than decreased myocardial performance. Specifically, acute severe fetal bradycardia from strong vagal stimulation alone, as might occur with brief head compression or umbilical cord compression, can give a lengthened PEP.

Many recording techniques have been described for clinical application of cardiac interval determination. The simplest of these is the "eyeballing" methods, or synchronizing a signal (usually the R wave) on an oscilloscope cathode ray tube (CRT) with a second cardiac signal such as fetal heart sounds or Doppler signal. The CRT method is accurate but fatiguing. As alternatives, a number of recorders have been developed that provide permanent records of various fetal cardiac intervals.[282]

One clinical technique for determining PEP is based on the use of a specially filtered Doppler signal reflected from the fetal ventricular waves. Despite glowing reports from other institutions,[487, 518] we found it difficult to keep the fetal aortic or pulmonic valve in sharp Doppler focus. Indeed, it is not clear as to which fetal heart valve is being monitored. However, valve opening can be identified, the only measure needed for PEP is that from the Q or R wave to the Doppler signal of Ao (or R − Ao).

Another technique we attempted was that proposed by Weissler for adults. It requires simultaneous measurement of fetal pulse, ECG, and heart sounds (PEP = R → S_2 − ejection time or R → S_2 minus scalp pulse, Fig. 11-9). We found that the fetal scalp pulse is sometimes modified by many unrelated factors, and after much work, we abandoned the method.

In chronic fetal sheep preparations, we measured the interval between the R wave and the upsurge recorded by a flow probe on either the pulmonary trunk or ascending aorta. Such an interval approximates "PEP." We observed that interval of R-opening of ventricular waves (R − Po) was decreased during early hypoxemia but that it lengthened with asphyxia (pH 6.91, P_{O_2} 7 torr, and P_{CO_2} 74 torr, Fig. 11-10). Presumably, these PEP changes were the effect of initially stress-elevated catecholamine levels that increased cardiac performance; cardiac performance decreased when asphyxia occurred. The sheep fetus may be more prone to excrete catecholamines under stress than the primate fetus. The relationship in fetal sheep between heart rate and PEP (R to pulmonary trunk or R to ascending aorta) is presented in Figure 11-11. For any one fetus, there appears to be a relationship between heart rate and "PEP," but there are wide ranges when comparing PEP intervals at any given heart rate among different fetuses.

Wolfson et al.,[764] using an "interactive computer routine," demonstrated a linear

Fig. 11-10. Values of interval between R wave of fetal ECG and upswing of flow probe placed on a sheep fetus's (chronic preparation) pulmonary trunk (Rudolph's laboratory) according to heart rate.

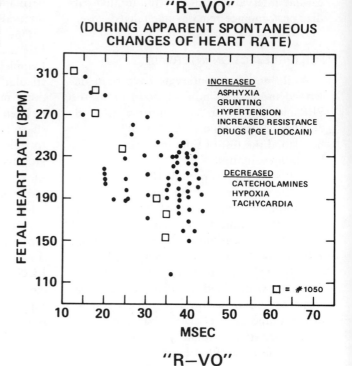

Fig. 11-11. Intervals of R wave of ECG to flow probe on either ascending aorta or pulmonary trunk of chronic sheep fetuses in good condition (R-Vo). The squares are one particular fetus. Other values demonstrate wide ranges of heart rate for no apparent reason.

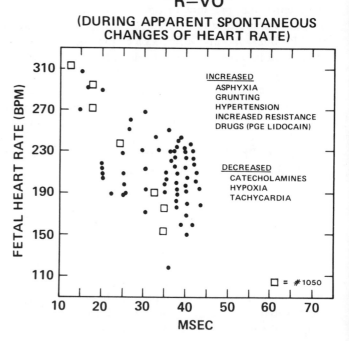

correlation between PEP and gestational age between the 20th week and term in normal human fetuses. This relationship was apparently true even when allowances were made for the slowing of the FHR which occurs over this developmental period.

R − S$_2$ INTERVAL

Two fetal cardiac signals that have always been easy to obtain are fetal R wave (scalp or abdominal) and fetal heart sounds (S$_1$ and S$_2$) (Fig. 11-8). While R − S$_1$ interval does not consistently follow the PEP and isovolumetric contraction time changes, there is a close relationship. Unfortunately, the fetal S_1 signal is often prolonged and diffuse. Since $S_1 - S_2$ remains relatively constant during severe labor-induced bradycardias, we have focused on the $R - S_2$. (The $R - S_2$ interval represents a composite as IVC and VET may change in opposite directions.) Clinically, it appears useful (Fig. 11-7).

R — PL INTERVAL

Another cardiac interval useful in interpreting fetal cardiovascular change is the time required for an arterial pulse to reach a peripheral point. This distal point may be fetal scalp, leg, or placenta, but the placental Doppler pulse is easiest to obtain. From such measurements, we can also estimate the relative degree of hypertension, since, with an increase in the mean blood pressure, pulse wave transmission time (Tx of Fig. 11-8) along the artery is decreased.

The $R - Pl$ provides a method to circumvent the "false positive" PEP finding with the relatively innocuous vagal bradycardias as it combines the PEP interval with arterial pulse-wave velocities. This time interval is determined in human fetuses from the R wave of the ECG to the arrival of the Doppler pulse wave at a peripheral site (Fig. 11-4). While the fetus is small, its umbilical circulation is relatively long, and it makes an ideal location for measurement of the pulse-wave transmission time by measuring from the R wave to placental "pulse" (Figs. 11-8 and 11-12–11-14). Pulse-wave velocity is increased by age, hypertension, valsalva maneuver, and is faster in the peripheral arteries, but it is reduced with decreased cardiac performance.[579] PEP is *increased* in hypertension because afterload is increased, but at the same time, pulse-wave transmission time is *decreased* by hypertension, tending to negate the overall effects of hypertension on the measurement of cardiac performance. Thus, the R-to-placental pulse $(R - Pl)$ provides an index of cardiac performance which has, in theory at least, greater applicability for the fetus than other electromechanical intervals.

Since hypotension (increased afterload) is so common in the fetal bradycardias occurring during labor, we have invested considerable effort in the $R - Pl$ determination of the intrapartum fetus. As with all other indicators of fetal cardiovascular function, we tested our theories first in the fetal sheep.

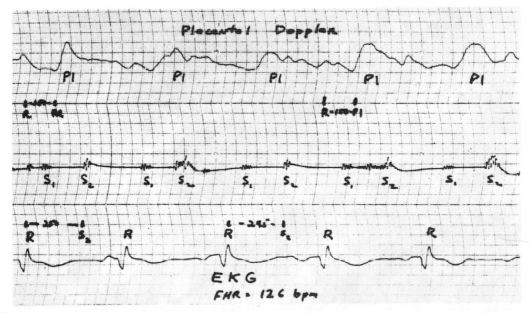

Fig. 11-12. Simultaneous recordings of fetal ECG, phonocardiogram, and filtered placental Doppler signal. Numbers refer to time intervals from R wave to fetal S_2 and to placental signal.

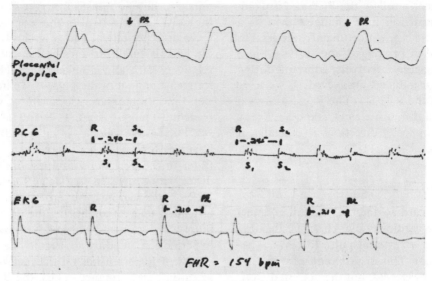

Fig. 11-13. Simultaneous fetal EKG, heart sounds (PCG), and placental Doppler pulse.

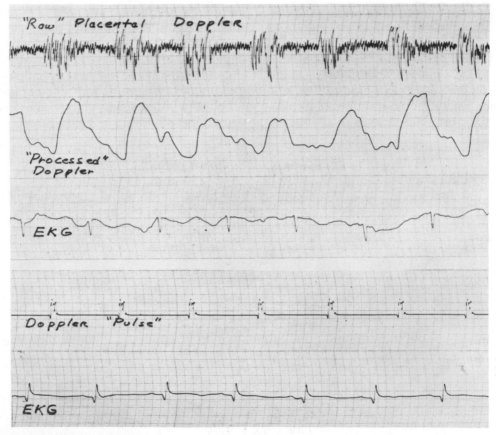

Fig. 11-14. Two recordings of placental Doppler with filtering and as converted to a pulse. Upper recording shows unfiltered and processed Doppler.

FETAL SHEEP—TECHNIQUE FOR R − PL INTERVAL

A chronic fetal sheep preparation from Rudolph's laboratory, whose recording is presented here, was 130 days gestation and in its third postoperative day. Catheters had been placed in the fetal aorta, and IVC and an umbilical flow probe (Clark electromagnetic flow transducer) had been placed around the common umbilical artery (Fig. 11-15). As shown in Figure 11-16, the animal, on its first postoperative day, showed no evidence of asphyxia, but on the second day, the fetus had an unexplained acidemia (pH 6.85) and hypoxemia P_{O_2} (7 torr) and hypercarbia (74 torr). Despite these most abnormal blood gas findings, indicative of severe asphyxia, the fetus' R-to-umbilical probe interval (R − Um) was unchanged from the previous day. The preparation was of no use for the original study and therefore the fetus was subjected subsequently to excessive uterine contractions, infusions of lactic acid, and maternal hypoxia. Despite its apparent asphyxia, the fetus withstood these additional stresses as well as had any other fetus in the laboratory. It finally expired only when the fetal P_{O_2} reached 4 torr and after some 3 hr of continued excessive stress. This observation suggested that this indicator of cardiac function may be a more accurate indicator of fetal cardiovascular reserve than do blood gases.

Four other sheep fetuses in Rudolph's laboratory were followed as they began to deteriorate. As asphyxia occurred (pH 7.11 and P_{O_2} 10 torr), the R − Um lengthened. As progressive asphyxia and severe bradycardia occurred, the R − Um intervals became markedly prolonged. During infusions of various catecholamines, the R − Um interval improved (shortened) briefly, then lengthened as cardiac vascular failure occurred.

HUMAN INTRAPARTUM R − PL DETERMINATIONS

In a human fetus, the placental Doppler is determined through localization of the placenta with an ultrasonic scan and the fetal placental "pulse" with the hand Doppler. After localizing the typical placental soufflé of the fetal circulation, the time interval is determined from the fetal R wave of the fetal ECG to the beginning of the placental "pulse" (R − Pl) (Figs. 11-8, 11-9, 11-12, and 11-14). This interval can be determined with

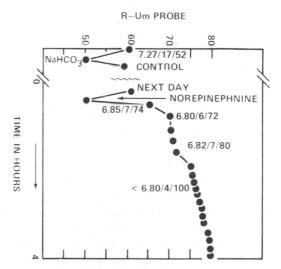

Fig. 11-16. Values of interval from R wave of ECG to flow probe on umbilical artery of a fetal sheep (chronic preparation) in Rudolph's laboratory. The next day, the fetus demonstrated asphyxia, but R-Um values were only slightly increased until severe asphyxia occurred (pH = 6.82, P_{O_2} = 7 torr, P_{CO_2} = 80 torr).

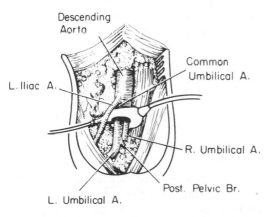

Fig. 11-15. Diagrammatic representation of electromagnetic flow transducer in place around the common umbilical artery (common umbilical A). A catheter has also been inserted into a branch of left iliac artery (L iliac A). (From Berman, W., et al.: *J Appl Physiol* **30:** 1056, 1975. Reproduced with permission.)

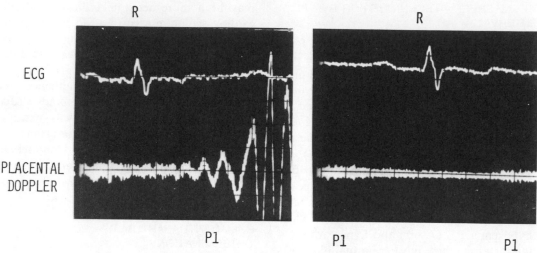

Fig. 11-17. Photograph of dual-beam oscilloscope showing fetal ECG and placental Doppler. At times the latter is easily observed (on left) and at others, despite audible placental "pulse," is difficult to visualize (on right).

the "eyeballing" technique (Fig. 11-17), using an oscilloscope which is synchronized with the fetal R wave and which displays the placental pulse. The position of the placental pulse on the abscissa of the screen then indicates the R-to-Pl interval. This interval also can be continuously recorded with a commerically available recorder (RSR Recorder—Berkeley BioEngineering). Because the fetal placental soufflé "disappears" so often during uterine contractions, we have essentially limited our observations to uterine asystole.

As observed in R − Pl measurements of more than 250 human fetuses, each fetus seems to have its "own" R-to-Pl interval which becomes readily apparent with a few minutes of recording. We have also recorded this interval in two fetuses whose pH's (scalp) decreased to below 7.20. In one case, the R-to-Pl interval had increased 0.13 sec and the fetus was delivered immediately by cesarean section. Its cord artery blood was 7.01 and the fetus required vigorous resuscitation. In the other, the interval had increased 0.05 sec and again the infant was delivered by cesarean section. This infant, however, had a cord artery pH of 7.21 and was in good condition.

The R-to-Pl intervals have been determined in 34 other cases in which there was

consideration of fetal distress because of apparent fetal heart rate abnormalities. While there is a slight increase in RPL intervals with bradycardia in some, and a decrease in others, none of these were considered to show abnormal values. None of these fetuses had abnormal scalp pH's and all were born in good condition.

The question continues to arise with me as to which is the better indicator of fetal health—blood gases, systolic time intervals, or FHR patterns. If the fetal brain continued to function better in asphyxia than does the fetal heart, the answer is probably systolic time intervals. While Myers' recent studies[492] of cerebral palsy in monkey fetuses suggest that it may be brain lactic acid accumulation and not the cardiac performance or absolute degrees of asphyxia which is important in subsequent CNS function, we continue cautiously to explore these techniques.

At the University of Southern California, PEP has been studied extensively in primate fetuses during both the antenatal and intrapartum periods.[357, 487] Findings from this work are somewhat different from ours. Acidemia caused PEP interval to increase in monkey fetuses; in human fetuses, PEP was likewise lengthened during fetal acidemia in labor and with antenatal chronic fetal distress. For unknown reasons, the PEP during asphyxia were not different than those during hypoxia. As would be expected, PEP was not appreciably affected by heart rate during the antenatal period, since presumably they are not concerned with the baroreflex. By contrast, the Canadian group has found that the PEP usually shortens with chronic asphyxia.[49a]

Our studies of human fetuses have been severely limited by the few occurrences of acidemia. Of the fetuses with both abnormal heart rates and scalp blood pH studied over the past seven years, only one had normal PEP or R − S_2 intervals; the others had either shortened or prolonged intervals as compared with our control values.

In studies of our normal human fetuses, R − S_2 intervals changed with bradycardia in the antenatal period, remained relatively constant during brief bradycardias in the intra-

partum period, and were markedly prolonged with true asphyxia. On the other hand, PEP remained relatively constant over wide ranges of heart rate in the antenatal period, but changed with fetal heart rate in the intrapartum period. As noted, these PEP changes probably reflect the different etiologies of most bradycardias in the two periods.

We have not ignored other indicators of fetal distress, such as scalp pH, and refrained from interfering because "cardiac performance" was normal. The main value of fetal systolic time intervals determination would appear to be to check those fetal heart rate patterns which appear to be worrisome. Despite having used fetal systolic time intervals for more than 7 years, we are uncertain of the technique's precision in evaluating fetal health. This is mostly because we had only nine cases in which there was proven acidemia in which we simultaneously determined

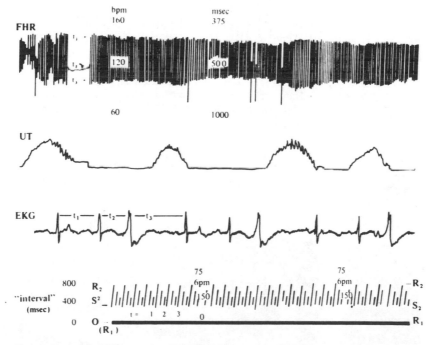

Fig. 11-18. From a Berkeley RSR recorder. Fetal monitoring recording (FHR and uterine tension) of the fetus with PVCs with representative EKG and R − S_2 interval recording. With "interval" recordings, R wave of EKG starts records at zero (0), then skips to time of second heart sound ("S_2") and marks until next R wave occurs. Thus, O − S_2 = R − S_2 and O − R = R − R interval. As with FHR recorder, it is possible to read either R − R intervals or FHR from interval recordings. While it is possible to determine R − R intervals (T_1, T_2, T_3) from any FHR, EKG, and "interval" recordings, it is only the latter which show the physiologic effects of PVCs on ejection times (changing R − S_2 intervals). (From *Crit Rev Bioeng* **2**: 149, 1975. Reproduced with permission.)

systolic clinical intervals. While eight of the nine cases demonstrated abnormal values, the degree of abnormality of the interval determination did not correlate well with the degree of fetal illness. It still is impossible to predict what systolic time interval change might occur in fetal distress because of the variables (cardiac hypoxemia, changes in pre-load and afterload, cardiostimulatory activity) which may occur in the different types of fetal malfunction recognized clinically as fetal distress.

Obviously, we hope that determination of fetal electromechanical (systolic) intervals will provide back-up data for interpreting apparently abnormal FHR patterns. With

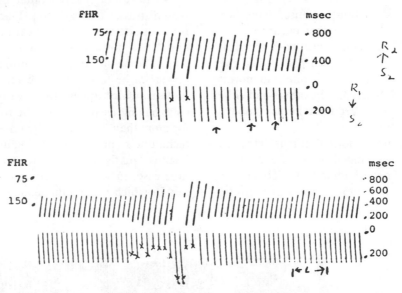

Fig. 11-19.   Also from RSR recorder of FHR showing BBV at arrows. With change in heart rate, there is a lag (L) in R − S_2 to catch up with R − R interval. However, with BBV, the R − S_2 interval precedes the R − R change. This demonstrates that fetal stroke volume changes with BBV. The "x" indicates recording errors.

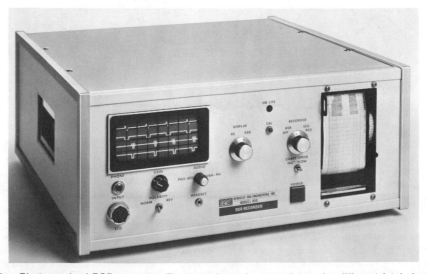

Fig. 11-20.   Photograph of RSR recorder. The four-channel scope shows the different fetal signals (as ECG & placental pulse) and their derived pulse. Recording shows cardiac intervals, heart rate (R − R interval), and uterine contraction (marker).

this goal in mind, we have attempted to design a recorder that can measure all of these various intervals and also serve as a routine fetal monitor.[281] If, for instance, an abnormal FHR pattern should occur, it would be possible to measure the $R - S_2$ (Fig. 11-18) and perhaps $R - Ao$ (PEP), and if these were abnormal, the $R - Pl$. Presumably, it would be possible to determine whether abnormal intervals reflected decreased cardiac performance or fetal hypertension. Figure 11-18 is a recording from the "RSR" recorder showing continuous $R - S_2$ interval determinations of a fetus with PVC. Figure 11-19 shows effect of BBV on $R - S_2$ intervals.

Our tentative conclusion from laboratory data and reports is that no matter how ominous the FHR recording or scalp pH may be, if the systolic time intervals are normal, the fetus is satisfactorily coping (at least from a cardiovascular standpoint) with its intrauterine environment. By contrast, if other indicators of fetal well-being are normal, but the systolic time intervals are abnormal, fetal cardiac dysfunction is occurring and disaster may be just around the corner. Since human intrapartum fetal asphyxia is rare, and we are for many reasons unable to study these cases without treating them. It may therefore be years before this hypothesis is proved or disproved in human beings. As with other electronic fetal heart rate techniques, my present justification for fetal cardiac recordings is based upon a few anecdotal case histories.

CHAPTER 12

Interesting FHR Patterns

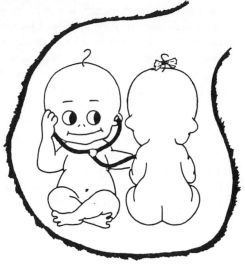

Everyone studying FHR recordings has conjured up some intrauterine mechanism which would explain the apparent deviation from the normal or ordinary. However, as continuing experience is gained in classifying these unusual FHR patterns and their fetal outcome, it has become apparent (to me at least) that our knowledge of fetal physiology is inadequate to explain their occurrence. Instead, like human geneticists, obstetricians may be forced to determine "empiric risks" for various FHR patterns, as to the probability of fetal asphyxia being present or developing with each type of FHR pattern. Having thus suggested that attempts at discussion of a physiological basis for many FHR patterns are hopeless, permit me to attempt to explain several of the more interesting patterns that I have seen.

Abruptio Placentae

Abruptio placentae has been the most difficult pattern for us to interpret (Fig. 12-1). Often, the uterine tension is increased and contractions occur at such a frequency as to produce a "saw-tooth" pattern. However, in our experience, FHR pattern abnormalities often occur too late to allow for effective fetal therapy. In our cases of abruptio, FHR analysis has not often allowed the delivery of a severely stressed newborn. Such newborns are usually well, or stillborn, unless the dying fetus has been rescued. We have no explanation for our failure to find an "impending" pattern of fetal asphyxia in cases of abruptio.

Overshoot

The occurrence of tachycardia after bradycardia, we have termed "overshoot." We have suggested that such an FHR pattern (Fig. 12-2) represents excess levels of catecholamines or sympathometric stimulation in response to a severe hypoxic episode (Chap. 8).[280] Others feel that such a pattern is evidence of a highly aroused and responsive fetus. The difference in viewpoints is perhaps explained by acknowledging that brief tachycardia (accelerations) before and after the abrupt bradycardia (Fig. 10-7), or "shoulder," is a healthy sign and may reflect nothing more than partial cord compression or vagal stimulation.

158

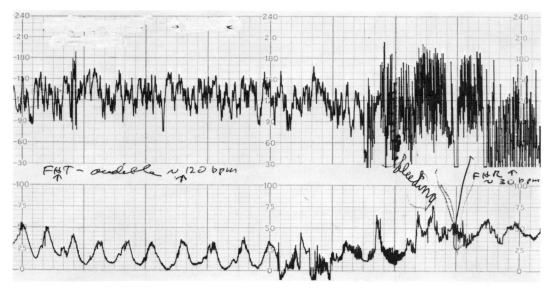

Fig. 12-1. FHR (Doppler) recording of an 1850-g human fetus showing the typical "saw-tooth" pattern of abruptio placentae prior to any external bleeding. When external bleeding occurred, FHR was abruptly 30 bpm and delivery occurred 20 min later (stillborn infant).

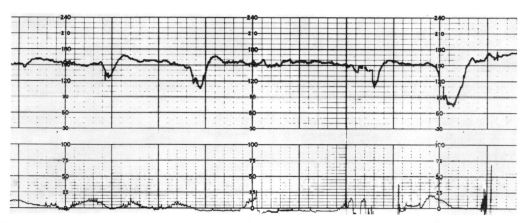

Fig. 12-2. Fetal heart rate recording demonstrating "overshoot" (and improperly applied external uterine tension sensor). Since overshoot was considered ominous, fetus was delivered 18 min later with an Apgar 1 and 5 and requiring resuscitation. Paper speed 3 cm/min.

Undershoot

The occurrence of decelerations after acceleration (brief tachycardia–bradycardia; lambda) has perhaps two different etiologies, depending on the severity of the bradycardia. Where the bracycardia is moderately severe, the pattern probably reflects partial, then complete, funis compression (Chap. 8). When mild, the brief subsequent bardycardia is per-

haps the baroreflex secondary to the tachycardia pressor response (Chap. 9). These fetuses are in good condition (Fig. 12-3).

Partial Heart Block

The rare congenital lesion of the fetal heart associated with heart block can be sometimes diagnosed by strip chart recordings (Fig. 12-4). P waves occur at the expected heart rate,

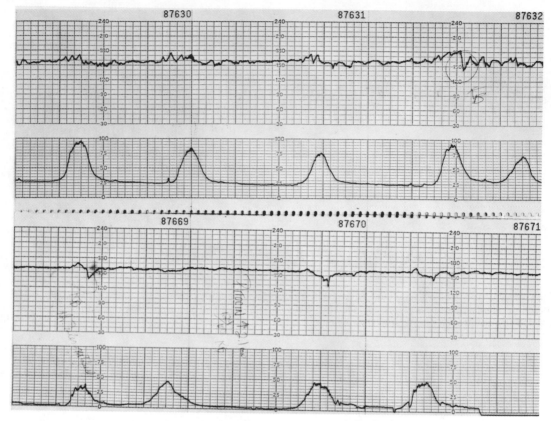

Fig. 12-3.   Recording demonstrating bradycardia after acceleration, or undershoot.

but R waves are at a reduced frequency. Since the Doppler transducer can easily pick up the beating auricle, the FHR determined with Doppler will be different than that with the scalp ECG.

"Cycling" Base Line Patterns

Kates and Schifrin[397] have described a FHR pattern which was previously considered to be increased BBV, but actually represented a status epilepticus activity (Fig. 12-5). The spiking pattern occurs in cycles, was unresponsive to oxygen or change in position, and the subsequent newborns usually had seizure activity despite good Apgar scores. (When seizures are induced in sheep, the FHR pattern is one of severe bradycardia secondary to the associated hypertension.) We have seen a slower "cycling" FHR pattern associated with a fetus having CMV

infection with mild hydrocephalus (Fig. 12-6).

Bradycardia After Fetal Hemorrhage

The sheep and human fetus respond to massive blood loss with bardycardia[279] (Fig. 12-7). Gabbe and associates[219] reported in 1975 an initial fetal tachycardia which probably occurs in the less severe cases. An interesting feature of Figure 12-7 is the stronger maternal ECG (of the scalp electrode) when compared to the dying fetus (and therefore her heart rate is counted by the fetal monitor). I have unfortunately seen one further case which had a fetal scalp ECG complex of lesser voltage than that of its mother and no FHR could be picked up by the Doppler. An emergency cesarean section was done, but even though there was an occasional newborn

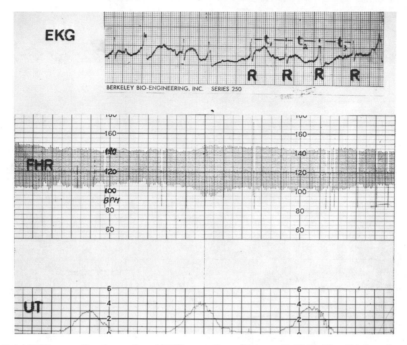

Fig. 12-4.   Fetal EKG recording (upper) and FHR recording of fetus with PVC. R − R interval varies markedly, as does instantaneous FHR.

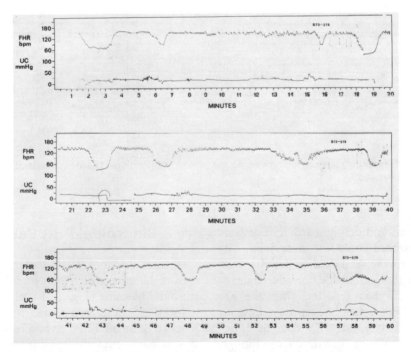

Fig. 12-5.   An FHR recording of apparent seizures activity *in utero,* showing loss of BBV and cycles of brief accelerations (courtesy of B.S. Schrifrin, M.D.).

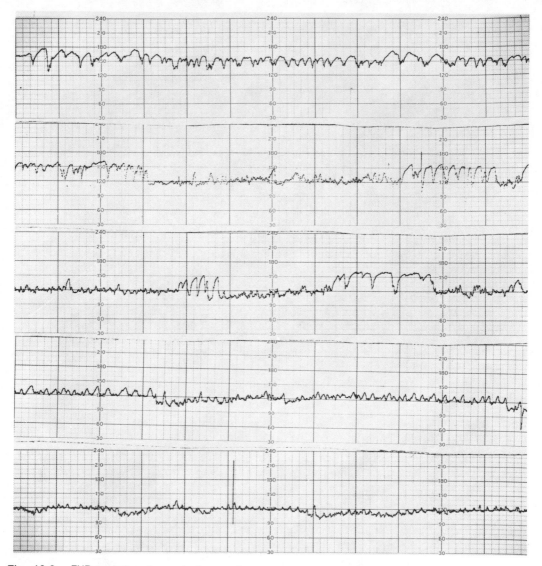

Fig. 12-6. FHR recording demonstrating varying patterns of accelerations. Newborn had mild hydrocephalus due to CMV and expired.

QRS complex, and despite cardiac resuscitation, the newborn could not be revived. Apparently when the fetal cardiac activity is so reduced, the fetus should be considered dead. Indeed, Myers has reported that the asphyxiated monkey fetus' heart may show no mechanical activity, but QRS complexes occur at 60 bpm as long as 35 min. Even though resuscitation is still possible, the newborn monkey shows severe cerebral dysfunction.

Sinusoidal FHR Pattern

A rare, ominous FHP pattern is the "sinusoidal," consisting of an undulating or sinusoidal baseline (Fig. 12-8). Modanlou and associates[480] described a case associated with a severely anemic and hypotensive newborn due to massive fetomaternal transfusion. This pattern has been previously associated with severe anemia in Rh-isoimmunization. How-

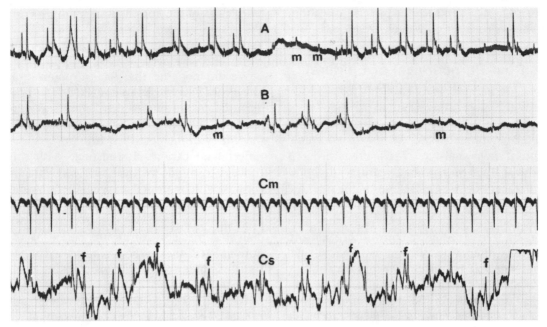

Fig. 12-7. Fetal scalp ECG recording of a 1950-g fetus dying from blood loss. An amniocentesis had been attempted and an umbilical vein on the placental surface had been lacerated. In A, the maternal R of scalp recording is of much less relative voltage than the fetal R wave. In B, the fetal R wave is infrequent. At C, the fetal monitor counted only the maternal R wave (Cm) but a small low voltage R wave (f) was still present. A, B, and Cs are fetal scalp ECG pickups. Cm is maternal chest lead.

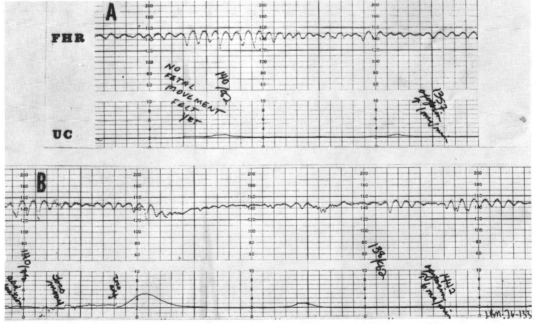

Fig. 12-8. This represents an FHR tracing obtained with an ultrasonic Doppler-type transducer. Panel A shows the baseline FHR pattern obtained prior to oxytocin stimulation. Note the sinusoidal FHR pattern and minimal uterine activity. Panel B shows a continuation of the sinusoidal pattern and late deceleration of the FHR following oxytocin-induced uterine contraction.

ever, Kubli[416] reported the pattern to occur in a more diverse group. Such a pattern is usually seen shortly prior to fetal death.

Post-Paracervical or Epidural Block Bradycardia

We[286] have shown that if the amount of anesthetic used in the paracervical block (PCB) is limited (i.e., 200 mg of lidocaine) and if no vagal-type FHR bradycardia is present, then *no* fetal bradycardia will follow a paracervical block. If these simple rules are violated, then post-PCB fetal bardycardia occurs with a high frequency. As shown in Figure 12-9, through unknown mechanisms, there is often a decrease in maternal vaginal and femoral blood volume pulses. Cibils[107] has demonstrated that the effect is one of local anesthetic on the uterine blood supply.

A number of unexplained fetal deaths have occurred after PCB. The accepted explanation for these deaths is the presence of toxic fetal levels of the anesthetic agent, by way of absorption through the uterine artery. (This appears to be much more frequent with the use of bupivacaine.)

We did not find that fetal atropinization uniformly prevented the post-PCB fetal bradycardia. According to the concepts as outlined in Chapter 8, this observation implies that many of the post-PCB fetal bradycardia reflect fetal cardiac dysfunction. With this concept in mind, we treat such fetal bradycardias with maternal oxygen therapy and the lateral position and allow the fetus to recover *in utero*. On two occasions, when we delivered the fetus during the period of abnormal FHR, the newborn required exchange transfusions to reduce its toxic serum levels of lidocaine.

While FHR abnormalities following paracervical block have been discussed much, those following epidural anesthesia are largely ignored. The probable explanation is

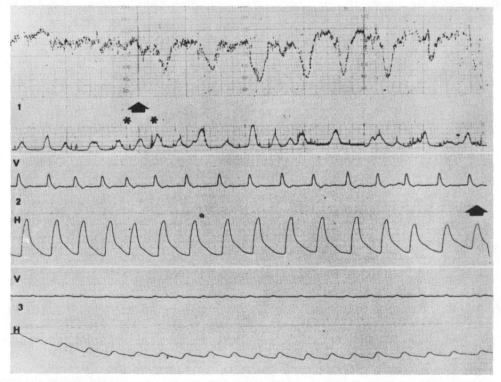

Fig. 12-9. Simultaneous FHR tracings and vaginal (V) and hallux (H) maternal pulses. (The arrow of No. 2 corresponds to the arrow of No. 1.) After a paracervical block (* *), late FHR deceleration occurred along with marked decrease in maternal and vaginal pulses.

that FHR abnormalities after various types of epidural anesthesia are almost always benign in regard to the fetal welfare, in contrast to those associated with PCB. Nevertheless, fetal bradycardia of a spectacular degree sometimes occurs after epidural anesthesia (Fig. 12-10) apparently related to uterine hypoperfusion. Unlike those associated with PCB, such epidural bradycardias are usually released by the maternal lateral position.

Fetuses Dying from Asphyxia

One type of FHR recording which no one enjoys obtaining is that of the dying fetus.

Figure 12-11 is that of a 690-g fetus with abruptio. The upper recording (with Doppler) shows late decelerations, but the latter (middle) showed severe abrupt, or just the reverse of the way it should occur. The terminal event was as expected (lower tracing) with loss of BBV and bradycardia.

Figure 12-12 is a disastrous case of a "postdate" fetus and a bloody aminocentesis. After the aminocentesis, there was (738) one late deceleration, but the gravida was supine and hyperventilating and all appeared well 2 hr later (748) with apparent FHR accelerations. One hour later (774), normal FHR and move-

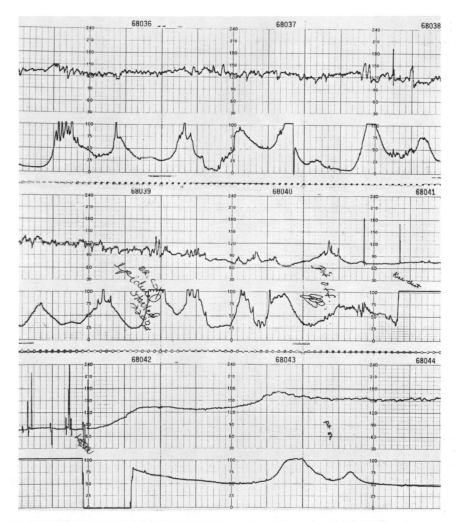

Fig. 12-10.   FHR tracing showing fetal bradycardia after an epidural anesthetic (Lidocaine) at 68039. Oxytocin infusion was stopped and patient was placed in knee-chest position. FHR gradually recovered.

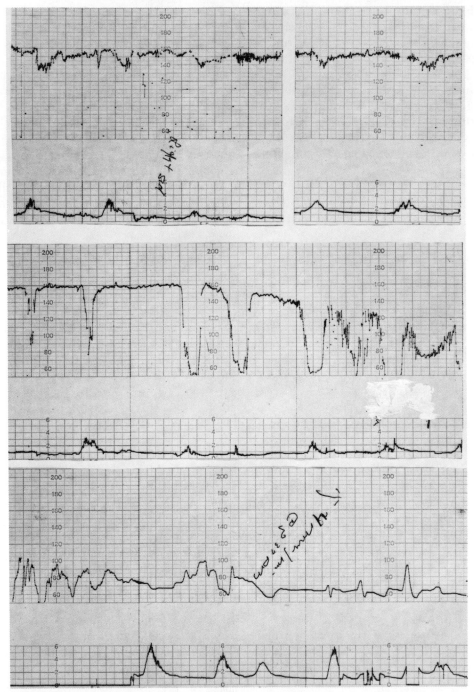

Fig. 12-11. A dying 690-g human fetus from probable abruptio. Upper FHR recordings are from an external Doppler recording showing "late decelerations." Latter (middle) recording is from a scalp ECG pickup showing vagal abrupt bradycardia and lower recording is terminal event with loss of BBV. Paper speed 1 cm/min.

ments appeared to be occurring, but over 15 min time, the fetus "expired." An emergency cesarean section was done as the scalp tracing (strip chart) showed fetal ECG complexes at

30 bpm. A complete abruptio was found; the placenta had been implanted on the posterior uterine wall and was intact. Apparently the abruptio was present prior to the aminocen-

tesis and was responsible for the bloody tap. The newborn had an occasional ECG complex recorded, but could not be revived.

Figures 12-13 and 12-14 are multiple FHR recordings of a severely growth retarded fetus, first at 34 weeks (A) showing abrupt bradycardia (X) with uterine contraction (during an OCT). At 35 weeks (B), the decelerations were less abrupt (Z) and there were no accelerations of the FHR. At 36 weeks, B scan suggested fetal growth retardation and as shown in Figure 12-14, there was a ques-

tionable late deceleration (A), then a sustained bradycardia which recovered (X), followed by fetal death 10 min later (B). At delivery, there was no amniotic fluid and the 1150-g fetus was estimated to be 38 weeks gestation. Postmortem exam showed normal urinary tract and poorly developed brain. Often, the absence of amniotic fluid is associated with abrupt FHR decelerations (Chap. 15), but this fetus failed to produce the typical vagal FHR pattern (except at 34 weeks, Figure 13, "X").

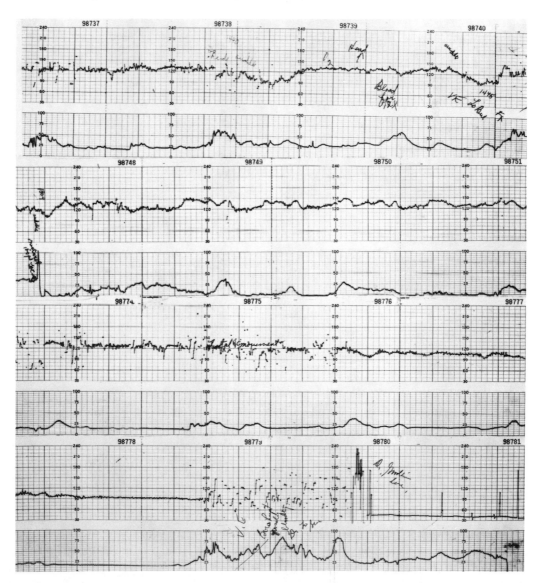

Fig. 12-12. A 3810-g post date fetus dying from an apparent abruptio. See text for details. Paper speed 3 cm/min.

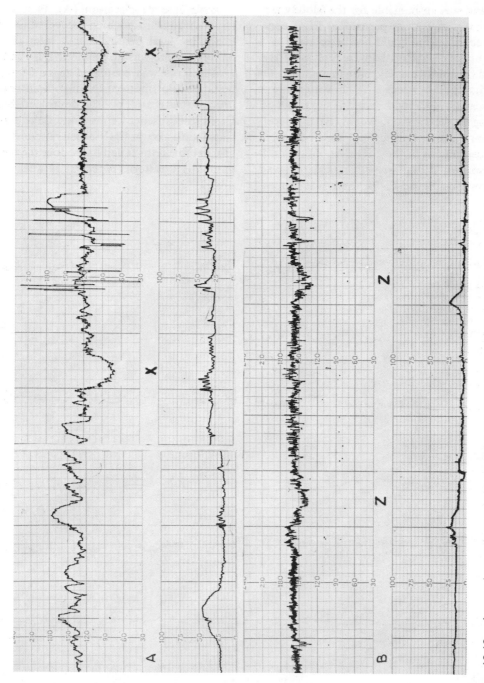

Fig. 12-13. A severely growth-retarded fetus which showed relatively "mature" FHR pattern at 34 weeks. See text for details. FHR recordings with external Doppler. Paper speed 3 cm/min.

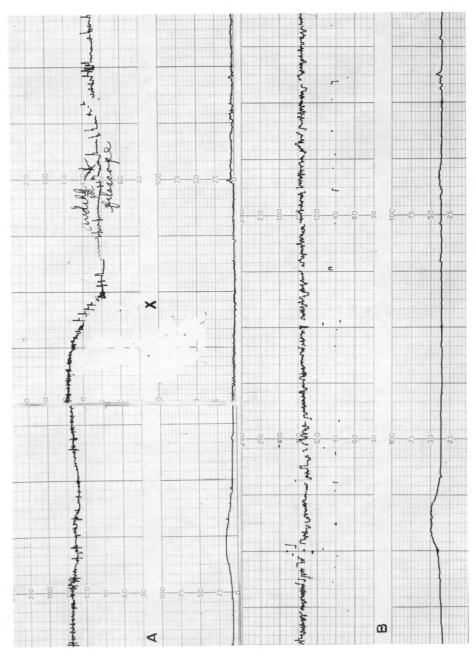

Fig. 12-14. Same fetus as Fig. 12-13, but at 35 ard 36 weeks gestation when it expired. Recordings with external Doppler at 3 cm/min.

Constant Ejection Times

During the intrapartum period (in contrast to the antenatal or newborn period), during acute bradycardia, the interval between the first and second fetal heart sounds ($S_1 - S_2$) remained relatively constant. As shown in Figure 12-15, the $S_1 - S_2$ intervals were constant over ranges of 142 bpm (1) to 64 bpm (5). But in the immediate newborn period, bradycardia is associated with changing systolic intervals, suggesting that stroke volumes do increase. There are at least two explanations for the changing stroke volumes in the newborn period. One is that the bradycardia of the intrapartum fetus is often secondary to hypertension (and that of the newborn is not) or that cardiac performance is increased in the newborn period, perhaps related to increased oxygen tensions.

False Positive FHR Tracing

We frequently find abnormal FHR tracings which cannot be confirmed either by systolic time intervals or scalp pH due to a closed cervix or technical difficulties. When the FHR pattern persists, a stat cesarean section is often done. Figure 12-16 shows such a case in which the obstetrician was certain he would find a funis occlusion because of the ominous FHR pattern. Instead, at cesarean section, the cord was free and the fetus was in excellent condition. In the nursery, the newborn's heart rate pattern was perfectly normal. The bradycardia with loss of BBV implies fetal cardiac dysfunction and not vagal activity, which is difficult to explain in a healthy fetus.

Exercise Tolerance Test (ETT) of the Fetus

Believing that maternal exercise steals blood flow from the uterus, we tested many of our high-risk gravida with the standard Master's two-step test. Figure 12-17 shows loss of fetal movements and BBV after such maternal exercise, suggesting fetal compro-

Fig. 12-15. Simultaneous intrapartum fetal EKG and heart sounds (PCG). 1–5 represent the intrapartum period, when $S_1 - S_2$ and $R - S_2$ remained relatively constant over range of FHR from 64 to 142 bpm; 6–10 represent the same individual at 2 h of age. At this time, $S_1 - S_2$ and $R - S_2$ intervals change with heart rate. (Same as Fig. 11-5).

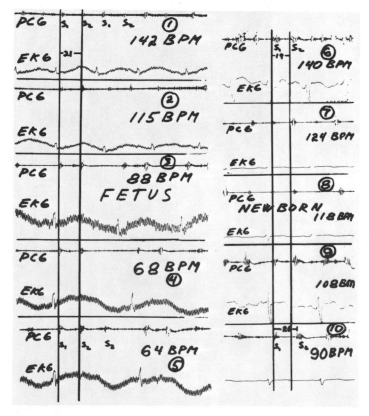

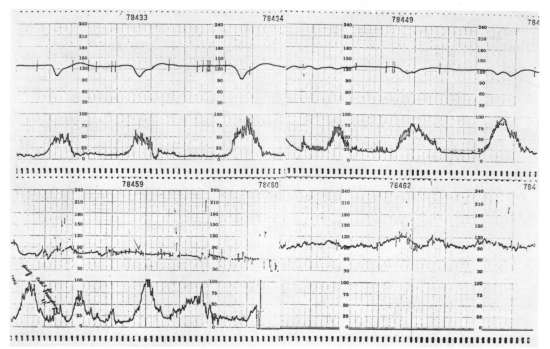

Fig. 12-16. FHR tracing showing bradycardia with loss of BBV, then severe bradycardia (459). At 460, apparent "normal" FHR but was actually maternal as fetus had died.

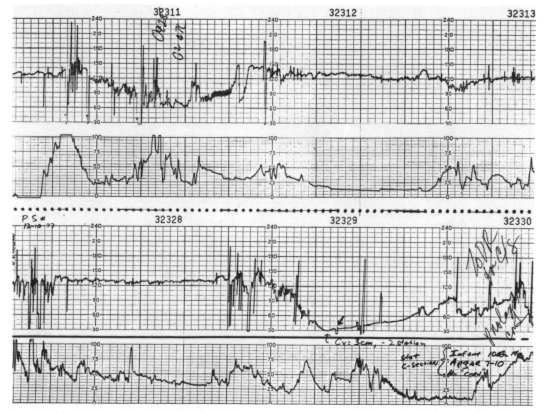

Fig. 12-17. False positive FHR tracing showing severe bradycardia with apparent uterine hypertonus in upper recording. Lower recording shows marked bradycardia (arrow) with loss of BBV. A prolapsed funis was presumed, but none was found at cesarean section.

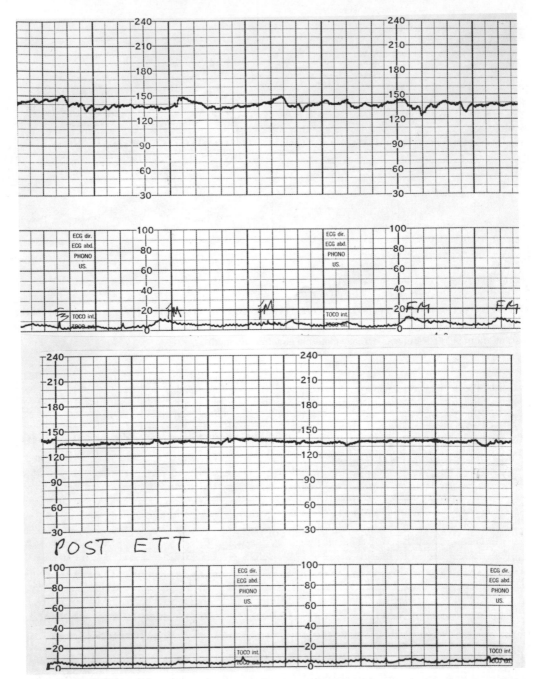

POST ETT

Fig. 12-18. An FHR recording before an antenatal two-step exercise tolerance test (upper). Lower shows marked loss of BBV and no fetal movements (FM).

mise. However, all other tests of fetal well-being (OCT, estriol, and HPL) were normal. The fetus tolerated labor without event and was normal at birth.

The gravida reported that any physical activity on her part was associated with decreased movements, suggesting that the positive ETT was real. Whether increased maternal activity would have eventually compromised the fetus is conjecture, but seems

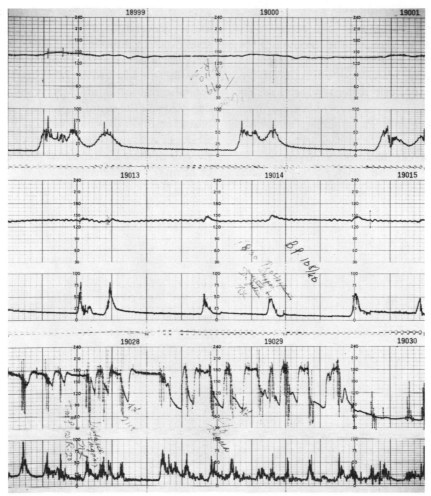

Fig. 12-19. Anencephalic fetus with intrapartum death.

reasonable. Nevertheless, such positive ETT tests have, in our experience, proved unreliable for reasons that are not understood.

Fetal Scalp Pickup of Maternal ECG

As noted above, the automatic gain control will sometimes increase until an R wave is found, adequate to trigger the pulse detector of a fetal monitor. Figure 12-18 is such a case. The FHR was very ominous, with decelerations and loss of BBV (78433). The FHR then decreased and was lost (78459). After a few minutes, the typical *maternal* heart rate pattern of good BBV at 110 bpm was recorded (78462). The physician incorrectly assumed

that a miracle had occurred and did a stat cesarean section, only to deliver a stillborn infant. In this case, the Doppler failed to detect a FHR prior to the cesarean section. I have learned through sad experience that Doppler pickup of FHR is very accurate and when absent (despite an apparent fetal scalp ECG pickup), the fetus is "dead."

The Anencephalic Fetus

Most anencephalic fetuses show loss of BBV, although I have seen two recordings of such fetal anomalies which demonstrated at least minimal BBV. Figure 12-19 is of a 36-week anencephalic fetus whose labor was induced with oxytocin and prostaglandin E_2

(dinoprostone). While the FHR recording demonstrated loss of BBV and apparent absence of vagal activity, the terminal FHR tracing (19029 of Figure 12-19) showed abrupt and severe episodes of abrupt bradycardia. This latter FHR pattern (which I usually ascribe to vagal activity) obviously may have other mechanisms. Presumably, the chemoreceptors within the heart itself can evoke this type of bradycardia during asphyxia.

Atropine may be deleterious to a fetus without higher brain centers. In both sheep fetuses decerebrated at the supracollicular level and in human anencephalic fetuses, atropinization is associated with cardiovascular failure. Most writers describe how anencephalic fetuses as an experiment of nature demonstrate the significant role of the higher brain centers in the configuration of the usual FHR. In addition, I believe they demonstrate the role of these higher centers in the function of normal vagal activity.

CHAPTER 13
Fetal Incubator Studies

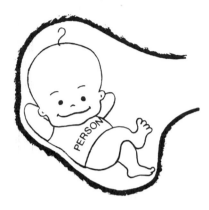

Cutaneous respiration has been an occasional topic of scientific inquiry since Gerlach's studies in 1851,[224] with even such scientific luminaries as Krogh studying[415] and speculating over its possible medical application. As an undergraduate student in J. Percy Baumberger's laboratory at Stanford University, I helped measure the transfer of both carbon dioxide and oxygen through the skin of an adult's finger. With a finger immersed in a warm physiologic saline solution, Professor Baumberger[41] demonstrated that both oxygen and carbon dioxide tension of the surrounding immersion salt solution came into rapid equilibrium with the individual arterial CO_2 and O_2 tension. He showed that this was an accurate method for continuously measuring arterial P_{O_2} and P_{CO_2}. Since the fetus is similarly surrounded in a warm, physiologic salt solution (amniotic fluid), we calculated *what* oxygen tension of the amniotic fluid would be required to supply all of the fetal oxygen requirements if there were no placental respiratory function. Based on Clement Smith's data,[636] we determined that it would require approximately 3 atm (45 lb/in.^{2}) in the surrounding fluid to satisfy the oxygen needs of a fetus.

On my return to Stanford University as an assistant professor, I immediately sought the advice of Professor Baumberger. Although he had long since retired, he and I proceeded to build a "fetal incubator." In fairness to Professor Baumberger, he sensed that cutaneous respiration had no serious medical applications, but I fearlessly plunged ahead. Within a year's time, we had constructed a stainless-steel chamber which held 20 liters of Whites or Hanks embryonic solution (Fig. 13-1); it had multiple viewports, electrical outlets, and techniques for sampling. We found that under 3 atm of oxygen, the fetal incubator could maintain an extrauterine rabbit fetus (without its placenta) with a beating heart for up to 8 days duration.

Most of the fetuses that we studied were rabbits, but we also used hundreds of mice, a few pigs, dogs, cats, and unfortunately, we studied some 40 human fetuses. Most of the human fetuses were from hysterotomies done for therapeutic abortion, although six were from apparent spontaneous abortion. The incubator attracted a great deal of lay attention and I foolishly cooperated with national magazines, television shows, radio, and local newspapers. The incubator was also finan-

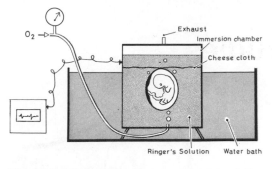

Fig. 13-1. Schematic diagram of fetal incubator. Oxygen pressure within incubator is 3 atm.

cially supported by a foundation which was interested in the fate of the premature infant.

In a few years time, we described fetal movements and responses to stimuli which were similar to those of the Japanese investigator, Chie Mori,[481] as viewed with a hysteroscope, which are also now being confirmed with both the fetoscope and ultrasound. We noted that an immature second trimester human fetus swallowed, nodded its head frequently, and rolled its body ("righting movements") constantly. If stabilized, the fetus had many less movements than when allowed to float freely in the immersion fluid. These fetuses responded to tactile and light stimuli with flinching, excreted urine, and tracheal fluid, and swallowed their own weight in amniotic fluid every 18 hr. We further showed that barbiturates protected the fetus against both hyperoxia and hypoxia. Our studies with rabbit fetuses clearly demonstrated that the fetal lung had a high fluid excretion rate and could excrete such materials as bilirubin, electrolytes, and sugar. Despite what I thought were many interesting observations, the scientific community was never enthused about the incubator and considered it only a laboratory gimmick. I thought its greatest potential was as a device to keep the immature fetus alive or as a resuscitator of a depressed, immature fetus.

The largest immature human fetuses (approximately 400–500 g) performed best and on five occasions, I was given (with parental permission) immature human fetuses, after they had been pronounced dead by the neonatologist. The fetuses were quickly placed in iced saline and transferred to the laboratory where they were immersed in White's solution and gradually warmed in the hyperbaric oxygen chamber. All five fetuses revived with heart rates of up to 190 bpm and three began active body movements of swallowing, nodding, and turning. One fetus had a heart rate for 5 days. Death in these fetuses, as with all others, was associated with infection and hypercarbia. The apparatus had many problems, but I was convinced that given more financial support, they could be solved, but this optimism was brought to a halt by the local Pro-Life group.

In my initial report, I had described how we had opened the fetuses' chests (thoracotomies) in order to prove that the fetus' heart was beating. There were a number of reasons for this procedure which laymen (particularly the Pro-Life group) found to be offensive and intolerable. In the early 1960s, as now, it was commonly believed that a fetal heart could produce an ECG long after it had ceased to beat and only by opening the chest could I prove that such fetuses indeed had beating hearts. In addition, as a house officer, I had witnessed and participated in many open heart cardiac massages, as that was the accepted procedure in my hospital when patients appeared to have died. In those very few cases in which the patient recovered, I recall none having any memory of pain associated with their resuscitation. In addition, the immersion fluid of the fetal incubator usually contained barbiturates, was run at a temperature of 30°C, (hypothermia) and was generally an anesthetic-type condition. We never did thoracotomies, of course, when the immersed fetus showed any signs of life. When Doppler FHR monitors became available, we were most happy to dispense with the thoracotomies, as then we could demonstrate a beating heart without jeopardizing the fetus. In all, approximately 20 human fetuses had thoracotomies, and some lived for as long as 17 hr after the procedure. Prior to beginning these studies with the human fetuses, I had sought local legal advice and was told that fetuses delivered because of a therapeutic abortion did not have the rights of a human and therefore were not covered by the various ethical and moral codes.

I had become known to Pro-Life because I had foolishly answered an inquiry from one of their local officers about whether the immature fetus could feel pain, had responses, and so forth. (We still receive requests from similar groups.) I sent them my reprints and also described in great detail about the fetus's response to stimuli. The result of their reaction to my studies at Stanford University forced me to close the laboratory and I nearly lost my medical license. The State Legislature passed a law forbidding such "research" and granting agencies withdrew support, refused me further funds, and even publicly denied that they had ever supported the "fetal incubator."

It now seems, in retrospect, that the studies should not have included human fetuses, but unfortunately, they performed better in the incubator than any other species. If it is unacceptable to immerse and study nonviable human fetuses from therapeutic abortions, I still believe that the immersion technique has something to offer the sick neonate.

As shown in Figure 13-2, immersion of the sick neonate was described a century ago and apparently was used at intervals in Europe.[242] The value of immersing a fetus would be to remove excess carbon dioxide, for it has been repeatedly demonstrated that an individual's CO_2 tension can be brought to nearly any level if he or she is immersed in a salt solution. If the salt solution is warm and agitated and contains considerable carbon dioxide, the

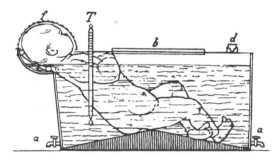

Fig. 13-2. Tubwarmer after Winchel: aa—drains; b—window; d—opening for adding water; T—thermometer; f—opening for the infant's head.

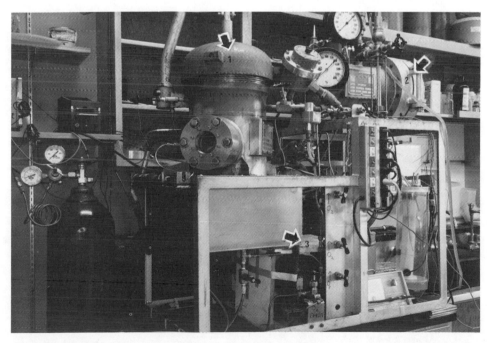

Fig. 13-3. Photograph of "fetal incubator." 1—main immersion chamber; 2 and 3 are reserve tanks.

data from the studies of warm mineral baths show that the individual takes on a considerable carbon dioxide load through the skin. On the other hand, if the immersion solution contains excess buffers and is free of carbon dioxide, the same individual will have his CO_2 lowered to nearly dangerous levels. For years, I have stood ready with a warm immersion chamber to aid the sick neonate with elevated CO_2 tensions. As yet, I have had no call for my service by any neonatologist.

In retrospect, the incubator was a most unfortunate concept for it apparently gave impetus to the Pro-Life movement at a critical time in their development. The need for observing human fetal movements can now be met with the newer ultrasonic apparatus. However, fetal responses and excretion still require extrauterine study. Cutaneous respi-

ration still should be evaluated in the small neonate with hypercarbia.

Another Point of View

Given the problems that neonatologists have in assuring normal development in the newborn under 800 g, it was clearly naive to believe that we could design an immersion fluid adequate to support such a fetus. Furthermore, our monitoring techniques were inadequate. Despite our repeated efforts at modifying conditions within the immersion chamber, as Dawes had observed, the condition of these fetuses were substantially different than those *in utero*. Dawes believed that even for experimental study, the hyperbaric immersion chamber was not an acceptable alternative. One area in which our hyperbaric chamber excelled was preservation of viable hearts and kidneys. Isolated pig hearts would continue to beat for more than 4 days.

CHAPTER 14

In Utero Breathing

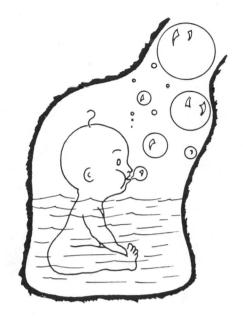

Historical Aspects

"Fetal breathing *in utero* serves to strengthen and prepare the diaphragm and chest muscles for function of respiration, but these movements are not strong enough to suck amniotic fluid further than the pharynx where it is generally swallowed. If one carefully observes the umbilical region of a thin woman, pregnant and near term, one may discover fine rising and falling movements of the abdominal wall. They occur 60–80/min and are intermittent and are most pronounced in the region of the child's chest." So stated DeLee[153] in his early 20th-century American obstetrical text. Ahlfeld, as quoted by DeLee, had carefully studied (Fig. 14-1) these abdominal wall movements in pregnant women and became convinced that they were due to minute fetal breathing efforts. Using a cardiograph, he was able to show that when the *in utero* fetal chest expands, its abdomen contracted, and vice versa. Subsequent American textbooks suggested that such observations were probably inaccurate and the conclusion was generally reached that the human fetus *in utero* was apneic, unless stimulated, although as noted in a review by

Duenhoelter and Pritchard,[169] several investigators (1930 1940) agreed with Ahlfeld's 19th-century conclusions.

In 1969, Jost and Quilligan[388] demonstrated that *in utero* sheep fetuses display REM (rapid eye movement) sleep patterns which were associated with marked activity of their cardiovascular systems. Unfortunately, they did not measure tracheal pressures and although we had observed in the chronic fetal sheep preparation shallow, rapid fluctuations of tracheal pressure, we were unable to satisfactorily record fetal EEG's. Dawes' laboratory in England was able to put everything together and showed convincingly in the chronic fetal sheep preparation that these rapid, shallow fluctuations of tracheal pressure were correlated with REM activity of the fetal cortex.

One type of *in utero* breathing that has long been recognized by both laymen and physicians is the fetal hiccup. While it had been described in the obstetrical literature as early as 1880 by Mermann,[470] it was Ahlfeld[9] who described the pattern of the human fetal hiccup in detail. Fetal hiccups occur at a frequency of 10–30 per minute, are often regu-

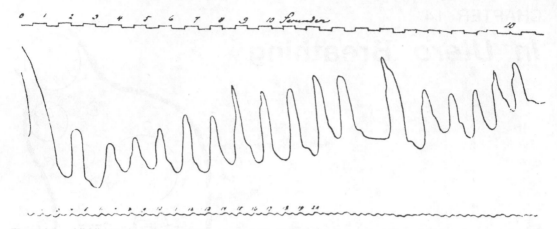

Fig. 14-1. Middle tracing demonstrates movements of fetal chest recorded through the maternal abdominal wall with the use of a glass funnel and kymograph: fetal chest wall movements averaged 54 per minute. Top recording shows time in seconds. Bottom tracing demonstrates maternal radial pulse. (After Ahlfeld, F.: Die intrautorine Taetigkeit der Thorax-und Zerchefellmuskulatur. *Intrauterine Atmung Monatsschr Geburtschilfe* **21:** 143, 1905.)

lar, visible through the abdominal wall, and at times apparently "audible" to the keen observer. Such *in utero* hiccup was described to occur as early as the fifth month of pregnancy and with most fetuses had a definite cyclic pattern of activity.

Clinical Application

Following Dawes' description of sheep fetal breathing, there occurred an outburst of clinical reports, mainly from the British Isles. But from a practical standpoint, clinical measurements of fetal breathing activity depends on the availability of a high resolution ultrasonic scanner (Fig. 14-2). A few years ago, I sought to apply the A-scan technique to the detection of fetal breathing. It seemed to be a simple method to master but was obviously inaccurate in our hands (see Case History section).

Others have trained themselves to "hear" fetal breathing with the standard FHT doppler instrument.

Using the intrapartum scalp blood pulse recorder in the late 1960s, we soon learned to recognize fetal alpha waves (Herring Breuer waves) as fluctuations of the baseline which are indicative of fetal CNS breathing activity (Fig. 14-3). Our interest waned in this indicator of fetal brain respiratory activity for it

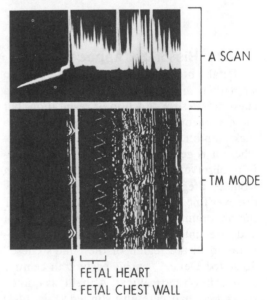

Fig. 14-2. A-scan utlrasound of fetal chest. Time–motion (TM) mode demonstrates both fetal heart motion and chest wall motion. (From Fox, H.E. and Hohler, C.W.: In *Ultrasonography in Obstetrics Gynecology*, R.E. Sanders and A.E. James, Eds. Appleton-Century-Crofts, New York, 1977. Reproduced with permission.)

soon became apparent that such fetal breathing (alpha waves) was directly correlated with a degree of "reactivity" of the FHR pattern (Chapter 9). While studies of fetal breathing activities are obviously of academic interest, they seem to have little direct clinical application. For it now appears that the same information regarding the state of fetal arousal (health) may be obtained from the degree of reactivity of the FHR pattern or even more simply, by asking the gravida how active is her fetus.

There are, however, at least two clinically significant fetal breathing patterns (grunting and gasping). Fetal grunting may be a deleterious cardiovascular activity in terms of its associated decreased cardiac performance. Fetal gasping in the presence of meconium in the amniotic fluid (Chapter 20) may be related to the subsequent development of meconium aspiration.

Not unexpectedly, drugs markedly influence fetal breathing activity, just as they do arousal levels. In a chronic fetal sheep preparation, sedatives, especially barbiturates and general anesthetics, markedly diminish fetal respiratory motions, and all other signs of

increased fetal arousal levels. On the other hand, isoproterenol causes the sheep fetus to take large gasps, and, to a lesser degree, so do sodium cyanide, lactic acid, and doxapram. While drugs may be used purposefully to induce apnea (Chapter 20), the drug "induction" of breathing can only be condemned.

The possibility that the fetal lung can serve as an organ of excretion and absorption is one that we have studied,[258] as did Adams *et al*.[2a] In rabbits,[248] we observed that the fetal alveolar membrane appeared to excrete bilirubin, chloride and urea, and to absorb glucose. I was unable to confirm these observations in the fetal sheep. In human fetuses with renal agenesis, we have found a high concentration of urea in the scant amount of amniotic fluid available in these cases, suggesting some sort of nonrenal fetal excretion (skin, cord, lung, etc.). There is no apparent clinical implication for fetal lung alveolar function, except to note that it probably ex-

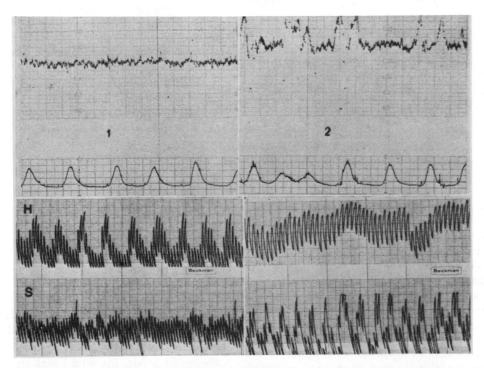

Fig. 14-3. Simultaneous cardiotocogram and hallux (H) and fetal scalp (S) pulse recordings during relatively silent (1) and responsive (2) fetal phases are seen. Hallux pulse (H) demonstrates fluctuating base-line seen in many parturients, waves which are correlated with maternal breathing. In "active" fetuses, similar baseline fluctuations are seen, suggesting fetal breathing or movement.

ists. For instance, the newborn with a hypoplastic lung secondary to a diaphragmatic hernia is otherwise "normal" and not at special risk of being stillborn. Since the *in utero* fetus is required to maintain the proper placental gradients despite wide changes in maternal colloid osmotic pressure and with immature renal function, I have considered that osmoregulation may be a function of the fetal alveolar membrane. In fetal sheep, we found that with reduced plasma COP, lung excretion was increased.

Another Point of View

The British school holds that the measurements of human fetal breathing is of clinical value.[346] As reviewed by Manning of Los Angeles,[460] there are three patterns of breathing movements *in utero*. The most common is a small-amplitude chest movement that increases to a peak level of activity and then gradually subsides and is associated with fetal movements. The second type is large amplitude chest movements interspersed with the small-amplitude activity. Fetal movements are less common apparently with this type of activity. The third is the hiccups which are isolated, large amplitude, and sometimes exceedingly fast movements. These patterns may apparently all occur independently or in various combinations. Boddy of England has attempted to correlate human fetal well-being with these types of fetal breathing activity. As might be expected, those fetuses which showed apnea throughout most observations were in poor condition more frequently than those demonstrating breathing activity. Those showing mixed patterns, which he defined as fetal breathing movements during less than 50% of the observation time, together with isolated, deep, prolonged chest wall movements, was also associated with a high degree of fetal distress in labor. Maternal drugs such as diazepam, sparine, amytal, methyldopa, all suppress fetal breathing even when maternal sedation is minimal.[61a] Manning believes that fetal breathing activity is an accurate index of the fetal condition. He cautions, however, that any clinical application must await extensive clinical research. This is especially so since fetal breathing has no known function, other than practice for extrauterine life.

Unfortunately, investigators of fetal breathing have not rigorously compared this parameter with that of fetal movement. In part, this may reflect the fact that ultrasound stimulates the fetus. Fetal movements then are very common during an ultrasound examination and may give a false impression of the degree of fetal respiratory motion.

Lewis and Trudinger[435] have linked the maternal sensation of fetal hiccups with fetal observation through a real-time ultrasonic scanner. They describe the "hiccupping" movement as often violent, often jolting the whole fetus. Such fetal hiccups are interspersed between rapid fetal chest wall movements, which are not felt by the mother.

Duenhoelter and Pritchard[169] concluded in their 1977 review that it is not clear whether monitoring fetal breathing will provide an index of fetal well-being. They also questioned whether induction of fetal apnea is ever of value, a concept I believe is "proven" (Chapter 20).

A more important clinical question than *in utero* fetal respiratory motion is, perhaps, what initiates effective newborn breathing. Harned has recently reviewed the subject and still apparently agrees with Burn's older view, that at the time of birth the central respiratory neurons received massive nonrespiratory neuron activity which initiates rhythmic activity in the respiratory center itself. Our studies of 1969 demonstrated that a host of various stimuli appeared to initiate regular breathing in newborn sheep. These stimuli include cold, asphyxia, acidemia, and perhaps even noise.

From a clinical standpoint, the importance of *in utero* fetal breathing is related only to the possible occurrence of meconium aspiration. Monitoring of fetal breathing adds no clinical information to that obtained by the FHR monitor or maternal diaries of fetal movements.

Case No. 14-1

An unregistered gravida at term with a history of decreased fetal movements was examined, and no FHT were heard. While searching for the fetal heart with ultrasound on the M mode, the fetal heart appeared to be beating very slowly, but there also appeared to be fetal "respirations" at approximately 70–80 cycles/min. An amniocentesis produced heavily stained fluid and an immediate cesarean section was done. The fetus was stillborn and macerated. Apparently, the movements of the maternal aorta "bounced" the fetus at a frequency somewhat different than that of the maternal heart rate. In our inexperience, we interpreted this movement as that of fetal respirations.

The use of ultrasound for determining fetal breathing activity is still a research technique.

CHAPTER 15
Amniotic Fluid

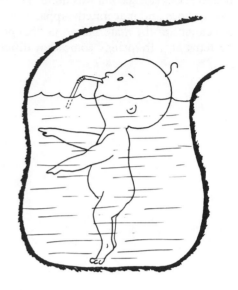

Historical Aspects

It was Hippocrates who postulated that amniotic fluid was a product of the fetal kidneys. In the early 20th century, DeLee[152] administered methylene blue to gravida in labor and while finding the fetal urine stained, noted that the amniotic fluid was clear. He concluded that the fetus did not void (an observation which may be true in stressful labor). Holtermann[348] performed a similar study and made the same conclusion, and for decades it was assumed that fetal urine was not a contributor to amniotic fluid. In 1963, Thomas *et al.*[696] was apparently the first to record a common observation, mainly that with injection of contrast media into either the uterine arteries or amniotic sac, the fetal kidneys excrete the radioopaque dye. The association of oligohydramnios with renal agenesis was noted by Atospa-Sison[24] in 1936 and was popularized by Potter in 1946.[537] The relationship between fetal kidneys and amniotic fluid was somewhat confused by reports of hydramnios with renal agenesis.

In early pregnancy, Van Wagenen and Newton showed that removal of the fetus in

pregnant monkeys resulted in a transudate of maternal plasma filling the amniotic sac (and the contents being delivered at term).[713a] More extensive studies were made in monkeys by Berkman[44a] who postulated that in early pregnancy the amniotic fluid (but not the cells) represented a maternal transudate. The ability to detect fetal enzymes in amniotic fluid in early pregnancy (for genetic studies) seems to argue against this concept (Tables D-68–D-75).

Studies by Hutchinson[366] have suggested that the umbilical cord contributes large quantities of water to the amniotic fluid. Reynolds[568] proposed that the fetal lungs were a source of fluid. The fetal salivary glands, buccal mucosa, and skin are also theoretical sources.[608a]

It was the classical isotope studies of Vosburgh[719] that demonstrated that the amniotic fluid is not a static reservoir, but represents a continuous exchange between the gravida and her fetus. (Such informative studies are now no longer possible.) The turnover is so rapid that an error of 1% could increase amniotic fluid volume 1 liter every 10 days.[341] It is confusing why gravida with ruptured membranes lose, on a chronic basis, only a few ounces a day. Apparently, one concept (rapid exchange) deals with molecular diffusion and the other (slow exchange) with bulk flow.

Taussig[678] suggested that the fetus swallows amniotic fluid as most any amniogram will demonstrate. Pritchard[551a] showed in 1966 that the term fetus swallowed approximately 500 ml of fluid a day, approximately equal to its urine output.

While yellow amniotic fluid was noted more than a century ago in cases of hydrops fetalis, it was Bevis[51] who related the severity of the hemolytic disease to the bilirubin-like pigments in amniotic fluid.

The cellular elements of amniotic fluid were studied by Robin in 1904. Prenatal sex determination was first made by Bosa and Fanard in 1951,[64a] followed by Makowski et al. in 1956.[458]

In 1961, Fuchs and Philips[215] obtained karyotypes from amniotic fluid and Nadler's laboratory has systematically described multiple enzymes (Tables D-67–D-75) present in amniotic fluid, useful for genetic diagnosis.

Amniotic Fluid

AMNIOTIC FLUID VOLUME

Amniotic fluid volume in late pregnancy is apparently kept in proper balance by fetal voiding and swallowing. Serious fetal abnormalities or illness are frequently associated with abnormal amounts of amniotic fluid. Excess amounts of amniotic fluid are seen with defects of fetal swallowing as occur with brain defects, gastrointestinal lesions, and fetal heart failure. Oligohydramnios may be found in cases of renal agenesis and/or dysplasia, urinary tract obstruction, and the chronic leakage of amniotic fluid. Aside from these lethal fetal defects, which are probably responsible for the abnormal amniotic fluid volume, "secondary" anomalies indirectly associated with decreased amniotic fluid, such as hypoplastic lungs and limb abnormalities, are important to the fetus' extrauterine survival.

OLIGOHYDRAMNIOS

Reduced amounts of amniotic fluids may be associated with cases of severe in utero growth retardation (IUGR). When it can be sampled, the fluid demonstrates abnormalities of color and content. The creatinine and urea contents may be markedly elevated and the fluid shows a high Δ450 value. The lack of fluid in growth-retarded fetuses may itself be deleterious to the welfare of the fetus. Freeman and James[206] believed that funis compression is more likely to occur under these circumstances of reduced amniotic fluid volume, which may actually lead to added stress or to fetal death.

Thomas and Smith[697] have ascribed the newborn pulmonary hypoplasia associated with oligohydramnios to the consequences of external (uterine) compression upon the fetal thoracic cage. (Why this fetal compression does not occur in pregnancies with normal amounts of fluid is unclear.) In cases of newborn pulmonary hypoplasia, the pulmonary abnormality appears to be a defect of late development, as the bronchi and bronchioles are adequately developed. Incomplete lung development similar to that seen in oligohydramnios are also found in cases of diaphragmatic hernia and thoracic deformaties such as Jeune's thoracic dystrophy syndrome.[697] Potter herself believes[537] that the clinical association of absent amniotic fluid and pulmonary hypoplasia indicates the importance of the fluid in development of the lungs. Duenhoelter and Pritchard[169] likewise found that significant amounts of amniotic fluid is exchanged through the tracheal–bronchial tree is evidenced by absorption through the fetal alveoli in apparently normal human fetuses. From our fetal incubator studies,[247] (Chapter 6) we reported significant fetal breathing activity in rodents and absorption and excretion through fetal alveoli. However, current thinking is that while the fetus breathes in utero, the amounts of fluid exchanged through its trachea is insufficient to play a significant role in lung development. A compelling argument for the lack of significance of amniotic fluid, and the importance of amniotic volume, in fetal lung development is the report of normal pulmonary development in cases of tracheal agenesis or obstruction.[195]

In addition to the pulmonary abnormalities associated with the reduced amounts of amniotic fluid are those of the fetal face and limbs. The typical fetus with oligohydramnios (Potter's syndrome) has a flat nose, aberrantly flattened ears, talipes equinovarous, and limbs that tend to wrap around themselves.[537] In those cases of reduced amniotic fluid associated with chronic leakage in which a band of amnion may form, amputation of extremities, and even the nose are seen.[30, 701] On our service, approximately one to two cases of limb amputations in otherwise normal infants are delivered per thousand deliveries. These fetal amputations are generally associated with chronic leakage of amniotic fluid and gravida with prolonged rupture of the membranes should be warned of this risk. We have sought to diagnose such limb amputations in utero in these cases of chronic fluid leakage by a roentgenogram, but to date have been unsuccessful even when a limb amputation was present. Because of secondary effects, absent amniotic fluid can then have ominous significance for the fetus, even when its' urinary tract is apparently normal.

In cases of fetal growth retardation associated with oligohydramnios, fetal death is an increased risk. I do not accept the concept that actual funis occlusion is more likely,[206] but rather that the absence of amniotic fluids indicates just long-standing fetal illness. If funis occlusion risks were related to the relative absence of amniotic fluid, the incidence of silent fetal death would be inversely related to amniotic fluid volume and this is not so. For instance, fetuses with Potter's syndrome do not have an appreciably high stillborn rate although neonatal mortality is 100%. McLain[498] demonstrated that chronically distressed fetuses swallowed amniotic fluid at a faster rate than did normal fetuses. Chronically ill (growth-retarded) fetuses often have little or no respiratory reserve and therefore are likely to succumb to even minor stress. The abrupt and severe vagal bradycardia (variable decelerations) frequently seen in these fetuses admittedly can represent funis compression, but even more likely is that such fetal heart rate patterns reflect low metabolic reserve and hypoxia (or even asphyxia).

The argument for fetal death from chronic asphyxia rather than funis occlusion is based on observations of the FHR patterns of such fetuses in their terminal phase (Chapter 12). It is with embarrassment that we can report these cases, for we literally allowed the fetuses to die in utero. Their FHR patterns showed occasional severe abrupt bradycardia (variable decelerations), but were mostly characterized by a nonreactive pattern suggestive of chronic asphyxia, and their terminal phases were not typical of funis compression (see Case History).

In growth-retarded human fetuses, we have attempted to instill normal saline into the amniotic space and thus create an artificial amniotic fluid hoping to "prime the well" of the amniotic sac, but to date, have been without success. Tyson et al.[709] have shown that prolactin content in amniotic fluid is extremely high. Perhaps when the significance of this prolactin is understood, it may be possible to medically treat cases of oligohydramnios and reverse the problems associated with reduced amounts of fluid. We demonstrated[254] that the human amnion responds to oxytocin and digitalis (as does the toad bladder) with changes in pore size and electrical potential. I attempted to alter amniotic volume with small but continuous amounts of oxytocin without success in gravida undergoing saline abortions. It is probable that I used the wrong hormone for prolactin has now been shown to control the salmon's gill osmoregulators, and it seems possible that this ancient hormone may do likewise with the fetal membranes. To date, we have not been able to demonstrate a deficiency of maternal prolactin levels in cases of growth-retarded fetuses, but such negative findings may reflect only our poor methodology. The concept that creation of an amniotic volume may be the essential feature of fetal growth-retarded fetuses is one that seems worthy of further pursuit. The reduced in utero fetal space only compromises the already chronically ill fetus, provides no nutrition, and may even increase the risk of funis compression.

HYDRAMNIOS

The occurrence of hydramnios is like that of oligohydramnios, a worrisome sign as regards fetal welfare. By tradition, acute hydramnios supposedly has a more ominous fetal implication than does a slowly occurring hydramnios. In approximately 25% of the cases with hydramnios, major fetal anomalies are present. The most well-known associations are anencephaly and meningocele. Actually, anything which interferes with fetal swallowing (including brain or gastrointestinal defects, or even a severe hair lip), along with chronic illness, can be associated with hydramnios. Acute hydramnios can be seen in the twin transfusion syndrome, with the maternal syndrome (Chapter 5), with diabetic pregnancies, or in cases of fetal heart failure.

Despite the advances in ultrasonography, the amniogram continues to be an important diagnostic test in gravida with hydramnios. In addition to making obvious the hydropic fetus, or those unable to swallow (contrast media in stomach within 2 hr), it provides a hint at some general illnesses (or states of health) that such fetuses may have. Radioactive contrast media injected into the amniotic space carries a small risk of induction of labor,[257] but it is essential to determine the fetal rate of swallowing. The "rapid" swallower is often difficult to discern as "he" may appear to swallow less because the contrast media itself is bitter. His rate of swallowing may also depend on his arousal level or on how the solution "tastes." In general, contrast media can be seen as early as 1 hr after injection in the rapid swallower's small intestine. The slow swallower, however, may not have contrast media in its small intestine for a matter of days. While there is concern now about the ultimate fate of such fetuses because of the apparent antithyroid effects of such iodinated contrast media, we still perform such fetal swallowing studies whenever

there is a hint of abnormal amounts of amniotic fluid. We have attempted to discern such fetal abnormalities as tracheo-esophageal fistula, but failed even when it was present.

Another test which we find useful in gravida with hydramnios is maternal HCG levels. When placental mass is increased, it apparently may be the etiology of the excess fluid, and maternal HCG levels are often markedly elevated (Chapter 5). This seems to be part of the "Ballantyne's triple edema" syndrome (maternal, fetal, and placental edema plus hydramnios) and in my experience suggests the only chance for fetal survival is immediate delivery. When fetal movements are diminished and FHR patterns are normal (NST or OCT), but fetal swallowing is absent, the fetus may be in heart failure and hydramnios (instead of pulmonary edema). We have used digitalis therapy in an attempt to correct this condition. The dose is critical as fetal death may occur after direct fetal injection of toxic amounts. Unfortunately, maternal digitalization or diuretic therapy has been of no benefit. In two cases, we did inject the pediatric dose of digitalis into the fetal buttock and in one there appeared to be a marked improvement in the hydramnios and fetal activity. Both fetuses died *in utero* 2 days after their "treatment."

TWIN TRANSFUSION SYNDROME

Likewise, in cases of the twin transfusion syndrome, we have attempted digitoxin therapy but instead of attempting to correct a heart failure, the dose of digitoxin was designed to sacrifice the smaller fetus. While the larger fetus may obviously receive part of the dose given to the small fetus (they have in part a common circulation), it appeared that the risk was worthwhile as the situation was truly desperate. As Benirschke has suggested,[44] unless one of the twins dies or they are delivered, both are due to an *in utero* death because of heart failure in one and hypoxia in the other. Now that our neonatal colleagues are doing so well with 1 kg and larger newborns, it may be better management to deliver such fetuses even when only of 28-week pregnancies.

Thus, the ill fetus may be associated with either abnormally large amounts or small amounts of amniotic fluid. The difference between these degrees of amniotic fluid volume apparently relate to relative fetal cardiovascular function and to how much fluid the fetus swallows. In cases of erythroblastosis fetalis, infants of diabetic mothers, and those of the twin transfusion syndrome, there is a suggestion of heart failure plus the obvious problem of decreased fetal swallowing (oligopsia). On the other hand, possibly in an effort to obtain more nutrients, the chronically stressed fetus engages in increased swallowing (polyopsia) and therefore has decreased amounts of amniotic fluid.

THERAPEUTIC AMNIOCENTESIS

Amniotic fluid is generally regarded as a constantly changing fluid, and has its obstetrical value only as a source of sampling and the fact that its volume, within limits, has little influence on fetal welfare. There is admittedly much clinical support for this view.[605] In midtrimester, nearly all of the amniotic fluid can be removed without seemingly endangering the fetus' health. On several occasions, in pregnancies of 20 to 26 weeks gestation with "hourglassing" of the membranes through an incompetent cervical os, we have removed abdominally 150–200 ml of fluid (this allows the membranes to be "stuffed" back through the cervix). Providing that amnionitis and/or labor do not occur, the pregnancies proceeded uneventfully after the cerclage, for the amniotic fluid volume was quickly reformed. However, it is in the third trimester that I believe amniotic fluid volume per se is important to the otherwise normal fetus.

I have already noted our failure to increase amniotic fluid volumes with medical therapy (low dose oxytocin, digitalis, etc.), or by infusions of either balanced salt solutions or nutrients. We have also failed to improve fetal welfare in cases of hydramnios by repeated or chronic taps of the amniotic sac. In my experience, infection and/or labor complicates their management. However, Pitkin[545] has managed successfully such cases with chronic drainage. Perhaps "prolactin-like" stimulation may be of aid in the future.

CLINICAL OBSERVATIONS

The twin transfusion syndrome with hydramnios is one that I fail to understand. I can visualize why a small artery-to-vein shunt in the placentas of identical twins leads to heart failure, polycythemia, or anemia. However, we recently had a case of identical twins deliver at 36 weeks in which a major umbilical arterial branch of one twin was intertwined on the placenta with a major umbilical vein of the other twin. In this example of major arterial–venous cross circulation, both twins were normal with absolutely no evidence of the twin transfusion syndrome.

There is one clinical observation, which in my teaching experience, requires emphasizing again and again. If membranes are artifically ruptured and no amniotic fluid is found, the fetal situation is ominous. Either renal agenesis, severe postmaturity, or dysmaturity is present. In the majority of cases with true absence of amniotic fluid, abnormal FHR patterns will occur and prompt some sort of response. If fetal abnormality has been previously considered, this response will perhaps be more appropriate. The usual situation is that after failing to find amniotic fluid, the obstetrician convinces himself (herself) that the membranes have previously ruptured and therefore fails to take advantage of this very significant sign of chronic fetal distress. Such situations are fortunately rare (1–2 per 1000 births), but correct interpretation of this sort of event, in my opinion, distinguishes the true specialists. On the other hand, hydramnios is so obvious after rupture of the membranes, that we seldom fail to recognize that the fetus is high risk.

In performing amniocentesis, occasionally one obtains dark brown ("tobacco juice") fluid. After midpregnancy, this sort of amniotic fluid indicates fetal death[244] and is a useful confirmatory test for fetal demise. However, the aspiration of such dark amniotic fluid in the early second trimester has no special significance as regards fetal health. We have found such fluid on numerous occasions when performing saline abortions,[254] and when doing amniocentesis for chromosome analysis. In the later group, the fetuses were normal. As Seller[624] has suggested, the fluid color is probably due to old hemoglobin. On two occasions, we have removed by hysterotomy the 14-week fetus and its membranes intact, only to see the chorionic sac still present and filled with such "tobacco juice" fluid with a relatively clear inner amniotic sac. Amniocenteses at 14 weeks of pregnancy may then actually be a "choriocentesis." Sometimes the chorionic sac does not disappear at 8–10 weeks and its presence or rupture at 20–24 weeks often leads to clinical confusion (Chapter 22).

Case Histories

The commonly accepted mechanisms of amniotic fluid formation have failed to explain a number of the cases that we have seen.

Case No. 15-1

A newborn was delivered at term by repeat cesarean section. As part of an ongoing study, amniotic fluid was obtained at the time of delivery which had essentially normal chemical values. Demonstrating considerable skill, the neonatal team diagnosed a tracheoesophageal fistula and before the newborn was 4 hr of age, the defect was surgically repaired. Unfortunately, it was not until the child was 36 hr of age that it was noted the child had no kidneys (renal agenesis). At postmortem examination, the child's lungs appeared to be normally developed. Its normal newborn lung was difficult to understand for it was doubtful whether as a fetus it could have "breathed" adequately with its tracheoesophageal fistula. For, presumably, the tracheoesophageal fistula allowed G.I. fluids to maintain lung development and form am-

niotic fluid. It had immediate respiratory difficulty as a newborn.

Case No. 15-2

A growth-retarded fetus (1.6 kg at term) with hydramnios was delivered with a large (1.1 kg) placenta. The case was even more striking because the mother demonstrated the "maternal syndrome" with massive edema, but the fetus (not its placenta) was literally just the opposite for it appeared to be dehydrated. This exception to the triple edema syndrome of Ballantyne was perhaps explained at postmortem examination when a "parachute anomaly" of the fetal mitral valve was noted. Apparently, the fetus had right-sided heart failure with a large, edematous placenta (hyperplacentosis). The placenta (or umbilical cord) appeared to be the source of the hydramnios and maternal edema. Support for this concept came from finding that the maternal levels of HCG were elevated markedly. Why this particular fetal heart anomaly was associated with such an hydropic placenta is not clear.

Case No. 15-3

An anomaly which in my experience is limited to the Mexican–American population was seen in four cases. Ballantyne's syndrome appeared at around the 31st week of pregnancy and the fetus demonstrates scalp edema on ultrasonic scanning (Fig. 15-1). These gravida previously have had normal pregnancies. The maternal HCG levels are elevated, but the estriol and oxytocin challenge tests are within normal limits for this period of gestation. To date, I have been unsuccessful in convincing the responsible physicians in the four cases to deliver the fetus immediately. Instead, because of absence of laboratory abnormalities and marked prematurity, all four fetuses were allowed to die *in utero*. Extensive postmortem studies of these hydropic fetuses, their hydropic placentas, serum, and hemoglobins, have not suggested an etiology. One affected gravida has had a subsequent normal preg-

Fig. 15-1. An ultrasound picture of unexplained fetal hydrops (scalp edema), hyperplacentation and hydramnios. (Courtesy of A. Curtis, M.D.)

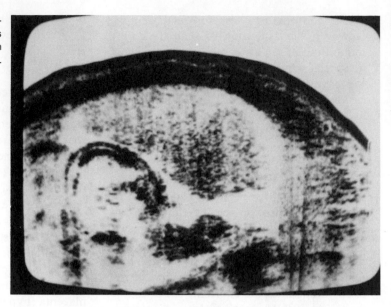

nancy. The placenta in these cases was similar from an histological standpoint to that seen in erythroblastosis fetalis.

Case No. 15-4

One that already has been alluded to or that seen with the growth-retarded fetus without amniotic fluid. Our first impression in these cases has been that they represent "Potter's syndrome," which in two cases has, from the fetus' standpoint, been a disastrous impression. Both of these fetuses demonstrated no amniotic fluid or urine on ultrasonic scanning and had apparently normal fetal movements virtually up until the time of their deaths. Their FHR recording did demonstrate the abrupt-type bradycardia (variable deceleration). The FHR in the terminal phases became nonreactive. We made our decisions for delivery too late in both cases and delivered a 1.1 and a 1.2 kg stillborn fetus whose gestational ages appeared to be between 36 and 37 weeks. Despite the features of a typical Potter's syndrome, both stillborns had normal urinary tracts. As has been previously discussed, I believe that the absent amniotic fluid reflects the fetus' chronic distress with increased swallowing. It would seem that intraamniotic infusions of nutrients, besides expanding the deficient amniotic space would be theoretically of benefit.

Whether immediate delivery at some point during their last 2 weeks would have been wise, as they appeared to have hypoplastic lungs and very immature cerebral cortexes, is doubtful. They were not, in other words, the typical type-2 growth-retarded fetus.

Case No. 15-5

Perhaps the most interesting case I have seen with hydramnios was one associated with a "thanatophoric dwarf."[280] Actually, as six letters to the editor after our paper indicted, it was not a thanatophoric dwarf, but a new variety of fetal dwarfism stated by Gorlin of the University of Minnesota to be a form of "dysostotic dwarfism." This was this woman's second such infant (Fig. 15-2). While hydramnios is common in the "short-limbed dwarf," its etiology is unknown. As shown in Figure 15-2, this fetus swallowed, it had anomalies of the urinary tract, the amniotic fluid L/S was greater than 1 at term, its lungs were hypoplastic, and there was no obvious lesion of its umbilical cord or placenta which could explain the hydramnios. However, the amniotic fluid was stained, suggestive of possibly an esophageal source for the excess fluid. In sheep fetal studies,[275] I became convinced that eructation was a source of amniotic fluid. Since we had fairly well ruled out all other sources of the hydramnios in this short-limbed dwarf, I believe that eructation may likewise be a source of amniotic fluid in the human.

Another Point of View

The University of Southern California faculty have argued that it is funis compression which endangers the fetus with oligohydramnios. I regard their arguments unconvincing as all of their cases also involve chronic fetal hypoxia and/or growth retardation. Odendall[511] found an increased incidence of all types of FHR decelerations during labor in growth-retarded fetuses. He was unable to understand the higher incidence of early decelerations, believing that such FHR represented not hypoxia but head compression. My argument is that mild vagal bradycardia (early decelerations) may represent hypoxia, then such FHR patterns are understandable in the growth-retarded fetus (chronic fetal distress). My views for the role of hypoxia would be stronger if all growth-retarded fetuses showed evidence of decreased oxygenation by having elevated hematocrits. Unfortunately, such infants born in California (unlike those delivered in Colorado) usually have normal cord blood hematocrit levels. Regardless of the mechanisms, the obstetrician must keep in mind that the fetus with oligohydramnios has a higher risk of dying *in utero*.

Our European colleagues[329, 607] have been much bolder than we have in attempting supplemental fetal feedings by amnio-infusions. Evidently the problems of infection and premature labor have prevented such therapy from being used routinely in growth-retarded fetuses. Heller[329] of Frankfurt/Main reported that intrauterine amino acid feeding in four cases of fetal dysmaturity (all demonstrating abnormal HPL and estriol levels, biparietal diameters, and FHR patterns) reversed the signs of decreased placental function. Two hundred and fifty milliliters

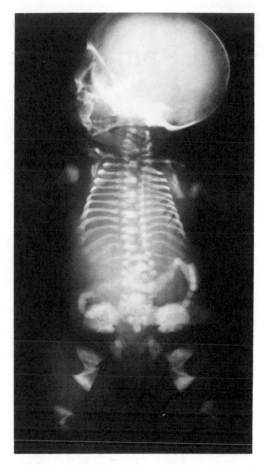

Fig. 15-2. A stillborn thanatophoric-like dwarf with contrast media in its intestine. (From Goodlin, R.C., and Lowe, E.W.: Unexplained hydramnios associated with a thanatophoric dwarf. *Am J Obstet Gynecol* **118**, 873, 1974. Reproduced with permission.)

containing 5.36 ml of amino nitrogen was infused into the amniotic sac without event. The amino acids disappeared much faster from the amniotic fluid than could be accounted for by diffusion, suggesting that the fetus consumed the nutrients.

CHAPTER 16
Fetal Pain

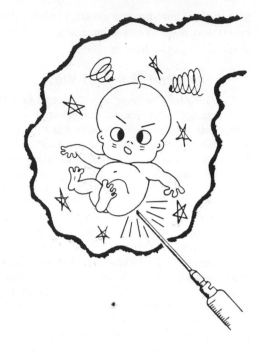

I have been thinking and writing about fetal pain for more than a decade, and now (totally unrelated to my efforts) it has become a popular topic with pseudopsychiatrists and, in my opinion, misguided obstetricians. Leboyer's "nonviolent" approach to delivery is difficult to accept, for it is the intrapartum, not the newborn period, which is filled with pain and stress for the infant. In my view, only a completely anesthetized fetus would be free of such painful intrauterine stimuli prior to birth. The obvious benefit which comes from such a so-called nonviolent delivery is the bonding allowed between the newborn and its mother.[407] Such bonding can be accomplished after any type of delivery except when general anesthesia is used.

Psychiatrists, i.e., colleagues, tell me that theories of birth pain related to subsequent psychopathology are generally held in disrepute because of lack of supporting data. There is perhaps a slight disagreement as some psychoanalysts believe there is a "birth process" occurring in the process of psychotherapy, but it does not necessarily refer to fetal pain or birth trauma that the individual may have suffered. The "primal screaming therapy" plan of Arthur Janov, as it relates to possible residual effects of birth pain or trauma, is likewise usually discounted in academic circles. Otto Rank spoke about birth being a traumatic event because it left behind a wiseful and idyllic world which, as we noted in Chapter 1, probably is not accurate from either a physiologic or a psychological aspect. We then have little support from psychiatry for our concern over fetal pain.

Although they were writing in a different time period, the early French writers spoke of "sufferance" of the fetus during labor. It still seems to be a most appropriate and modern term. Our regard is so low for the severity of newborn pain that circumcisions are routinely performed without any type of pain relief, and indeed, stressful and complicated surgery of the newborn often does not include significant pain relief. It is even more unusual for concern to be expressed over "fetal pain." An obvious exception has been Sir Albert Liley of New Zealand, where he used multiple fetal x-ray films during labor and described rather "frantic" fetal movements at the time of uterine contractions. These he believed were characteristic of a human being in severe pain, as the fetus threw its arms and legs about and appeared to actively resist each contraction with various contortions of its body.

We discovered during the performance of hundreds of amniocenteses that the healthy near term fetus responds to needle sticks (much as does any extrauterine human being) with movement and FHR change. Prior to performing the amniocentesis, we had in some cases recorded fetal heart rates for up to 5 min time. If we obviously stuck the fetus with the needle during the amniocentesis, we invariably found that the FHR abruptly changed. This was usually FHR acceleration, but sometimes a deceleration occurred in those fetuses that seemed less aroused. On the other hand, we found no constant changes of FHR when there was no apparent "feel" of puncture of the fetus with the needle, suggesting (to us) that these fetal responses were those of the pain of a needle stick. This experience is somewhat different than those of Ron and Polishuk[581a] who found FHR changed with the amniocentesis if the fetus was in good health regardless of whether the needle apparently stuck the fetus. The suggestion is that a fetus reacts to any threat to its environment or responds to maternal anxiety. A healthy fetus, in our experience, responds to being stuck by a needle both with changes in heart rate and fetal movements. In the absence of these changes and absence of clear evidence that the fetus has been stuck, we were unable to reach any conclusion as to the state of fetal health.

The occurrence of *in utero* human crying (vagitus uterinus) is sufficiently rare that when it occurs, it is often considered to be worthy of a case report. Apparently the feature that is rare is the presence of air in the fetal trachea, for after the procedure of air amniogram, "fetal crying" is often an annoying feature, even with apparently normal and nonstressed fetuses. (There is no way to prove this point, but presumably the normal fetus is frequently "crying *in utero*," but only the presence of air within the uterus makes it obvious.) According to those using air amniograms, it is often necessary to caution the mother to assume the sitting or upright position (post air amniogram) for several hours after the amniogram so that air will be kept away from the fetal larynx; otherwise, the annoyance for the gravida of hearing her unborn fetus cry.[42a] It therefore seems reasonable to assume that fetuses are often as uncomfortable (enough to cry) *in utero* as *extra utero*.

In early labor, the well *in utero* human fetus will often respond with movement or FHR change to an extrauterine sound stimulus, but commonly as labor progresses, it no longer will react.[276, 380] This is likely not a case of fetal "habituation" to a stimulus, but a result of overwhelming painful stimuli distracting the fetus from responding to the extrauterine sound stimulus. One of my interpretations of intrapartum FHR acceleration patterns is that they represent a fetal response to pain which is often later overridden by strong stress-induced vagal activity. As noted in Chapter 9, FHR changes are common when a scalp electrode or scalp sampling is done, suggestive of fetal pain response.

The newborn who demonstrates depression is usually considered to be suffering from brain edema or metabolic acidosis. When we studied the immediate newborn of mothers who had received only caudal or no drugs with responses to a loud noise stimulus in the nursery, the earliest any of the 20 newborn infants clearly responded was 18 min after delivery. These same infants did respond to head compression or nasopharyngeal suction with pronounced bradycardia. On the other hand, when five newborns were studied who had been delivered of elective cesarean section under caudal anesthesia, they responded within 3 min to the same sound stimulus. It seems entirely reasonable to me that the newborn, after a long and painful period of a crushing *in utero* existence, will seem like an adult similarly stressed, depressed, or withdrawn immediately after delivery. On the other hand, when spared these times of travail, as by elective cesarean section, it should respond to sound stimulus.

There are obviously at least two methods to avoid this period of travail for the fetus during the period of its birth. One is maternal systemic (and therefore, fetal) pain relief as was common for the parturient (and her fetus) during the 1920s and 1930s, termed "twilight sleep." With such depressive pain relief drugs, it would be necessary to have techniques to reverse their effects after birth and for many, the narcotic antagnoist Naloxone seems to be effective. The other method to avoid this period of painful birth would be to deliver everyone by elective cesarean section.

As suggested in Chaper 1, the psychiatric or neurological demonstration of birth pain is lacking. Neither is there apparent newborn data which separate birth trauma from birth pain. But my basic concept that the fetus is a person and has a psyche, and that it often responds as in pain, leads me to believe that a "humanistic" birth process should include efforts to provide a painless birth (for the fetus).

Another Point of View

The only other paper[443] concerned with fetal pain during parturition is that by the famous New Zealand obstetrician, A. W. Liley. He notes that while the fetus responds with violent movement to needle puncture, we are, nevertheless, not entitled to assert that the fetus feels pain. He also suggests that the immediate newborn probably does not (in contrast to all other times) cry for fun or joy; that pain relief in childbirth is traditionally concerned (worldwide) only with maternal pain, and reports that the first sleep of neonates is more profound than any subsequent sleep. He argues, however, that it would seem prudent to consider the possibility that birth is a painful experience for a baby. As noted in Chapter 20, the current trend is toward delivery of the alert and crying newborn. Maternal pain relief of any sort is often considered detrimental to the immediate adjustment of the newborn.

CHAPTER 17

Maternal–Fetal Acidosis

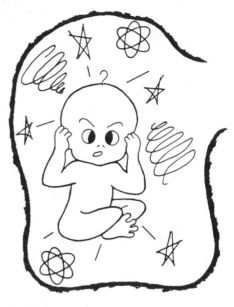

Historical Aspects

The scientific studies of fetal distress began nearly a century ago, in 1884, with Cohnstein and Zuntz's acid–base analysis of newborn animals.[115] In 1929, Siendentroph and Eissner,[631] using the hydrogen gas electrode, studied the acid–base status of the human newborn in 94 cases. Eastman,[175] in 1932, was apparently the first to correctly recognize the acid base significance of newborn asphyxia. His observations were confirmed by the 1937 Japanese studies of Noguchi,[508] who used the micro-pH electrode. From such investigations, it became apparent that the normal fetus maintained certain gradients with its mother and had a lower oxygen tension and a higher hydrogen ion and carbon dioxide concentration than its mother. With fetal asphyxia, these gradients were exaggerated. The observed increases in levels of lactic and pyruvic acids in the asphyxiated neonate were assumed to represent prior fetal anaerobic glycosis.[603]

In 1957, Irwin Kaiser and I[390] reported the results of giving ammonium chloride to nearly 200 apparently normal gravida at term. (In this time period, edema of pregnancy was considered to be a "disease" and was commonly treated with the diuretic, ammonium chloride.) Nearly all of the newborns studied showed an increased hydrogen ion concentration in their cord bloods (Fig. 17-1), with six newborns having such exaggerated responses as to show laboratory evidence of asphyxia. In addition to increased hydrogen ion concentrations, these six neonates had an increased CO_2 tension (P_{CO_2}) and lactic acid concentration while oxygen values were lower than controls (Table 17-I). The only apparent etiology for these laboratory findings was the change in maternal acid–base status that was induced by ammonium chloride administration. Clinically, while three of the six neonates were cyanotic, all did well without resuscitative efforts. Because of the apparent innocuous nature of this type of fetal acidosis, Kaiser[391] subsequently concluded that fetal acidosis could represent anything from an essentially benign condition (secondary to maternal acidosis) to

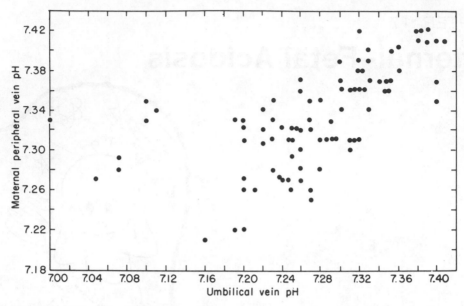

Fig. 17-1. A plot of umbilical vein pH (taken before newborn's first breath) versus maternal "arterialized" peripheral vein, of pregnancies given ammonium chloride. The six values to the left were those newborns who did not maintain the usual maternal–fetal pH gradient.

a serious morbid state (secondary to fetal asphyxia).

Relationship Between Maternal Acidemia and Fetal Asphyxia

The maternal ammonium chloride studies raised the question of why maternal acidemia can cause fetal acidemia, hypercarbia, and hypoxemia (in Tables 17-I and 17-II), and why these abnormalities occur only in selected fetuses. If fetal P_{CO_2} is increased by maternal acidemia, the decreased fetal oxygen concentration could be explained by the Bohr effect; and with a decreased oxygen content, anaerobic glycolysis would increase fetal lactic acid levels. The elevated fetal CO_2 (hypercarbia) may therefore be the essential abnormality (rather than the hypoxemia).

FETAL HYPERCARBIA

There are several possible mechanisms for the occurrence of fetal hypercarbia in the face of maternal acidosis. The mother with acidemia may herself have an increased P_{CO_2}, therefore the increased fetal P_{CO_2} may simply represent the equilibrium of CO_2 across the placenta; or the elevated fetal P_{CO_2} could

Table 17-I. Six Infants with Umbilical Vein pH Less than 7.15 of Mothers Receiving NH₄Cl

pH	CO$_2$ content	P_{CO_2}	Hemo-globin	O$_2$	O$_2$ (% sat.)
	Maternal peripheral vein at delivery				
7.30	18.7	37.7	12.9	11.0	72
(7.37)	(20.2)	(34.1)	(12.0)		
±.04 [b]	±2.6	±4.8	±1.3		
	Umbilical vein				
7.08	20.4	55.5	15.9	7.6	35.2
(7.34)	(22.9)	(41.6)	(15.3)	(12.7)	(62)
±.05	±2.8	±6.8	±0.8	±	±13
	Umbilical artery				
6.99	21.6	80.5	15.2	2.7	13.1
(7.28)	(25.4)	(52.9)	(15.3)	(5.6)	(29.0)
±.07	±2.5	±8.5	±0.9	±2.0	±10.0

[a] Values in parentheses are normal values.
[b] Standard deviation.

result from the maternal hydrogen ion (H$^+$) effect on the fetal H_2CO_3/HCO_3 equilibrium. I had observed[238] a constant bicarbonate gradient across the human placenta which suggests that since the fetal hydrogen ion concentration is always maintained above the maternal value, the fetal P_{CO_2} values would not be determined by maternal P_{CO_2} levels, but by the maternal bicarbonate and hydrogen ion concentration. This concept of a

Table 17-II. Six Infants with Umbilical Vein pH Less than 7.15 of Mothers Receiving NH₄Cl

Na (meq/liter)	K (meq/liter)	Ca, Mg (meq/liter)	Cl (meq/liter)	HCO₃ (meq/liter)	Lactic acid (meq/liter)	PO₄ (meq/liter)
		Maternal peripheral vein at delivery				
138.9	3.9	5 4	103.1	17.7	3.6	2.0
(137.8)[a]	(4.2)	(5.3)	(104.6)	(16.8)	(3.6)	(1.9)
±3.0[b]	±0.7	±0.4	±3.3	±2.0	±1.8	±0.3
		Umbilical vein				
138.3	5.4	5.9	102.9	18.4	7.4	3.3
		Umbilical artery				
139.0	5.3	5.7	104.2	19.4	9.1	3.7
(138)	(5.5)	(5.6)	(105.3)	(20.2)	(6.6)	(3.1)
±3.5	±1.3	±0.4	±2.9	±2.8	±3.9	±0.4

[a] Values in parentheses are normal values.
[b] Standard deviation.

"constant" transplacental bicarbonate gradient is consistent with the findings of Chang and Wood.[96] These investigators noted that the correlation coefficient between maternal and fetal P_{CO_2} was lower than that between maternal and fetal base excess, bicarbonate, and total CO_2.

Another possible explanation for fetal hypercarbia and hypoxemia during maternal acidemia is that the placental gas transfer is reduced, as described by Blechner et al.[58] in acute human acidemia. There may be some mechanism within the placenta (similar to the kidney) which seeks to maintain the proper fetal pH–P_{CO_2} relationship during fetal acidemia by decreasing umbilical capillary perfusion and thus elevating the fetal P_{CO_2}. This mechanism would likewise reduce fetal oxygen supply. However, studies in pregnant sheep and goats, unlike the acute human studies, have not shown any decrease in uterine or umbilical blood flow simply on the basis of increased hydrogen ion concentration. Since there appear to be several mechanisms by which maternal acidemia could produce fetal hypoxemia, they could all operate in varying degrees, producing inconsistent fetal effects.

Acute Versus Chronic Fetal Acidemia

The ammonium chloride studies suggest that the fetus appears able to tolerate the abnormal blood gases in chronic maternal acidemia. With a rapid onset of maternal acidemia, the fetus does poorly. This is seen in the many case reports of fetal death during maternal ketoacidosis and in the laboratory with acute acid loads in pregnant sheep. Given that the fetus then may be at increased risk with at least a subacute maternal acidemia, the question resolves around what can be done for the fetus' welfare. Rooth and others[583] have demonstrated that it is possible to decrease fetal hydrogen ion concentration by a treatment of the mother with bicarbonate. As these authors later noted, "the treatment of maternal metabolic acidosis by alkalizing agents in those cases where it is excessive should not only increase the maternal-fetal pH, but should also improve fetal oxygen supply." Such treatment would then offer the fetus increased oxygen in addition to that provided by oxygen administration directly to the mother.

MATERNAL SODIUM BICARBONATE INFUSIONS

Sodium bicarbonate has been infused into fetal sheep by Assali's laboratory[382] and by Helligiers and his associates.[330] Contrary to that found with maternal therapy, infusion of bicarbonate directly into the fetus has a wide spectrum of action, for it can either aggravate abnormal fetal blood gases or partially improve them. This difference in therapeutic response may be determined by whether the fetal acidemia is associated with a decrease in cardiac output (which may be improved by correcting the acidemia). Even in the healthy sheep fetus, direct infusion of bicarbonate into the umbilical circulation may increase fetal CO_2 tension and lower O_2 tension.

At one time, we measured routinely maternal pH and lactic acid levels during the intrapartum period. We used venous blood from the dorsum of the hand as it is virtually arterialized in the pregnant woman. Like so many studies that one undertakes, 3 out of the first 100 parturients had unexplained elevated blood lactic acids and lowered pH's. We did not find our next case until we had studied more than 500 parturients. Obstetricians commonly believe that they keep their laboring patients in good balance, but in case an unexpected maternal acidemia occurs, there are at least theoretical reasons to correct the maternal pH with bicarbonate.

At one time, Rooth[582] believed that maternal pH controlled fetal pH and all that was required during labor was to monitor and treat the mother's acidemia. This concept is obviously no longer held, but there still may be merit in treating fetal acidemia by maternal infusion, either intravenously or within the amniotic fluid. The acceptable methods of *in utero* treatment of fetal acidemia include maternal oxygen therapy, inhibition of uterine contractions, maternal lateral position, and maternal glucose infusions. These are discussed in greater detail in Chapter 20 and protocol P-IX. The following is a case history concerning maternal acidemia and probable fetal acidemia treated by maternal bicarbonate infusions.

Case No. 17-1

J.S. was a 23-year-old, G4-P2-1-0-2, who was followed in the Sacramento Medical Center High Risk Obstetrics Clinic because of Class C diabetes mellitus. Her prenatal course was complicated by poor diabetic control and failed clinic appointments. She presented to labor and delivery at 35 weeks of pregnancy with complaints of difficult breathing and decreased appetite. Estimated fetal weight was 4 lbs. Moderate uterine con-

tractions were noted to occur every several minutes, but the cervix was only a fingertip dilated, posterior and 25% effaced. A urinalysis showed only 3+ glucose and moderate acetone, the WBC was 17,900 with 90% total neutrophils, and a hemoglobin was 13.0 g%.

Both maternal cardiac and fetal monitoring were instituted shortly after admission. Part of the external fetal monitor tracing is shown in Figure 17-2. The tracing is initially characterized by late decelerations and maternal hyperventilation. When this FHR pattern was noted, the patient was given intravenous sodium bicarbonate and preparations for cesarean section were made. As the patient's diabetic ketoacidosis improved, contractions subsided and the frequency and intensity of late decelerations diminished. Several hours after admission, late decelerations were no longer noted in the FHR recording, but there was apparent loss of beat-to-beat variability, perhaps related to the sedation the patient had received (Fig. 17-2).

Approximately 12 hr after admission, the patient left the hospital against medical advice. She subsequently underwent an uncomplicated repeat cesarean section and tubal ligation at approximately 37½ weeks of pregnancy and the infant did well.

The opportunity to obtain a series of such cases is limited and the proper course of events would be to do a controlled study. Bicarbonate will decrease fetal hydrogen ion concentration when given to the mother and it probably crosses the placenta. It seems a logical adjuvant for a diabetic ketoacidosis when the patient is pregnant and fetal distress is suspected or when profound maternal acidemia exists.

Other Points of View

While sodium bicarbonate has often been given to correct base deficit associated with metabolic acidosis in various clinical situations, its use has come under considerable criticism. Bicarbonate infusions have been challenged in newborn resuscitation, treatment of newborn respiratory distress, salicylate poisoning, chronic renal failure, diabetic ketoacidosis, and cardiac arrest in adults.[184] The basic concern is

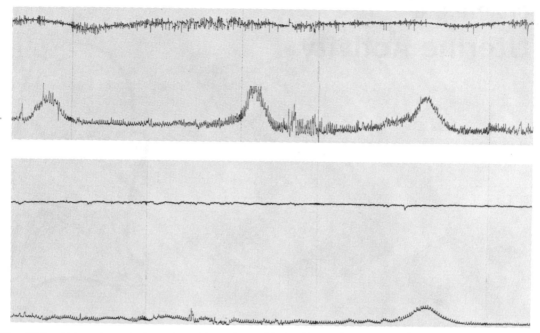

Fig. 17-2. External monitoring of gravida in ketoacidosis. Upper FHR shows "late decelerations." After bicarbonate therapy and diazepam, lower tracing was obtained (note loss of BBV). (From Goodlin, R.C., and LoBuc: *J Reprod Med* **20**: 101, 1978. Reproduced with permission.)

that bicarbonate generates carbon dioxide which diffuses easily into cerebral spinal fluid creating a paradoxical cerebral acidosis. It is presumed by some that this occurs in the fetal compartment with maternal correction of the acidemia by bicarbonate.

Longo and Power[452a] have shown in pregnant sheep that the bicarbonate ion apparently does not effectively cross the placenta, but that CO_2 as a gas does so rapidly. (If accurate for humans, bicarbonate therapy would not be logical.)

In a review of the etiology of the fetus with a false acidemia (reflecting maternal acidemia)

Roversi and associates[586] note that several investigators have shown that artifically induced maternal acidosis causes a shift of the fetal acid–base balance in the same direction. He suggests that such secondary fetal acidosis during maternal metabolic acidosis is not harmful and that Motoyoma *et al.*[486] actually suggest that such fetal acidosis could favor oxygenation.

Others have considered direct therapy to the acidotic human fetus. Lippert described[450] in 1972 a device (hypodermic needles in the form of the Junge cork screw scalp electrode) for use of direct fetal scalp injection in cases of fetal acidosis.

CHAPTER 18

Uterine Activity

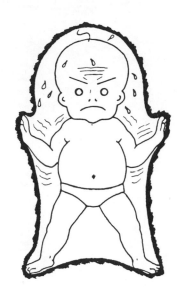

"By means of the woman's efforts, which, in strong labor pains, was equal, upon an average, to the weight of 470 pounds; the said head was compressed and moulded." So wrote Laurence Sterne in *Tristram Shandy* in 1759. As Reynolds, Harris, and Kaiser[570] noted in 1954, Sterne's authority for such a statement is unknown (and inaccurate), for it was more than 100 years later before the first instrument was developed for measuring uterine forces.

Historical

More than 100 years ago, Schatz placed balloons within the uterus in the extraovular space to record intrauterine pressure.[608b] These water-filled balloons were connected to kymographs (Fig. 18-1) providing recordings that were used in many American obstetrical textbooks until recent times. In 1927, Wieloch studied drug effects on uterine activity using the same transabdominal technique.[570]

The modern understanding of uterine activity began with the work of Reynolds and the South American group of Alvarez and Caldeyro-Barcia.[13] Reynold's group was to provide us with the concepts of uterine pacemaker, fundal dominance, uterine tone, and contractions of varying intensity. These ideas spilled over into clinical obstetrics as uterine hypotonic and hypertonic uterine dysfunction, dyscoordinate uterine contractions, and so forth.[570]

Internal intrauterine studies were advanced in 1936 by Moir's[477] canalization of umbilical vein after delivery of the infant. Williams[750a–751] (England), in 1951, and Carey (Baltimore), in 1952, independently inserted transcervical catheters through a Drew–Smyth catheter, introducing the clinical technique for recording intrauterine pressures.[570]

In 1896, Schaeffer applied external tocodynamometry to studies of uterine activity,[570] a technique further developed by Moir[477] and Embrey.[188a] Electrical recordings of uterine activity was originally proposed by Polaillon in 1880.[534a]

Uterine Activity

As demonstrated by the Montevideo group, uterine activity during the first 30 weeks consists mostly of small and frequent contrac-

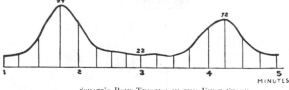

SCHATZ'S PAIN TRACING IN THE FIRST STAGE.

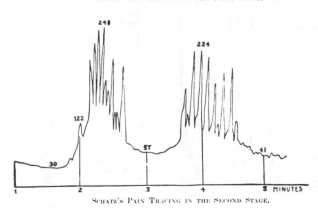

SCHATZ'S PAIN TRACING IN THE SECOND STAGE.

Fig. 18-1. From DeLee's 1920 *Principles and Practice of Obstetrics* of Schat's recording of uterine contractions in first and second stage of labor. Note how DeLee refers to contractions as "pains." (Reproduced with permission from W. B. Saunders.)

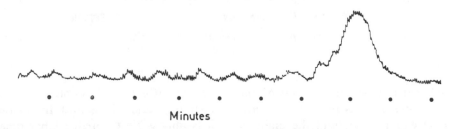

Minutes

Fig. 18-2. External recording of antenatal uterine contractions. The dots represent "Alvarez" waves. At the right, a Braxton–Hicks contraction. (From Fenning, G.: *Am J Obstet Gynecol* **43**: 791, 1942. Reproduced with permission.)

tions. The contractions (Braxton–Hicks) then begin to increase in intensity. While the uterus is flaccid between Braxton–Hicks contractions, runs of minimal contractions of 2–5 torr occur (Fig. 18-2), which are termed "Alvarez waves" after Professor Alvarez of Montevideo. These Alvarez waves are thought to represent isolated contractions of small segments of the myometrium.[198] With present-day recordings, they are often confused with fetal movements as both may be associated with acceleration of FHR. These contractions serve to form a lower segment and "ripen" the cervix prior to the onset of labor (Fig. 18-3), with gradual development to the degree seen in what is recognized as labor.

As labor progresses, the intensity and frequency of the contractions increase, as does the resting tone. The techniques for measuring uterine activity are, like most subjects discussed in this monograph, debatable. The measurement of uterine work or activity after rupture of membranes may be imprecise. We showed that with placement of multiple open-end catheters and miniature pressure transducers in different areas within the amniotic space after rupture of the membranes, values ranging between 50% and 200% of one another were registered during the same uterine contraction. This variation in pressure recordings has been demonstrated in Cincinnati[505] in a more elegant manner. Lindgren[446,]

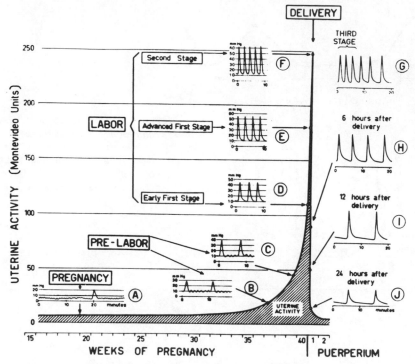

Fig. 18-3. Uterine activity throughout pregnancy, delivery, and postpartum. (From Caldeyro-Barcia, R., and Poseiro, J.: *Ann NY Acad Sci* **75**: 813, 1959. Reproduced with permission.)

[447] showed that if adequate amounts of amniotic fluid were present, pressure measurements were equal throughout the amniotic cavity during a contraction, even with rupture of the membranes. This Stockholm investigator, however, observed that pressures "operating" on the fetal vertex were often much greater than those measured within the amniotic cavity. It seems clear that the principles of a hydraulic space, particularly Hill's force–velocity equations for a single-chambered pump, are violated once the membranes rupture. Yet, Barclay *et al.*[34] and Seitchik *et al.*[622] treat the amniotic space after membrane rupture as if it is a closed, vascular space suitable for the same sort of calculations that are used with cardiovascular work.

The uterine activity as measured either by the external or internal technique, will vary throughout labor, although generally increase in intensity as labor progresses. The contractions may be extra strong (hypersystole), weak (hypotonic), too frequent (polysystolic), or too infrequent (asystolic). Sometimes a coupling occurs (bigemini). In any one case, it is impossible to predict labor times from the recording, although there is an obvious correlation in any large group of parturients between their degrees of uterine work and length of labor. As observed by Hendricks and Mowad,[337] maternal position and many drugs have an unpredictable effect on uterine activity during labor.

There are patterns of uterine activity such as increase in tonus and polysystole, which are much more frequently associated with abnormal FHR responses. The pattern of abruptio placenta seems to be fairly consistent in that it shows markedly increased tonus and contractions so frequent that they appear to be saw-toothed in fashion. Such patterns of uterine activity then can alert one that FHR abnormalities are likely without ever using a fetoscope or heart rate monitor.

For monitoring, I have argued that the internal versus the external technique is of advantage only as far as patient comfort is concerned, that the values obtained with the open-end catheter at an unknown level and amounts of anniotic fluid, and the potentially isolated space within the uterus, do not lend themselves to precise measurements.

It is a difficult concept to sell (particularly to house officers), but I further argue that the only measurement of uterine work which has clinical value is "the progress of labor." Provided that cephalopelvic disproportion can be ruled out, and the FHR recordings remain "normal," almost no measurement of uterine tension should be taken as indicating that contractions are "adequate," if cervical dilatation and descent of the presenting part fail to occur. There are obvious exceptions, such as uterine tetany or the saw-tooth uterine activity pattern, but repeatedly, cesarean section has been planned for failure to progress, when all that was required was a bit more oxytocin stimulation. Those believing in the precision of the internal technique suggest that certain intrauterine pressures (60–80 torr) should not be exceeded. Williams[570] suggested that intrauterine pressures above 80 torr were invariably associated with fetal bradycardia and probable fetal distress. Indeed, as discussed in Chapter 19, inhibition of excessive uterine activity is an old and useful technique in the treatment of fetal distress.

What then is the usefullness of measurements of uterine activity during labor? Several years ago I worked with an automated oxytocin apparatus from England and concluded that intrauterine pressures were imprecise indicators of effective labor in the individual case. The Cardiff group believe otherwise, but a well-trained labor room observer with careful attention to uterine activity (by palpation) does far better than the monitor. We continue to record activity without FHR monitors, but only as an aid to interpreting the various FHR patterns.

Hendricks and associates[336] have demonstrated that in human gravida a rise in amniotic fluid pressure is associated with similar rise in myometrium, uterine vessels, and even cerebral spinal fluid. But as shown in Figure 18-4, in Rudolph's laboratory we noted that while changes in amniotic fluid and maternal and fetal vessel pressures were similar, they were not exactly in phase. To me, this suggests that myometrial contractions independently affect fetal and maternal vessels and amniotic fluid pressures.

Another Point of View

Those advocates of electronic fetal monitoring would have us believe that "failure to progress" can be diagnosed from combining the Friedman curve (cervical dilatation versus time) and the recording of intrauterine pressure (using an open-ended intrauterine catheter). Given a secondary arrest of labor and "adequate" uterine activity (three contractions in 10 min of 40–50 torr), a diagnosis can be made of failure to progress which should not be treated by oxytocin. (These limits vary according to the institution.) In other words, the electronic monitor can provide a diagnosis as to whether adequate uterine work is occurring.

Others suggest that there is an optimal amount of oxytocin which should be infused, arguing that with excess doses, uterine activity becomes less efficient. Cases have occurred in which reduction of the oxytocin infusion rate dose produced progress in labor which had not occurred when larger amounts of oxytocin were used.

Donati et al.[159] suggest that current uterine work indices, the Montevideo unit [maxima of the pressure signal (torr) of all uterine contractions during 10-min interval] and the Alexandria unit (Montevideo unit multiplied by mean value of duration of contraction) are inadequate. They offer, instead, 25 parameters to summarize all aspects of the uterine contraction waveform.

Mendez-Bauer and colleagues[470a] have reported on the effects of the standing position (monitoring FHR and uterine tension) as compared with the supine position in 20 parturients. These investigators reported that uterine contractions were stronger in 75%, that uterine "activity" increased in 50%, and that there was less pain in parturients in the standing position. The therapeutic use of the maternal standing position, except for "walking" in early labor, in my opinion, does not exist. McManus and Calder[499] disagree, for they randomized 40 gravida undergoing induction of labor into either

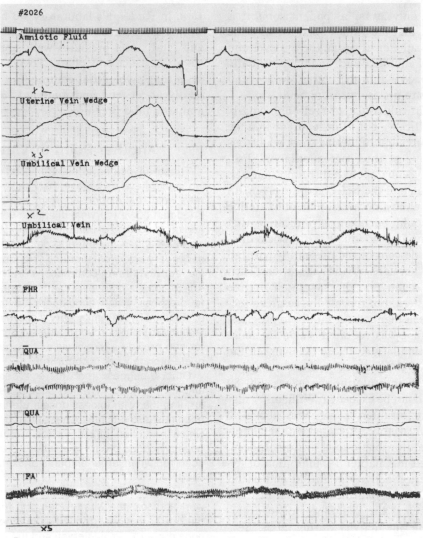

Fig. 18-4. Recording of a chronic fetal sheep preparation with catheters in amniotic space, "wedged" in maternal uterine vein and umbilical vein, and umbilical vein and fetal aorta. A flow probe was placed around the umbilical artery. With uterine contractions, unequal pressure effects were observed. The catheters were checked and flushed for accuracy.

a recumbent group or an upright group. No differences were found between the groups in length of labor, mode of delivery, oxytocic, or analgesic requirements.

It was Williams and Stallworthy[751] who introduced, in 1952, the transcervical catheter for measurement of tocography, and it is obvious that the technique has provided a very useful tool to obstetricians worldwide. The care which most investigators take to position the level of the intrauterine pressure transducer at the bedside suggests that most authorities consider it a precise technique for indicating intrauterine pressure.

Like so many techniques in obstetrical use, the intrauterine pressure apparatus has not been proven of value by a controlled study in managing the intrapartum gravida. One unfortunate feature is to directly relate increased intrauterine pressure to increased uterine activity. Paul, for instance, speaks of increased uterine activity during maternal seizures, because the intrauterine pressure recordings are of greater value.[528b] Presumably, the same sort of reasoning suggests that intrauterine activity is also increased during maternal sneezing, coughing, laughing, voiding, or defecating (as pressure readings are higher).

CHAPTER 19

Premature Labor

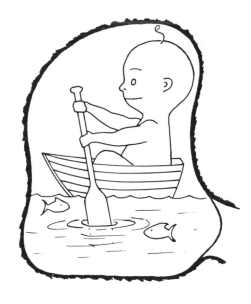

Winston Churchill is said to have arrived two months premature. Isaac Newton was likewise born prematurely and was reported to be so small and puny that he was not expected to live. One can only speculate on what these two men might have accomplished if they had had the advantages of a full nine months *in utero*. The techniques of the modern neonatal nursery can hardly equal what Dr. Dafoe accomplished in a country farmhouse in 1934, when he delivered and cared for the Dionne quintuplets, whose total newborn weight was only 6.1 kg.

Premature infants still contribute a disproportionate percentage to individuals with cerebral dysfunction. Even in 1978, Fitzhardinge's group[526] reported a 30% incidence of cerebral dysfunction in newborns weighing 1000 kg. While profound changes have occurred in the care and treatment of the prematurely born infant, obstetrics has made very little progress in the prevention of premature labor.

Premature Labor

The prevention of premature labor is, from the standpoint of improving perinatal mor-

bidity and mortality, the number one unsolved problem of American obstetrics (Fig. 19-1). We are still uncertain as to the mechanisms which maintain the fetus *in utero* or initiates the birth process.

MAINTENANCE OF PREGNANCY

The local progesterone inhibition theory (of uterine contractions) of Csapo has been (at least partially) accepted by most investigators, although there is still lack of agreement as to how the theory applies in clinical problems. Csapo[132] has restated his theory that "pregnancy is maintained as long as the intrinsic myometrial stimulant (such as prostaglandin) and the suppressor (such as progesterone) are in regulatory balance." In rodents and rabbits, there is no doubt that systemic progesterone therapy will inhibit the onset of labor and the fetuses will actually be absorbed rather than be delivered. In humans in premature labor, serum levels of progesterone are indeed reduced.[695]

LABOR

In humans, the effects of inhibitory systemic progesterone therapy is less clear, al-

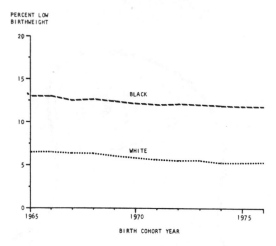

Fig. 19-1. Incidence of birthweight under 2500 g in California. (1965–1976 source, State of California, Department of Health, Maternal and Child Health, Birth Cohort Records.)

though Johnson[384] of Johns Hopkins has suggested that 17-hydroxy progesterone caproate is effective in treating theatened abortions and premature labor. In my experience, progesterone is best used in the treatment of painful Braxton–Hicks contractions or in threatened abortions. (In the latter, it will often "successfully" turn an inevitable abortion into a missed abortion.)

There has also been disagreement as to whether a decrease in serum progesterone levels occurs before the onset of term labor in humans and the current compromise theory is that there is an increase in the progesterone binding substance (perhaps produced by the fetus) before the onset of labor which effectively reduces the serum levels of progesterone surrounding the placenta.

The use of prostaglandins in therapeutic abortions has suggested that they play a role in the onset of labor and indeed, it appears that the synthesis of arachadonic acid by the fetal membranes is the basic biochemical mechanism in the initiation of most labors at term.[536] Phospholipase A2 catalyzes the release of arachadonic acid (the precursor of prostaglandins) from glycerophospholipids. Phospholipase A2 is located in the lysosomes of the fetal membranes. Like other steroids, such as estradiol-17 beta and glucocorticoids,

progesterone may likewise maintain the decidual lysosomes and its effective withdrawal allows the phospholipase enzymes to become active.

There is general agreement that high estrogen levels provide for the inhibition of uterine contractility, perhaps because of their effects upon calcium within the myometrial cells. This estrogen effect upon calcium appears to be counteracted by progesterone.

Several years ago we noted that the fetal membranes functioned much like the toad bladder with hypertonic solution of intraamniotic saline, i.e., oxytocin and digitalis increased the bulk transfer of sodium. This apparent effect of oxytocin on amniotic cell pore size seemed to be more than an isolated observation. The increased decidual destruction seen microscopically after oxytocin (with saline) I interpreted as a result of increased bulk transfer of hypertonic sodium solution.[254] We also demonstrated that a wide variety of agents, when injected into the amniotic sac, produced second trimester abortion.[261] Many of these were related parasympathomimetic agents and I have since championed the role of acetyl-choline in the onset of labor. Prolactin (the ancient hormone controlling salt transfer in fish gills) may be concerned with maintaining pregnancies as it is found in exceedingly large concentrations in amniotic fluid, perhaps controlling the pore size of the amnion.[387]

FETAL ANOMALIES AND LENGTH OF GESTATION

Anomalies of the brains of fetal calves,[350] fetal lambs,[55] and fetal humans[458a] are associated with prolonged pregnancies. Unlike pregnant farm animals with such anomalies, the pregnant human with an anencephalic fetus has normal secondary pregnancy changes and eventually goes into labor. The cow, for instance, with such a fetus, fails to develop her breasts or ligaments as normally occurs during gestation.[350] The human fetus with isolated adrenal hypoplasia appears to have prolonged gestation,[512] but I know of three newborns in whom the fetal pituitary was absent and who had normal gestational times. The newborns demonstrated adrenal failure. Johnson[383] has reported similar cases. The Dallas group[536] has suggested that the fantastic growth of the fetal adrenal (fetal zone) is a response to prolactin levels. They also postulate that the three prototypes for prolonged gestation in humans (fetal adrenal hypoplasia, fetal anencephaly, placental sulfatose deficiency) are all associated with an inability to produce adequate quantities of estrogen, apparently required for creating a "reactive" uterus.

It was Hippocrates who first suggested that the signal for the onset of labor comes from the fetus and nothing published since his writings have proven that it is otherwise. The onset of labor must then always be viewed from the interests of the fetus and when abnormalities of gestation occur, our first task must be to rule out fetal anomalies or illness.

ONSET OF PREMATURE LABOR

Oxytocin, while obviously capable of initiating labor in high doses, is considered to have an insignificant role in the onset of spontaneous term labor,[226] for it appears to act in physiologic doses only (or best) on a "reactive" uterus. The human fetus produces oxytocin and at term, along with the production of the progesterone binding substance,[536] it may excrete increased amounts of these and other substances to bring about the onset of labor. As noted in Chapter 6, increased serum levels of oxytocin (and prolactin) associated with orgasm or breast massage may be a factor in the onset of labor in the face of a reactive and ready uterus. (The proposed lack of a role for oxytocin is difficult for me to completely accept because alcohol is an effective agent for at least the temporarily inhibiting of labor and its action supposedly is that of an inhibitor of maternal oxytocin release.)

Analysis of amniotic fluids of women in premature labor and those at term have failed to consistently demonstrate alterations from normal amniotic fluids except for increased levels of prostaglandin, particularly F_2.

Whether this rise in amniotic fluid F_2 levels is the effect of uterine activity or the cause of the premature labor is debatable. Oxytocin, estrogen, and progesterone levels in amniotic fluid during labor are seemingly within normal limits.

CLINICAL EXPERIENCE

There are clinical situations in which the onset of premature labor seems to have an obvious etiology. Easiest to understand is overdistention of the uterus, such as with hydramnios or plural pregnancy, and the other is with amnionitis or, more properly, chorioamnionitis. The overdistention of the uterus presumably increases the relative mass of the membranes versus that of the placenta and local progesterone level and there is also often an increased intraamniotic pressure. In agreement with this concept is the observation of Von Bilderbeck who found a mean duration of pregnancy in singletons of 40 weeks, in twins of 37 weeks, and triplets of 35 weeks.

In the case of deciduoamnionitis that initiated premature labor, this could be explained by disruption of the decidual lysosomes with release of their enzymes and the production of prostaglandins. Such disruption of the lysosomes within the membranes and decidua could also explain how "stripping membranes" or even the infusion of normal saline in the extraovular space also initiates labor. Decidual disruption may also explain premature labor in women with premature separation of the placenta. There are other clinical associations with premature labor which are more difficult to understand. Honnebier noted a prematurity rate of 56% with various serious congenital anomalies, excluding anencephaly. Anencephalic fetuses with hydramnios had an average duration of gestation of 36.2 weeks. As noted, pregnancies with anencephalic fetuses and no hydramnios tend to be postmature.

Placental size is correlated with prematurity. Kloosterman found that even allowing for shortened gestation that placentas were smaller. Räihä[561] and Kauppinen[400a] found a positive correlation between maternal heart volume (or blood volume) and length of gestation. And the male fetus is born prematurely more often than the female. The sex ratio is lowest at 41 weeks of pregnancy.[408]

TOCOLYTIC DRUGS (Table 19-I)

In 1948, Ahlquist postulated the likelihood of two types of receptors in smooth muscles with opposite effects, which he labeled alpha and beta receptors. It generally is considered that there are both alpha and beta receptors within the myometrial cells of the uterus with the betamimetic drugs causing uterine relaxation and the alphamimetic drugs producing uterine contraction. The use of various betamimetic drugs to inhibit premature labor is widespread, but the American experience is limited to isoxsuprine except for various research protocols. Many of the currently used bronchodilators (terbutaline, orciprenaline) that are betamimetic are useful in inhibiting uterine contractions. There is no doubt that betamimetic drugs can inhibit uterine contractions, but whether they decisively stop premature labor or just make premature labor more prolonged (over weeks) is debatable. However, these agents are clearly useful in prolonging pregnancy where premature labor seems inevitable, where the addition of 48–72 hr will allow time for fetal maturation of lungs and presumably liver.

The various betamimetic drugs are listed in Table 19-II. Most of them have varying

TABLE 19-I. Drugs Used to Stop Labor

Alcohol
Aminophylline
Amyl nitrate
Analgesics
Antiprostaglandin (Table 19-II)
Analgesics
Beta-mimetic drugs (Table 19-III)
Diazoxide
Epinephrine
General anesthesia
Isopatin
Lututrin
Magnesium sulfate
Papaverine
Sedatives

TABLE 19-II. Betamimetic Drugs on Agonists Used in Pregnant Women

Isoxsuprine (Vasodilan)
Ritodrine (Premar)
Fenoterol (Berotec, Partusisten)
Salbutamol (Ventolin)
Orciprenaline (Alupent)
Isoproterenol (Isuprel)
Buphrenine (Nylidrin)
Terbutaline (Brethine)

degrees of maternal cardiac effects, particularly hypotension. There occasionally may be times when this hypotension and decreased uterine profusion would be deleterious to the fetal welfare; usually with the use of betamimetic drugs there is a fetal tachycardia. The occurrence of fetal bradycardia under such circumstances suggests an adverse effect on the fetus, as hypoperfusion of the placenta is presumably occurring. None of these bronchodilators (or even alcohol) have been released for use in the United States for inhibition of premature labor, although their use is apparently approved in gravida with asthma.[290]

Our own hospital experience is limited to alcohol with occasional uses of isoxsuprine and where asthma is "suspected," orciprenaline, terbutaline, or isoxsuprine are used.

The use of alcohol was first apparently described by Leland in 1920 and by Belinkoff in 1950. Fuchs brought it to our attention in 1967.[217] Our success rate in inhibiting premature labor for at least 48 hr with intravenous alcohol approaches 80%, but its use has low acceptance by both the labor room staff and the patients. Occasionally, there are objections to alcohol for religious reasons, but mostly it is because of the headaches, nausea, vomiting, gastritis, and inebriation that occurs after adequate therapeutic levels have been achieved. It is also considered bad obstetrics to deliver a "drunk" fetus as the premature's liver is immature and the excess prolonged levels of alcohol in the very immature newborn may lead to fetal acidosis, or "floppy newborn syndrome." Increased levels of alcohol in the amniotic fluid may likewise interfere with fetal lung surfactant materials if the fetus should gasp *in utero*.

Another group of agents used as inhibitors for premature labor are those which appear to inhibit prostaglandin synthesis (Table 19-III) and which are widely used for complaints of arthritis, such as aspirin, salicylic acid, naproxen, ibuprofen, and indomethacin. All of these drugs appear to interfere with the synthesis of prostaglandin E_2, F_2, and arachadonic acid.[437] Women who are arthritics and are pregnant and are being treated with one of these inhibitors of prostaglandin do have longer gestations. Gravid given aspirin because of severe rheumatoid arthritis have slightly longer gestation periods. These drugs also prolonged the time of labor for therapeutic abortions and indomethacin has been described as a successful inhibitor of premature labor in humans.

The major concern with the inhibitors of prostaglandin (or prostaglandins themselves) is that while they may inhibit uterine contractions, they can also be harmful. While arresting premature labor, they may also close the fetus' patent ductus arteriosis. They may also interfere with the newborn coagulation and immunologic processes and pulmonary vascular resistance. There is at the moment a general feeling that none of these prostaglandin inhibitors should be used in pregnant women until there has been a thorough investigation of their possible detrimental effects, both on the mother and the fetus.

Another type of uterine inhibiting agent is diazoxide. This drug is a smooth muscle, F_2 inhibitor, a hypoglycemic agent, and may also inhibit cyclic AMP. It is a powerful inhibitor of uterine contractions and a strong hypotensive agent. Apparently the hypotensive aspects of the drug are tolerable when given as an infusion. Adamsons and Myers[5] have reported excellent results both with its use as an agent for treating hypertension and for premature labor.

A different category of inhibitor of premature labor are those drugs affecting calcium metabolism, such as isopatin (Vrbanic) and magnesium sulfate (Harbert). Magnesium sulfate has long been used in American obstetrics for a variety of illnesses, treatment of hypertension, increasing renal function, anticonvulsant, and perhaps least of all, as an inhibitor of premature labor. Steer and Petrie[658] have suggested that it is more effective than alcohol in stopping premature labor. Since it is so widely used in women in labor who have toxemia, it has been difficult to accept that it has a profound inhibitory effect on uterine contractions. Isopatin has been tested by Vrbanic and colleagues[720] in combination with alupent. They found the best tocolytic effect with least side effects with combination of these two drugs. The numbers of controlled studies done because of the reluctance on the part of the pharmaceutical drug industry to be involved are limited.[291a] There is a suggestion that all of these drugs can inhibit labor for 2 or 3 days, but prolonged inhibition is rare. In three medical centers, Laverson *et al.*[424] compared ritodrine with ethanol and showed that both could prolong pregnancies for significant lengths of time, 30 plus days for ritodrine and 21 days for alcohol. In looking through these investigators' protocol, it is apparent that they really did not attempt to inhibit the cases in which premature labor had obviously occurred, that is, anyone above 4 cm or with ruptured membranes. The use of fluid for blood volume expansion to inhibit pituitary oxytocin release, bed rest, tranquilizers to control anxiety, have in many cases shown results comparable with all of these drugs.

CLINICAL APPLICATION

The prevention of premature labor is considered in Chapter 18; in brief, it includes expansion of maternal blood volume, physi-

TABLE 19-III. Antiprostaglandin Drugs (Prostaglandin Synthesis Inhibitors)

Aspirin
Fenoprofen (Nalfon)
Flufenamic acid
Ibuprofen (Motrin)
Indomethacin (Indocin)
Naproxen (Naprosyn)
Phenylbutazone

cal and emotional risk, and education of gravida about the early signs of premature labor. This latter point is important, as the best results are always found when the tocolysis score is low. In gravida at high risk for premature labor (Protocol P-35), we recommend bed rest, avoidance of infections (crowds, venereal diseases), "orgasm" (Chapter 6), and frequent vaginal examination after 26 weeks to detect early labor. For those with past second trimester abortions, even with a history of apparent labor, we urge cervical cerclage.

A tocolysis has been developed by Gruber and Baumgarten (Table D-45). Unfortunately, most women that we have referred have a score of greater than four, I can think of only two justifications for the inhibition of premature labor. One, to inhibit uterine contractions while draining off amniotic fluid in case of massive hydramnios, and the other is to "mature" the fetus so that the incidence of RDS is reduced. It is always a concern in any given case as to whether the uterus really "does know best" when it is attempting to rid itself of its contents. We have been caught in the trap of trying to inhibit labor in women who, in retrospect, had obvious amnionitis, small-for-age fetuses, abruptio, or fetal anomalies incompatible with life. The routine inhibition of all cases of apparent premature labor should be avoided and every effort should be made to individualize every case. Unfortunately, we are prone to make the incorrect decision when we obtain a battery of tests, as ultrasound, hormone levels, and revision of the history of LMP. For us, only the amniotic fluid L/S ratio has really stood the test of time as indicating fetal maturity.

Since prematurity remains the major prevailing cause of perinatal deaths, it seemed appropriate to make an all-out effort to test some of the available medical protocols designed to inhibit premature labor as well as to mature the fetal lungs in women with premature labor. We had planned to test the protocols in a double-blind fashion, but restrictions on human experimentation at our hospital made this impractical. Instead, the patient and her mate were told that the protocols were experimental and required to give permission for medical experimentation if they wished to participate in the study. We expected that the control group would consist of the women who declined to participate in the study as well as those who, for one reason or another, were not placed on the protocol.

Doing our best to explain the protocol to the gravida (and the father), she was admitted to the study if the following criteria were filled:

1. If the gravida willingly agreed to participate in the study.
2. If membrane rupture was for less than 48 hr. (We are still confused about whether rupture of the membranes accentuates fetal lung maturity, although the 1977 report of Thibeault and Emmanovilides[695] indicates that it does.)
3. That the fetus was apparently healthy.
4. That there were no obstetrical or medical conditions which contraindicated continuing the pregnancy, that amniotic fluid was negative either for bacterial counts greater than 10^3/ml, or leukocytosis.
5. That the pregnancy be more than 27, or less than 34 weeks, and that the estimated fetal weight be more than 800 g and less than 1900 g.
6. That the tocolysis score be 5 or less.
7. If there was a history of findings of cervical incompetence and if membranes were intact that a cerclage be done instead of use of the protocol. (Even if membranes are "hourglassing" through the cervix.)

Our therapy in this particular study consisted of bed rest, limited pelvic examinations, tranquilizers, expansion of the patient's blood volume with Ringer's lactate, antibiotics, and steroids (dexamethasone 12 mg × 2 d or betamethasone 6 mg × 2 d) and 9½% intravenous alcohol, or isoxsuprine or metaproteranol to inhibit labor.

We considered our "therapy" successful if delivery was prevented for 48 hr. If the estimated fetal weight was greater than 1200 g or if the amniotic fluids showed a mature L/S ratio following therapy, labor was induced 72 hr after beginning the protocol. While more than 100 gravida were admitted to the study, most cases were excluded for analysis for features such as their newborns weighed more than 1800 g, or that they were discharged as never having been in premature labor.

Out of this relatively large group, we were left with only 20 cases of apparent "success." One of the many ego-deflating experiences that occurred was the demonstration of our inability to accurately estimate fetal weights. Nearly one-third of the newborns weighed more than 1800 g (and were excluded) and presumably did not much benefit from our active interference with nature. In addition, about one-fourth of the cases in retrospect had neither been in premature labor nor had rupture of the membranes.

The use of steroids was based upon the classical work of Liggins and Howie[439] and recent studies suggest that it requires no apologies.[33a] Antibiotics were administered because of my conviction of the significant role of deciduitis in premature labor and neonatal morbidity. Bobitt and Ledger[63] have recently recognized this mechanism. Tranquilizers were for inhibition of norepinephrine and may have increased protection levels, recently suggested by Hauth et al.[324] as being beneficial in the prevention of the respiratory distress syndrome (RDS). We also avoided the use of drugs such as meperidine, antihistamines, and vasoconstrictors and repeated vaginal examinations because of their suspected role of stimulating uterine contractions.

When we matched our 20 successes with 20 nonstudy, the incidence of severe RDS was markedly reduced (0 vs. 4 cases). Also, the nonstudy group contained two cases of necrotizing enterocolitis and one case of intraventricular hemorrhage. The neonatal death rate was 0 for the study group and 3 for the nonstudy.

Using an exercise heard again and again in obstetrics, we began treating all cases (Protocol P-VI), believing that our preliminary results showed that it would not be ethical to withhold therapy in future cases of premature labor at 28–32 weeks.

Case No. 19-1

A 30-year-old white P 1-0-1-1 was admitted at 31 weeks with premature rupture of her membranes. Three days later, after bed rest and hydration, her hematocrit was found to have dropped from 32% to 23%. After 3 units of packed red cells, her hematocrit was 29%. Fifteen days later, she delivered a 1480-g infant that did well. Extensive hematologic studies for the etiology of her anemia were all negative.

This gravida was severely hypovolemic and while most pregnant women will reduce their hematocrits when placed at bed rest, this was an exaggerated case. We have other such cases of hemoconcentration which became obvious after bed rest for premature labor. These cases illustrate (to me) the association between reduced blood volume and premature labor as well as the benefit of bed rest.

Another Point of View

Concern for potential adverse effects on both mother and child of steroid therapy has been repeatedly expressed, but as noted by Treusch[705a] and Mead and Clapp[468] despite widespread use, it has not been associated with documented problems. The possibility of fetal abnormalities awaits years of follow-up, as illustrated by the DES problem.

Bobitt and Ledger[62] have reexamined the problem of amnionitis in the etiology of premature labor. They suggested that past studies may have been incomplete and suggest that the role of unrecognized amnionitis be reevaluated, Listeria monocytogenes is an uncommon pathogen in humans, but has an apparent predilection for the fetus or immunosuppressed adult. As reported by Ahlfors and associates,[11] the premature newborn in the Sacramento area has had an unusually high infection rate with this bacteria. Such neonates had clinical courses much like that described with β-hemolytic streptococcus. The interesting feature of the Listeria monocytogenes infections is that most of the mothers began premature labor with intact membranes and/or a fever. It may be that like with cattle, Listeria monocytogenes penetrates the intact amnion and induces premature labor (or abortion) in humans.

In a recent symposia held at the University of California at San Diego, Ronald Chez[103] reviewed the problem of premature labor in America. Premature labor occurs only in 10% of pregnancies, but accounts for 75% of perinatal morbidity. He claims that 20% of the cases are treatable. Ethanol, which suppresses oxytocin and vasopressin, has a 65–70% rate of effectiveness. Chez suggests that its use is associated with a decrease in the newborn respiratory distress syndrome. The beta-mimetics increase maternal cardiac output, but may cause hypotension, glycogenolysis, lipolysis, tachycardia, nausea, and tremor. The antiprostaglandins may cause headaches, gastrointestinal problems, coagulopathy abnormalities, decreased renal blood flow, and even closure of the ductus arteriosus of the fetus.

Chez rates the effectiveness of various therapies as bed rest alone as 40–70%, ethanol as 65–70%, beta-mimetics as 90%, and antiprostaglandins as 80%.

Zlatnik and Fuchs[768a] published an analysis of the Cornell prematurity experience and found that only 20% of women in whom premature labor was diagnosed would be candidates for suppression of premature labor. Exclusion was based on fetal size, premature rupture of the membranes, plural pregnancies, etc. (many of which we no longer consider to be contraindications). Hendricks[338] observed that perinatal mortality rates for prematures varies markedly (as New York City versus Chapel Hill) and the selection of inhibition of labor versus neonatal care will be determined much by one's own hospital's experience.

Fuchs[216, 217] has suggested that the role of prostaglandins may all be secondary in the onset of premature labor.

CHAPTER 20
Diabetes Mellitus in Pregnancy

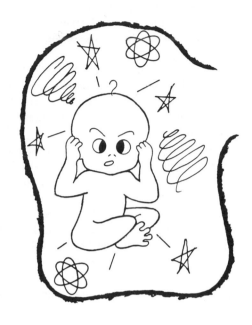

The perinatal mortality rate associated with diabetes has decreased remarkably over the last generation but still remains approximately twice as high as in the nondiabetic pregnancy. The reasons for this decrease are probably the same as those for the nondiabetic pregnancies; that is, better techniques for contraception, the availability for therapeutic abortion, fetal and neonatal intensive care, and probably changing concepts in the goals of diabetic management. The value of intensive antenatal fetal surveillance (OCT, estriol) has yet to be proven, but is now part of our dogma.

In Europe, it has been apparently easy to achieve a respectable rate of perinatal mortality in the pregnant diabetic.[190b, 532] Now, from the University of Southern California, comes a report by Gabbe *et al.*[219] that demonstrates that equally good perinatal mortality rates can be obtained in America with large populations of indigent patients.

The Gabbe report is somewhat difficult to evaluate since they introduce both hospitalization, after 32–34 weeks, and daily measurements of maternal estriol excretion and weekly OCT tests. At the same time, they apparently maintained tight control of the maternal diabetes. Since tight control of the maternal diabetes and hospitalization are the features in common with the protocols of the excellent results obtained in Europe, it would seem that these are important factors in achieving low perinatal mortality rates. It will, however, be years before the roles of "tight" blood sugar control and hospitalization versus careful fetal surveillance (33–36 weeks) can be evaluated in the achievement of good perinatal mortality rates.

The increased perinatal mortality rates are related to increased rates of stillborns and neonatal deaths, the fetal macrosomia leading to obstructed vaginal delivery and subsequent brachial plexus paralysis, the newborn morbidity associated with hypoglycemia and hyperbilirubinemia, and also the increased risk of congenital malformations.

The most striking congenital malformation seen in the infant with diabetes is caudal regression syndrome. This also occurs in the nondiabetic, but clearly is much more common in the insulin-dependent gravida. In my experience, I have seen it occur in one pregnancy, skip two pregnancies, and recur in the fourth pregnancy.

The problems of neonatal hypoglycemia

were seemingly solved by the Cleveland group[618] by the use of maternal intravenous fructose instead of dextrose solutions. The concept being that insulin was not directly used in the hydrolysis of the carbohydrate. This technique was gradually abandoned when it was shown that the newborns of such treated mothers still had a high incidence of neonatal hypoglycemia.

The problems of hyperbilirubinemia are often related to the macrosomia and bruising of the child and to the polycythemia (erythroblastosis) that many of these newborns display. Macrosomia of the fetus is a problem for which we have no solution and we often turn to cesarean section because of our inability to diagnose or to prevent its occurrence. Macrosomia appears to be particularly common in the mild gestational diabetic and is unfortunately often unrecognized until the newborn shoulders fail to deliver.

The increased rate of stillborns among infants of diabetics is often suggested to be related to the unrecognized hypoglycemia. As noted in Chapter 2, gravida with islet cell tumors of the pancreas and frequent hypoglycemia have no increased rate of stillborn infants. I have always considered a more likely etiology of stillborns are the challenges in osmoregulation that the fetus faces in the diabetic mother. Considering the fact that she may have hypoglycemia, abnormalities of albumin, etc., her fetus is constantly facing changing maternal osmolality and osmolarity gradients. Since blood hypertonicity is associated with a high mortality in the adult, it seems that its occurrence in the fetus might likewise be lethal.

The plans for management for the gravida with diabetes are outlined in protocols P-15 and P-16 and P-I. Upon arriving in Sacramento, I discovered that our high-risk clinic consisted mostly of abnormal oral glucose tolerance tests. Since it is my impression that roughly 70% of such gravida will have abnormal oral glucose tolerance tests, I simply reduced the attendance of our high-risk clinics by about two-thirds by declaring these women not at high risk. Actually, the woman with gestational diabetes is class A diabetic,[474a]

and as shown by Kaltreider years ago, is only high risk when the pregnancy becomes postmature. These authors also showed that about 9% of gravida with first trimester abnormal GTT later show overt diabetes. We do make every effort to control these women's obesity through diet (and it almost always fails) and to make certain that their pregnancies do not continue past their due date. The incidence of macrosomia (fetal) is high in these women and since many of them are candidates for elective postpartum tubal ligation, we often include in their delivery a cesarean section as a "bonus" both for the patient and her newborn, as well as for ourselves.

Although there is lack of confirmation of its value, we treat gravida with abnormal glucose tolerance tests with 100 mg of vitamin B_6 a day.[43, 656] Most such tests in our experience have "reverted" to normal values after one month of vitamin B_6, but the fetuses still have macrosomia.

For our insulin-dependent gravida, we have been forced to treat these patients on an outpatient basis. We begin our "careful" antenatal fetal surveillance at about 28 weeks, obtaining baseline estriols and HPL values (Protocol P-16). We have hopefully also obtained baseline fetal sonograms to indicate both the EDC and whether fetal growth is appropriate in the second trimester. The cardinal points of our outpatient management of these women is to divide their feeding into four times a day with the last being the late bedtime snack. We also divide their semi-long-acting insulin between doses in the morning and in the late afternoon. Surprisingly, we can obtain fasting blood sugars often below 120 mg% and no blood sugar above 160 mg% with this sort of management. We do fetal heart rate monitoring (nonstress tests or, if no contractions, OCT's) starting about the 32nd week. It would appear that the fetuses are much more active, and many of these women are much more likely to have uterine contractions in the late evening. While at one time, we performed routine amniocentesis or amnioscopy to check for amniotic fluid staining and it appeared to be a useful technique, I subsequently had two fetuses die within 24 hr of having had a normal amniocentesis and therefore abandoned routine amnioscopy in the diabetic gravida. The most important fetal surveillance test of all, of course, is the record of fetal movements. These diabetic patients do develop a variety of the "maternal syndrome" with edema, hydramnios, and decreased fetal movements. When this occurs, the fetus is usually not swallowing and in great jeopardy, and the pregnancy should be terminated.

Because pregnancy is never good news for diabetics as her control always becomes more difficult, because of the higher perinatal mortality risk and the risk of continuing deleterious genes (probably one related to late-onset diabetes), it seems that these patients should be encouraged to limit family size and be offered elective sterilization.

Another Point of View

Merkatz[306, 469a] of the MacDonald House in Cleveland considers the gestational diabetic to have increased perinatal mortality rates. He claims that by careful antenatal screening, approximately 2% of all gravida will be judged to be gestational diabetics. Unlike many, because of their ability to prevent fetal macrosomia, the Cleveland group will allow the pregnancies of gravida with diabetes to go as long as 42 weeks. There seems to be general agreement that the data of Hagbard[309] regarding the perinatal mortality rates of deaths from prematurity and from stillborns crossing at 37 weeks should now be ignored. Instead, fetal illness or maturity should determine the time of delivery.

Despite the fact that Eastman[752] (Williams' *Obstetrics,* 11th ed.) suggested that the main objective in the management of pregnancy complicated by diabetes was "rigid control of the disease," few agree on what constitutes rigid control. Duhring[170] still raises the spector of starvation ketosis (too tight control?) and its deleterious effects on intellectual development of the child.[105, 659] Bruksch[81a] has pointed out that no control study exists showing the prospective comparison of "loose" versus "tight" control in pregnancy complicated by diabetes.

CHAPTER 21

Immunological Aspects of Pregnancy

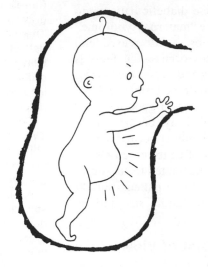
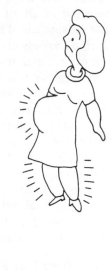

The Problem

Although the fetus has different histocompatibility antigens than its mother, it is not rejected. This immunological paradox was first noted by Medawar[469] and has yet to be satisfactorily explained. The uterus has been considered to be an immunologically inert organ and the fetus to be antigenically immature. Maternal immune responses are suppressed, particularly the lymphocytic function.[201] Unfortunately, this depression is not sufficient to prevent the various isoimmunization problems of pregnancy. There are several substances that appear in increased amounts during pregnancy which appear to reduce maternal immunologic responses. These include estrogen/progesterone, HCG, HPL and fetoprotein, and placental glycoproteins.[201] However, these seem insufficient and the blocking antibody concept is again attracting attention. Such "blocking antibodies" would be absorbed onto the placental antigens, thereby "hiding" paternal antigens from the maternal immune system.[193, 577] Deficiency of such "blocking antibodies" could explain diseases mostly restricted to first pregnancies, such as EPH gestosis or even spontaneous abortions.

Abortions

In cases of spontaneus abortions, ABO & Rh blood group differences have been reported to be related and by others to be unrelated.[377] In our studies of inbred strains of mice, fertility and pregnancies were no different than in outbred mice. One difference was that with strong H-2 differences in the parents, the fetuses and their placentas were slightly but significantly larger (showing the effects of "heterosis"). I had begun these mice studies expecting to find major differences in the degree of fibrinoid degeneration at the placental site between pregnancies of inbred (and histocompatibility the same) parents and those of outbred strains. After much effort and considerable disappointment, I concluded that there was none. The demonstration by Bresnihan et al.[72] that lymphocytotoxic antibodies are higher in pregnant women with systemic lupus erythematosus having spontaneous abortions again suggests that immunologic factors may well be involved in maintenance of pregnancy.

Clinical Aspects of Immunological Differences

Several years ago we became interested in the "postpartum chill" and tried to explain its occurrence on the basis of fetal–maternal transfusions.[252] We were able to show that the occurrence of such chills was directly related to the amount of fetal blood transfused into the mother during labor and to the maternal–fetal differences in blood group types. Such fetal–maternal transfusions (and chills) are more frequent after epidural anesthesia and in the immediate postpartum chill. Although a mother has less mixed lymphocyte response to her own child's lymphocytes than another child's, those with severe chills had a higher stimulation response. In those women with severe childbirth chills, her newborn was much more likely to have an "ABO incompatibility" type jaundice. While I still am uneasy whenever a gravida demonstrates such chills, because to me it indicates a significant fetal–maternal transfusion and the probability of newborn jaundice, most all other obstetricians ignore its occurrence other than asking for more warm blankets for the postpartum patient. In cases of severe fetal–maternal antenatal transfusions, if the fetus and mother have significantly different blood groups, a history of unexplained maternal chills can usually be obtained.

ERYTHROBLASTOSIS FETALIS

Historical Aspects

The major events leading to the discovery of the etiology and prevention of erythroblastosis have occurred within one generation. Ballantyne[33] of England described the clinical entity of hydrops fetalis in 1892. In 1940, Landsteiner and Wiener[420] described the Rh antigen on red blood cells. In 1946 Wallerstein[725] performed an exchange transfusion for erythroblastosis. Allen, Diamond, and Vaughn demonstrated that hyperbilirubinemia lead to kernicterus in 1950.[27a] In 1956, Bevis[51] reported on the significance of increased pigments in the amniotic fluid of a fetus with erythroblastosis. Levine[432] in 1958 demonstrated that ABO incompatibility protected against Rh sensitization. In 1960 Gorman, Freda, and Pollack[294] in New York began a program to prevent Rh sensitization with passively administered Rh antibody. Liley[441] of New Zealand reported in 1963 the first successful intrauterine transfusion. Thus, between 1940 and 1963, the eiology, its therapy, and prevention had all been discovered for erythroblastosis.

Clinical Management of Erythroblastosis

The treatment of fetal anemia relative to isoimmunization has been largely solved since the introduction of routine Rh immune globulin in the 1960s. On our own service, we attempt to make certain that every Rh negative postpartum patient having delivered an Rh positive is given adequate amounts of Rh immune globulin (Protocol P-28). Unfortunately, we sometimes fail. Sometimes the gravida's blood type is incorrectly determined (as Rh positive), other times we fail to recognize the excessive fetal–maternal transfusion, and in some cases we have failed to administer the "vaccine" after abortions or amniocentesis. While isoimmunization is rare in the Rh negative D^u positive patient having an Rh positive child, it does occur. Our blood bank colleagues will not let us administer the Rh immune globulin to these D^u positive women. In order to protect our patients, it is essential that the Rh negative patient's prenatal record be flagged in such a manner that none of the obstetrical staff can miss the fact (the patient must be so informed and her risks explained so that she also may look out for her own welfare).

At delivery (or after abortions or fetal manipulations) the patient's blood should be checked for significant fetal–maternal transfusion. This can be determined by finding a "mixed field" when cross matching with the Rh immune globulin or with any of the modifications of the Kleihauer–Betke test for fetal red cells. We have been alerted to several cases of fetal–maternal transfusions by patients whose blood types apparently changed from Rh negative D^u negative to Rh negative D^u positive in the postpartum period. When for one reason or another Rh immune globulin has not been given within 3 days of delivery, it should probably be given even up to 10 days after the event.

The antenatal management of the Rh negative gravida is outlined in Protocol P-28. Several points should probably be emphasized. Antibody screens should be obtained in each trimester and probably after the 36th week of pregnancy. For one reason or another, we have seen stillborns or severely sensitized newborns delivered of supposedly unsensitized women. Either the initial antibody screen was in error or a relatively large fetal–maternal transfusion occurred in the antenatal period, so that significant but unknown maternal sensitization occurred. Repeated antibody screens throughout pregnancy seem to be the only answer to preventing this rare but serious problem.

Once sensitizing has occurred and the antibody is known as one that can produce fetal disease (Tables D-106) and the paternal type is positive, maternal titers should be checked repeatedly until a significant level occurs (1:8 in our laboratory). We then turn to repeated amniocentesis.

I began performing diagnostic amniocentesis in 1955. At first, we (Dr. George Janda and I) looked at many different substances in the amniotic fluid. Because Dr. S. Schwartz at the University of Minnesota was an expert in bilirubin and Bevis had shown that coproporphyrin was elevated in the amniotic fluid of affected fetuses, we selected this marker. It took us nearly 6 years to collect a significant sample size and the paper was nearly two years in publication.[239] In the meantime, the technique of Liley's[441] was given the priority (it deserved). We had cautioned that multiple amniotic fluid tests were necessary at a time when Liley's technique of single test at Δ450 was considered infallible. I still cling to the belief that one amniotic test is seldom if ever justification for therapeutic intervention unless the fetus is mature.

Certain other pitfalls have occurred in my experience. The amniotic fluid staining may decrease, not because the fetus is mildly affected, but because its erythropoietic mechanisms are depleted (and it is on the verge of death). Another error is to stop performing amniocentesis because repeated amniocenteses have suggested that the fetus is at worst only mildly affected. Instead, in gravida with elevated titers, amniotic analysis should be repeated until the L/S is mature and the pregnancy should be terminated whenever induction of labor can be easily accomplished. To do otherwise is to miss the rare case in which significant fetal anemia occurs late in the pregnancy.

When severe fetal disease is present, I favor termination of the pregnancy. Our neonatologists now have at least a 50% survival as early as 28 weeks (1000-g fetus) and the alternative of intrauterine transfusions is a very dangerous procedure for even the healthy fetus. When severe erythroblastosis was a common event on our service, I saw several cases in which intrauterine transfusion was refused (either because the physician thought fetal hydrops was present or because the patient declined the procedure). Immediate delivery of such fetuses produced severely affected newborns. On several occasions the newborn was salvaged with expert neonatal care. A controlled study has never been done, testing the value of intrauterine transfusion. Years ago, Walker et al.[724] of Scotland showed that even where previous pregnancies had resulted in a stillborn, subsequent delivery of a live fetus at equal gestational periods occurred in one-fifth of the cases. Amniotic fluid analysis is far from precise and to subject a fetus to the hazards of intrauterine transfusion in the absence of a prior fetal death, I believe, is never indicated.

When a prior fetal death has occurred, one should always warn the gravida of the symptoms of the "maternal syndrome." I first learned of this process from I. Kaiser at the University of Minnesota. When I reviewed subsequent cases of stillborns from erythroblastosis, in Minneapolis, it became apparent to me that such a fetus never died *in utero* without considerable warning to its mother (and physician).

The full-blown mirror (maternal) syndrome consists of the following: (a) decreased fetal movements, (b) maternal "hydrops" or extensive edema and (c) maternal pruritus. It was from this syndrome that I first appreciated the significance of decreased fetal movements for these unfortunate gravida would often claim "that her fetus was about to die" based on prior experience with a stillborn (whose movements decreased sometimes weeks before *in utero* death occurred). In some cases of the mirror syndrome the maternal pruritus was almost intolerable. (I never learned what agent was responsible for the maternal symptoms.) The edema and mild hypertension often lead to a diagnosis of toxemia. On several occasions, when amniotic fluid had been heavily stained and there had been a prior fetal death and the fetus was immature, we refrained from terminating the pregnancy as long as fetal movements appeared "normal." This policy never let us down. Unfortunately, once the full blown "mirror syndrome" develops, the fetus is hydropic and in my experience, can not be salvaged.

Part of the maternal syndrome of fetal hydrops is elevated HCG titers and large thecaluteal cysts. On at least two occasions, I have seen cases where at the time of cesarean section, such cysts (and the ovary) were removed in the impression that that the patient had some sort of a dreadful tumor. In the five cases of maternal syndrome that I have measured HCG titer, they were markedly elevated. Postpartum, like with hydated mole, such cysts enlarge markedly with resulting patient discomfort and even asietes.

It is indeed fortunate that such cases are now very rare. However, among people of Southeast Asia, such processes still occur due to fetal hydrops secondary to alpha thalasemia (Barts hemoglobin).[298] We have had two such cases among immigrants from Malay. There is apparently no antenatal technique to diagnose such fetal disease in these gravida prior to the development of fetal hydrops.

A number of routines have been attempted to reduce the maternal antibody response to her Rh positive fetus. Because we found that progesterone reduced H-2 antibody formation in pregnant mice, we attempted a controlled study with progestational agents in sensitized women.[287] The results appeared to be encouraging, but the "disease" disappeared. Now promethazine is recommended for similar reasons.[305] Others used various steroids. At times, maternal exchange transfusions or plasmophoresis have been used. One puzzle has been the persistence of the Rh titer, in the absence of repeated stimulation (long intervals between pregnancies).

In the days before electronic fetal monitoring, Rh sensitization provided the best intellectual discussion (especially with pediatricians) available for practicing obstetricians. While the prevention of erythroblastosis due to Rh D antigen is one of the greatest triumphs of medicine, its victory cost us a truly rewarding and stimulating topic. Many questions went unanswered, such as what caused the fetal hydrops (it was not simply the anemia) or how the fetal bilirubinoid material reached the amniotic fluid, or the mechanism for the fetal anemia, or how best to do an intrauterine transfusion. As a topic, fetal monitoring is in no way its equal.

Another Point of View

Hamilton[316] has challenged the concept that premature delivery may be as good as intrauterine transfusion for the fetus of the severely Rh sensitized patient. He claims that in his institution (St. Louis University School of Medicine) that the fetal mortality rate for each intrauterine transfusion is only 2.2% versus 20% as often reported in the literature. While admitting that the results with hydropic fetuses are poor, he claims that intrauterine transfusion permits delivery of the more mature baby requiring much shorter hospitalization to reduce costs.

Gusdon and Witherow[305] suggest that promethazine hydrochloride ameliorates the effects of erythroblastosis in fetuses whose mothers are sensitized. His own study fails to conclusively show that amelioration of the erythroblastosis has been achieved in these newborns, but he believes there are individual cases which have apparently benefited. (As noted by Walker, there are always cases of erythroblastosis which even without therapy do much better than expected.) Rubenstein et al.[587a] had suggested that promethazine therapy during pregnancy may decrease the neonatal number and function of T-cells and the possibility remains that there may be an induction of fetal immunoincompet-

ence. Recently, Graham-Pole et al.[295] has reported on eight patients with severe Rh isoimmunization who were treated by intensive plasmaphoresis, using a continuous-flow cell separator. The plasmaphoresis was started at 16–27 weeks of gestation and continued until the delivery of the fetus. In seven out of eight cases, the anti-D concentration fell during the period of plasmaphoresis. Their findings suggest that plasmaphoresis may reduce fetal hemolysis in some cases.

CHAPTER 22
Intrapartum Factors

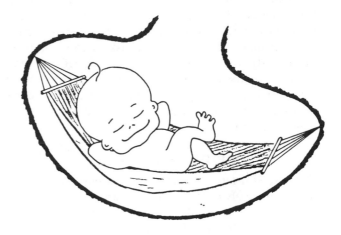

Introduction

It is assumed that primitive women survived the hazards of childbirth because of the relative lack of both infections and interference with natural processes. However, the perinatal mortality rate was known to be very high[152]: The great obstetrical physicians of the past, Soranos (Rome 98–138 A.D.) or Pare (France 1510–1590) or Smellie (England 1697–1763) were almost totally concerned with maternal welfare. The 19th-century British physicians, E. Kennedy (fetal heart rates), Little (the relationship between birth trauma and cerebral palsy), and Ballantyne (maternal and fetal factors causing neonatal mortality) were among the first to emphasize the obstetrician's role in achieving optimal fetal outcome. The history of the development of intrapartum fetal monitoring is outlined in Chapter 7. It has been our major fetal area of interest over the past generation. The present chapter concerns intrapartum fetal topics which have been largely neglected and are still in the formulative stages. For that reason, considerable laboratory work is described in order that the reader may better understand the basis for my views.

If during prenatal care our *in utero* patients have been properly studied and screened (Chapter 7), labor and delivery for them should pose no special risks. This reassuring statement assumes that certain rare fetal accidents will not occur, such as prolapsed umbilical cord or abruptio placentae, and that we can avoid iatrogenic-induced stress. Such rare *in utero* accidents often have no practical prophylaxis and are best managed by good luck and careful intrapartum care. Iatrogenic factors are, on the other hand, a very difficult problem to control. We obstetricians are overtrained to care for the normal parturient (in America at least), and our long and continuing problem has been the application of high-risk techniques to the low-risk parturient. It is not necessarily true that if electronic fetal monitoring, anesthesia, operative delivery, and so forth, are of benefit for the high-risk parturient, such procedures will likewise benefit the low-risk patient. During the early 20th century, American obstetrics had the worst maternal mortality record of any developed nation,[18a] and it was necessary during the 1940s to redefine good obstetrical care. The use of accouchement force, high forceps, general anesthesia, version and extraction, and so forth, were abandoned in the interest of improving maternal and perinatal mortality rates. Our own hospital has now added midwives and home-style deliveries to complement the normal obstetrical and intensive care program. Further efforts are continuing to define optimal care of all parturients, considering their wishes and their risk factors. While only a short time ago we envisioned all parturients in labor being extensively monitored, it now appears that we should retreat and that most parturients of the future will labor under "natural" conditions.

Maternal Position

A stressful fetal situation which occurs in many medically controlled labor wards is the maternal supine position, which is often iatrogenic. Our first rule is to make certain that every parturient is in the lateral position. Very often the pregnant uterus of the supine parturient will, during a contraction, foolishly cut off its own uterine artery blood supply as well as decreasing the return blood flow to the maternal heart (Poseiro effect, Chapter 10) (Fig. 22-1). This problem of supine hy-

potension is aggravated by the presence of conduction-type anesthesia. Indeed, I sometimes think that my major contribution to patient care in the labor ward is rolling the supine parturient onto her side. They have been placed supine for reasons such as watching television, allowing the conduction anesthesia to spread evenly, allowing for easier vaginal exams or monitoring of the fetal heart, and so forth. I find it difficult to understand, but it requires constant attention in order to avoid this very simple problem of the supine parturient.

Uterine Activity

After making certain that maternal position is optimal during labor, care should be taken to assume the same for the intensity of uterine contractions. For any given parturient, it is not obvious what degree of uterine intensity or contractions will be deleterious, but in retrospect, many apparent abnormal FHR patterns can be corrected by reducing uterine contraction intensity. Adamsons and Myers[4] report that the intervals between contractions and resting tone are the important

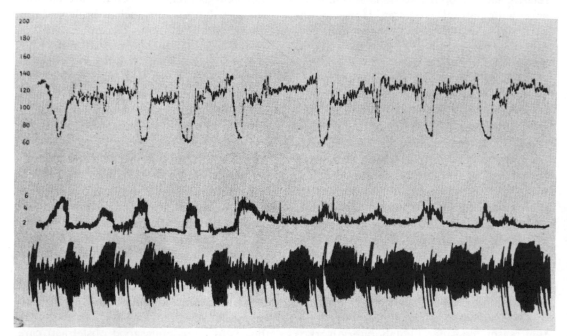

Fig. 22-1. FHR recording and maternal big toe pulse showing loss of pulse height with uterine contractions (Poseiro effect).

features. The critical levels they note are $1\frac{1}{2}$-min intervals and resting intrauterine pressures of 25–35 torr. Reduction of uterine contraction intensity can be accomplished by a number of simple techniques, such as decreasing the rate of oxytocin infusion, inhibiting uterine activity with beta-2 mimetic drugs or with various anesthetic agents such as chloroform or halothane, or by changing uterine activity by changing maternal position. Obviously, the simplest and safest technique should be used first, and on our service, it usually means decreasing the oxytocin infusion rate or rolling the parturient to the other side.

The reasons for poor correlation between excessive uterine activity and apparent fetal distress is a puzzle, but it is generally true that at some excessive degree of uterine intensity, the FHT pattern will be abnormal (Chapter 18). The extremes are illustrated by the dysmature fetus who will demonstrate abnormal FHR patterns with most any uterine contraction in contrast with the fetus whose mother has uterine tetany and still maintains apparently normal FHR patterns. This apparent riddle of poor correlation is probably due to a lack of our basic knowledge of the factor controlling placental perfusion and lack of agreement on what constitutes an abnormal FHR pattern. While there is no strict definition, I accept Sureau and his European colleagues[673] concept that any bradycardia associated with uterine contraction is probably "undesirable." Such a concept does not imply that the fetus is at any particular risk simply because it has a type I bradycardia but that it would be a more healthy situation *in utero* if no slowing of the fetal heart occurred. Confusion arises because those FHR patterns which are accepted universally as being ominous (late decelerations or severe abrupt with loss of beat-to-beat variability) are rare. The usual clinical situation is to ponder over severe vagal abrupt bradycardia (variable) with at least normal BBV which some people consider relatively benign and others, like myself, often consider as worrisome. If in retrospect the fetus had acidemia,

then one tends to classify the fetal heart rate as ominous and its associated uterine contraction as too stressful. On the other hand, if there were no acidemia, the clinical conclusion is usually the opposite, in that the fetus tolerated the bradycardia and that such an FHR pattern is indeed not worrisome.

Another reason that we are unable to define which degree of intensity of uterine contraction will result in fetal distress is perhaps the concept of "respiratory and nutritional reserve" of the placenta.[206] Most placental transport mechanisms have considerable resistance to acute stress, as suggested by any of the various placental function tests (NST, OCT, HPL, estriols, oxytocinase—Tables D-5–D-17). With abnormalities of any or all of these tests, lesser uterine contractions may evoke abnormal FHR patterns, confirming the impression of decreased placental reserve. However, this relationship is far from constant and only a clinical trial of labor will demonstrate any particular fetus' "placental reserve." As stated previously, almost by definition, any well-nourished fetus demonstrating normal fetal activity in the antenatal period has placental function adequate for most any normal labor.

When uterine blood flow is monitored during uterine contractions in sheep, monkeys, or humans, it would appear that many times the blood flow decreases before a rise occurs in amniotic fluid pressure (uterine contraction) (Fig. 10-2). It is unknown whether umbilical blood flow decreases in the absence of cord compression during uterine contractions. Since uterine perfusion is decreased with contractions and usually evokes no fetal bradycardia, it is difficult to understand the common situation causing type I bradycardia (Chapter 8).

In those parturients where we have monitored the maternal big toe pulse (hallux) and presumably were indirectly measuring lower aorta flow, we found that during uterine contractions there was many times a marked decrease in the hallux pulse (Poseiro effect, Chaps. 8 and 10). One interesting observation was that in only about 65% of the time where uterine contraction appeared to compress the aorta (as the toe pulse decreased markedly) was there an FHR response.[265] An obvious explanation is that these nonaffected cases in whom uterine blood flow was decreased represented those uteri which receive a sufficient blood supply from the ovarian anastomoses. Therefore, such uterine blood supplies are not subjected to the aortic constriction which occurs at the level of the fourth lumbar vertebra. Another possible explanation of the variable effects of decreased uterine blood flow has been suggested by Novy and associates,[510a] who surprisingly demonstrated that in pregnant monkeys uterine blood flow actually *increases* during uterine contractions. This concept is foreign to the usual clinical impression, but it is conceivable that placental hypoperfusion still occurs, as there may be a redistribution of blood flow during the contraction so that less of the flow goes to the uterine spiral arteries and more to the myometrium.

Drug Therapy for the Intrapartum Fetus

A significant portion of this chapter on intrapartum care of the fetus will be concerned with those circumstances in which drugs may be administered to the mother for fetal benefit. In Chapter 16, the philosophy of fetal pain relief was presented and the concept of treating fetal pain during birth will not be discussed again. There are, however, many other fetal conditions besides pain which may benefit from intrapartum drugs. These include (1) *in utero* resuscitation, (2) treating maternal acidemia, (3) protection against asphyxia, (4) prevention of meconium aspiration, and (5) preventing reduced cardiac output and umbilical flow during times of fetal distress. In all, I attempt to discuss our previous relevant laboratory and clinical experience.

IN UTERO RESUSCITATION

On our own service, true intrapartum fetal asphyxia occurs approximately 3 per 1000 deliveries and for a number of reasons I continue to believe that such an hypoxic or acidemic fetus should only be resuscitated extra uterine. For while I cannot prove it, I have the impression that some stillborn fetuses delivered on our service died in the absence of any acute uterine activity. While observing ongoing chronic fetal sheep studies in Rudolph's laboratory, it became obvious (to me, at least) that many otherwise healthy fetuses did not recover completely *in utero* from an acute, severe asphyxial insult. Several times, after an acute study involving some degree of fetal asphyxia performed in a chronic fetal sheep (who had been in good condition) preparation, the fetus would unexpectedly die within the next few hours, after their apparent biochemical recovery. While agreeing that the laboratory is different than the labor ward, I still have this fear that human fetuses will react similarly to brief asphyxia; and therefore cannot accept that an episode of suspected fetal asphyxia should be treated with anything other than immediate delivery (in an otherwise previously healthy and term size fetus).

MATERNAL ACIDEMIA

A form of intrapartum monitoring which I used to believe was important was that of recording maternal blood pH values (easily obtained from veins on dorsum of hand). Our studies[236, 237] suggested that maternal acidemia leads to fetal acidemia and hypoxemia (Chap. 17). Indeed, Rooth wrote[582] that the determination of maternal pH was sufficient for monitoring fetal pH and therefore the occurrence of fetal asphyxia. My early studies suggested that at least 1% of parturients have unexplained acidemia. When correlated with cord blood studies, there was an associated fetal acidemia and hypoxemia (Chap. 17). It has been my assumption that a fetal acidemia secondary to maternal acidemia is less ominous than that fetal acidemia secondary to hypoxemia (asphyxia). Nevertheless, optimal intrapartum care still includes the prevention of any fetal stress. We have not, however, treated unexplained maternal acidemia routinely with bicarbonate therapy.

INCREASED NEWBORN RESUSCITABILITY AFTER ASPHYXIA WITH DRUG THERAPY

This topic is discussed in detail since its concepts are rejected by the obstetrical and anesthesia communities at large. I hope that the reader will not dismiss these data, for recent work[493, 493e] from Myers' laboratory has fully supported my views on this controversial topic. There is "logic" in purposefully delivering a sedated or narcotized newborn!

In our laboratory we[259] have studied pregnant rabbits at term which were treated with a drug or a placebo prior to the introduction of fetal asphyxia. After 25 min of asphyxia, the fetuses were delivered and resuscitated with either tracheal intubation or hyperbaric oxygen. Success of resuscitation as well as other end points were evaluated. The drugs were of seven types: antacids, antihistamines, antimuscarinics, dextrose or fructose, narcotics, sedatives, and tranquilizers. In these rabbits, at least one drug from every group produced significantly increased rates of successful resuscitation after specific asphyxial stress, with sodium bicarbonate, scopolamine, dimenhydrinate, pentobarbital, and morphine being the best in their respective groups. Of all the drugs, scopolamine, dimenhydrinate, and dextrose appeared to offer the highest rate of resuscitability, although the differences between drugs were not large.

The studies suggest that at least three protective mechanisms against asphyxia are involved—the reduction of fetal acidemia, stimulation of glycolysis, and the introduction of fetal hypometabolism and inactivity. The antimuscarinic drugs may also prevent deleterious vagal reflexes in newborns, as they probably do in adults under stress. Combining various effective drugs did not increase the resuscitation rate above that of the individual drugs alone. Unlike the studies of Meyers, we made no follow-up evaluation of CNS function. While hyperglycemia may improve cardiovascular resistance to asphyxia, it may be harmful to subsequent CNS development (Chap. 23).

There is nothing new in the concept that maternal medication may protect her fetus in times of stress.[334, 411] In evaluating various obstetric analgesia regimens, Snyder[641] described the protective effects of pentobarbital and morphine in fetal and newborn rabbits subjected to asphyxia, and Balfour et al.[32a] demonstrated that paraldehyde and ether prolonged the time to the last gasp in anoxic newborn rats. Miller and Miller[473] concluded that pentobarbital prolonged the survival of newborn guinea pigs exposed to anoxic environment by depression of their oxygen uptake. Broom[78a] demonstrated that pentobarbital increased anoxic survival in adult rabbits by increasing the body-cooling rates. Quastel[558] suggested that sedatives reduce the oxygen requirements of the brain and also impede a step in ATP synthesis. Dawes et al.[139] believe that the reasons for prolongation of asphyxial survival of sedated newborns are related to reduction in the rate of brain ATP utilization and decreased acid production, as well as direct action of the agents on the individual cells; but Dawes concluded that for actual asphyxia, the protective effents of pentobarbital are small, and the subsequent difficulties encountered in caring for sedated newborns does not commend it for practical obstetric use. Campbell et al.[90] reported increased resuscitability with pentobarbital in rabbits but stated that their interpretations should not be applied to humans.

Antimuscarinic drugs provide inhibition of vagal reflexes both in mother and fetus, as well as a dry newborn respiratory tract. Von Steinbuchel[716] introduced scopolamine in 1902 as a preanesthetic for obstetric patients, and the subsequent relevant literature, as well as his own studies, were reviewed by Snyder in 1949.[641] Snyder concluded that there was no evidence of fetal injury in humans or experimental animals, even when massive doses of scopolamine were used. Atropine, which gave comparable results in our rabbit studies, may be the obstetric antimuscarinic drug of choice because of its lack of amnesic effect. On theoretical grounds, Klaus[406] criticized the obstetric use of atropine because of possible inhibition of fetal asphyxial protective reflexes, but, as noted here, atropine and scopolamine increased fetal asphyxial survival.

Dawes *et al.* demonstrated in sheep and monkey fetuses that infusions of glucose and sodium bicarbonate during birth asphyxia can prolong newborn survival by maintaining higher blood pH and glucose levels. Glucose alone was found by Romney and Gabel[580] to have therapeutic significance for the human fetus when administered during labor in the presence of fetal distress, but recent studies by Myers[492] have suggested that hypoxic hyperglycemia is deleterious to future cerebral function. In support of tranquilizers, Frice has recommended the "lytic cocktail" (meperidine hydrochloride, chlorpromazine and promethazine) for the prevention and treatment of surgical shock.

These observations from many different laboratories and from various time periods provide support for the concept that maternal drugs may protect (to a degree) the asphyxiated fetus from CNS damage, although they may further depress cardiovascular function.

In the clinical situation, there is fear of adding the depressive effects of drugs to the depressive effects of asphyxia. While the newborn with a low Apgar score from maternal drugs may require active resuscitation, such a newborn's cerebral function is no more endangered from these drugs than if he were recovering from a general anesthetic. Indeed, as noted, his brain is protected to a degree from asphyxia. Myers' monkeys studies[492] have reinforced our observations with rabbits. There are no human data on the long-term cerebral development effects of intrapartum sedation, but the extensive and classic work of Myers with primate fetuses tested with variable degrees of asphyxia should be enough to demonstrate the value of sedation during fetal hypoxemia.

PROPHYLAXIS OF MECONIUM ASPIRATION

Aspiration of meconium is considered to be a significant cause of newborn respiratory morbidity. Since the occurrence of meconium aspiration is dependent on fetal or newborn

gasping, induced fetal apnea may be prophylactic in times of fetal stress. To test possible techniques for inducing fetal apnea, laboratory and clinical studies of the breathing activity of fetal sheep, rabbits, and humans are reported.

Laboratory Studies

Fetal sheep of 105–140 days were studied in Rudolph's laboratory with the usual catheter in fetal carotid artery, right ventricle, trachea and amniotic cavity. In four out of seven fetuses, only negative tracheal fluid deflections (gasping) were recorded. In three out of seven, positive tracheal deflections (grunting) occurred as well as gasping. These grunting breathing movements were associated with fetal cardiovascular changes (Figs. 22-2 and 22-3). All breathing activity ceased when the mothers were given therapeutic levels of pentobarbital, morphine, diazepam, and were reduced with atropine or scopolamine.

Pregnant rabbits were sacrificed on the 28th day of gestation with an injection of intravenous air. Five minutes prior to her death, the doe was given either normal saline, sodium pentobarbital, atropine, morphine, or diazepam intravenously. As soon as the animal expired, the intact uterine horns with fetuses were delivered and immersed in warm saline. Saturated solutions of India ink were injected immediately into the various amniotic sacs, a technique introduced by Becland in 1813! Subsequent studies of the lungs' "staining index" of the stillborn fetuses from India ink, whose mothers had received one of the drugs was 0.8, while those which had received normal saline was 2.8. Thus, these "depressive" drugs had reduced the amount of fetal gasping (and aspiration) of fetuses dying of asphyxia. The most effective drugs in inducing fetal apnea were pentobarbital and diazepam.

Clinical Application

It is generally agreed that meconium staining of the amniotic fluid is sometimes associated with fetal hypoxemia or acidemia, al-

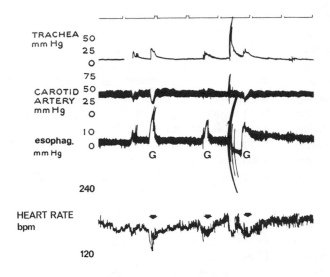

Fig. 22-2. Fetal sheep 118 days, with catheter in trachea, carotid artery, and esophagus. With fetal grunting, bradycardia and hypotension occurred.

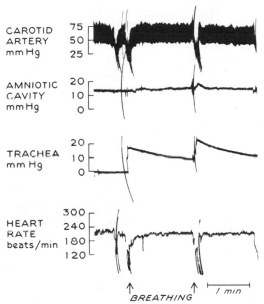

Fig. 22-3. Fetal sheep 127 days with catheter in trachea, amniotic cavity, and carotid artery. With fetal grunting, positive deflections, hypotension occurred.

though the relationship is unclear (Chapter 8). Meconium-stained amniotic fluid occurs in 16% of our parturients and their newborns subsequently have a relatively good initial Apgar score. Barring other problems, such as cardiovascular insult such as follows tracheal lavage or actual meconium aspiration, the newborn usually does well.

Because meconium aspiration obviously represents the sum of two separate fetal occurrences, namely, *in utero* defecation and gasping, its subsequent development may be

avoided either by preventing situations that introduce meconium into amniotic fluid or by inhibiting fetal breathing: although it would be desirable to avoid the mostly unknown situations that stimulate fetal defecation of meconium into the amniotic fluid (they appear to be largely vagal in origin and in the laboratory are usually prevented by atropine) such occurrences are relatively common and perhaps not completely avoidable. To prevent meconium aspiration, it seems more practical to inhibit fetal breathing by maternal medication, and if human fetuses respond like sheep or rabbits, narcotics, tranquilizers, or atropine would be appropriate drugs.

There is a widespread belief among both medical personnel and lay people that maternal sedation or narcosis is deleterious to the fetus. However, it can be demonstrated in the laboratory that a sedated or narcotized fetus is able to withstand limited asphyxia better and both fetal and newborn apnea are of advantage in cases of meconium in the nasopharynx. Meconium in a newborn's airway can produce "airblock syndrome," or obstructive respiratory distress unless removed prior to aspiration. Assuming that means for resuscitation are at hand at the time of delivery, purposeful sedation of a fetus may be indicated in high-risk pregnancies. There is no logic in allowing a stressed fetus to gasp or to metabolize faster.

In fetal sheep, gasping occurs without recognizable alterations in FHR pattern. This suggests that efforts to prevent fetal gasping (aspiration) cannot wait until worrisome FHR patterns occur, but must be used on a prophylactic routine basis if *in utero* meconium aspiration is to be prevented.

Induction of Fetal Apnea—Clinical Application

An animal's physiologic responses are not usually detrimental to itself for the species would be unlikely to survive. But because most mammals are meant to spend only a fraction of their life *in utero,* it is always possible that an extrauterine response could have selective advantages from an evolutionary standpoint and still be deleterious if enacted during fetal life. Besides prolonged bradycardia, gasping may be another such response.

My assumption is that while breathing activity is normal in the fetus (Chapter 14), when it includes gasping of meconium-stained amniotic fluid, it can be pathologic. Since commonly used maternal medications can inhibit fetal gasping, bradycardia, and

reduce metabolic needs, the responses are jointly presented and discussed.

For two years at the Santa Clara Valley Medical Center, an obstetrical effort was made to prevent every case of meconium aspiration. If amnioscopy were not possible, the protocol called for rupture of membranes early in labor and if meconium were present, to "sedate" the fetus. Fetal sedation was considered adequate (to the point of fetal apnea) if FHR recordings became "nonreactive" (Chap. 9) with decreased beat-to-beat variability and if the mother appeared well-sedated. Commonly used drugs were diazepam, pentobarbital, alphaprodine HCl, and meperidine HCl.

If for any reason the above routine were considered inadequate to have prevented fetal gasping, the mother was given up to 10 mg diazepam intravenously immediately prior to expulsion of the fetus. (This was prior to our concern for newborn effects of diazepam.) Its purpose was to induce newborn apnea so that tracheal aspiration could be more efficient in removing meconium that otherwise may have been in distal air passages. The newborn nasopharynx was aspirated prior to delivery of the shoulders. A pediatrician was present at all deliveries when meconium staining was diagnosed and performed newborn tracheal toilet when indicated.

Our meconium aspiration studies included 2056 deliveries during the time period with 243 cases of meconium staining of the amniotic fluid recognized. As so often happens in applying varying protocols, in only 148 cases was there sufficient concern or awareness by the staff to follow the meconium protocol for fetal sedation. No cases of meconium aspiration were diagnosed in the nursery in this group, although meconium was found three times (2%) below the newborn's vocal cords. Among the 95 newborns who received no specific fetal sedative therapy, meconium was noted below the fetal vocal cords in seven newborns (7%) and two of these were later diagnosed as having mild meconium aspiration.

During this same period, 13 newborns were referred to our hospital's newborn intensive care unit with a diagnosis of severe meconium aspiration of whom three died. None of their mothers had received more than meperidine 75 mg or diazepam 15 mg during their labors. Thus, it appeared that fetal sedation had some value in terms of reduced mortality.

The neonatologists objected very strongly to the use of diazepam as outlined in this protocol.[128] Newborns whose mothers have received a large dose tend to be "floppy," although the degree of floppiness cannot be correlated with serum levels of diazepam and "Letter to the Editor" in *Lancet* contests this point.[255a] I believe the drug to be especially useful for maternal seizure prevention[426a] and object to their restriction, but obstetricians must cooperate with those who care for our newborns. The Brazelton score and wideawake newborns are very much a part of our current nursery environment. Thus, while it is possible to demonstrate that the safest state for the intrapartum fetus is the anesthetized one, our attitudes will not allow us to use this information.

While the guinea pig is supposedly the only mammalian fetus which regularly defecates *in utero,* the same is often true of the postmature human fetus with its high frequency of meconium-stained fluid. Perhaps if all human newborns were as "mature" as is the newborn guinea pig at birth, they all would likewise be regularly defecating *in utero.* The point is that many of the early fetal breathing studies were done with guinea pig fetuses and they do gasp *in utero,* apparently with amniotic fluid frequently laden with feces. The guinea pig, however, seems to suffer little in terms of meconium aspiration. Obviously, there is some other protective mechanism from meconium aspiration than fetal apnea.

PREVENTION OF FETAL BRADYCARDIA (DECREASED UMBILICAL FLOW)

In fetal sheep, we have observed a particular type of fetal breathing response which is detrimental to the umbilical blood flow and is associated with an abrupt FHR bradycardia. Since abrupt heart rate patterns are usually considered benign in the intrapartum human fetus, it seems appropriate to once again note the pathophysiology of fetal sheep grunting now that we are discussing intrapartum management.

Laboratory Studies

The present analysis is based on the review of multichannel records from Rudolph's laboratory of fetal sheep studies (0.8 gestation) which include arterial pressure, heart rate, aortic, pulmonary or umbilical flows, and tracheal and amniotic fluid pressure.

In the chronic fetal sheep preparation, fetal breathing can be categorized into three different groups according to changes of tracheal pressures: (1) mild gasping or sighing (-1 to -7 mmHg), (2) regular gasping (-7 to -20 mmHg), and (3) grunting (+changes). The patterns may be mixed and may indeed reflect various stages of fetal health; but since grunting is the only breathing pattern to be related to fetal cardiovascular responses, it will be described in detail.

During fetal grunting and increased tracheal or intrapleural pressure, there is a simultaneous and proportional increase in fetal vena cava and peritoneal pressure, systolic arterial pressure, and umbilical vein pressure. There is an associated abrupt bradycardia and decrease in cardiac output and *umbilical* flow.

As Dawes and his associates[130] in England noted, umbilical flow is passive and is relatively nonresponsive to drugs. This suggests that umbilical flow is dependent only on cardiac output, mean arterial pressure, and pressure within the umbilical vein. Many periods of bradycardia in fetal sheep are secondary to fetal hypertension, which is a fortunate safeguard when fetal cardiac output falls, as the rise in mean systemic pressure maintains umbilical flow. However, a rise in umbilical vein pressure is consistently associated with a fall in umbilical flow, and it is the rise of this pressure during grunting that may make this breathing activity deleterious.

For, with repeated episodes of decreased umbilical flow (as can also occur in umbilical cord compression), fetal asphyxia may occur.

Survey of the recordings from Rudolph's laboratory suggested no clear-cut correlation between fetal blood gases, anniotic fluid pressure changes, other breathing activity, and the initiation of grunting. However, one fetus is illustrative of the possible deleterious effects of grunting. On its third post-surgical day, it was noted to have frequent episodes of grunting with associated abrupt falls of heart rate and umbilical flow (Fig. 22-4). Its distal aorta P_{O_2} fell from 19 to 9 torr as the periods of bradycardia became more frequent. With atropinization, a fetal tachycardia and increased umbilical flow occurred with a rise in P_{O_2} to 18 torr. The fetus was dead the next day, apparently from infection. Nevertheless, this case suggests that atropine can overcome the detrimental effects of grunting (valsalvaing) with its associated bradycardia. In the newborn, grunting is of advantage during hypoxia as it increases pulmonary vein P_{O_2} and presumably, fetal grunting (with its decreased umbilical vein P_{O_2}) represents an inappropriate use of this newborn response.

In our prior description of fetal grunting,[275] we recognized the associated bradycardia and probable decrease in cardiac output. It was only with the availability of acute determination of umbilical flow in Rudolph's laboratory that the possible detrimental effects of grunting and its bradycardia were appreciated. Whether abrupt human fetal deceleration (variable deceleration) should be prevented by atropinization on the assumption that atropine may prevent the decreases in fetal cardiac output has been debated.[525, 765b] However, the knowledge that abrupt decelerations of fetal heart rate may

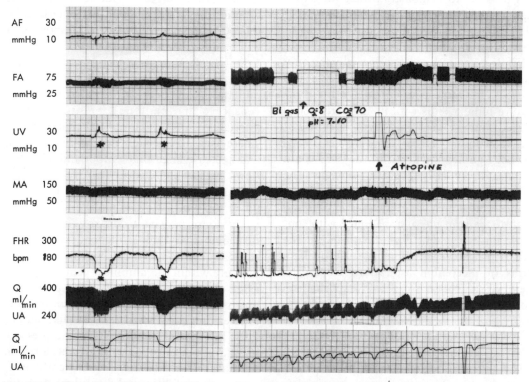

Fig. 22-4. Recording of "grunting (*)" sheep fetus (MA—maternal aorta; FA—fetal aorta) which turned into profound bradycardia. After atropine, FHR improved as did blood gas values. Note bradycardia with grunting (*). (From Goodlin, R.C.: *Obstet Gynecol* **48**: 1976. Reproduced with permission.)

represent grunting and decreased umbilical flow would seem to speak in favor of atropine or sedation. As mentioned above, the abrupt bradycardias may also reflect the fetal hypoxia–asphyxial response.

Because the adult diving reflex includes bradycardia, carcass, gut, and skin vasoconstriction, and constant stroke volume, it has often been compared to the fetal hypoxic reflex, despite the very different biochemical means by which diving animals and fetuses cope with distress (Chapter 8). Such reflexes obviously serve the diving seal well, but the fetal baroreceptor–bradycardia response may be self-destructive, mainly because umbilical flow may be compromised. From a phylogenetic standpoint, the diving and baroreflexes occurring in different species of fish. Perhaps the fetus inappropriately employs this ancient reflex.

In the hypoxic fetus, the carcass, skin, and intestinal constriction is apparently initiated by the aortic chemoreceptors via the aortic nerve, its severity is determined both by P_{O_2} and P_{CO_2} levels and it is maintained by the fetal catecholamine response. The hypertension reflects the generalized vasoconstriction and appreciably aids flow through the "nonreactive" umbilical circulation, but the hypertension also initiates the baroreceptor reflex which reduces heart rate proportional to the rise of blood pressure. While the fetal baroreflex appears late in *in utero* development, it is easily evoked. Atropine abolishes the bradycardia, the undesirable fetal feature of the hypoxic reflex, but leaves untouched the useful features (if not excessive) of hypertension and vasoconstriction.

In institutions where psychoprophylaxis is practiced and maternal hyperventilation and alkalosis are common, FHR decelerations occur less frequently during the first stage. The fetal baroreflex concept offers an explanation for lack of bradycardia since alkalosis (low P_{CO_2}) reduces vasoconstriction, thus reducing the episodes of secondary hypertension and resulting bradycardia following fetal stimulation by uterine contractions. While alkalosis may reduce the frequency of early decelera-

tions, it prevents the development of the desirable selective vasoconstriction and thus less blood will be diverted to the umbilical and cerebral circulation during times of fetal stress.

Fetal hypertension can occur through a variety of situations, including changes in fetal arousal level, fetal grunting, as well as the so-called fetal "head compression" associated with uterine contractions. Depending on the presence or absence of increased peripheral resistance and the cardiac performance, such fetal bradycardias may (or may not) be associated with reduced cardiac output and umbilical flows.

As discussed in Chapter 8, fetal bradycardia may be secondary to increased peripheral resistance (the bradycardia) or it may reflect direct central vagal stimulation. Likewise, fetal hypertension may be secondary to increased peripheral resistance, or it may reflect direct midbrain stimulation. Fetal cardiac performance can also be adequate for the situation and increase stroke volume during the bradycardia, or it may not be adequate. With those acute and severe bradycardias, usually stroke volume is not increased, as suggested by relatively constant $S_1 - S_2$ intervals (Chaps. 9 and 11). In the last situation, atropinization is of benefit since it abolishes the bradycardia and maintains cardiac output (Fig. 20-4). Obviously, the healthy fetus tolerates decreased umbilical flow and respiratory exchange, but the compromised fetus may not.

Avoiding Fetal Bradycardia— Clinical Application

As a clinical trial, an attempt was made to prevent the repeated occurrence of fetal intrapartum severe abrupt bradycardias (type I deceleration) with atropine, as long as the scalp pH values were above 7.20. A type I deceleration was considered severe if there was a decrease in FHR of more than 60 bpm, a FHR below 60 bpm, or if a bradycardia lasting longer than 60 sec was exceeded (the rule of "60"). If the bradycardia could be improved by other therapy, such as decreasing the oxytocin infusion rate, oxygen therapy, or changing maternal position, atropine was not used.

Atropine was administered to the fetus through either the maternal paracervical area or intravenously without any obvious benefit of one route over the other in terms of primarily fetal (and no maternal) atropine effects. Others have administered atropine directly into the fetal scalp, but the placental transfer of atropine is such that the maternal compartment must be filled if a therapeutic level is to be maintained in the fetus. By injecting into the maternal compartment, the risk of fetal overdosage is avoided. Figure 22-5 is a recording of a case in which the fetus was treated with atropine and had a satisfactory outcome. The patient was a 19-year-old parturient, para 0-0-0-0 at term with fetal bradycardia observed when she was 6 cm

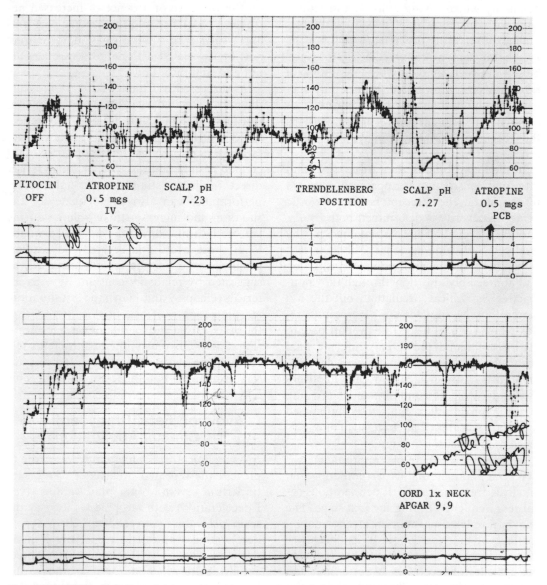

Fig. 22-5. FHR recording of fetus with severe vagal type bradycardia, which persisted despite stopping oxytocin, Trendelenberg position, and oxygen. Atropine was given in paracervical area. Tachycardia with minimal decelerations occurred. (From Goodlin, R.C.: *Obstet Gynecol* **48:** 117, 1976. Reproduced with permission.)

dilated. The bradycardia did not respond to discontinuation of oxytocin infusion, change in maternal position, or administration of oxygen. Scalp pH's were 7.23 and 7.27. Atropine 1.0 mg was given in the paracervical area in divided doses. The fetus responded with a tachycardia, and the fetus was delivered 2 hr later in good condition (umbilical artery pH 7.32). We have similarly treated more than 50 other fetuses and they have done well (no umbilical artery pH less than 7.23).

There were two other cases (out of more than 150) in which the bradycardia was not modified by atropine, and despite normal scalp pH, the babies were delivered by cesarean section for impending fetal distress. A failure of atropine therapy is shown in Figure 22-6. The fetus was postmature and showed vagal type bradycardia. A scalp pH (08116 of Fig. 22-6) was 7.22 and the gravida was given atropine 0.4 mg I.V. A questionable FHR atropine effect occurred (loss of BBV). However, when the gravida was 9+ cm dilated, severe vagal-type bradycardia returned (08126 of Fig. 22-6) with loss of BBV (a very ominous FHR pattern). Forty minutes after the scalp pH of 7.22, a 4020-g depressed newborn was delivered who had an umbilical artery pH 6.84! The newborn had immediate

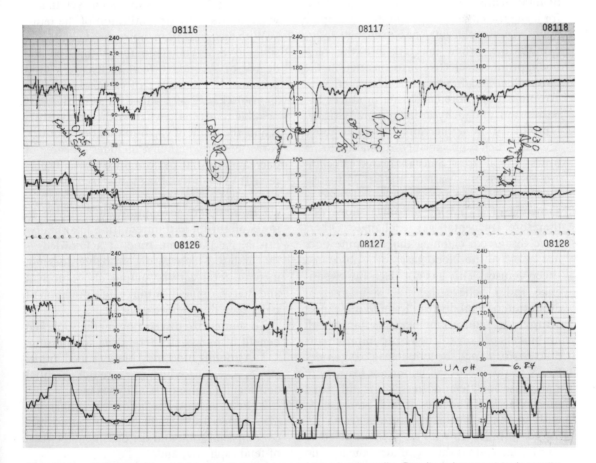

Fig. 22-6. FHR recording of fetus showing severe vagal-type bradycardia. Despite subsequent tachycardia, vagal activity continued. Newborn had severe acidemia (pH 6.84).

seizure activity, but by 8 hr of age was doing well. There was no explanation for this newborn asphyxia, although there was a loose nuchal cord. I would like to think that this atropine therapy "failure" represented an inadequate drug dose and effect.

The fetal baroreflex should at least be partially reduced by inducing maternal hyperventilation because of the diminishing effects of hypocarbia on fetal selective vasoconstriction (Chap. 8). While hypocarbia does diminish the incidence of abrupt fetal bradycardia in the laboratory, we have not found maternal hyperventilation to be nearly as effective as atropinization in the labor room in abolishing type I dips.

A final argument for atropine during times of fetal distress is illustrated in Figure 10-1, for it suggests that during fetal stress, atropine may increase placental gas exchange. Norepinephrine, when injected into the fetal body, produces selective vasoconstriction, the baroreflex, and bradycardia. However, with atropinization, norepinephrine produces hypertension, and tachycardia, not bradycardia! Umbilical flow is therefore increased above normal which is presumably of benefit during times of fetal stress. Since increased catecholamine levels are part of the fetal distress response, atropine appears to be indicated as a means of increasing umbilical flow, and therefore, placental gas exchange. Others have disagreed, claiming that atropine does not improve the blood gases of asphyxiated sheep fetuses. This has not been my experience and I believe that it is a manner of definition of fetal distress. I would not expect atropine to reduce umbilical resistance with umbilical cord obstruction or to improve cardiac performance, or to increase oxygen delivery to the uterus, all important features of some cases of "fetal distress." It is only used prophylactically in cases of fetal bradycardia with impending fetal hypoxemia (from reduced umbilical flow). This point needs to be emphasized—that the use of atropine is in no way an attempt at "*in utero* resuscitation."

Discussions with other obstetricians have indicated that many believe fetal vagal function is beneficial (and atropine harmful) during the stress of birth, despite the fact that they recognize vagal activity as sometimes being detrimental during other stresses, such as surgery. The concept that the baroreflex could be detrimental to a fetus and for the human race to have survived, seems to many of my colleagues to be incompatible. More important than this "back to nature" argument are the obscuring effects of atropine on FHR interpretation.

Since 1967, we have considered the presence of what is now termed "beat-to-beat variability," the single most important FHR pattern parameter of fetal well-being. To deliberately smooth over the FHR recordings with drugs and to obscure this parameter appears to be a regressive step, yet this is what occurs with atropinization of the fetus.

With atropinization, however, it is still possible to estimate sympathetic tone by the degree of secondary fetal tachycardia (and presumably the degree of catecholamine response) (Fig. 22-7). Most importantly, it is possible to estimate whether the bradycardia is only the result of vagal stimulation (entirely corrected) or whether it includes a degree of decreased cardiac performance (partially corrected). The latter diagnostic test, plus the prophylactic benefits of maintaining umbilical flow, makes atropinization desirable in times of abrupt and unremitting fetal bradycardia. At the same time, it acknowledges that induced tachycardia probably does not increase fetal cardiac output above normal and that atropine may make interpretation of FHR recordings more difficult.

To summarize this section on the supposed benefit of purposeful fetal drug suppression:

1. Atropinization may prevent fetal grunting/bradycardia which is a rare but potential detrimental cause of fetal hypoxemia;

2. Fetal narcosis/sedation/tranquilization may protect (to a slight degree) against meconium aspiration and the detrimental effects of fetal asphyxia; and,

3. Fetal narcosis may relieve fetal pain (Chap. 16).

The disadvantages of fetal drug therapy

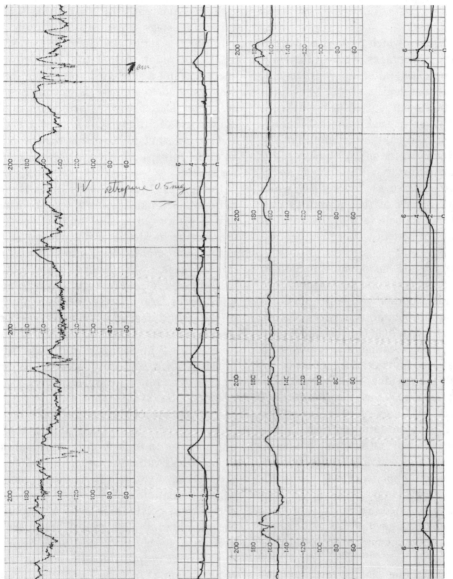

Fig. 22-7. FHR recording showing moderate vagal activity. After atropine, only accelerations remained (plus loss of BBV and tachycardia). Umbilical artery pH was 7.19.

are:

i. FHR recordings may be more difficult to interpret.

ii. The sedated fetus may have low Apgar scores, require resuscitation, and be a nonresponsive or "floppy" newborn.

AMNIONITIS

In those cases in which there is prolonged rupture of the membranes, we treat the gravida with ampicillin (after appropriate culture). The neonatologists object when they believe the treatment is used in the absence of maternal fever, as such maternal therapy confuses their own culture techniques of the newborn. However, too many viable size infants die in the nursery with group B *Streptococcus, Listerosis,* or *Escherichia coli,* while awaiting the results of the newborn's culture for me not to believe that this form of prophylaxis is of benefit to both mother and newborn.

When the gravida has obvious amnionitis as evidenced by fever and leukocytosis, we have treated the mother with very high doses of intravenous ampicillin, as the drug reaches the amniotic fluid in high concentrations. An argument against treating amnionitis with systemic maternal antibiotics is that the drugs do not reach the decidua in sufficient quantities to be effective. We use a technique that was described by Carey of New Zealand in the 1950s, infusing the antibiotic (usually ampicillin) through an intrauterine catheter, achieving very high amniotic fluid levels of the antibiotic. Our experience is limited to 15 cases, but such intraamniotic therapy has, in my experience, resulted in dramatic improvement of the maternal symptoms and has resulted in the delivery of infants in good condition.

If gravida have unexplained fever, an amniocentesis is always worthwhile. We have cultured out of amniotic fluid such bacteria as *Clostridia, Proteus,* and *Staphylococcus* in gravida with no other symptoms.

THE SECOND STAGE OF LABOR

The duration of the second stage of labor has been subjected to arbitrary rules ever since the availability of the obstetrical forceps. Hellman and Prystowsky[331] ascribed to the great obstetrical authorities of the past (Hunter, Osborne, and Denman) the banishment of forceps to shorten the second stage of labor, although Denman did establish a 6-hr limit. Apparently the 2-hr rule for duration of second stage arose with Hamilton, who published a series of papers from 1853 to 1871. He reported that in 1500 deliveries, there was not a single stillborn when forceps were applied to shorten the second stage. It was after DeLee's recommendation in 1920 for the use of prophylactic forceps to shorten the second stage of labor that the acceptance of outlet forceps occurred with American obstetricians.

In their 1952 review of the Johns Hopkins material, Hellman and Prystowsky concluded that a prolonged second stage of labor increased the incidence of postpartum hemorrhage, puerperal febrility, and infant mortality. However, I was taught as a house officer in the mid-1950s that, barring maternal exhaustion or fetal distress, there was no limit on the second stage of labor, as long as "progress" was occurring. From a practical standpoint, after 2 hr of the second stage, we, as house officers, somehow managed to detect fetal bradycardia and usually mercifully terminated labor at this point.

The concept of the detrimental effects of prolonged fetal bradycardia during the second stage as an indication for termination of labor is still valid. As noted in Chapter 10, the acute severe vagal bradycardia is common with full dilatation of the cervix, particularly with a tight pelvic floor and with rupture of the membranes. This sort of bradycardia is presumed to be associated with decreased fetal cardiac output and often leads to a mild fetal acidemia. In fact, I consider the fetus "at risk" whenever these second stage FHR patterns occur, even when the cervix is not completely dilated. This at risk concept does not imply that a midforceps operation is indicated, only that delivery should be accomplished as soon as an easy outlet forceps may be done. On the other hand, in the absence of such second stage FHR patterns, it seems safe and prudent to wait (as long as true progress is occurring) for an easy and simple delivery.

Any discussion of the second stage of labor presumes that its definition is precise. In reality, the cervix is often dilated 10 cm and is not fully retracted. Whether such cervical "lips" or "rims" mean that the second stage has not begun is a subject of frequent debate on our service. If the cervix must be completely retracted, then many parturients labor and deliver with virtually no second stage. For some, cervix can often be palpated just before the fetal head delivers. (The occurrence of "second stage" FHR patterns (Chapter 9) may be a more accurate definition).

Optimal Modes of Delivery

The Collaborative Study,[211] as well as smaller, detailed investigations,[173] have suggested that certain fetuses with operative procedures are at increased risk of subsequent cerebral dysfunction or decreased performance. Included among these would be the IUGR fetus, the premature, the surviving twin, the postmature, or macrosomic fetus, the breech presentation, the fetus delivered by midforceps operation, the fetus delivered after treatment of secondary arrest, the fetus of the gravida with toxemia or with hypoglycemia or with Rh incompatibility, the fetus born after prolonged labor or short labor, the fetus whose placenta has an abnormality such as previa or abruptio or cord prolapse, and so forth. The point of such a list is to emphasize that many different factors have been reported to be associated with subsequent neurological dysfunction besides fetal asphyxia or breech presentation. To offer cesarean section to one group (or list of obstetrical abnormalities) and not the entire group, seems illogical.

PREMATURITY

From a clinical standpoint, the problems of prematurity have several partial solutions. As noted repeatedly, gravida at risk (prior premature delivery, those with vascular disease, cervical factors, pyelitis; see Table D-

(42) should avoid hard physical work, emotional stress, orgasm, and have an expanded blood volume. If premature labor occurs prior to 34 weeks of pregnancy, labor should be inhibited, chorioamnionitis treated with antibiotics, and fetal lungs "matured" with steroids if the L/S is below 1.5. Delivery should probably be accomplished by cesarean section if optimal newborn development is to be achieved (Chapter 19).

Delivery of the Small Fetus

Perhaps as important as the problems of pulmonary maturity are those related to the mode of delivery of the fetus weighing less than 1300 g. For the small fetus in the breech presentation, abdominal delivery appears best, but for the same size fetus in vertex presentation, we are undecided. Since a classical type of uterine incision is almost always required at this stage of pregnancy, we allow the gravida the option of either abdominal or vaginal delivery (after explaining the relative risks). We site Stewart's data[666] from England in support of delivery by cesarean section. On the other hand, the maternal risks of a classical section, because of the probable presence of chorioamnionitis or weaker scare, are significant. At the same time, the 1000–1300-g fetus in the vertex presentation often does well as a newborn, but unfortunately it may also be bruised or otherwise severely stressed by vaginal delivery. (Sometimes abdominal delivery of these small fetuses is also a traumatic experience, especially if attempted through a lower segment section.) In the less than 1-kg newborn, the occurrence in the nursery (it hardly ever occurs intrapartum) of intraventricular hemorrhage with subsequent hydrocephalus is frequent. However, the stresses of labor in these small fetuses can remotely cause cerebral bleeds.

Even when we have proclaimed that abdominal delivery of the small fetus shall be the "rule" of our service, review of our records shows that cesarean section only because the fetus was immature was seldom used. Sometimes the gravida declined after explanation of the risks and newborn prognosis, other times serious chorioamnionitis was present (and maternal risks appeared to be too great) and in others, by the time that inevitable labor was obvious, vaginal delivery appeared imminent.

The management problem is even more difficult when the fetus weighs less than 800 g. Such newborns do very poorly with a high incidence of neurological impairment among survivors despite great efforts and expense on the part of the neonatologists. When we have not actively resuscitated the smaller than 800 g newborn in the delivery room, an occasional one has survived on its own, only to develop intraventricular hemorrhage and hydrocephalus subsequently. The thought that our benign neglect was in part responsible for such an unfavorable outcome, compels us to active care, with the result that our intensive care nursery is often filled with relatively hopeless cases (in terms of ultimate survival of a normal child) of newborns weighing less than 800 g. One technique which should probably be abandoned is to routinely deliver the small fetus by forceps. This is usually accomplished under regional anesthesia and the subsequent "low" forceps is often far from gentle, producing severe forceps marks on the small and fragile vertex.

CESAREAN SECTION

Cesarean sections on our service are done as rapidly as possible and preferably under general anesthesia. Eight years experience with maternal pulse monitoring has demonstrated (to me at least) that the maternal supine position on the firm operating room table produces varying degrees of aortal occlusion (Fig. 22-8). While the maternal lateral position or devices designed to displace the uterus have been tried, I still believe that the best technique is one which delivers the infant in the shortest time after the skin incision. Our technique is to use a low transverse abdominal incision, cutting down in the midline immediately. The subcutaneous tissue is then spread with right-angle retractors. The peritoneum is often opened by blunt dissection with a Kelly clamp. We rarely find it necessary to tie bleeders prior to the uterine incision. With this technique of blunt dissection in primary cesarean section, the infant can easily be delivered in less than 5 min time and the gravidas have done well.

Another Point of View

OBSTETRICAL INTERFERENCE

Richards has recently reviewed the induction and acceleration of labor with its apparent benefits and complications. Jeffcoate and Scott,[378] for instance, have reported that induction rates of 20–50% are occurring in some British maternity units and that these units give the best maternal and fetal results. But, as noted repeatedly, perinatal mortality rates are decreasing worldwide under many different circumstances. Richards[575] observes that these improvements in perinatal rates are probably occurring because of more optimal maternal reproductive age, legal abortion, and improvement in general health.

One of the popular arguments for elective induction is the avoidance of postmature fetuses being stillborn. However, in the United Kingdom, despite widespread use of induction, the incidence of problems associated with postmaturity have not decreased.[359] Nor does a high induction rate necessarily reduce this incidence of night time complicated deliveries.[116] Williams[755] has suggested that the night time load is reduced, but apparently this reduction reflects mostly normal pregnancies. Then too, everyone from house staff to nurses aids recognized that elective induction increases hospital costs with its pumps, monitors, and increased need for pain relief and additional staff.

The obstetrical complications for inductions are many. In some British hospitals, the commonest indication for cesarean section is failed induction.[575] There is usually an increased rate of forcep deliveries, probably because of the availability of staff with its increased rate of epidural anesthesia. The British Births Survey suggests that trauma is increased for both mother and child with elective induction. Maternal infections are likewise more likely after inductions.

Newborn depression, jaundice, and respiratory problems are more common after induction of labor. This is perhaps related to providing maternal pain relief, or labor that is abnormally

Fig. 22-8. Pulse recordings during cesarean section. F, finger; V, vaginal; T, hallux (big toe); 1, control period (chart speed 2.5 cm/min); 2, brachial BP 70/20, infused saline; 3, BP 90/60; 4, uterine incision with vaginal movement; 5, delivery of head with partial return of vaginal and hallux pulses; 6, delivery of newborn with Apgar 2, maternal pulses returning to normal height (chart speed 2.5 mm/min.) (Reproduced with permission of *Obstet Gynecol,* 1972).

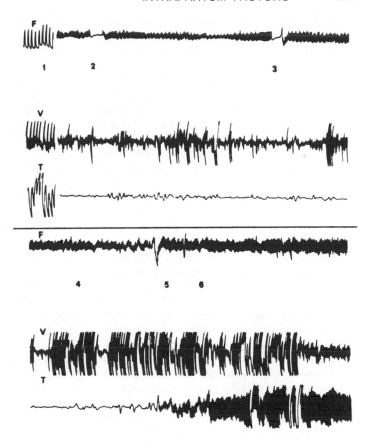

accelerated or the increased incidence of prematurity. The occurrence of neonatal jaundice with induction is perhaps related to fetal bruising and drugs used with epidural anesthesia or to lack of proper fetal inductions of enzymes associated with spontaneous labor.[213a] Then too, mother–infant separation is apparently more common in induced labors.[575]

Another series of related studies concerning obstetrical intervention was by Chambers and colleagues[95] of two hospital groups in Wales. They were unable to demonstrate that use of prenatal estrogen analysis or ultrasonography reduced perinatal mortality. Likewise, they were unable to show improvements in perinatal mortality with elective induction. This latter is especially important as one of the coauthors was A. C. Turnbull. Turnbull designed the "Cardiff infusion pump" which automatically controlled oxytocin infusion for (elective) induction of labor.

On our service, I argue for widespread induction of labor because our senior staff disappears in late afternoon in both the labor wards and

nursery and because it evens out the work load during the week for the hospital staff. With small obstetrical units like ours, there are tremendous "valleys and peaks" in work loads and numbers of deliveries. The peak times are when we are more likely to provide less than optimal care (more postpartum hemorrhages, more misdiagnoses) or be out of supplies. However, the house staff clearly prefers to let "nature take its course" as the work load is less, and perhaps iatrogenic complications are reduced.

MECONIUM ASPIRATION

The problem of meconium aspiration is still present. Gregory *et al.*[300] studied 1000 newborns who had an unbelieveably high incidence of meconium aspiration at the University of California, San Francisco. They demonstrated that immediate endotracheal aspiration reduced by a marked degree the incidence of serious subsequent neonatal problems. Carson and others[91] from the University of Colorado showed a similar improvement with suctioning of the nasopharynx prior to delivery of the newborn's shoulders. We have routinely suctioned newborns as recommended by both the Colorado and San Francisco groups. Unfortunately, since we no longer induce fetal apnea, we still have cases of moderate to severe meconium aspiration occur among our newborns. In addition, newborn endotracheal lavage often seems to be a traumatic and dangerous procedure. We have witnessed cardiac arrest and general depression of those sometimes already stressed newborns. Meconium-stained fluid is now associated on our service with low 5-min Apgar scores, not (I believe) because of intrapartum events, but often because of prophylactic therapy in the immediate newborn period (Fig. 22-9).

An entirely different approach is taken by O'Driscoll *et al.*,[513] who showed in 1000 deliveries that meconium never appeared intrapartum after clear amniotic fluid had been demonstrated. Thus, meconium-stained fluid always made itself evident with the rupture of membranes and meconium staining was not a product of the stresses of labor, but of pregnancy. They also conclude that the introduction of fetal heart rate monitors into routine clinical practice may have been premature, since most fetal distress occurs in the antenatal period. While sharing their views on the importance of antenatal versus intrapartum fetal monitoring, I have seen many cases (Chap. 10) in which meconium staining occurred not before, but during, labor.

THE COUNTERCULTURE GROUP

The counterculture aspect of obstetrical care is perhaps best expressed in America by the International Childbirth Education Association. In a 1973 paper by Doris Haire, she argues against the basic concepts of what many of us consider to be the essence of regionalized obstetrical care.[312] Among those features coming under her fire are the university hospital obstetrical services (versus the small neighborhood hospital), the "judicious use" of obstetrical drugs, induction of labor, use of ultrasound, and fetal monitoring in general. It seems obvious that small obstetrical units should have better perinatal rates, not because of the type of obstetrics practiced, but because of the type of patient they serve. University hospitals have the high-risk obstetrics.

The problem of drug testing for obstetrical patients is a serious one. The U. S. Food and Drug Administration does not require that drugs used during labor have long-term safety demonstrated prior to their general release. One could assume that since most of the drugs used have been on the market for a number of years, if any produced detrimental effects, this would have become apparent by now. However, the 1973 report of the alcohol syndrome by Jones and Smith[386] questions this logic. The dreadful effects of chronic alcoholism on newborn de-

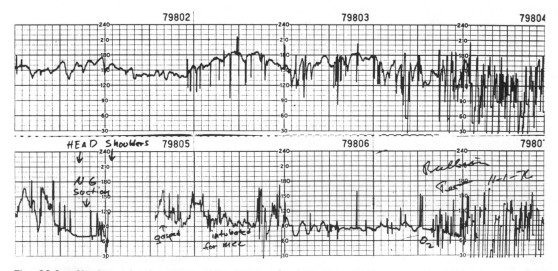

Fig. 22-9. Newborn showing prolonged bradycardia associated with attempts at tracheal suction for mild meconium aspiration. Initially, newborn appeared in good condition, but after lavage, required intensive care. (Same as Fig. 10-10.)

velopment is now apparent and presumably has always been so. How this common syndrome, arising from a common drug, could have been missed for so long in the American literature is indeed a mystery. Presumably, at this very moment, the same sort of detrimental effects could be occurring with some of the other less commonly used intrapartum drugs. On the other hand, the almost instantaneous publishing of poorly designed drug studies demonstrating possible harm to the fetus by otherwise distinguished medical journals seems to be a "cross" that all obstetricians must bear.[184a] The number of drugs from diuretics to aspirin that have been reported to be deleterious and then later found to have a questionable relationship is indeed confusing. Unless we wish to return to the preanesthesia days when labor was for some "travail," then there appears to be no immediate solution to the possible detrimental effects of intrapartum drugs on the newborn's development. However, it is obvious that obstetricians should begin to look at the possible deleterious effects of intrapartum drugs on the fetus in longer terms than whether they may depress the initiation of respiration.

Differences in interpretation on the effects of general anesthesia on fetal well-being are shown by a recent paper on Timor-Tritsch and associates.[699] They recorded FHR patterns during general anesthesia for cesarean sections, some done for fetal distress. They reported that many of the abnormal FHR patterns decreased, presumably because of decreased uterine contractibility associated with general anesthesia. They did not consider the alternative (as noted above) of the probable benefit of anesthesia on fetal asphyxial responses.

Taylor,[678] of Cambridgeshire, noted that general anesthesia (atropine, thiopentone succinylcholine) during cesarean section tended to reduce FHR decelerations. He concludes that delay up to 10 min in delivering the infant does not depress the newborn. Both Crawford[125] and Cohen[111] suggest that optimal time in delivering an infant after a general anesthetic should allow time (7–10 min) for the barbiturate to partially clear from the fetal circulation. Crawford[127] was to modify his recommendation to suggest that time elapsed between incision of the uterus and delivery of the infant was more closely related to depression of the newborn than the time between induction of anesthesia and incision of the uterus.

Myers'[492] report about the detrimental effects of hyperglycemia during asphyxia has caused us to reevaluate the routine use of intravenous fluids during labor. Perhaps most parturients should be allowed to go dry!

As Desmond[154] has noted, intrapartum sedatives, narcotics, tranquilizers, anesthetics (general and regional), all depress the newborn suckling and responsive reflexes. However, it has not been demonstrated that there is any untoward drug effect on a newborn's subsequent development. Children of the affluent tend to do better in our society than do those born of poor parents. Yet, because of the nature of private versus charity obstetrical practice in America, it is the children of the affluent who were much more likely to have been "drugged" as fetuses and newborns. To many it appears that obstetrical medication presents a recognizable hazard to the development of newborn infants. If and when this is demonstrated, our current obstetrical practices will be significantly changed. We should not panic however, just because neonatologists have new techniques (toys?) which can demonstrate that minimal use of intrapartum drugs affect such newborn responses as reaction to a pin prick at three days of age. The introduction of electronic fetal monitoring and its techniques should have taught obstetricians that all new gadgets are not necessarily an advance in patient care. The proof of the supposedly harmful effects of intrapartum drugs must await long-term controlled studies.

BONDING

In a 1977 guest editorial, Sloan[634] of New York Medical College suggested that childbirth is "no disease to be cured," but rather a series of "tasks to be accomplished." He challenges the concept of routine deep nasopharyngeal suctioning, slapping, bright lights, low room temperatures and so forth. Sloan claims that "too sudden and early separation" of mother and newborn can lead to a poorer growth weight pattern, lower I.Q., lesser vocabulary, weaker intellect, and increased infection rate. While he supplies no references or data, if his statements are accurate, then the answer is obvious. Since all workers in the health field are committed to avoiding every one of the deleterious effects he blames on early mother–infant separation, we should bring about a bonanza in human welfare by not separating a mother and her newborn under any set of circumstances. We can all agree that it is not enough to deliver a "good baby," but to deliver a "good person." If this can all be accomplished in the delivery room, obstetrics must then be the most important of all medical professions.

A serious study about early separation was that by Beusel *et al.*[691] In the follow-up study of children admitted to the special care nursery, a significant difference between the histories of the "abused" and "nonabused" infants was that the mothers of abused suffered from medical illnesses during pregnancy and the puerperium. These maternal illnesses presumably prevented maternal–newborn interaction along with other factors. While such maternal–newborn separation (as occurs with maternal infection) may be unavoidable, these affected newborns should be considered as high risk for child abuse.

Our neonatologist (B. Goetzman) has stated that if only wanted children were born, our neonatal unit would be nearly empty. As discussed in Chapter 1, I believe that maternal attitudes, emotions, and anxiety influence her fetus's personality. Thus, while the tranquil mothers "bond" well, and have good relationships with their infants, the relationship was in part determined during pregnancy. On the other hand, the gravida poorly adapted to her pregnancy is high risk for premature labor and even at term has a less tranquil fetus. Bonding (it seems to me) is unlikely by itself to overcome this poor gravida–fetus relationship. In humans, the effects of maternal bonding have not been tested in a truly controlled study.

BREECH DELIVERY

In 1974, Brenner *et al.*[70] sounded the alarm on the perils of breech vaginal delivery. Based upon an analysis of 30,359 deliveries at the MacDonald House in Cleveland (1962–1969), they found that congenital abnormalities complicate breech presentation in 5% of the cases versus 2.1% in nonbreech presentations. A more important finding was that perinatal mortality for breech presentation for vaginal delivery was 3.2% and zero for cesarean section. Immediately, in clinics everywhere in America, cesarean section became the preferred mode of delivery for breech presentation.

The USC group in Los Angeles County Hospital began a randomized study of breech presentation comparing cesarean section versus vaginal delivery.[116a] Their criteria for allowing breech vaginal delivery were very restrictive (frank breech with large pelvis as demonstrated by x-ray pelvimetry). As probably luck would have it, those mothers undergoing cesarean section in the USC service suffered serious complications.

We are fortunate to have on our service some gravida who "insist" on vaginal deliveries with breech presentation. If their pelvis is normal by roentgenogram and if they accept the slight increased risk of CNS abnormalities in their child, we are pleased to agree with their demands. However, I remain convinced that we should not allow vaginal delivery of the "tiny" (900–1250 g) breech. Even if the child is born in good condition, the soft tissue trauma associated with breech delivery can be overwhelming for the tiny neonate.

AMNIOTIC FLUID INFECTION

Naeye and Peters[501a] have continued to analyze the Collaborative Project data, collected between 1959 and 1966, relative to the amniotic fluid infections (syndrome). They found that the syndrome was the most frequent cause of perinatal death (6.17 per 1000 births). The mortality rates declined after midgestation, but a second peak of fetal infections was found after 37 weeks gestation. The amniotic fluid infection syndrome was positively correlated with poverty, lack of prenatal care, or adequate weight gain. These authors suggest that there may be an antimicrobial factor in amniotic fluid, which is lacking in certain gravida and which explains the occurrence of the amniotic fluid infection. I am convinced that our premature labor protocol (Protocol P-V) using antibiotics is helpful in these patients.

In California at least, Chicano and Vietnamese gravida are often malnourished, poor, and fail to attend antenatal clinics. Yet, their newborns are relatively large and their perinatal mortality rates are good. Perhaps genetic factors are more important than prenatal care or nutrition in determining perinatal mortality rates. In the past, Naeye's study group was chiefly black, and from the ghetto of the inner city.

Just to demonstrate that controversy surrounds nearly every topic discussed in this section, Seppala and associates[625] suggest that the presence of meconium in amniotic fluid may have some fetal benefits. Mainly, that meconium has oxytocin-like activity and that its presence in amniotic fluid leads to shorter labors!

CLINICAL CASES NO. 22-1

With a university hospital service of approximately 1600 deliveries a year, we have a dreadful perinatal rate of approximately 50 per 1000. As previously noted, this reflects (I hope) the large number of transfers to us of gravida in labor prior to the 30th week of pregnancy or gravida with fetal deaths. Indeed, one county in Northern California has reduced its stillborn rate to essentially zero by transferring all such cases to our hospital.

We encourage gravida with prior cesarean sections or breech presentation to deliver vaginally if certain criteria can be met. We do only 5–7 cesarean sections a year for acute fetal distress. Nevertheless, our cesarean section rate is approximately 11%. This high rate is explained by our efforts to deliver the tiny premature or SFD fetus by classical cesarean section, to attempt to prevent prolonged labor (acute phase longer than 18 hr), and the fact that many women with prior cesarean sections or breech presentation request delivery by cesarean section. Our midforceps rate is 7%. Unless the gravida requests otherwise, all women in labor are electronically monitored and receive intravenous fluids. Approximately 6% of the fetuses have at least one scalp pH.

Adjacent to our delivery room is a beautifully furnished homestyle room with a queen size conventional bed. Approximately 350 women have given birth in this alternate birth facility (15 per month), the majority under the supervision of a certified midwife. No fetal monitoring is done, no intravenous fluids or significant pain relief is used. The women are discharged home often after only 6 hr. Home visits are made by nurse practitioner for the first 5 days postpartum. Only 3% of the newborns have been readmitted, mostly for hyperbilirubinemia. The perinatal mortality rate has been zero (and with luck we hope that it continues). Only 50% of the primigravida remain low risk (Goodwin score less than 1) and stay in the program, but 85% of those having had a previous normal pregnancy are able to do so. Among the 360 gravida registering and delivering in the home style program, four eventually had a cesarean section and two were delivered by midforceps.

Only a huge series will prove the safety of the alternate birth center. One disappointing feature of our home style program is that the individualized nursing care has made its costs equal to those of a physician-managed delivery.

CHAPTER 23

The Obstetrician's Role in the Occurrence of Cerebral Palsy

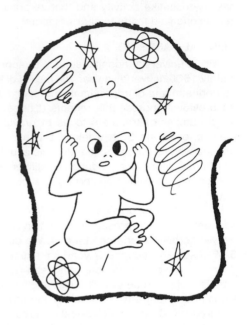

It is uncertain at which stage DNA replication ceases in the human brain, but it is probably by six months after birth. The cerebellum is somewhat later in reaching its cellular maturity than is the cerebrum.[343] Since dividing or immature cells are more sensitive to asphyxia, cases of true fetal distress at term or in the newborn are more likely to produce damage in the cerebellum than in the cerebrum. Cerebellum dysfunction has been the clinical picture seen by most observers since the time of Little's first descriptions in 1847.[451]

Etiology—Historical Aspects

A complication which obstetricians consider more terrible than fetal death is the occurrence of cerebral dysfunction or cerebral palsy (CP) in any child whom he or she has delivered. More than a century ago, Little[451] proposed that parturition was a significant cause of subsequent cerebral palsy in the child. He found an association of abnormal parturition, difficult labor, premature labor, asphyxia neonatorium, and cerebral palsy. Most obstetricians of his day objected to Little's concept, for they believed[632a] that it was unfair to be held responsible for the occurrence of cerebral palsy, citing many case histories of infants that were markedly depressed at the time of birth, but who had subsequent normal development. Sigmund Freud, in the late 19th century, also objected to Little's concepts, instead proposing that most cases of cerebral palsy or dysfunction represented prenatal developmental defects. The subsequent arguments as to the etiology of cerebral palsy vacillated between the concepts of Little and those of Freud, with most discussants agreeing that there was some validity in the extremes of both viewpoints.

There is no doubt that actual obstetrical trauma such as the grotesque misuses of the obstetrical forceps, can produce newborn cerebral damage which leads to subsequent cerebral dysfunction. And even the most enthusiastic advocate of obstetrical trauma as a major cause of cerebral palsy agrees that there is poor correlation between the condition of the term-size infants and whether they subsequently develop cerebral palsy. It is possible to argue rather convincingly with supporting data that either parturition is a significant cause of cerebral palsy or that *in utero* or neonatal events outside the time of parturition are the most frequent etiological factors.[290]

During the early 1950s, Eastman,[176] as professor of obstetrics at the Johns Hopkins University and author of the Williams' *Textbook of Obstetrics,* began searching for "new avenues for obstetrical research." The research problems relative to maternal death had been solved and Eastman apparently believed that the relative lack of research problems was why obstetrics was failing to attract the better medical students. Professor Eastman also had an abiding interest in the etiology of CP and in his famous "Mount Everest *In Utero*" address,[177] stated that "knowing as we do that intrauterine anoxia actually kills such a large number of infants, would it not be logical to believe that sometimes a degree of anoxia may not be quite sufficient to kill the infant but enough to inflict irreparable injury to the cerebrum?" This concept had been voiced before and since, but never as well and remains a widely held concept, though still unproven. While Eastman probably hoped for an outpouring of obstetrical research interest in CP, his question instead evoked widespread legal interests.

Eastman knew (as indicated from his own references) that his view on sublethal damage contradicted much of the published literature. Many studies have suggested the transient nature of perinatal results and the importance of environmental versus biological events in the subsequent development of cerebral dysfunction. Papers in America as well as Europe have attested to the difficulty of correlating the condition of the newborn with his subsequent development,[105, 161, 163, 165, 507, 744] and animal experiments had suggested that the normal fetus responds to asphyxia in an "all-or-nothing phenomenon," as most monkey newborns exposed to asphyxia either recovered or died despite rather precise protocols for the duration of stress and timing of the resuscitation.

An important paper in the controversy about the etiology of CP was that of Lilienfeld and Parkhurst.[445] They studied the incidence of various perinatal complications among 561 children with cerebral palsy using information that had been derived retrospectively from birth certificates. They found the "observed to expected ratio" of cerebral palsy to be very high among conditions that are normally associated with prematurity, such as placenta previa, breech, and abruptio placentae. On the other hand, there was a low incidence of "observed to expected ratio" in those in which the child was obviously at term, such as dystocia. The authors offered no controls for birth weight, although they recognized that cerebral palsy occurred at a much higher incidence among children who were born prematurely. Indeed, Eastman himself acknowledged that prematurity was present at least in 30% of the cases that developed cerebral palsy. These older investigators speculated on the relationship of the CP and prematurity. They hardly considered that it might represent inadequate neonatal care!

Following Eastman's statements and with his encouragement, the National Institute of Health sought to determine the etiology of cerebral palsy, choosing to monitor in great detail 50,000 pregnancies and the subsequent children through school age. With typical American confidence, it was expected that if enough money and time were expended, the etiology of most cases of CP could be determined, and therefore subsequently prevented. This study is now in its final stage with many of the children old enough to vote in state elections, but even yet, not all of the data have been analyzed. However, it does appear to support the concepts of Sigmund Freud. This has been shown in at least three reports from the Collaborative Project,[105, 163, 507] which, for unknown reasons, have been largely ignored by our pediatrics and neurological colleagues.

Recent Studies

In a conference involving the directors of the Collaborative Project, Drage *et al.*[163] reported that the condition of the term infant was poorly correlated with subsequent development of cerebral palsy. Furthermore, Niswander and colleagues,[506, 507] in a most significant study, compared the infants born of mothers who had been in shock from abruptio and placenta previa or where there had been prolapse of the umbilical cord with those infants of normal mothers and pregnancies. At ages of eight months and 4 years, despite the fact that the initial Apgar scores had been very different, they could find no difference in performance between survivors of the two groups. These unexpected results have not generally been accepted by most of the American authorities. (There were cases lost to follow-up because of deaths and a minimal difference could be shown with special tests.) Nevertheless, it is a definitive answer in the sense that it represents studies of the infants at the time of birth and subsequent development and it once again demonstrates that in the human fetus, the all-or-nothing concept is usually operative.

Another important paper for this argument was that of Churchill et al.[106] also using data of the Collaborative Project. This project, you will recall, was undertaken to determine the etiology of cerebral palsy. Churchill and colleagues studied infants weighing less than 2 kg from the Collaborative Study. Forty-four had spastic diplegia at 1 year of age, and all were preterm. Of all the possible newborn variables, only a low hematocrit was correlated, suggesting that many of these cases might result from intraventricular hemorrhage occurring sometime in the nursery. There were no clearcut obstetrical factors which were responsible for the development of these most unfortunate cases.

Curron's[134] monograph on fetal monitoring reviews both the American and English literature. He notes that every obstetrician's intuition tells him that adequate oxygenation is essential for the proper health of the newborn. But he suggests there is no evidence "that this need be so" and that either the fetus is fit to withstand delivery and survive as a normal human being, or it dies. In other words, he supports the "all-or-nothing" con-cept. Curron further indicates that it is probably events prior to the onset of labor which determines whether a fetus will subsequently have cerebral palsy and not the intrapartum factors.

Scott[620] has provided a long-term follow-up of severely asphyxiated infants resuscitated (and rescued) at birth. They all were judged to have "Apgar 0" or failed to establish spontaneous breathing by 20 min of age. Fifty percent of the infants did not survive despite modern resuscitative efforts including alkali infusions. Of the survivors, only 25% demonstrated neurological handicaps at 3–7 years of age. Of this group, most had prolonged partial in utero "asphyxia" rather than the acute variety. The acute, brief, but total asphyxia had a high immediate perinatal mortality rate, but the survivors were apparently normal. (Again, the all-or-nothing concept.) However, the devastating CNS effects of repeated episodes of hypoxemia (partial asphyxia) in fetal monkeys[490] and human fetuses[620] with its associated brain edema is still an unsolved therapeutic problem.

Durech and associates,[172] from the University of Alabama, studied 20 infants who had demonstrated signs of "asphyxia" at birth (Apgar less than 3). Among this small group of "asphyxiated" newborns, only those with evidence of intrauterine growth retardation demonstrated cerebral abnormalities at ages of 14–40 months.

Summary of Literature Review

The number of studies such as these are nearly without end and the message seems to be clear (although each investigator writes as if he has discovered something new!). Obstetrical factors around the time of parturition seem to have only a minor role in the development of most cases of cerebral palsy. It is events occuring during other times in in utero life that set the stage for development of later cerebral palsy. The factors responsible for the dysmature newborn seem to be especially important and the need for obstetricians to prevent such cases seems clear.

The Immature Newborn

The subsequent neurological development of the tiny premature (less than 1200 g) has been most unsatisfactory in the past, as these infants had a high degree of cerebral dysfunction or outright cerebral palsy. As the neonatologists have given more attention to newborn nutrition, their blood glucose levels, temperature, blood gas levels, and psychological support, the neurological outcome has been markedly improved. Recent studies indicate that the occurrence of subsequent cerebral palsy is minimal in these tiny newborns and that intelligence as measured by I.Q. tests is essentially equal to that of term newborns. Grassy[297] reported on 28 infants who weighed less than 1 kg at birth. At 4 years, the survival rate was 29% and only 30% had neurologic abnormalities. Reports from other centers (San Francisco, Denver) suggest even better results.

The prematures of the 1950s undoubtedly included many cases of what is now considered the dysmature or small-for-gestational-age (SGA) fetus. As discussed below, the recent Swedish studies[310, 599] would indicate that such SGA newborns contribute 20–30 times the rate of subsequent cerebral palsy as do the term infants. The other aspect of the relationship between "low birth weight" and cerebral palsy is indicated by recent follow-up studies[455] of children whose birth weights were less than 1.5 kg. As noted by the Denver group, the outlook for these infants born in the mid-1960s was dismal and probably with better care is now a much more hopeful situation. Even the extremely small premature who spent days on assisted ventilation apparently is now able to perform at levels that are comparable to those of the term newborn.

A major unsolved problem for the tiny premature is the occurrence of intracranial hemorrhage and its severe central nervous sequelae. Intraventricular hemorrhage originating from the terminal veins is a condition apparently restricted in the human to the premature newborn. The condition can occur prior to birth; however, it usually occurs hours to days into the neonatal period. The availability of the CAT scanner has caused a reevaluation of the condition for apparently significant intraventricular bleeds can occur with minimal acute or remote symptoms. It has been suggested that intraventricular hemorrhage develops as a consequence of necrosis of the subependymal germinal matrix located in the region of the terminal veins. The thinness of the walls of the intracranial veins and the lack of any surrounding cerebral tissue support has been accepted as an explanation in the occurrence of such hemorrhages when circulatory abnormalities lead to increases in venous pressure. The implication is that whatever the initial underlying basis for the intracranial hemorrhage, major subsequent disturbances in the fetus or newborn's cardiovascular function must occur and therefore play a significant role in its occurrence.

In the past, the occurrence of intraventricular hemorrhage (IVH) in the newborn appeared to be significantly correlated with subsequent CNS dysfunction. Many of our small prematures have developed this dreadful complication with hydrocephalus and CNS dysfunction. Some, however, are circumventing these abnormalities despite an early grim prognosis. I have argued that such cases of IVH are generally the responsibility of the neonatologists, but as shown with one case of prematures with twin transfusion syndrome, this is not always so. About the only contribution that obstetrics can make to avoid this dreadful complication is to deliver all fetuses at risk by cesarean section. How we would determine the risk factors is unclear. Enthusiasm for the ultimate outcome of such tiny newborns is not universal, as was indicated by Fitzhardinge et al.[204] but in general, there is much optimism. If it can be assumed that the optimism is justified, then it would appear that the previous poor experience with a premature newborn represented not problems related to parturition, but related instead to neonatal care. In other words, it would now appear that most cases of cerebral palsy are related to factors prior to the onset of birth or after the onset of birth. Hence, my present view that intrapartum electronic monitoring, intrapartum of any sort for that matter, will not really significantly reduce the problem of cerebral palsy as I (and most obstetricians) had believed in 1968. The apparent need now is to turn toward the fetal problems of the antenatal period.

The SGA Newborn

Hagberg et al.[311] have reported that between the years 1954 and 1970, the incidence of cerebral palsy in a district of Sweden decreased from 2.2/1000 to 1.3/1000. The decrease in rate was limited to those infants who developed diplegia and were under 2.5 kg at birth. Unfortunately, for those individuals whose in utero histories suggested placental dysfunction or dysmaturity, the incidence of cerebral palsy did not improve. Sabel et al.,[599] in a study of children with major CNS sequelae, such as cerebral palsy, psychomotor retardation, sensory–neural hearing defects born from a single Swedish hospital, found a 20-fold increase of these abnormalities in the infant which had been diagnosed as having in utero growth retardation at birth. These authors suggested that finding such a high rate of infants with uterine undergrowth indicates some sort of metabolic disorder which rendered the fetus vulnerable to the stresses of labor.

Cerebral Palsy—Its Prevention

What then should be the obstetrician's views on how he or she can prevent the occurrence of cerebral palsy? No one would argue that the available data indicate that it is only the gross or inadequate obstetrical management which can ever be held responsible for intrapartum factors to be the cause of the case of cerebral palsy. The argument comes over what is gross management. Such obstetrical factors, in my opinion, do not include the subtle abnormalities that can be discerned only with electronic fetal monitoring. Factors may include excessive and prolonged stimulation, prolonged maternal hy-

potension, or the heroic rescue of a fetus who is about to die from asphyxia. Avoidance of such events involves nothing more than following common delivery room surveillance and refraining from rescuing the essentially dead fetus.

It is unfair that the obstetrician is held responsible for most cases of cerebral palsy. The general health of the fetus is more important than what happens during labor, and fetal health has not been our major concern. (Since we incorrectly assume credit when all goes well, it could be argued that we should assume the "blame" when matters go badly.)

LABORATORY STUDIES

Certain lessons about prevention of cerebral palsy can be learned from the laboratory. In utero fetuses, whether they be dogs, cats, mice, rabbits, or monkeys, can, in the laboratory, be demonstrated to be protected from asphyxial brain damage by adequate blood levels of sedatives, narcotics, or tranquilizers, and the avoidance of hyperglycemia. The sedated fetus becomes a sedated newborn and may require special care in the nursery because of recurring apnea and floppy newborn syndrome. But this sort of care is something that most nurseries can easily master, and the drugs which produce the apnea spells or heavy sedation also, in all probability, protected it to at least some small degree from asphyxia. For several years I have attempted to convince my colleagues of the usefulness of purposeful fetal sedation and apnea through selective maternal medications during labor (Chapter 22). These drugs (narcotics, tranquilizers, sedatives) should reduce the incidence of meconium aspiration as they do induce fetal apnea, and at the same time, they should protect the brain against some degree of asphyxia. To date the results of my efforts are a failure as neonatologists, anesthesiologists, and other obstetricians are strongly aligned themselves against such purposeful sedation of any fetus/newborn. They relate the problems of dealing with the heavily sedated newborn as far as nursery care goes, its feeding habits, and they also believe that tracheal toilet at birth is capable of preventing meconium aspiration.

Myers recently suggested that in the monkey the occurrence of subsequent cerebral palsy can be correlated with fetal serum lactic acid levels which reflects, in addition to the degree of asphyxia, the levels of blood glucose prior to the onset of asphyxia. In his study of monkey fetuses and newborns, Myers[493] showed that the pretreatment with infusions of glucose or normal feeding prior to 14 min of circulatory arrest, causes them to suffer a breakdown of the blood–brain barrier and to develop subsequent brain edema. This hyperglycemia is associated with marked accumulation of lactate in brain tissues. Myers also showed that magnitude of oxygen deprivation significantly affects the degree and distribution of brain pathology. He found that at 25% oxygen saturation, the cardiac performance was reduced, producing bradycardia and hypotension. An equally important finding was that oxygen saturation must be reduced even further before nervous system function is affected. (An explanation is then found for the apparent "all-or-nothing" phenomenon, i.e., the heart fails before the brain.)

HUMAN STUDIES

An important paper from an obstetrical standpoint on the etiology of cerebral palsy is that of Durkin et al.[173] (1976) from the University of Wisconsin. They analyzed the gestational, parturitional, and neonatal histories of 281 severely mentally retarded individuals with cerebral palsy. As with most every retrospective study since Little,[451] they found an increased incidence of past histories of prematurity, older and younger mothers, breech deliveries, SGA, prolonged labor, and twins. Unlike other studies, they also discovered an increased incidence among postmature pregnancies and in large-for-gestational-age fetuses. Durkin and associates also suggest that disseminated intravascular coagulation (DIC) due to a prenatal death of a twin may have been the cause of brain damage in several of their cases. (Melnick[468a] in 1977 has

calculated the risk of such DIC in twin pregnancies as about 1 in 600.) Among the Wisconsin data, it is not possible to determine whether the risk of CP in breech deliveries is greater than that associated with their premature pregnancies.

From this Wisconsin study, which found that one-third of the cases had no apparent significant past history, one-third with problems not usually associated with a bad outcome, and only one-third with either multiple or severe complications, the obstetrician's role in preventing CP is obviously very limited. Certainly little can be done to prevent fetal DIC from a dead twin or to improve the outcome in the infertile patient. We could offer all gravida with SFD fetuses, breech presentations, twins, postmature, prolonged labor (over 24 hr), abnormal bleeding, and premature labors a cesarean section. Assuming that avoidance of labor were 100% effective in preventing CP (especially difficult to accept as for such etiologies as the TORCH syndrome), the incidence of cerebral palsy among the Wisconsin study would only have been reduced by one-third. To compound the problem of the obstetrical prevention of CP by offering only those with breech presentation delivery by cesarean section and to ignore all of these other apparent etiologies (post-datism, macrosomia, prematurity) will not solve the "CP" problems. On the other hand, to employ cesarean section for such loose indications is to expose a high percentage of our obstetrical patients to the risk of surgery and to destroy the art of obstetrics.

Obstetrical Prevention of Cerebral Palsy

SUMMARY

For an individual obstetrician to prevent CP requires a bit of luck. If his or her fetal patients are normal and healthy, it will probably be easy to believe that he or she practices safe and good obstetrics. On the other hand, if many of his or her fetal patients are growth-retarded, have viral infections, premature or postmature labor, this same obstetrician will probably be judged to practice "poor" obstetrics and require much legal support and postgraduate education. However, about all he can do prophylactically is to have a high rate of cesarean sections, a good neonatal back-up, and a good lawyer. All other measures, such as increasing or reducing intrapartum maternal drugs, preventing hyperglycemia, allowing only "easy vaginal" deliveries, or using electronic fetal monitors, will probably be of little help.

Case History No. 23-1

A 22-year-old white female with one prior abortion had a severe fever from "Montezuma's revenge" at about the time of conception. Her labor at 35 weeks was unusual in that she delivered a small fetus papyraceus and then was allowed to continue in labor. After oxytocin stimulation, delivering by breech presentation was easily accomplished of a microcephalic newborn.

The child showed no signs of birth asphyxia and did satisfactorily in the nursery. It later showed cerebral palsy and mental retardation. A malpractice suit was lodged, claiming that the child should have been delivered by cesarean section. In favor of this argument was that the newborn had suffered a fractured humerus (easy delivery?). Maternal x-ray pelvimetry had subsequently showed a contracted pelvis. I argued in vain that the CP (and microcephaly) probably resulted either from the maternal fever or DIC associated with the second twin (fetus papyraceus). It took the jury only a short time to award the child $1,750,000.00 in damages.

Case History No. 23-2

A 16-year-old, para 0-0-0-0 had an uneventful pregnancy except postdatism. She was induced at 42½ weeks of pregnancy and during the terminal phases of labor, the FHT patterns appeared to be abnormal. A stat section wasn't possible, and a difficult midforceps delivery was done of a 4460 g child with Apgars of 6 and 8. The cord pH was 7.28, the newborn had a "staring gaze," and neurologically appeared to be depressed. The

infant did very poorly in the nursery with lack of sucking, high-pitched cry, and demonstrated seizure-like activity. The neonatologist's impression was cerebral abnormality secondary to asphyxia and birth trauma. However, a computerized axial tomography (CT) scan showed a large porencephalic cyst which provided an obvious antenatal etiology for the infant's CNS disease. At 2 weeks of age, the infant was noted to have optic atrophy and at 3 weeks began to suck, and was discharged to a nursing home. The child subsequently required a ventricular peritoneal shunt for expanding hydrocephalus. Subsequent hospital and clinical records ascribed its CNS disease due to asphyxia, despite the fact there was never any acidemia or that there was a congenital porencephalic cyst. The mother has now filed a huge malpractice suite.

The case is an example of congenital factors causing apparent birth trauma and cerebral palsy.

Another Point of View

The concept of the "all-or-nothing" rule as regards the stress of asphyxia on the intrapartum fetus has not been accepted by most American studies which suggest that the converse is true, that the occurrence of fetal or newborn asphyxia is directly related to the subsequent development of cerebral palsy.[120, 218] As noted previously, this point of view is more or less the common dogma both in American obstetrical textbooks and in American courts of law.

Admittedly, it is difficult to explain why, if intrapartum asphyxia kills the fetus, a "little asphyxia" does not produce brain damage. As we discussed previously, one explanation that has been demonstrated repeatedly in the laboratory is that asphyxia kills the intrapartum fetus not by brain damage, but by cardiovascular failure. The fetal brain may be as or more resistant to asphyxia than is the fetal cardiovascular system. Another reason is that when CP is from oxygen lack, it arises not from asphyxia, but repeated episodes of moderate hypoxia—a fortunately rare situation in the labor ward.

Lilienfeld and Parkhurst's study of children born in New York State in the 1930s and 1940s was a significant study and had a major impact upon American views. They, like many older studies, generally found that prematurity and various maternal complications were associated with the subsequent development of cerebral palsy. These investigators were usually unable to decide whether the correlation between the maternal condition (toxemia, abruptio placentae, heart disease, placenta previa, and so forth) and cerebral palsy was a direct one or whether the relationship was secondary through the common association with prematurity. In Eastman's extensive and exhaustive analysis of 753 children with cerebral palsy, he noted that extreme prematurity was a significant factor in the development of these cerebral problems. He ascribed the tendency of the small premature to develop cerebral damage to neonatal hypoxia, incomplete development of the CNS pyramidal tracts, or hypernatremia. But Eastman further concluded that hypoxia or ischemic hypoxia (resulting from pressure of a contracted pelvis or forceps, or decreased uterine blood flow) was even a more significant factor in the etiology of cerebral palsy.

From another exhaustive literary study of cerebral palsy, Schwartz,[616] in 1961, suggested that birth trauma was the predominant cause of cerebral palsy. Courville,[120] a neuropathologist, championed the concept that cerebral lesions were probably due to "anoxia at the time of birth and to disturbance of circulation incident thereto." Courville suggested that the motor disturbances of cerebral palsy (or defects in motor development) are the result of "birth injury." He notes that the term "birth injury" is an extremely poor one, failing to define the mechanism responsible for CNS injury. Courville believed that if the recognized condition (such as toxoplasmosis, kernicterus, and metabolic disorder) could be excluded that most of the CNS deformities resulted from disorders of circulation of the fetal brain, either before or during the birth process. While this viewpoint could include the dysmature or small-for-dates fetus, it is apparent that Courville did not consider the now-recognized significant group of *in utero* environmental factors in his otherwise monumental text.

Towbin[703] wrote that direct trauma to the brain, such as tearing of the corpus callosum, may occur during delivery and lead to subsequent cerebral damage. Also, lacerations and hematomas on the brain, with or without associated skull fracture, occur in rare instances.

However, in 1970, he was to write that the commonly held concept of birth injury may be in error in a significant degree, that there is pathological evidence that a major portion of CNS lesions present at birth are due to a latent process having origin prenatally and may be well advanced prior to labor.

There have been several prospective epidemiological studies of perinatal mortality and morbidity, all performed at great effort and cost. The largest was the Collaborative Perinatal Project in the United States which registered in the years 1959–1966, 60,000 pregnancies. The British National Child Development Study involved 14,000 newborns. Several "at risk" registries in Britain, as well as the national study, suggested that there is no sequelae of hypoxia births, only death. Indeed, Knox and Mahon[409] suggested that such registries were a waste of time and money. And, as noted, although the purpose of the Collaborative Project in America was to determine the etiology of cerebral palsy, the massive study failed to incriminate obstetric practice except for the rare case of true birth trauma.

Stembera and colleagues[662] reported at the Fourth European Congress of Perinatal Medicine on their definition of risk fractors for perinatal death and morbidity (cerebral palsy, minimal brain damage, etc.). These Czechoslovakian investigators briefly reviewed the 12 different scoring systems proposed in Europe. Their own scoring index included the patient's education, social standing, endocrine abnormalities, and so forth. When they included the newborn risks, they noted that the higher the score, the more likelihood of perinatal death. The morbidity or cerebral problems were most likely to occur when the score was only moderately elevated. They concluded that if essentially zero morbidity and mortality were to be achieved among the Czechoslovakian prenatal patients, 43% of all pregnancies would be at risk. By selecting the top 7% of the high-risk pregnancies, only 23% of the perinatal morbidity and mortality would have been identified prenatally. We again come to the observation that if pregnancy high-risk criteria are broad enough to include all perinatal and subsequent problems, only a small majority of gravida remain at low risk. In order to define the problem to "not overtreat" and to still have high-risk factors have a major impact on perinatal rates, it will require more knowledge than is now available.

In a series of well-defined studies, Ginsberg and Myers[228] exposed monkey fetuses to varying degrees of fetal hypoxia through maternal carbon monoxide inhalation. After delivering the fetuses by cesarean section, the newborns were ventilated until they were able to breath on their own. Out of nine fetuses exposed to this hypoxic stress, only one had neurological damage. The others were either normal or died. Whether all of the newborns would have died without the supportive ventilation immediately at birth is not known. As a believer in the "all-or-nothing" phenomenon, I prefer to believe that at least the animal which developed neurological damage would have died without the assisted ventilation at the time of its birth.

In 1975, Quilligan and Paul[560] suggested that fetal monitoring could appreciably reduce the incidence of CP. Unfortunately, they offered no data to support this hope.

McManus and associates[499] have recently published, "Is Cerebral Palsy a Preventable Disease?" It is a retrospective analysis of the obstetrical histories of two groups of children with cerebral palsy as compared with the total population of a Canadian province. In one group, their success in obtaining past obstetrical records was 58/126 (46%) and in the other, 38/46 (82%), or overall, 58%. Undaunted, they proceeded to analyze their cases and review the literature. They even discuss a case where the fetal heart rate was "lost" for 45 min. Throughout, they cite references and refer to their own data, confusing cerebral palsy which occurs in the term newborn with that in the dysmature and premature infant. Not unexpectedly, they conclude that "in the last 10 years, methods of prevention (of cerebral palsy) have become available." The authors suggest that obstetricians are not aware of the problems of cerebral palsy and that changes in remuneration and more regionalization may decrease the incidence of cerebral palsy.

In California, we are very much aware of the problem of cerebral palsy, if only through the huge malpractice suits that are occurring. Maternal and newborn transport is very much a part of our lives and the cesarean section rate is climbing to levels of approximately 20%. Whether all this will improve our rate of cerebral palsy or lessen the malpractice suits is unknown.

Sarnatt and Sarnatt[608] studied the clinical and electroencephalographic changes of 21 human newborns afflicted with varying degrees of hypoxia (Apgar less than 5 at 5 min). Their major interest was in categorizing the stages of newborn encephalopathy (three stages). Of the 21 newborns, 12 were found to be normal at "six plus" months of age, 4 had died, 3 showed spastic diplegia, and 2 demonstrated retarded development. Considering the fact that they only studied those surviving the neonatal period, the results would indicate at least mild support for the "all-or-nothing" phenomenon. Others will probably disagree.

An important paper on the development of mental processes is that by Friedman and Sachtleban.[212] Using data from the Collaborative Project, they studied the long-term effects on individuals delivered by midforceps or following labors characterized by prolonged decelerations, secondary arrest of dilatation, or arrest of descent. They demonstrated apparent deleterious effects of all these factors with the worse combination being midforceps after secondary arrest. They were unable to answer whether cesarean section after abnormal labor prevented problems of subsequent neurological development.

Such pediatric neurologists as J. Keith Brown of the Royal Hospital for Sick Children of Edinburgh believe that 50% of all cases of cerebral palsy are still preventable and that 50% of all cases are related to perinatal events (not necessarily intrapartum events). In Scotland, so many cases of dyskinetic CP (due to hyperbilirubinemia) and to diplegia (due to prematurity) have been prevented that the incidence of CP is now 1/1000 deliveries (a 60% improvement). This is so significant a drop in numbers of cases of cerebral palsy in Scotland that therapists dealing with these children are feeling their jobs threatened (J. Keith Brown, personal communication).

Using the data from the Collaborative Project referred to so often in this text, Nelson and Broman[504] came to essentially opposite conclusions from those previously reported. These authors concluded that some pregnancies become special risk only during labor. That perinatal complications, particularly those associated with asphyxia, were more common in children who eventually showed severe motor and mental disabilities. They also found that more than 80% of the neurologically handicapped children weighed more than 2500 g at birth. As reported by Friedman and Sachtleban,[212] they found that lowest FHR in the second stage of labor, arrested progress of labor, and use of midforceps discriminated between those children with neurological abnormality and the control group.

It is indeed strange that when the serious complications (as abruptio) are studied, the "all-or-nothing" rule seems to hold. On the other hand, when those minor conditions which I, at least, considered insignificant as to future neurological development (such as arrested labor) are investigated, the "all-or-nothing" rule apparently is not operative. Myers' concept of repeated episodes of mild hypoxia producing brain edema may indeed be accurate for the human.

Adamsons and Myers[5] have proposed that in monkeys, asphyxia sufficient to elicit late decelerations of FHR was insufficient to produce CNS dysfunction. However, the studies were conducted under pentothal anesthesia, which as the authors admit, may have selectively protected the brain from asphyxial damage.

Myers has reviewed[492, 493] his years of experience in producing CP in monkeys. As previously noted, he believes that the most critical issue in determining whether brain damage occurs during oxygen deprivation is the animal's prior history of food intake. He found that the carbohydrate-deprived hypoglycemia animal is markedly less vulnerable to brain damage than is the animal exposed to normal high carbohydrate loads prior to exposure to anoxia. Thus, our policy of maintaining relative hyperglycemia during labor with intravenous infusions may actually be detrimental to those fetuses subsequently exposed to hypoxia. In addition, Myers has shown that whenever a starved fetus (or any animal) is exposed to asphyxia and circulatory arrest, damage is usually restricted to the nuclear structure of the brain stem. On the other hand, repeated exposure only to hypoxia (for 20-30 min) leads to brain edema, occurring several hours after reoxygenation. If the hypoxia is accompanied by hypercarbia, there is damage to gray matter with the edema. With hypercarbia (and hypoxia), only white matter is damaged. In my experience, neonatologists do not accept this "edema" concept, being unwilling to treat hypoxic newborns for cerebral edema (as with steroids).

Sabata et al.[597, 598] of Prague have argued that intrapartum glucose infusions improve the fetal situation. They claim that SGA newborn has greater "energetic" reserves after intrapartum glucose infusions and lower free fatty acids. It is especially interesting in view of Myers[492] work demonstrating the deleterious effects of lactic acid, that Sabata found in the term fetus intrapartum glucose infusions lower newborn lactic acid. The opposite was true in the SGA and premature (that glucose infusions increased fetal lactic acid levels). This was even more so with fructose infusions.

An entirely different etiology than asphyxia for CP is that caused by CMV. In addition to the obvious defects of microcephaly, intracranial calcification, and bilateral deafness, approximately 1/900 of all newborns may subsequently have I.Q. and other mental defects due to silent CMV infections. Alford et al.[11] believe that many children have minor but significant forms of brain damage due to CMV. Likewise, subclinical congenitally acquired toxoplasmosis, rubella, syphilis, and natally acquired HSV can also produce silent CNS involvement in early life which can lead to a wide array of neurologic problems. Thus, while it is common practice to assume that cerebral dysfunction represents a perinatal asphyxial insult, this may often not be the case.

It should also be noted that some do not accept that the SFD newborn has a worse CNS prognosis than does the premature of equal weight.[184, 737] One explanation for confusion is that intracranial bleeding may occur and be unrecognized in some nurseries. Also, the incidence of child abuse and neglect is high among survivors of having been very low birth weight,[156] perhaps because of disruption of early infant-maternal bonding by neonatal intensive care. Larroche and Korn[423] of Paris believe that the brain of the intrauterine deprivation (chronic fetal distress) newborn has developed normally; that their brain lesions occur in the neonatal period.

An example of severe fetal asphyxia associated with apparently normal subsequent infant development was reported by Cohn et al.[113] Through a series of mistakes, a 1630-g human fetus was left inside an intact amniotic sac for approximately 76 min after delivery. At 25 months of age, the infant's development was slow, but progressive. Presumably, the hypothermia the newborn endured through its first 75 min of extrauterine life prevented serious neurological damage.[473]

CHAPTER 24

Parturitional Position and the Water Bed

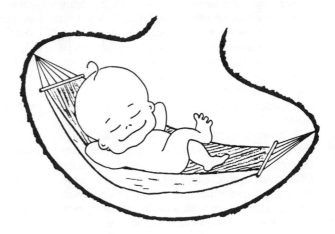

Introduction

A recent review by Atwood[25] simply points out the obvious—that parturients have labored and delivered in virtually all positions, including the head down position. The birth stool is perhaps the oldest parturitional posture aid. It was known to exist in Egypt in 2500 B.C., was described in the Bible, was recommended by Soranus, and was widely used throughout Europe until the 17th century. It was apparently the 17th-century French obstetrician Mauriceau who substituted the bed for the birth stool in order to apply the Chamberlen obstetrical forceps. At the end of the 19th century, especially designed tables were introduced to accommodate the obstetrician.

There are a number of various positions that the parturient may assume while in the bed. The squatting position is said to enlarge the pelvic outlet to some extent and is claimed by some to provide for easier delivery than does the recumbent position. The maternal sitting position is apparently recommended by no one as it allows absolutely no exposure of the perineum. The knee–elbow position has been recommended by Moir[478] as useful

in certain breech deliveries. The lateral position is considered to be an advantage when the obstetrician has little or no assistance. These include the absence of aortocaval compression, good control of the fetal head or the perineum, and natural drainage of the maternal pharynx if emesis should occur.

The lithotomy position is widely used in America, but one of its main problems is considered to be aortocaval compression. (Actually, with the fetal head deep in the pelvis, no position seems completely superior as regards aortocaval compression.) Its use is usually accompanied by positioning of the parturient's legs in stirrups, which often can be a nuisance, in order to achieve the optimal position, and sometimes are a source of discomfort to the parturient. The mother also has a difficult time observing the delivery of her infant and if emesis occurs, the position does not provide for easy drainage. Many gravida now strongly object to being strapped into such a bed.

Maternal Position

It is debatable which is the best maternal position during parturition to achieve shorter labors, optimal fetal outcome, and maternal welfare. If the parturient is to have epidural anesthesia, or other significant pain relief, it would appear obvious that she should be in bed. If the patient is in bed, then she should be in the lateral position. There are midwives and obstetricians[470a] who are attempting to reverse the trend toward monitored labor and are recommending that women walk when in early labor and squat when in late labor. As with most any different obstetrical technique, its advocates claim that the walking–squatting parturient is in less pain, has shorter labors, and healthier newborns.

The Water Bed

Our own approach to the maternal position problem was to offer parturients a water bed. In 1972, a specially built bed was donated by Jobst to our obstetrical service. While the water bed has been considered a symbol of the present generation, it has also been a part of our therapeutic armamentarium since 1965 when Weinstein and Davidson[740] described the use of a fluid-support mattress for the prevention and treatment of decubitus ulcers. A medical water bed maintains the patient in a state of flotation with pressure of approximately 8 torr equally distributed over the surface of the body in contact with the mattress.

Our experience suggests that many supine parturients will demonstrate the "Poseiro" effect when supine (Chapter 9) with many having associated fetal distress and/or maternal hypotension. These deleterious syndromes can be completely circumvented by maintaining the parturient in a prone or semiprone position. However, nearly all gravida are unwilling to assume such a position during labor in a standard hospital bed, but when floated prone in a water bed, find it comfortable, especially if they have used such a bed throughout their pregnancy. Thus, the rationale for employing a heated water bed which achieves flotation of the prone parturient is that it allows an improved lower aortic blood flow; the associated improved patient comfort is an added bonus.

The parturient water bed (Jobst Institute, Inc., Toledo, Ohio) was a standard-size hospital bed with the addition of a water mattress (bladder) constructed of neoprene nylon material. A heater and circulation pump are used to maintain the bladder's temperature at approximately 34°C and a special pump and dumping valve are available for emptying and filling of the bladder in 60 sec. When the bladder was empty, the bed could be positioned in the Trendelenburg position. It has adjustable side wings for constricting the bladder width enabling the patient to be floated free of the bed's firm surface.

External monitoring of fetal heart rates was accomplished simply by placing an ultrasound transducer between the prone patient's abdomen and the bladder. No abdominal straps were necessary. It was occasionally possible to pick up fetal heart sounds and uterine contractions transmitted through the water-filled bladder, although a more pliable bladder well would perhaps allow better transmission of uterine sounds and pressure changes.

Application of the Parturient Water Bed

More than 200 parturients used the bed and their personal evaluation has been overwhelmingly favorable. The warmth of the mattress has been particularly pleasing and many appreciate being able to lie comfortably in the prone position. While nursing care and the administration of caudal anesthetics or intravenous fluid is considered by some to be hampered by the flotation of the patient, the dumping valve provides for quick conversion of the bladder to a standard foam rubber mattress.

In 20 patients, hallux blood volume pulse monitoring was accomplished and there was never any suggestion of a Poseiro or aortocaval compression during the time of uterine contractions when the parturient was in the semiprone position.

With the parturient prone, and using filtered underwater and cardiac microphones with the bladder, it was sometimes possible to record FHR, maternal pulse, and uterine contractions. Unfortunately, maternal movement produced so much noise that such recordings were usually impossible.

The reason that only one parturient water bed was manufactured was related to the associated nursing problems. The bladder was easily punctured by pins, the sheets tended to collect in the middle and amniotic fluid and other excrement was difficult to handle. With proper design and with suction pumps, these problems could hopefully have been solved.

The water bed did demonstrate that with gravida previously acclimatized to such a bed, labor was conveniently accomplished. Our observations suggested that compression of maternal vessels did not occur.

Intuitively, the pregnant prone abdomen, floating freely on a water bed seems to approximate the dependent abdomen (uterus) of four-legged pregnant animals, or of the effects of abdominal decompression.[124] In our alternate birth center, gravida are allowed to assume any position, provided the fetal vertex is "fixed" in the pelvis. Only 6% have elected other than the "queen size" standard bed. Many have indicated the main attraction of such a bed is that we allow their mate to share it with them!

CHAPTER 25
Third Trimester Bleeding

Placenta Previa

HISTORICAL

Until 1945, when MacAfee and Johnson[457] suggested delay in terminating pregnancies of women with placenta previa for the sake of the fetus (conservative management), the fetus' welfare in gravida with placenta previa was ignored. The worldwide introduction of the Braxton–Hicks version (tamponade of the placenta against the lower segment by extraction of the fetal leg) significantly reduced maternal mortality in 1910 to 7.6% in Europe and 3% in Chicago, but the perinatal rate was 65%! In 1927, Bill[54] of Cleveland recommended blood transfusions and immediate cesarean section in women who had apparent placenta previa. Since maternal bleeding often occurred prior to the 34th week, again the technique was directed strictly towards the maternal welfare and the perinatal mortality rates remained distressingly high.

With the introduction of the conservative management of placenta previa in women prior to their 35th week, gravida were placed at bedrest with blood transfusions administered as needed until they either had an "exsanguinating" hemorrhage or fell into obvious labor. Following the conservative therapy on our own service, we had women who in retrospect had no previa, but carcinoma of the cervix or bleeding varices of the vagina, and were treated by such management (much to our embarrassment). With the present improvement in neonatal care, there seems to be a definite tendency toward returning to Bill's concept of delivering the fetus whenever significant maternal hemorrhages occur. This return to older concepts is based on 20 years of experience with the conservative therapy in placenta previa which showed that many women go into labor a few days after having had a significant hemorrhage and our management had only added numerous blood transfusions without significant improvement in fetal maturity. There is also the risk of the fetus being stillborn with conservative management. Since we now attempt to avoid blood transfusions whenever possible, and it is noted that the neonatologists are doing much better with the immature newborn, it seems that for all concerned, the fetus is "better out than in."

In the discussions of placenta previa, it is often suggested that the fetus bleeds through

257

its disrupted placenta into its mother's birth canal. This assumption is made on finding unexplained newborn anemia and an apparent increase of hemoglobin F in the blood clots of women bleeding from placenta previa. The increased hemoglobin F in such vaginal clots probably reflects the fact that hemoglobin F is more resistant than hemoglobin A and is more likely to be found in higher percentages in old clots. The newborn anemia probably reflects tearing of the placenta at the time of the cesarean section. The risk of the placenta previa to the *in utero* fetus is decreased placental exchange (asphyxia), due either to maternal shock or partial separation of the placenta from the lower segment. We have noted an occasional case of fetal–maternal hemorrhage in such cases.

The availability of ultrasound has altered the management of gravida placenta previa more than any other modality since Bill's recommendation for blood transfusions and cesarean section. Our own experience with ultrasound has shown that it remains relatively imprecise as to the exact location of the placental edge (particularly partial previas) and the diagnosis should be confirmed by vaginal examination under operating conditions. The survey by Tatum and Mule at the Charity Hospital in New Orleans demonstrated that vaginal delivery has little to offer a fetus regardless of whether the placenta is only low-lying, partial, or incomplete. If one can palpate placenta in the lower segment, our management is to proceed immediately with a cesarean section in these women with bleeding greater than 500 ml.

Abruptio Placentae

THE PROBLEM

In diagnosing abruptio placentae, our service has a terrible record. For example, we have performed emergency cesarean sections when there is no placental separation and we have watched while fetuses *in utero* die in our labor wards from unrecognized abruptio (Chapter 12). Another unsolved problem on our service has been the gravida in her 26th–34th week of pregnancy who has vaginal bleeding with questionable pain and uterine tenderness, whose ultrasonic scan shows a fundal location of the placenta. It obviously is inappropriate to inhibit labor in cases of true abruptio placenta; yet, many of these "minimal bleeders" are apparently only small premature separations (marginal sinus rupture?) and the only real risk to the pregnancy is premature delivery.

Despite Niswander's conclusions[506, 507] from the Collaborative Project, my experience in reviewing charts for legal cases and those in our hospital, would indicate that abruptio may have a devastating CNS effect on the surviving newborn. In most cases of abruptio, it is an "all-or-nothing" phenomena (Chap. 23); either the fetus survives without ill effects, or it expires *in utero* or in the nursery. The one danger, of course, is that the obstetrician interferes and saves the dying fetus in cases of severe abruptio placenta, only to have the newborn survive with cerebral dysfunction.

CLINICAL MANAGEMENT

Based on our own experience, gravida beyond the 28th week with apparent abruptio should be delivered. In those cases where the mother has DIC, is in shock, and the fetus is dead, the diagnosis is obvious. However, when the diagnosis is questionable, we obtain ultrasonic scanning and perform amniocentesis. If the amniotic fluid appears bloody or "port-wine" in color, we assume there is an abruptio. The ultrasonic scan diagnosis of abruptio from a thickened placenta, despite Kobayoshi's findings, has been most misleading in my experience. Years ago, when I was developing the intravenous dye injection for placental localization,[239] we had two cases of suspected placenta previa which were actual cases of abruptio placentae. In these cases, we could see dye actually leaking extraovular and following the course of the maternal bleeding. The intravascular dye techniques are cumbersome and carry considerable risk to the mother, and therefore are not used anymore, but they certainly were a "neat" way to diagnose abruptio placentae.

Our use of the fetal heart rate monitor, as

noted in Chapter 12, has also been at times a disaster in cases of suspected abruptios. While the uterine contraction pattern may show a "saw-tooth" pattern with little uterine relaxation, this has not occurred consistently enough to be an accurate warning sign in gravidas with questionable abruptio placentae. In at least six cases, the fetal heart rate pattern has remained "normal" right up until near the time of fetal death. By the time that signs of fetal distress (severe vagal-type or late decelerations) have occurred, it has been too late to salvage a normal fetus.

The infants born of mothers with abruptio often have a stormy course in the nursery. In addition to recovering from their *in utero* stress, they frequently have absorbed a considerable amount of maternal blood, either in their trachea or esophagus, and must be observed very carefully. They can also show evidences of shock and sometimes even DIC. The prognosis for their development must always be guarded.

PROPHYLAXIS

A difficult question is the patient who has had a previous abruptio which has ended in some sort of a disaster who consults you about future pregnancies. The incidence of repeated abruptio placentae is exceedingly high (perhaps 10%) and we have virtually nothing to offer in the way of prophylaxis for future pregnancies when the women are without other obvious disease processes. If the patient has such things as diabetes, essential hypertension, renal disease, lupus, etc., it is pretty clear that one can say that the risks of repeated abruptio are high and the prognosis is rather grim. However, when there is no associated findings, we are at a loss as to what to tell these patients. We do recommend increased vitamins, folic acid, bedrest, fluids, tranquility, iron, and the avoidance of orgasm (Chapter 8).

When students ask why abruptio placentae occur and what can be done on a prophylactic basis, I explain to them that I have essentially nothing to offer. I am unable to explain why *all* placentas do not separate prematurely, why uterine spiral arteries do not frequently

burst with stress, or how fetuses can survive when 50% of their placental exchange has been acutely destroyed by separation. My favorite past theory about vena cava obstruction or maternal shock leading to premature separation apparently is no longer valid. Morris et al.[484] report that with the production of marked hypotension in gravida with severe hypertension with diazoxide, only one out of nine fetuses showed even minimal bradycardia. Hypotensive shock itself must then not often produce placental separation. And while Mengert[471a] found that occluding the vena cava produced partial separation, Vorherr claims[718] that the relationship between increased uterine venous pressure and abruptio placentae has not been clearly demonstrated.

In terms of perinatal mortality rates and subsequent newborn development, I believe that we fail more with severe abruptio than any other entity.

Another Point of View

An unusual and apparently often successful conservative type of therapy for placenta previa is the McDonald encirclement suture of the cervix. Apparently believing that the bleeding of placenta previa was from gradual placental separation, the technique was introduced by the Norwegian, Löuset,[453] in 1959. Continuing reports[715] from Scandinavia suggest improved perinatal rates with the "encirclage" suture in cases of placenta previa prior to the 34th week of pregnancy.

Crenshaw et al.,[129a] at Duke University, suggest after review of 106 cases of placenta previa, that only one-half of these patients can be treated expectantly. They found that 3% of the surviving infants had subsequent CNS impairment. They note that 6% of the newborns were anemic because of incision through the placenta at the time of cesarean section. From their review, these authors recommend that gravida with placenta previa be delivered by cesarean section if significant bleeding occurs after 32 weeks of pregnancy. On the other hand, Brenner,[71] also from North Carolina, and after reviewing an equal size series, recommends the conservative (expectant) management. Brenner admits that a higher rate of stillborns will occur, but suggests that overall perinatal rates are improved by the conservative management.

CHAPTER 26
The Perinatal Technician

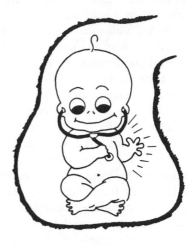

While intensive care for maternal illness is an established obstetric principle, clinical focus on the care of the fetus is a relatively recent development. The new field of fetology is developing rapidly and its practitioners apparently are not being limited to our specialty. Even though a subspecialty of Maternal–Fetal medicine has been formed by our own Board to offer expertise in this area, it still seems appropriate that the general obstetrician (as well as the specialist) should continue to be able to apply new fetal techniques in an efficient and low-cost manner. One way to accomplish this would be to have available "perinatal technicians," individuals who would monitor the fetus and immediate newborn, but would participate in its care only when appropriate to improving the records or as a "good samaritan." I believe that it is important for someone to be present who considers the "record" the important feature of parturition and who can not be used for urgent clinical matters.

The perinatal technician (PT) should preferably be a female with prior obstetrical experience so she can work without challenge in the labor ward and out-patient clinic. She should be able to relate easily with physicians and nurses, and to participate in both their learning and teaching exercises. In addition, she needs to have at least minimal mechanical ability so that she can aid in keeping the various types of fetal monitors, ultrasonic equipment, pumps, and resuscitative apparatus in operating condition. She also needs some technical training so that she can apply scalp electrodes, obtain scalp blood, and also aid in the resuscitation of the newborn. Above all, she should be trained as an objective interpreter of fetal recordings and of the various indices of fetal development.

In the antepartum period, the PT would serve as a record keeper, as an interpreter of the various FHR challenge tests, as an aid in performance of amniocentesis, and would participate in whatever additional studies may seem appropriate for high-risk fetuses. Ideally, the PT would be trained in sonography in order to determine biparietal and placental diameters and fetal movements. In the high-risk antepartum clinic, the PT acts as an interface between the hospital and clinic nursing staff and between the specialty areas.

For the intrapartum periods, the PT's major responsibility is to supervise the application of fetal monitors, to assure adequate supplies for recorders and fetal scalp sampling trays, and to interpret recordings in an objective manner. In the absence of an immediate obstetrician or midwife, she should (like other labor room nurses) be able to apply such fetal therapies as decreasing the oxytocin infusion, maternal O_2, changing maternal position, giving sedatives and tranquilizers, and preparing the patient for cesarean section. The PT should also be able to obtain fetal scalp blood.

During the immediate newborn period, the PT would be responsible for the resuscitation equipment and must be able to assist in the resuscitation of the newborn and to assist in its transfer to an intensive care unit.

When the PT is not otherwise involved, she should file and interpret records, and make certain that there is continuity of care between the outpatient clinics, delivery areas, and nursery in the care of high-risk or ill fetuses. It is also desirable that the PT participate in inservice training, journal clubs, and clinical research projects.

For 17 weeks we made an attempt to train and use such a perinatal technician in a small hospital (1000 deliveries per year) with a relatively high ratio of high-risk obstetric patients. The obstetric staff was comprised of interns and residents supervised by two full-time attending obstetricians. During four months there were only 131 deliveries whose labors were monitored by the PT and only once or twice a week did she function in the high-risk clinic as an aid with amniocentesis or an oxytocin challenge test. Nevertheless, even after this brief experience, the following observations or impressions were made: It is possible in a relatively short time to train a labor room nurse in the interpretation of fetal heart rate recordings to a degree that makes her an "expert" as much or more than anyone on the service. FHR stress tests required much less time to perform and were more accurate. Her attention to the fetal monitors assured that they functioned efficiently, and

record keeping improved immensely, as did attention to details of diagnoses and fetal well-being associated with various fetal heart rate patterns. The use of scalp pH determinations increased because of her suggestions or because there was a technician ready to assist in the collection of scalp blood. Such a technician was readily accepted by regular labor room nurses who apparently felt more comfortable in dealing with the needs and anxieties of labor patients than with the monitors.

With the employment of a perinatal technician, every effort was made to arrange for high-risk gravida to labor during her presence (which was also the time when the staff was available). At the same time, she was able to bring together specialists (anesthesiologists, neonatologists, endocrinologists) in discussion of specific problems not clearly appreciated by each specialty. Though not engaged to provide support and nursing care of parturients, she was actually a very reassuring factor to both the patients in labor and their families because of her ability to explain the equipment and remain enthusiastic, calm, and objective about its use.

In other hospitals, such perinatal technicians have performed and interpreted sonography efficiently and accurately. Obviously, the particular duties of a PT will be largely determined by the needs of her institution, but it seems important not to limit her role *a priori*. One of the unforeseen advantages we experienced with the use of a PT was a move toward more objectivity in record and laboratory interpretation. Thus, it seems important that the PT be independent of any particular physician or nurse.

One method of providing the general obstetrician and their patients with the techniques that are usually only available at selected centers seems relatively easily accomplished by obstetrical services employing perinatal technicians. (Modified from: Goodlin, R., and Crocker, K.: The perinatal technician. *J Reprod Med* **15**: 209, 1975.)

Epilogue

It is hoped that upon finishing this book, the reader will now agree with Ballantyne[33] in 1902 that antenatal care for the fetus is "a field sparsely settled, very vast and intensely alluring." DeLee[153] suggested in 1913 that with scientific study, means of cure, prevention, or amelioration of fetal diseases would be found. As noted repeatedly, significant advances have been made and perinatal rates are improving, but I remain concerned for the future. The vocal "Right to Life" groups in America are, in my opinion, about to effect a halt in the scientific study of the human fetus and the search for means to improve its *in utero* existence. It is one thing to be opposed to therapeutic abortion, but a very different and harmful stand to oppose all research on the human fetus (or even the primate fetus) because the unborn are "unable to give their informed consent." To see the thousands of therapeutic abortions occur and to be unable to use this material for research is, in my view, insane. Such a concept is much like the early Church's stand against dissection of the human body or autopsy.

If we are going to improve human fetal life, other than through serendipity and hope, it will be necessary to again undertake many careful (and humanistic) fetal investigations. Claude Bernard[48] wrote that "For direct applicability to medical practice, it is quite certain that experiments made on man are always the most conclusive. Nobody has ever denied it. . . First, have we a right to perform an experimental operation on man? Physicians make therapeutic experiments daily on their patients and surgeons perform operations daily on their subjects. Experiments, then, may be performed on man, but what are the limits? It is our duty and our obligation to perform an experiment on a person whenever it can save life, cure or gain personal benefits for the person. The principle of medical and surgical mortality, thus, consists in never doing on human beings an experiment which might be harmful to any extent, even though the results might be of great advantage to science, that is, to the health of others."

Sir Thomas Browne's words, "There are incurable diseases in medicine, incorrigible vices in the ministry and insoluble cases in law," suggest that our systems are far from perfect. But surely the day will again return when we can study the previable fetus condemned to die by its mother or by nature. It seems to me that as a specialty we must find an acceptable solution to improving fetal health and development, while protecting human rights. After all, future generations have the "right" to our increasing efforts to assure their optimal fetal health.

References

1. ACOG: Executive Board, Statement of Policy, May, 1977.
2. Abdul-Karim, R.: In *Progress in Perinatology,* H.A. Kaminetsky and L. Iffy, Eds., Stickley, Philadelphia, 1977.
2a. Adams, F.: *J Pediat* **63:** 881, 1963.
3. Adamsons, K.: *Contrib Gynecol Obstet* **5:** 40, 1975.
4. Adamsons, K., and Myers, R.: *Pediat Clin North Am* **20:** 465, 1973.
5. Adamsons, K., and Myers, R.: *Am J Obstet Gynecol* **128:** 893, 1977.
6. Adamsons, K., and Fox, H.: *Preventability of Perinatal Injury,* Liss, New York, 1975.
7. Adolph, E.F.: *Am J Physiol* **209:** 1095, 1965.
8. Ahlfeld, F.: *Monatsschr Geburtshilfe* **21:** 143, 1905.
9. Ahlfeld, F.: *Lehrbuch Geburtshilfe* **6:** 44, 1903.
10. Ahlfeld, F.: *Z Geburtschilfe Gynak* **69:** 91, 1911.
11. Ahlford, C.E., *et al.: Am J Dis Child* **131:** 405, 1977.
12. Ahlford, C.A., *et al.:* In *Intrauterine Asphyxia and the Developing Fetal Brain,* L. Gluck, Ed., Year Book, Chicago, 1977.
12a. Aladjem, S., *et al.: Br J Obster Gynecol* **84:** 487, 1977.
12b. Aladjem, S., and Brown, A.: *Perinatal Intensive Care,* C.V. Mosby, St. Louis, 1977, p. 150.
13. Alvarez, H., and Caldeyro-Barcia, H.: *Surg Gynecol Obstet* **91:** 1, 1950.
14. Anders, T.F., and Roftward, H.P.: *Neuropadiatrie* **4:** 151, 1973.
15. Anderson, W.A., and Harbert, G.: *Am J Obstet Gynecol* **129:** 260, 1977.
16. Anderson, H.T.: *Acta Physiol Scand* **58:** 263, 1963.
17. Anderson, H.T.: *Physiol Rev.* **46:** 22, 1966.
18. Ando, Y., and Hattori, H.: *Br J Obstet Gynecol* **84:** 115, 1977.
18a. Antler, J., and Fox, D.: *Bull Med Hist* **50:** 559, 1976.
19. Antonov, A.N.: *J Pediat* **30:** 250, 1947.
20. Assali, N.S., Bekey, G.A., and Morrison, L.W.: In *Biology of Gestation II,* N.S. Assali, Ed., Academic Press, New York, 1968.
21. Assali, N.S., Brinkman, C.R., and Nuwayhid, B.: *Am J Obstet Gynecol* **120:** 411, 1974.
22. Assali, N.S., and Vaughn, D.L.: *Am J Obstet Gynecol* **129:** 355, 1977.
23. Atkinson, S.M.: *J Reprod Med* **9:** 223, 1972.
24. Atospa-Sison, H.: *Am J Obstet Gynecol* **31:** 139, 1936.
25. Atwood, R.J.: *Acta Obstet Gynecol Scand Suppl* **57:** 1, 1976.
26. Aubury, R.H., *et al.: Clin Perinatal* **2:** 207, 1975.
27. Bachman, D.S.: *Pediat* **51:** 755, 1973.
28. Baillie, P., *et al.: J Physiol* **195:** 55, 1968.
29. Baillie, P., and Dawes, G.S.: *J Physiol* **218:** 635, 1971.
30. Bain, A.D., Smith, I., and Gauld, I.K.: *Br Med J* **5409:** 598, 1964.
31. Baker, C.I., and Rudolph, A.J.: *Am J Dis Child* **121:** 393, 1971.
32. Baker, C.I., and Barnett, F.: *J Pediat* **83:** 919, 1973.
32a. Balfour, W.N. *et al.: Physiologists* **2:** 5, 1959.
33. Ballantyne, J.W.: *The Diseases and Deformities of the Foetus,* Oliver and Boyd, Edinburgh, 1892.
33a. Ballard, R., and Ballard, P.: *Am J Dis Child* **130:** 982, 1976.
34. Barclay, M.L., DeHart, W., and Mercer, J.F.: *Am J Obstet Gynecol* **128:** 242, 1977.
35. Barcroft, J.: *Physiol Rev* **16:** 103, 1936.
36. Barcroft, J. and Barron, D.H.: *J Comp Neurol* **70:** 477, 1939
37. Barcroft, J. and Barron, D.H.: *J Exp Biol* **22:** 63, 1945.
38. Barcroft, J.: *Researcher of Prenatal Life,* Blackwell Scientific, Oxford, 1946.
39. Barcroft, J.: In *Marshall's Physiology of Reproduction,* Longmans Green, London, 1967, Vol. 2.
40. Battle, C.U., and Miller, G.: *Am J Obstet Gynecol* **108:** 485, 1970.
41. Baumberger, J.P.: *Manual of Field Physiology,* Stanford University Press, Stanford, 1954.
41a. Beltram-Paz, C., and Driscoll, S.: In *Pathology of the Human Placenta,* K. Benirschke and S. Driscoll, Eds., Springer-Verlag, New York, 1967.
42. Bendek, E.: *Obstet Ginec Lat Am* **14:** 255, 1956.
43. Bennink, H., and Schruers, W.: *Br Med J* **3:** 13, 1975.
44. Benirschke, K.: In *Fetal Growth and Development,* G. Waisman, and G. Kerr, Eds., McGraw-Hill, New York, 1968.
45. Berman, W., Goodlin, R.C., Heymann, M.A., and Rudolph, A.M.: *Pediat Res* **9:** 123 (Abstr.), 1975.
46. Berman, W., Goodlin, R.C., Heymann, M., and Rudolph, A.M.: *J Appl Physiol* **39:** 1065, 1975.
47. Berman, W., Goodlin, R.C., Heymann, M., and Rudolph, A.M.: *Circ Res* **38:** 262, 1976.
48. Bernard, C.: *An Introduction to the Study of Experimental Medicine,* McMillian, New York, 1927.

49. Berne, R.M., and Levy, M.N.: *Cardiovascular Physiology*, C.V. Mosby, St. Louis, 1967.

49a. Bernstein, A. *et al.*: *Am J Obstet Gynecol* **126**: 238, 1976.

50. Bernstein, R.L.: *Fetal Electrocardiography and Electroencephalography*, Thomas, Springfield, 1960.

51. Bevis, D.C.: *J Obstet Gynecol Brit Cwlth* **63**: 68, 1956.

52. Bieniarz, J., and Maqueda, E.: *Am J Obstet Gynecol* **100**: 203, 1968.

53. Bilderbeck, J., 1960, quoted by G.J. Kloosterman in Ref. 408.

54. Bill, A.H.: *Am J Obstet Gynecol* **14**: 523, 1927.

55. Binns, W., James, L.F., and Shupe, J.L.: *Ann NY Acad Sci* **111**: 571, 1964.

56. Bjerre, B., and Bjerre, I.: *Acta Paediat Scand* **65**: 577, 1976.

57. Blackfan, K., and Hamilton, B.: *N Engl J Med* **193**: 617, 1925.

58. Blechner, J., *et al.*: *Am J Obstet Gynecol* **121**: 789, 1975.

59. Blekta, M., *et al.*: *Am J Obstet Gynecol* **106**: 10, 1970.

60. Blumberger, K.: *Ergeb Inn Med Kinderheilkd* **62**: 424, 1942.

61. Boddy, K., *et al.*: *Br Med Bull* **31**: 3, 1975.

61a. Boddy, K.: In *Therapeutic Problems in Pregnancy*, P. Lewis, Ed., University Park Press, Baltimore, 1977.

62. Bobitt, J.R., and Ledger, W.J.: *J Reprod Med* **19**: 8, 1977.

63. Bobitt, J.R., and Ledger, W.J.: *Obstet Gynecol* **51**: 56, 1978

64. Boddy, K., Dawes, G.S., and Robinson, J.S.: In *Foetal and Neonatal Physiology*, K.S. Comline *et al.*, Ed., Cambridge University Press, 1973.

64b. Bradfield, A.: *Aust NZ J Obstet Gynecol* **1**: 106, 1961.

65. Bradley, R.M., and Mistretta, C.M.: *Physiol Rev* **35**: 1, 1975.

66. Brady, J., and James, L.: *Am J Obstet Gynecol* **84**: 1, 1962.

67. Brain, M.C., Kuah, K.B., and Doxon, H.G.: *J Obstet Gynecol Br Cwlth* **74**: 702, 1967.

68. Braine, M.D.S., *et al.*: *Monogr Soc Res Child Devel* **31**: 106, 1976.

69. Braundwald, E., Sarnoff, S.J., and Stainsby, W.N.: *Circ Res* **6**: 319, 1958.

70. Brenner, W.E., Bruce, R.D., and Hendricks, C.H.: *Am J Obstet Gynecol* **118**: 700, 1974.

71. Brenner, W.E.: *ACOG*, Chicago, May, 1977.

72. Bresnihan, B., *et al.*: *Lancet* **2**: 1205, 1977.

73. Brewer, T.H.: *Am J Obstet Gynecol* **83**: 1352, 1962.

74. Brewer, T.H.: *Medikon* **4**: 14, 1974.

75. Brinkman, C.R., III, Kirschbaum, T.H., and Assali, N.S.: *Gynecol Invest* **1**: 115, 1970.

76. Brinkman, C.R., III: *Clin Obstet Gynecol* **13**: 565, 1970.

77. Brinkman, C.R., III, *et al.*: *Am J Physiol* **223**: 1465, 1972.

78. *British Perinatal Mortality Survey: Perinatal Problems*, Livingstone, London, 1969.

78a. Broom, B.: *Nature (London)* **203**: 498, 1964.

79. Bross, I.D., and Natarajan, N.: *JAMA* **237**: 2399, 1977.

80. Brotanek, V., Hendricks, C., and Yoshida, T.: *Am J Obstet Gynecol* **105**: 535, 1969.

81. Brown, T., quoted by W.B. Bean: *Bull Hist Med* **51**: 75, 1977.

81a. Bruksch, L.W.: *Am J Obstet Gynecol* **130**: 240, 1978.

82. Burrow, G.N., and Ferris, T.F.: *Medical Complications during Pregnancy*, Saunders, Philadelphia, 1975.

83. Bustos, R., *et al.*: *J Perinat Med* **3**: 172, 1975.

84. Cahill, G.F.: *Pediatrics* **50**: 357, 1972.

85. Caldeyro-Barcia, R., and Poseiro, J.J.: *Ann NY Acad Sci* **75**: 813, 1959.

86. Caldeyro-Barcia, R., *et al.*: In *The Heart and Circulation in the Newborn Infant*, Grune & Stratton, New York, 1966.

87. Caldeyro-Barcia, R., *et al.*: *Maternal and Child Health Practices*, E.M. Gold, H.M. Wallace, and E.F. Lis, Eds., Thomas, Springfield, 1975.

88. California Department of Health: *Standards and Recommendations for Perinatal Care*, Berkeley, December, 1977.

89. California Department of Health: *Nutritional Management of Obese Pregnant Women*, Sacramento, October, 1977.

90. Campbell, A.G.M., *et al.*: *J Pediatr* **72**: 518, 1968.

91. Carson, B.S., *et al.*: *Am J Obstet Gynecol* **126**: 712, 1976.

92. Casalino, M.: *J Reprod Med* **14**: 249, 1974.

93. Chamberlain, R., *et al.*: *The First Week of Life*, Heineman, London, 1975.

94. Chamberlain, R.W.: *Pediatrics* **59**: 971, 1977.

95. Chambers, J., Lawson, G., and Turnbull, A.: *Br J Obstet Gynaecol* **83**: 921, 1976.

96. Chang, H., and Wood, C.: *Am J Obstet Gynecol* **125**: 61, 1976.

97. Chang, T., and O'Keefe, A.: *N Engl J Med* **296**: 573, 1977.

98. Chase, H.P., *et al.*: *Pediatrics* **52**: 513, 1973.

99. Chesley, L.C.: In *Pathophysiology of Gestation*, N.S. Assali, Ed., Academic Press, New York, 1972.

100. Chesley, L.C.: *Prog Clin Biol Res* **7**: 19, 1976.

101. Chesley, L.C.: In *Blood Pressure, Edema and Proteinuria in Pregnancy*, E.A. Friedman, Ed., Liss, New York, 1976.

102. Chesley, L.E.: *Hypertensive Disorders of Pregnancy*, Appleton-Century-Crofts, New York, 1978.

103. Chez, R.A.: In *Intrauterine Asphyxia and the Fetal Brain*, L. Gluck, Ed., Year Book, Chicago, 1977.

104. Churchill, J.A.: *Neurology* **15**: 341, 1965.

105. Churchill, J.A., Berendes, H., and Nemore, J.: *Am J Obstet Gynecol* **105**: 257, 1969.

106. Churchill, J.A., *et al.*: *Dev Med Child Neurol* **16**: 143, 1974.

107. Cibils, L.: *Am J Obstet Gynecol* **129**: 833, 1977.

107a.Clifford, S.H.: *J Pediatr* **77**: 1, 1970.

108. Cloer, E.N., *et al.*: *N Engl J Med* **287**: 1356, 1972.

109. Cloeren, S.E., Lippert, T.H., and Hinselmann, M.: *Arch Gynaekol* **215**: 123, 1973.

110. Cockburn, F.: In *Prevention of Handicap through Antenatal Care*, A.C. Turnbull and F. Woodford, Ed., Elsevier, Amsterdam, 1976.

111. Cohen, E.N.: *Anesth Analg* **41**: 122, 1962.

112. Cohen, W.R., Schifrin, B.S., and Doctor, G.: *Am J Obstet Gynecol* **123**: 646, 1975.

113. Cohn, H.E., Sacks, E.J., Heymann, M.H., and Rudolph, A.M.: *Am J Obstet Gynecol* **120**: 817, 1974.

114. Cohn, H.E., *et al.*: In *Circulation in the Fetus and Newborn*, L. Longo, Ed., Springer Verlag, Berlin, 1977.

115. Cohnstein, J., and Zuntz, P.: *Arch Ges Physiol* **34**: 173, 1884.

116. Cole, R.A., *et al.*: *Lancet* **1**: 767, 1975.

116a.Collea, J., *et al.*: *Am J Obstet Gynecol* **131**: 185, 1978.

117. Comline, R.S., and Silver, M.: *J Physiol* **156**: 424, 1962.

118. Comline, R.S., and Silver, M.: *J Physiol* **222**: 233, 1972.

119. Coen, R.W., *et al.*: *Pediatrics* **53**: 760, 1974.

120. Courville, C.B.: *Birth and Brain Damage*, Courville, Pasadena, 1977.

121. Cowett, R.M., and Oh, W.J.: *N Engl J Med* **295**: 1222, 1976.

121a.Cox, L.W.: *Lancet* **1**: 84, 1963.

122. Cox, L.W., *et al.*: *Br Med J* **2**: 1221, 1959.

123. Cox, L.W., and Aust, N.Z.: *J Obstet Gynecol* **1**: 99, 1961.

124. Coxon, A., and Haggith, J.: *J Obstet Gynecol Br Cwlth* **78**: 49, 1971.

125. Crawford, J.S.: *Br J Anaesthesiol* **28**: 146, 1956.

126. Crawford, J.S., *et al.*: *Br J Anaesth* **48**: 661, 1976.

127. Crawford, M.A.: *Lancet* **1**: 452, 1976.

128. Cree, J.E., Meyer, J., and Hailey, D.M.: *Br Med J* **4**: 251, 1970.

129. Cremer, M.: *Munch Med Wochnschr* **53**: 811, 1906.

129a.Crenshaw, C.: *Obstet Gynecol Surv* **28**: 461, 1973.

130. Crocker, E.F., Johnson, R.O., and Korner, P.I.: *J Physiol* **199**: 267, 1968.

131. Cruikshank, D.P.: *Am J Obstet Gynecol* **130**: 101, 1978.

132. Csapo, A.: *Am J Obstet Gynecol* **121**: 578, 1975.

133. Curet, L.B., *et al.*: *J Am Phys* **40**: 725, 1976.

133a.Curran, D.F.: *J Gen Physiol* **43**: 1137, 1960.

134. Curron, J.T.: *Fetal Heart Monitoring*, Butterworths, London, 1975.

134a.Dalessio, D.: *JAMA* **239**: 52, 1978.

135. Dalton, K.J., Dawes, G.S., and Patrick, J.E.: *J Physiol* **256**: 37P, 1976.

136. Dalton, K.J., Dawes, G.S., and Patrick, J.E.: *Am J Obstet Gynecol* **127**: 414, 1977.

137. Datta, S., and Brown, W.: *Anesthesiology* **47**: 262–276, 1977.

137a.Davis, A.E., III, *et al.*: *N Engl J Med* **297**: 144, 1977.

138. Dawes, G.S.: *Am J Obstet Gynecol* **84**: 1634, 1962.

139. Dawes, G.S., *et al.*: *J Physiol* **169**: 167, 1963.

140. Dawes, G.S.: *Foetal and Neonatal Physiology*, Year Book, Chicago, 1968.

141. Dawes, G.S., *et al.*: *J Physiol* **195**: 55, 1968.

142. Dawes, G.S., *et al.*: *J Physiol* **201**: 105, 1969.

143. Dawes, G.S.: In *Respiratory Gas Exchange and Blood Flow in Placenta*, L. Longo and H. Bartels, Eds., DHEW, Bethesda, 1972.

144. Dawes, G.S.: In *Foetal and Neonatal Physiology*, X. Comline *et al.*, Eds., Cambridge University Press, 1973.

145. Dawes, G.S.: *Pediatrics* **51**: 965, 1973.

146. de Castillo, D.: *Rev Clinic Esp* **6**: 166, 1972.

147. DeGeest, H.M., *et al.*: *Circ Res* **17**: 222, 1965.

148. de Hann, J., *et al.*: *Eur J Obstet Gynecol* **3**: 103, 1971.

149. de Haan, R., *et al.*: *Am J Obstet Gynecol* **127**: 753, 1977.

150. DeKergaredec, cited by L.M. Hellman, *J Obstet Gynecol Br Cwlth* **72**: 896, 1965.

151. Delgado, H., *et al.*: *Nutritional Impact on Women*, K.S. Moghissi and T. Evans, Eds., Harper & Row, New York, 1971.

152. DeLee, J.B.: *Am J Obstet Gynecol* **11**: 48, 1878.

153. DeLee, J.B.: *Principles and Practice of Obstetrics*, W.B. Saunders, Philadelphia, 1913.

154. Desmond, M.M.: *Anesthesiology* **40**: 111, 1974.

155. DeSnoo, K.: *Monatsschr Geburtsh Gynaekol* **105**: 88, 1937.

156. Dews, P.B., and Wiesel, T.N.: *J Physiol* **206**: 419, 1970.

156a.Dieckmann, W.: *Am J Obstet Gynecol* **18**: 227, 1926.

157. Dieckmann, W.J.: *The Toxemias of Pregnancy*, 2nd ed., C.V. Mosby, St. Louis, 1952.

158. Dobbing, J.: *Pediatrics* **53**: 2, 1974.

159. Donati, F., *et al.*: *J Perinat Med* **4**: 255, 1976.

160. Dong, E., Jr., and Reitz, B.A.: *Circ Res* **27**: 635, 1970.

161. Douglas, J.W.B.: *Br Med J* **1**: 1008, 1960.

161a.Downing, G., *et al.*: *Obstet Gynecol* **21**: 453, 1962.

162. Downing, S.E., *et al.*: *Am J Obstet Gynecol* **208**: 931, 1965.

163. Drage, J., *et al.*: *Pan Am Health Org* **185**: 222, 1969.

164. Drillien, C.M.: *Dev Med Child Neurol* **14**: 563, 1972.

165. Drillien, C.M.: *The Growth and Development of the Prematurely Born Infant*, Williams & Wilkins, Baltimore, 1964.

166. Driscoll, S.G.: *Pediatr Clin North Am* **12**: 493, 1965.

167. Dressendorfer, R.H.: *Phys Sports Med* **6**: 76, 1978.

168. Dudzinski, P.K., *et al.*: *J Urol* **106**: 621, 1971.

169. Duenhoelter, J.H., and Pritchard, J.A.: *Am J Obstet Gynecol* **129**: 326, 1977.

170. Duhring, J.L.: *Am J Obstet Gynecol* **128**: 613, 1977.

171. Dunn, J.M.: *Am J Obstet Gynecol* **125**: 265, 1976.

172. Durech, R., *et al.*: *Am J Obstet Gynecol* **119**: 811, 1974.

173. Durkin, M.V., *et al.*: *Eur J Pediat* **123**: 67, 1976.

174. Dyer, D.C.: *J Pharmacol Exp Ther* **175:** 565, 1970.
175. Eastman, N.J.: *Bull Johns Hopkins Hosp* **50:** 39, 1932.
176. Eastman, N.J.: *Obstet Gynecol Surv* **7:** 645, 1952.
177. Eastman, N.J.: *Am J Obstet Gynecol* **67:** 701, 1954
178. Eastman, N.J.: *Obstet Gynecol Surv* **11:** 624, 1955.
179. Eastman, N.J., *et al.*: *Obstet Gynecol Surv* **17:** 459, 1962.
180. Editorial: *JAMA* **68:** 732, 1917.
181. Editorial: *Br Med J* **2:** 4, 1971.
182. Editorial: *Lancet* **2:** 1349, 1972.
183. Editorial: *Lancet* **2:** 445, 1975.
184. Editoiral: *Lancet* **1:** 946, 1976.
184a.Editorial: *Lancet* **2:** 595, 1977.
184b.Eidelberg, E.: *J Neurosurg* **38:** 326, 1973.
185. Elder, M.G.L., *et al.*: *J Obstet Gynecol Br Cwlth* **77:** 481, 1970.
186. Eliakim, M., Sapoznikov, D., and Weinman, J.: *Am Heart J* **82:** 448, 1972
187. Ellis, H.: *Studies in the Psychology of Sex,* Random House, New York, 1940.
188. Elsner, R.W., and Franklin, D.L.: *Science* **135:** 941, 1966.
188a.Embrey, M.: *J Obstet Gynecol Br Emp* **47:** 371, 1940.
188b.Emerson, K., *et al.*: *Obstet Gynecol* **40:** 786, 1972.
189. Engen, T., *et al.*: *J Comp Psychol* **56:** 73, 1963.
190. Erkkola, R., *et al.*: *Acta Obstet Gynecol Scand* **55:** 441, 1976.
190a.Espinoza, J.: In *Perinatal Care,* S. Aladjem and A. Brown, Eds., C.V. Mosby, St Louis, 1977.
190b.Essex, N.: In *Therapeutic Problems in Pregnancy,* P. Lewis, Ed., University Park Press, Baltimore, 1977.
191. Faber, J.J.: In *Respiratory Gas Exchange and Blood Flow in the Placenta,* L. Longo and H. Bartels, Eds., DHEW, Bethesda, 1972.
192. Fanaroff, A., *et al.*: *Pediat Res* **9:** 395, 1975.
193. Faulk, W.P., and Jeannet, M.: In *Maternofoetal Transmission of Immunoglobulin,* W.A. Hemmings, Ed., Cambridge University Press, 1976.
194. Feder, H.W.: *J Pediatr* **89:** 808, 1976.
195. Feingold, M.J., *et al.*: *Am J Dis Child* **122:** 155, 1971.
196. Feldman, H.A.: In *Progress in Perinatology;* H. Kaminetsky and L. Iffy, Eds., Stickley, Philadelphia, 1977.
197. Felig, P.: *N Engl J Med* **290:** 1360, 1974.
198. Fenning, G.: *Am J Obstet Gynecol* **43:** 791, 1942.
199. Ferreira, A.J.: *Prenatal Environment,* Thomas, Springfield, 1969.
200. Finn, R., *et al.*: *Br Med J* **1:** 1486, 1961.
201. Finn, R., *et al.*: *Lancet* **2:** 1200, 1977.
202. Fitzhardinge, P.M., and Steven, E.M.: *Pediatrics* **50:** 50, 1972.
203. Fitzhardinge, P.M., and Ramsay, M.: *Dev Med Child Neurol* **15:** 447, 1973.
204. Fitzhardinge, P.M., *et al.*: *J Pediatr* **88:** 531, 1976.
205. Freeman, R., and Schifrin, B.S.: *Int Anesthesiol Clin* **11:** 69, 1973.

206. Freeman, R., and James, J.: *Obstet Gynecol* **46:** 255, 1975.
207. Freis, E., and Kenney, J.: *J Clin Invest* **27:** 283, 1948.
207a.Freud, S.: In *Collected Papers, Vol. 5,* Hogarth Press, London, 1950.
208. Freund, V., *et al.*: *Am J Obstet Gynecol* **126:** 206, 1977.
209. Freund, S. quoted by A. Lilienfeld and F. Parkhurst: *Am J Hyg* **53:** 262, 1961.
210. Friedman, W.F., *et al.*: *Prog Cardiovas Dis* **15:** 87, 1972.
211. Friedman, E.A., and Neff, R.K.: *Pregnancy Hypertension,* Publishing Sci., Boston, 1977.
212. Friedman, E.A., *et al.*: *Am J Obstet Gynecol* **127:** 779, 1977.
213. Friedman, L. A., and Lewis, P.J.: In *Therapeutic Problems of Pregnancy,* P.J. Lewis, Ed., Baltimore, University Park, 1977.
214. Friedman, W.R., and Roberts, W.C.: *Circulation* **34:** 77, 1966.
214a.Fries, M., and Woolf, C.: In *The Psychoanalytic Study of the Child, Vol. 8,* R. Eissler, *et al.,* Eds., International University Press, New York, 1953.
215. Fuchs, F., and Phillips, J.: *Nord Med* **69:** 572, 1961.
216. Fuchs, F.: *Am J Obstet Gynecol* **99:** 627, 1967.
217. Fuchs, F.: *Am J Obstet Gynecol* **126:** 809, 1977.
218. Fuldner, R.V.: *Arch Neurol Psychiat* **74:** 267, 1955.
219. Gabbe, S.G., *et al.*: *Am J Obstet Gynecol* **129:** 723, 1977.
220. Gabriel, M., Albonic, M., and Schulte, P.J.: *Pediatrics* **57:** 142, 1976.
221. Gant, N., and Worley, R.: In *Advances in Perinatal Medicine,* A. Goldstein, Ed., Stratton Int Med Book, New York, 1977.
222. Garrod, A.H.: *Proc Roy Soc London* **23:** 140, 1874.
223. Genesis 25:22 Holy Bible.
224. Gerlach, A.: *Arch Anat Physiol* **11:** 431, 1851.
225. Gessner, W.: *Zbl Gynak* **43:** 1033, 1919.
226. Gibbens, G.O.L.: *Br J Obstet Gynecol* **82:** 588, 1975.
227. Gibson, A.M.: *J Obstet Gynecol Brit Cwlth* **80:** 1067, 1973.
228. Ginsberg, J., and Myers, R.E.: *Neurology* **26:** 15, 1976.
229. Giroud, A.: *Nutrition of the Embryo,* Thomas, Springfield, 1970.
230. Glaze, H.J., Jr., and Dong, E., Jr.: *Mathematical Models for Heart Rate Responses to Vagal Nerve Stimulation,* Natl Tech Inf Service, Springfield, 1971.
231. Glick, G., and Braunwald, E.: *Circ Res* **16:** 363, 1965.
232. Gluck, L., *et al.*: *Am J Obstet Gynecol* **109:** 440, 1971.
233. Gluck, L.: In *Intrauterine Asphyxia and the Developing Fetal Brain,* L. Gluck, Ed., Year Book, Chicago, 1977.
234. Goldenberg, R., and Nelson, K.: *Am J Obstet Gynecol* **123:** 617, 1975.

235. Golditch, I.: In *Nutritional Supplementation and Outcome of Pregnancy;* Nat Acad Science, Washington, 1973.

236. Goodlin, R.C., and Kaiser, I.H.: *Am J Med Sci* **233:** 662, 1957.

237. Goodlin, R.C., and Kaiser, I.H.: *Univ Minn Med Bull* **28:** 29–35, 1957.

238. Goodlin, R.C.: *Obstet Gynecol* **10:** 299, 1957.

239. Goodlin, R.C., and Schwartz, S.: *Am J Obstet Gynecol* **84:** 808, 1962.

240. Goodlin, R.C.: *Am J Obstet Gynecol* **86:** 571, 1963.

241. Goodlin, R.C.: *Trans Am Soc Art Internal Organs* **9:** 348, 1963.

242. Goodlin, R.C.: *Minn Med* **46:** 1227, 1963.

243. Goodlin, R.C., and Herzenberg, L.: *Transplantation* **2:** 357, 1964.

244. Goodlin, R.C.: *Am J Obstet Gynecol* **88:** 1090, 1964.

245. Goodlin, R.C., and Dirkson, L.A.: *Am J Obstet Gynecol* **91:** 953, 1965.

246. Goodlin, R.C.: *Obstet Gynecol* **26:** 9, 1965.

247. Goodlin, R.C., and Lloyd, D.: *Biol Neonat* **8:** 274, 1965.

248. Goodlin, R.C., and Perry, D.: *Am J Obstet Gynecol* **94:** 268, 1966.

249. Goodlin, R.C., and Herzenberg, L.: *Am J Obstet Gynecol* **95:** 133, 1966.

250. Goodlin, R.C., and Lloyd, D.: *Third International Conference on Hyperbaric Medicine,* National Academy of Science, Washington, D.C., 1966, p. 125.

251. Goodlin, R.C., and Sohlberg, O.II.: *Pacific Med Surg* **75:** 54, 1967.

252. Goodlin, R.C., O'Connell, L.P., and Gunther, R.E.: *Lancet* **11:** 79, 1967.

253. Goodlin, R.C., and Lloyd, D.: *Biol Neonat* **12:** 1, 1968.

254. Goodlin, R.C., and Kresch, A.J.: *Am J Obstet Gynecol* **100:** 839, 1968.

255. Goodlin, R.C.: *Obstet Gynecol* **32:** 94, 1968

256. Goodlin, R.C.: *Obstet Gynecol* **34:** 109, 1969.

257. Goodlin, R.C., et al.: *Obstet Gynecol* **34:** 1, 1969.

258. Goodlin, R.C., and Rudolph, A.M.: *Am J Obstet Gynecol* **106:** 597, 1970.

259. Goodlin, R.C., and Lloyd, D.: *Am J Obstet Gynecol* **107:** 227, 1970.

260. Goodlin, R.C.: *Am J Obstet Gynecol* **106:** 940, 1970.

261. Goodlin, R.C.: *Am J Obstet Gynecol* **107:** 429, 1970.

262. Goodlin, R.C., and Fabricant, S.J.: *Obstet Gynecol* **35:** 646, 1970.

263. Goodlin, R.C.: *Obstet Gynecol* **36:** 944, 1970.

264. Goodlin, R.C.: *Int J Gynaecol Obstet* **8:** 189, 1970.

265. Goodlin, R.C.: *Am J Obstet Gynecol* **110:** 210, 1971.

266. Goodlin, R.C., Fabricant, S.J., and Keller, D.W.: *J Reprod Med* **7:** 75, 1971.

267. Goodlin, R.C.: *Obstet Gynecol* **37:** 698, 1971.

268. Goodlin, R.C.: *Lancet* **2:** 604, 1971.

269. Goodlin, R.C.: *Obstet Gynecol* **37:** 702, 1971.

270. Goodlin, R.C., and Horowitz, M.: *Am J Obstet Gynecol* **110:** 674, 1971.

271. Goodlin, R.C., Keller, D.W., and Raffin, M.: *Obstet Gynecol* **38:** 916, 1971.

271a.Goodlin, R.C., et al.: *Obstet Gynecol* **39:** 125, 1972.

272. Goodlin, R.C.: *JAMA* **220:** 1015, 1972.

273. Goodlin, R.C., Schmidt, W., and Creevy, D.C.: *Obstet Gynecol* **39:** 125, 1972.

274. Goodlin, R.C., Girard, J., and Hollmen, A.: *Obstet Gynecol* **39:** 295, 1972.

275. Goodlin, R.C., and Rudolph, A.M.: In *Physiologic Biochemistry of the Fetus;* A. Hodari and F. Mariona, Eds., Thomas, Springfield, 1972.

276. Goodlin, R.C., and Schmidt, W.: *Am J Obstet Gynecol* **114:** 613, 1972.

277. Goodlin, R.C., and Lowe, E.W.: *Obstet Gynecol* **43:** 22, 1974.

278. Goodlin, R.C.: *Obstet Gynecol* **43:** 157, 1974.

279. Goodlin, R.C., and Clewell, W.H.: *Am J Obstet Gynecol* **118:** 285, 1974.

280. Goodlin, R.C., and Lowe, E.W.: *Am J Obstet Gynecol* **119:** 341, 1974.

281. Goodlin, R.C., Lowe, E.W., and Douglass, R.: *Obstet Gynecol* **119:** 344, 1974.

282. Goodlin, R.C., et al.: *Obstet Gynecol* **46:** 69, 1975.

283. Goodlin, R.C.: *Am J Obstet Gynecol* **122:** 518, 1975.

284. Goodlin, R.C., and Crocker, K.: *J Reprod Med* **15:** 209, 1975.

285. Goodlin, R.C.: *Contrib Obstet Gynecol* **7:** 107, 1976.

286. Goodlin, R.C., Crocker, K., and Haesslein, H.C.: *Amer J Obstet Gynecol* **125:** 665, 1976.

287. Goodlin, R.C.: *Obstet Gynecol* **48:** 117, 1976.

288. Goodlin, R.C.: *Am J Obstet Gynecol* **125:** 747, 1976.

288a.Goodlin, R.C.: *Am J Obstet Gynecol* **125:** 704, 1976.

289. Goodlin, R.C.: *Contemp Obstet Gynecol* **8:** 21, 1976.

290. Goodlin, R.C.: *Obstet Gynecol* **49:** 371, 1977.

291. Goodlin, R.C., and Haesslein, H.C.: *Am J Obstet Gynecol* **128:** 440, 1977.

291a.Goodlin, R.C.: *Am J Obstet Gynecol* **128:** 129, 1977.

292. Goodwin, J.W.: In *Perinatal Medicine;* J. Goodwin et al., Eds., Williams & Wilkins, Baltimore, 1976.

293. Gordon, H.R., et al.: *Am J Obstet Gynecol* **122:** 287, 1975.

294. Gorman, J.G., Freda, V.J., and Pollack, W.: *Proc 9th Cong Int Soc Hematology* **2:** 545, 1962.

295. Graham-Pole, J., Barr, W., and Willoughby, M.L.: *Br Med J* **1:** 1185, 1977.

296. Grainger, R.G.: *Br Med Bul* **28:** 193, 1972.

297. Grassy, X.: *Clin Pediatr* **15:** 549, 1976.

298. Gray, G.R.: *Canad Med Assoc J* **107:** 1186, 1972.

299. Green, R., et al.: *Gyn Invest* **120:** 817, 1977.

300. Gregory, G.A., et al.: *J Pediatr* **85:** 848, 1974.

301. Gresham, E.L., et al.: *J Clin Invest* **51:** 1949, 1972.

302. Gresham, E.L., et al.: *Pediatrics* **50:** 372, 1972.

303. Gruenwald, P.: *Biol Neonat* **5:** 215, 1963.

304. Gultekin-Zootzmann, B.: *J Perinat Med* **3:** 135, 1975.

305. Gusdon, J.P., and Witherow, C.: *Am J Obstet Gynecol* **112:** 1101, 1973.

306. Gyves, M.T., et al.: *Am J Obstet Gynecol* **128:** 606, 1977.

307. Habichi, J.P., et al.: *Am J Clin Nutr* **26**: 1046, 1973.
308. Haesslein, H.C., and Goodlin, R.C.: *J Reprod Med* **14**: 8, 1975.
309. Hagbard, L.: *Acta Obstet Gynecol Scand (Suppl)* **35**: 1, 1956.
310. Hagberg, B., Hagberg, G., and Olow, I.: *Acta Paediatr Scand* **64**: 193, 1975.
311. Hagberg, B., et al.: *Pediatrics* **57**: 652, 1976.
312. Haire, D.B.: *Envir Child Health* **19**: 171, 1973.
312a.Hajeri, H., and Papiernik, E.: *Contr Gynec Obstet* **3**: 48, 1971.
313. Hall, M.H., et al.: *Br J Obstet Gynecol* **83**: 132, 1977.
314. Hall, M.H.: *J Obstet Gynecol Brit Cwlth* **79**: 159, 1972.
315. Hamburger, V.: In *Behavioral Embryology*; G. Gottlieb, Ed., Academic Press, New York, 1973, Vol. 1, p. 51.
316. Hamilton, L.A., et al.: *Clin Obstet Gynecol* **17**: 199, 1974.
317. Hammacher, K.: In *Intrauterine Danger to the Foetus*; R.J. Horsky and Z.K. Stembera, Eds., Excerpta Medica, Amsterdam, 1967.
318. Hammacher, K.: *Perinatal Medicine,* Verlag, Stuttgard, 1969.
319. Hanshaw, J.B.: In *Infectious Diseases of the Fetus and Newborn Infant*; J.S. Remington, and J.O. Klein, Eds., Saunders, Philadelphia, 1976.
320. Harris, R., and Mead, P.: *N Engl J Med* **296**: 454, 1977.
321. Harrison, R.S., Roberts, A., and Campbell, S.: *Br J Obstet Gynecol* **84**: 98, 1977.
322. Harter, C., and Benirschke, L.: *Am J Obstet Gynecol* **124**: 705, 1976.
323. Hauth, J., Whalley, F., and Cunningham, P.: *Obstet Gynecol* **48**: 75, 1976.
324. Hauth, J.C., et al.: *Obstet Gynecol* **51**: 81, 1978.
325. Haverkamp, A.D., et al.: *Am J Obstet Gynecol* **125**: 310, 1976.
326. Hay, D.: *J Obstet Gynaecol Br Cwlth* **80**: 280, 1974.
327. Hayashi, R., and Foy, M.: *Am J Obstet Gynecol* **122**: 786, 1975.
328. Hehre, F.W.: *Clin Anesthesiol* **10**: 81, 1974.
328a.Heldford, A.: *Am J Obstet Gynecol* **128**: 466, 1977.
329. Heller, L., Bode, H., and Warshaw, J.: *Adv Exper Med* **46**: 206, 1974.
329a. Helper, M.M., et al.: *J Psychosomat Res* **12**: 312, 1968.
330. Helligiers, A.E., and Armstead, E.E.: *Am J Obstet Gynecol* **105**: 786, 1969.
331. Hellman, L.M., and Prystowsky, H.: *Am J Obstet Gynecol* **63**: k223, 1952.
332. Hellman, L.M., et al.: *Am J Obstet Gynecol* **87**: 650, 1963.
333. Hellman, L.M., et al.: *Lancet* **1**: 1133, 1970.
334. Henderson, Y., and Radloft, E.: *Am J Obstet Gynecol* **101**: 647, 1932.
335. Hendricks, C.H.: *Clin Obstet Gynecol* **9**: 535, 1966.
336. Hendricks, C.H., Eskes, T.K., and Saamelik, K.: *Am J Obstet Gynecol* **83**: 890, 1962.
337. Hendricks, C.H., and Mowad, A.H.: *Am J Obstet Gynecol* **98**: 1091, 1967.
338. Hendricks, C.H.: *Am J Obstet Gynecol* **126**: 817, 1977.
339. Heston, L.L.: *Hosp Pract* **12**: 43, 1977.
340. Heymann, M.A., and Rudolph, A.M.: *Circ Res* **21**: 741, 1967.
341. Hibbard, B.M.: *Clin Obstet Gynecol* **5**: 1044, 1962.
342. Hibbard, E., and Smithells, R.: *Lancet* **1**: 1254, 1965.
343. Hill, D.E., et al.: *Biol Neonat* **19**: 68, 1971.
343a.Hill, R.M., et al.: *Clin Obstet Gynecol* **20**: 381, 1977.
344. Hobbins, J., and Mahoney, X.: In *Intrauterine Fetal Visualization*, M. Kaback and C. Valenti, Eds., Exerpta Medica, Amsterdam, 1976.
345. Hobel, C.J.: In *Management of High Risk Pregnancy*, W. Spellacy, Ed., University Park Press, Baltimore, 1976.
346. Hogg, M.I.J., et al.: *Br J Obstet Gynecol* **84**: 48, 1977.
347. Hoff, C.E., and Green, H.D.: *Am J Physiol* **117**: 411, 1976.
348. Holtermann, C.: *Zbl Gynak* **48**: 2536, 1924.
349. Hooker, D.: *The Prenatal Origin of Behavior,* University of Kansas Press, Lawrence, 1952.
349a.Holley, R.: *Brit J Med* **1**: 283, 1969.
350. Holm, L.W.: *Adv Vet Sci Comp Med* **11**: 159, 1967.
351. Hon, E.H., and Lee, S.T.: *Am J Obstet Gynecol* **86**: 772, 1962.
352. Hon, E.H.: *Am J Obstet Gynecol* **87**: 814, 1963.
353. Hon, E.H.: *Obstet Gynecol* **30**: 281, 1967.
354. Hon, E.H.: *An Atlas of FHR Patterns,* Harty, New Haven, 1968.
355. Hon, E.H., and Yeh, S.: *Med Research Eng* **8**: 14, 1969.
356. Hon, E.H., et al.: *Obstet Gynecol* **40**: 362, 1972.
357. Hon, E.H., et al.: *Obstet Gynecol* **43**: 722, 1974.
358. Honnebier, W.J., and Swab, D.F.: *J Obstet Gynecol Brit Cwlth* **80**: 577, 1973.
359. Howie, P.W., et al.: *Br. Med J* **1**: 150, 1976.
360. Hubel, D.H., and Wiesel, T.N.: *J Physiol* **206**: 419, 1970.
361. Hughey, M.J., et al.: *Obstet Gynecol* **49**: 513, 1977.
362. Humphrey, T.: In *Physiology of the Perinatal Period,* A. Stove, Ed., Appleton Century Crofts, New York, 1970.
363. Humphrey, T.: In *Third Symposium on Oral Sensaton and Perception,* J.F. Bosma, Ed., Thomas, Springfield, 1972.
364. Hunter, G.L.: *J Agric Sci* **51**: 325, 1958.
365. Hurley, L.S., et al.: *Teratology* **1**: 216, 1968.
366. Hutchinson, D.L., et al.: *J Clin Invest* **38**: 971, 1959.
367. Hytten, F.E., and Leitch, I.: *The Physiology of Human Pregnancy,* Blackwell, Oxford, 1971.
368. Hytten, F.E.: In *Hypertension in Pregnancy,* M.R. Lindheimer, A. Katz, and F. Zuspan, Eds., Wiley, New York, 1976.
368a.Hytten, F.E., and Thomson, A.M.: *J Obstet Gynaecol Br Cwlth* **73**: 714, 1966.

369. Iriuchyima, J., and Kumada, M.: *Jpn J Physiol* **14:** 479, 1964.
370. Irving, L.: *Science* **38:** 422, 1934.
371. Irving, L.: *J Appl Physiol* **18:** 489, 1963.
371a. Jacobson, H.N.: *N Eng J Med* **297:** 1051, 1977.
372. James, E., *et al.*: *Pediatrics* **50:** 361, 1972.
373. James, J.E.A., and Daly, M.: *J Physiol* **201:** 87, 1969.
374. James, L.S.: *Acta Paediat Suppl* **122:** 17, 1960.
375. James, L.S., *et al.*: *Am J Obstet Gynecol* **113:** 578, 1972.
376. James, L.S., *et al.*: *Am J Obstet Gynecol* **126:** 276, 1976.
377. Javert, C.T.: *Spontaneous and Habitual Abortion,* Blakiston, New York, 1957.
378. Jeffcoate, T.N.A., and Scott, J.S.: *Canad Med J* **80:** 77, 1957.
379. Joelsson, I., *et al.*: *Am J Obstet Gynecol* **114:** 43, 1972.
380. Johanson, B., Wedenberg, E., and Westin, B.: *Acta Otolaryng* **57:** 188, 1964.
381. Johnson, H.W.: *Am J Obstet Gynecol* **50:** 398, 1945.
382. Johnson, G., Brinkman, C., and Assali, N.: *Am J Obstet Gynecol* **112:** 1122, 1972.
383. Johnson, J.: *Pediatrics* **84:** 272, 1974.
384. Johnson, J.W.C., *et al.*: *N Engl J Med* **293:** 675, 1975.
385. Johnson, P., Robinson, J.E., and Salisbury, R.: In *Foetal and Neonatal Physiology;* K. Comline *et al.*, Eds., Cambridge University Press, 1973.
386. Jones, K.L., and Smith, D.W.: *Lancet* **2:** 999, 1973.
387. Josimovich, J., and Archer, O.: *Am J Obstet Gynecol* **129:** 777, 1977.
388. Jost, P., and Quilligan, E.T.: *SGI Society for Gynecological Investigation* Abstract **46,** 1969.
389. Kaiser, I.H., and Goodlin, R.C.: *Pediatrics* **22:** 1097, 1958.
390. Kaiser, I.H., and Goodlin, R.C.: *Am J Med Sci* **233:** 662, 1958.
391. Kaiser, I.H.: *Am J Obstet Gynecol* **77:** 573, 1959.
392. Kaiser, I.H.: *Am J Obstet Gynecol* **110:** 115, 1971.
393. Kaplan, S., and Toyama, S.: *Obstet Gynecol* **11:** 391, 1958.
394. Karn, M.N.: *Am Eng* **17:** 233, 1957.
395. Kasius, R., *et al.*: *Milbank Mem Fund Q* **33:** 230, 1955.
396. Kass, K.H.: *Progress in Pyelonephritis,* Davis, Philadelphia, 1965.
397. Kates, R., and Schrifrin, B.: *ACOG,* May 10, 1977.
398. Katona, P.G., *et al.*: *Am J Physiol* **218:** 1030, 1970.
399. Katz, L., and Feil, H.: *Arch Intern Med* **32:** 672, 1923.
400. Katzin, D.B., and Rubinstein, E.H.: *Am J Physiol* **231:** 179, 1976.
401. Kennedy, E.: *Observation on Obstetrical Auscultation,* Hodges and Smith, Dublin, 1833.
402. King, D.L.: *Radiology* **109:** 163, 1973.
403. Kirkpatrick, S.E., *et al.*: *Am J Phys* **231:** 495, 1976.
404. Kitahama, K., and Sasaoka, K.: *Jpn J Med Elect Biol Eng* **5:** 27, 1967.
405. Kitay, D.Z.: *Contrib Obstet Gynecol* **10:** 25, 1977.
406. Klaus, M.: In *Neonatal Respiratory Adaptation;* T. Oliver, Ed., USPH, Bethesda, 1963.
407. Klaus, M.H., and Kennell, J.H.: *Maternal-Infant Bonding;* C.V. Mosby, St Louis, 1976.
408. Kllosterman, G.J.: *Fourth European Congress of Perinatal Medicine,* Goerge Thieme, Stuttgart, 1975.
409. Knox, E.H., and Mahon, D.F.: *Arch Dis Child* **45:** 634, 1970.
410. Knutzen, V.K., and Davey D.A.: *S Afr Med J* **51:** 672, 1977.
411. Koleta, F.: *Cesk Gynek* **26:** 490, 1961.
412. Korner, A.F., and Colley, A.: *Child Dev* **39:** 1145, 1968.
412a. Korner, A.F.: *Am J Orthopsychiat* **4:** 608, 1971.
413. Korner, P.I.: *Physiol Rev* **51:** 312, 1971.
414. Korsch, B.M.: *Pediatrics* **59:** 1063, 1977.
415. Krogh, A.: *Skan Arch Physiol* **16:** 348, 1904.
416. Kubli, F.: *Z Geburtshilfe Perinatal* **176:** 309, 1972.
417. Kunzel, W., *et al.*: *J Perinat Med* **3:** 360, 1975.
418. Kurjak, A., and Barsic, B.: *Acta Obstet Gynecol Scand* **56:** 161, 1977.
419. LaCroix, G.E.: *Mich Med* **67:** 976, 1968.
419a. Laga, E.M.: *Pediatrics* **50:** 33, 1972.
420. Landsteiner, K., and Wiener, A.: *Proc Soc Exper Biol* **43:** 223, 1940.
421. Larks, S.D.: *Electrohysterography,* Thomas, Springfield, 1960.
422. Laros, R.K., and Sweet, R.L.: *Am J Obstet Gynecol* **122:** 182, 1975.
423. Larroche, J.C., and Korn, G.: In *Intrauterine Asphyxia and Development of the Brain,* L. Gluck, Ed., Year Book, Chicago, 1976.
424. Laversen, H.H., *et al.*: *Am J Obstet Gynecol* **127:** 837, 1977.
425. Lawrence, A.C.K.: *J Obstet Gynecol Brit Cwlth* **69:** 29, 1962.
425a. Lazard, E., *et al.*: *Am J Obstet Gynecol* **12:** 104, 1926.
426. LeBoyer, F.: *Birth Without Violence,* Knopf, New York, 1975.
426a. Lean, T., *et al.*: *J Obstet Gynec Brit Cwlth* **75:** 856, 1968.
427. Lechtig, A., *et al.*: *Am J Clin Nutr* **28:** 1223, 1975.
428. Ledger, W.L.: *Amnionitis, Endometritis and Premature Rupture of Membranes;* Upjohn, Kalamazoo, 1976.
429. Lee, S.T., and Hon, E.H.: *Obstet Gynecol* **22:** 553, 1963.
430. Lee, C.Y., *et al.*: *Obstet Gynecol* **48:** 19, 1976.
431. Levin, D.L., Hymen, A.I., Heymann, T.M., and Rudolph, A.M.: *J Pediatr* **92:** 265, 1978.
432. Levine, P.: *Hum Biol* **30:** 14, 1958.
433. Levy, M.N., and Zieske, H.: *Circ Res* **27:** 429, 1970.
434. Lewis, B.V.: *J Obstet Gynecol Brit Cwlth* **75:** 87, 1968.
435. Lewis, P.J., and Trudinger, B.: *Lancet* **2:** 355, 1977.
436. Lewis, M.: *Hum Dev* **16:** 108, 1973.

437. Lewis, R.B., and Schulman, J.P.: *Lancet* **2:** 1159, 1973.
438. Liggins, G.C.: *J Endocrinol* **42:** 232, 1968.
439. Liggins, G.C., and Howie, R.N.: *Pediatrics* **50:** 515, 1972.
440. Liggins, G.C., *et al.*: *J Reprod Fert Suppl* **16:** 85, 1972.
441. Liley, A.W.: *Br Med J* **2:** 1107, 1963.
442. Liley, A.W.: *Int J Gynecol Obstet* **8:** 358, 1970.
443. Liley, A.W.: *Aust NZ J Psych* **6:** 99, 1972.
444. Liley, A.W.: In *Intrauterine Fetal Visualization*; M. Kaback and C. Valenti, Ed., Excerpta Medica, Amsterdam, 1976.
445. Lilienfeld, A.M., and Parkhurst, F.: *Am J Hyg* **53:** 262, 1961.
446. Lindgren, L.: *Acta Obstet Gynecol Scand* **51:** 37, 1972.
447. Lindgren, L.: *Acta Obstet Gynecol Scand Suppl* **66:** 87, 1977.
448. Lindheimer, M.D., Katz, A., and Zuspan, F.: *Hypertension in Pregnancy,* Wiley, New York, 1976.
449. Limner, R.R.: *Sex and the Unborn Child,* Julian Press, New York, 1969.
450. Lippert, T.H.: *Am J Obstet Gynecol* **112:** 1112, 1972.
451. Little, W., quoted by N.J. Eastman: *Obstet Gynecol Surv* **17:** 459, 1962.
452. Lofebvres, J.: *Ann Med* **52:** 225, 1951.
452a.Longo, L.D., and Power, G.G.: *J Appl Physiol* **26:** 48, 1969.
452b.Longo, C.D., *et al.*: *Society for Gynecological Investigation* Abstract #10, Atlantic, 1978.
453. Löuset, J.: *Acta Obstet Gynecol Scand* **38:** 551, 1959.
454. Lubchenko, L.O., *et al.*: *Pediat* **32:** 793, 1963.
455. Lubchenko, L.O., Deliboria-Papadopoulos, M. and Searles, P.: *Pediatrics* **80:** 501, 1972.
456. Lubchenko, L.O., *et al.*: *Dev Med Child Neurol* **16:** 421, 1974.
456a.Lumley, J., and Wood, C.: *Clin Anes* **101:** 121, 1974.
457. MacAfee, C.H.G., and Johnson, R.: *J Obstet Gynecol Br Cwlth* **52:** 313, 1945.
457a.Maeck, J.: *Am J Obstet Gynecol* **106:** 553, 1965.
458. Makowski, D.L., Prem, K.S., and Kaiser, I.H.: *Science* **123:** 542, 1956.
458a.Malpas, P.: *J Obstet Gynecol Br Cwlth* **40:** 1046, 1933.
459. Mann, C.I., Pritchard, J.W., and Symmes, D.: *Am J Obstet Gynecol* **106:** 39, 1970.
459a.Mann, L., *et al.*: *Am J Obstet Gynecol* **84:** 428, 1973.
460. Manning, F.A.: *Postgrad Med* **61:** 119, 1977.
461. Martin, C.B., Jr., *et al.*: *Obstet Gynecol* **44:** 503, 1974.
462. Martin, J.D.: *Aust NZ J Obstet Gynaecol* **12:** 102, 1972.
463. Mathews, D.D.: *Br J Obstet Gynecol* **84:** 108, 1978.
464. Masters, W.H., and Johnson, V.E.: *Human Sexual Response,* Little, Brown, and Co., Boston, 1969.
465. Mata, L.J., *et al.*: *Proc Western Hemisphere Nutrition Cong III,* Futura, Mt. Kisco, 1972.
466. Mayer, P.S., and Wingate, M.B.: *Int J Gynaecol Obstet* **14:** 329, 1976.
467. Mead, P.B., and Harris, R.: *Tex Med* **70:** 59, 1974.
468. Mead, P.B., and Clapp, J.F.: *J Reprod Med* **19:** 3, 1977.
468a.Melmick, L.: *Lancet* **2:** 167, 1977.
469. Medawar, P.B.: *Symp Soc Exp Biol* **7:** 320, 1954.
469a.Merkatz, I.: *Am J Obstet Gynecol* **128:** 615, 1977.
470. Mermann, J.: *Central Gyn* **337:** 1880 (quoted by DeLee, 1913).
470a.Mendez-Bauer, C.: *J Perinat Med* **2:** 89, 1975.
471. Metcalfe, J.: *Presentation CURI* November, 1976.
471a.Mengert, W.F., *et al.*: *Am J Obstet Gynecol* **66:** 1104, 1953.
472. Meyer, C.M.: *Gynaecologia* **161:** 110, 1966.
473. Miller, J., and Miller, F.: *Am J Obstet Gynecol* **84:** 44, 1962.
474. Minkowski, A., *et al.*: In *Falkner Human Development,* Saunders, Philadelphia, 1960.
474a.Misenhimer, H., and Kaltrieder, D.: *Obstet Gynecol* **33:** 642, 1969.
475. Mitchell, M.D., *et al.*: *Br Med J* **2:** 1183, 1977.
476. Mocsary, P., and Gaal, J.: *Am J Obstet Gynecol* **106:** 407, 1970.
477. Moir, J.C.: *Trans Edinb Obstet Soc* **92:** 93, 1934.
478. Moir, J. Chasser: *Monro Kerr's Operative Obstetrics,* 7th ed., Williams & Wilkins, Baltimore, 1974.
479. Mondanlou, H.D., *et al.*: *Am J Obstet Gynecol* **127:** 861, 1977.
480. Mondanlou, H.D., *et al.*: *Obstet Gynecol* **49:** 537, 1977.
481. Mori, C.: *Jpn J Obstet Gynecol* **3:** 374, 1956.
482. Morris, J.A., *et al.*: *Obstet Gynecol* **49:** 675, 1977.
483. Morris, J.A.: personal communication.
484. Morris, N., *et al.*: *Lancet* **2:** 481, 1956.
484. Morris, A., *et al.*: *Obstet Gynecol* **49:** 675, 1977.
485. Morton, N.E.: *Ann Hum Genet* **20:** 125, 1955.
486. Motoyama, E.K., *et al.*: *Anesthesiology* **28:** 891, 1967.
487. Murata, Y., and Martin, C.: *Obstet Gynecol* **44:** 224, 1974.
488. Myers, R.E.: *Pan Am Health Organ Sci Pub* **185:** 234, 1969.
489. Myers, R.E., *et al.*: *Am J Obstet Gynecol* **109:** 248, 1971.
490. Myers, R.E.: *Am J Obstet Gynecol* **112:** 246, 1972.
491. Myers, R.E., Mueller-Heubach, E., and Adamsons, K.: *Am J Obstet Gynecol* **115:** 1083, 1973.
492. Myers, R.E.: In *Intrauterine Asphyxia and the Developing Brain,* L. Gluck, Ed., Year Book, Chicago, 1977.
493. Myers, R.E.: In *Advances in Perinatal Neurology,* R. Korobkin and C. Guilleminauh, Ed. Spectrum, New York, 1978.
493a.Myers, R.E.: *Am J Obstet Gynecol* (in press).
494. McBurney, R.D.: *West J Surg Obstet Gynec* **55:** 363, 1947.
495. McCrann, D.J., and Schrifrin, B.S.: *Clin Perinatol* **1:** 229, 1974.
496. McCullough, R. *et al.*: *Arch Envir Health* **32:** 36,

1977.

497. McKay, D.G.: *Obstet Gynecol Surv* **27**: 399, 1972.

498. McLain, C.R.: *Am J Obstet Gynecol* **86**: 1079, 1963.

499. McManus, T.J., and Calder, A.A.: *Lancet* **1**: 72, 1978.

500. Naeye, R.L., *et al.*: *Pediatrics*, **52**: 494, 1973.

501. Naeye, R.L.: *JAMA* **238**: 227, 1977.

501a.Naeye, R.L., and Peters, Y.: *Pediatrics* **61**: 171, 1978.

502. National Research Council: *Recommended Dietary Allowance*, 8th ed., Natl Acad Science, Washington, 1974.

503. Neel, J.: *Am J Hum Gnet* **14**: 353, 1962.

503a.Neligan, G., *et al.*: *Clin Devel Med* **61**: 223, 1976.

504. Nelson, K.B., and Broman, S.H.: *Ann Neurol* **2**: 371, 1977.

505. Neuman, M.R., *et al.*: *Gynecol Invest* **3**: 163, 1972.

506. Niswander, K.R., Gordon, M., and Drage, J.S.: *Am J Obstet Gynecol* **118**: 935, 1974.

507. Niswander, K.R., Gordon, M., and Drage, J.S.: *Am J Obstet Gynecol* **121**: 892, 1975.

508. Noguchi, M.: *Jpn J Obstet Gynecol* **20**: 218, 1937.

509. Novy, M.: In *Respiratory Gas Exchange and Blood Flow in the Placenta*, L. Longo and H. Bartels, Ed., DHEW, Pub. 73-361, Bethesda, 1972.

510. Novy, M.J., *et al.*: *Prostaglandins* **5**: 543, 1974.

510a.Novy, M.J., *et al.*: *Am J Obstet Gynecol* **122**: 419, 1975

511. Odendall, H.: *Obstet Gynecol* **42**: 187, 1976.

512. O'Donohoe, N.V., and Holland, P.D.: *Arch Dis Child* **43**: 717, 1968.

513. O'Driscoll, S., *et al.*: *Br Med J* **2**: 1451, 1977.

514. O'Gureck, J., *et al.*: *Obstet Gynecol* **40**: 356, 1972.

515. Oldenburg, J.T., and Macklin, M.: *Am J Obstet Gynecol* **129**: 425, 1977.

516. Okada, D.M., *et al.*: *Am J Obstet Gynecol* **127**: 875, 1977.

516a.O'Reilly, R., and Taber, B.: *Obstet Gynecol* **51**: 590, 1978.

517. Organ, L.W.: *Can Med Assoc J* **98**: 199, 1968.

518. Organ, L.W., *et al.*: *Am J Obstet Gynecol* **115**: 369, 1973.

519. Osofsky, H.: In *Intrauterine Asphyxia and the Developing Brain*, L. Gluck, Ed., Year Book, Chicago, 1977.

520. Owen, J.R., *et al.*: *Arch Dis Child* **47**: 107, 1972.

521. Packard, V.: *The People Shapers*, Little, Brown & Co., Boston, 1977.

522. Page, E.W., and Christianson, R.: *Am J Obstet Gynecol* **125**: 740, 1976.

523. Palmquisth, H.: *Child Dev* **46**: 292, 1975.

524. Palmrich, A.H.: *Z Geburtsch Gynik* **138**: 304, 1953.

525. Parer, J.T.: *Gynecol Invest* **8**: 50, 1977.

526. Pape, K.E., Buncic, S., and Fitzhardinge, P.M.: *J Pediatr* **92**: 253, 1978.

527. Parmelee, A.H., and Haber, A.: *Clin Obstet Gynecol* **16**: 376, 1973.

528. Paul, R.H., *et al.*: *Am J Obstet Gynecol* **123**: 206, 1975.

528a.Paul, R.H.: *Postgrad Med* **61**: 160, 1977.

528b.Paul, R.H., *et al.*: *Am J Obstet Gynecol* **130**: 165, 1978.

529. Payne, G.S., and Bach, L.M.N.: *Biol Neonat* **8**: 308, 1965.

530. Pearson, J., and Weaver, J.: *Br Med J* **1**: 1305, 1976.

531. Pecoradi, D., and Trovati, G.: *Clin Exper Obstet Gynecol* **2**: 1, 1975.

532. Pedersen, J.: *The Pregnant Diabetic and Her Newborn: Problems and Management*, Williams & Wilkins, Baltimore, 1976.

533. Peiper, A.: *Geburt Mschr Kinderheilk* **29**: 236, 1924.

534. Pockett, E.M.C., and Cole, T.J.: *Br Med J* **1**: 7, 1977.

534a.Polaillon, J.: *Arch Physiol Norm Pathol* **7**: 1, 1880, quoted in Ref. 570.

535. Pope, A.: *An Essay on Man*, Epistle II, 1704.

536. Porter, J.C.: *Research Planning Workshop on Human Parturition*, DHEW 76-1101, Bethesda, 1975.

537. Potter, E.L.: *Am J Obstet Gynecol* **51**: 885, 1946.

538. Potter, E.L.: *J Obstet Gynecol Brit Cwlth* **25**: 3, 1965.

539. Poseiro, J.J., *et al.*: WHO Publication #185, Washington, 1969.

540. Power, G.G., Hill, E.P., and Longo, L.D.: In *Respiratory Gas Exchange and Blood Flow in the Placenta*; L. Longo and H. Bartels, Eds., DHEW 73-361, Bethesda, 1972.

541. Power, G.G., and Longo, L.D.: *Am J Physiol* **225**: 1490, 1973.

542. Pion, R.J., and Reich, L.A.: *The Female Patient* **3**: 85, 1977.

543. Pitkin, R.M., *et al.*, Committee on Maternal Nutrition: *Obstet Gynecol* **40**: 773, 1972.

544. Pitkin, R.M.: *Obstet Gynecol* **43**: 157, 1974.

545. Pitkin, R.M.: *Am J Obstet Gynecol* **121**: 724, 1975.

546. Pitkin, R.M.: *The Female Patient* **2**: 38, 1977.

547. Pitkin, R.M.: *Med Clin North Am* **61**: 3, 1977.

548. Preyer, R.W.: *Spezielle physiologic des embryo*, Leipzig, 1885.

549. Pritchard, J.A., *et al.*: *N Engl J Med* **250**: 89, 1954.

550. Pritchard, J.A.: *Obstet Gynecol* **25**: 289, 1965.

551. Pritchard, J.A.: *Anesthesiology* **26**: 393, 1965.

551a.Pritchard, J.: *Obstet Gynecol* **25**: 606, 1966.

552. Pritchard, J.A., and Stone, R.: *Am J Obstet Gynecol* **99**: 754, 1967.

553. Pritchard, J.A., Cunningham, F.G., and Mason, R.A.: *Gynecol Invest* **6**: 5, 1975.

554. Pritchard, J.A., and Pritchard, J.A.: *Am J Obstet Gynecol* **123**: 543, 1975.

555. Prochownick, L.: *Zbl Gynak* **13**: 577, 1889.

556. Prochownick, L.: *Zbl Gynak* **41**: 785, 1901.

557. Putz, T., and Ullrich, O.: *Arch Gynaekol* **171**: 14, 1941.

558. Quastel, J.: *Anesth Analg* **31**: 151, 1952.

559. Quilligan, E.J.: *Postgrad Med* **61**: 115, 1977.

560. Quilligan, E.J., and Paul, R.: *Obstet Gynecol* **45**: 96, 1975.

561. Räihä, C.E.: *Adv Pediatr* **15**: 137, 1968.

562. Ravelli, G., Stein, Z.A., and Susser, M.W. *N Engl*

J Med **2:** 349, 1976.

563. Redman, C., Beilin, L., and Bonner, J.: *Lancet* **2:** 753, 1976.

564. Regan, J.A.: *Perinatal Care* **1:** 8, 1977.

565. Reinold, E.: *Contrib Gynecol Obstet* **1:** 102, 1977.

566. Reitan, J.A., *et al.*: *Anesthesiology* **36:** 76, 1972.

567. Renou, P.: *Aus N.Z. J Obstet Gynecol* (Abstract #8) **15:** 122, 1975.

567a.Renou, P., *et al.*: *Am J Obstet Gynecol* **126:** 470, 1976.

568. Reynolds, S.R.M.: *Nature* **172:** 307, 1953.

569. Reynolds, S.R.M.: *Am J Obstet Gynecol* **70:** 148, 1955.

570. Reynolds, S.R.M., Harris, J.S., and Kaiser, I.H.: *Clinical Measurements of Uterine Forces in Pregnancy and Labor*; Thomas, Springfield; 1954.

571. Reynolds, S.R.M., and Paul, W.N.: *Am J Physiol* **193:** 249, 1958.

572. Reynolds, S.R.M.: *Am J Obstet Gynecol* **83:** 800, 1962.

573. Reynolds, S.R.M.: *Obstet Gynecol* **32:** 134, 1968.

574. Reynolds, W.A., *et al.*: *Am J Obstet Gynecol* **104:** 633, 1969.

575. Richards, M.P.M.: *Early Human Dev* **1:** 3, 1977.

576. Robertson, A., and Karp, W.: *South Med J* **69:** 1358, 1976.

577. Rocklin, R.E., *et al.*: *N Engl J Med* **295:** 1209, 1976.

578. Rockwood, A.C., and Falls, F.H.: *JAMA* **81:** 1683, 1923.

579. Rodbard, S.: *Israel J Med Sci* **4:** 1115, 1968.

580. Romney, S., and Gabel, P.: *Am J Obstet Gynecol* **96:** 698, 1966.

581. Ron, M.: *Obstet Gynecol* **48:** 456, 1976.

581a.Ron, M., and Polishuk, W.: *Br J Obstet Gynaecol* **83:** 768, 1976.

582. Rooth, G.: *Lancet* **1:** 290, 1964.

583. Rooth, G., *et al.*: In *Respiratory Gas Exchange and Blood Flow in the Placenta*; L. Longo and H. Bartels, Eds., DHEW 73-361, Bethesda; 1972.

584. Rosa, P.A., and Fanard, A.E.: *Int J Sexol* **4:** 160, 1951.

585. Ross, H.J.S.: *Aust NZ J Obstet Gynaecol* **1:** 104, 1961.

585a.Rosso, P., and Winick, M.: *Pediatric Annalis* **2:** 33, 1973

586. Roversi, G.D., *et al.*: *J Perinat Med* **3:** 53, 1975.

587. Rubens, R.: *Br J Obstet Gynecol* **84:** 543, 1977.

587a.Rubenstein, A., *et al.*: *J Pediat* **89:** 136, 1976

588. Rubsamen, D.: *Ob Gyn News*, June, 1977.

589. Rudolph, A.M., *et al.*: *Pediatr Res* **5:** 452, 1971.

590. Rudolph, A.M., and Heymann, M.A.: *S Afr Med J* **47:** 1859, 1973.

591. Rudolph, A.M., and Heymann, M.A.: *Foetal and Neonatal Physiology*, Comline *et al.*, Eds., Cambridge University Press, 1973.

592. Rudolph, A.M., and Heymann, M.A.: *Ann Rev Physiol* **36:** 187, 1974.

593. Rudolph, A.M.: *Congenital Heart Disease*, Year Book, Chicago, 1974.

594. Rudolph, A.M., and Heymann, M.A.: *Am J Obstet Gynecol* **124:** 483, 1976.

595. Ruttgers, H., and Kubli, F.: *Geburtsh v Fravenheik* **31:** 654, 1971.

596. Ryder, G.H.: *Am J Obstet Gynecol* **46:** 867, 1943.

597. Sabata, V., *et al.*: *Biol Neonat* **22:** 78, 1973.

598. Sabata, V., and Pribylova, H.: In *4th European Congress of Perinatal Medicine*, Z.K. Stembera, *et al.*, Eds., Thieme, Stuttgart, 1975.

599. Sabel, K.G., *et al.*: *Pediatrics* **57:** 652, 1976.

600. Sadovsky, E., *et al.*: *Lancet* **1:** 1141, 1973.

601. Sadovsky, E., and Weinstein, D.: *Israel J Med Sci* **13:** 295, 1977.

602. Sadovsky, E., and Polishuk, W.: *Obstet Gynecol* **50:** 49, 1977.

603. Saling, E., and Schneider, D.: *Br J Obstet Gynaecol* **74:** 799, 1967.

604. Saling, E.: *Foetal and Neonatal Hypoxia*, Williams and Wilkins, Baltimore, 1968.

605. Saling, E.: *J Perinat Med* **1:** 142, 1973.

606. Salk, L.: *World Mental Health* **12:** 1, 1960.

607. Salvadori, B.: *Therapy of Feto-Placental Insufficiency*, Springer-Verlag, New York, 1975.

608. Sarnatt, H., and Sarnatt, M.: *Arch Neurol* **33:** 698, 1976.

608a.Schatz, F.: *Arch Gynak* **3:** 58, 1900.

609. Schift, D., *et al.*: *Pediatrics* **48:** 139, 1971.

610. Schifrin, B.S.: *JAMA* **222:** 196, 1972.

611. Schifrin, B.S., and Dame, L.: *JAMA* **219:** 1322, 1972.

611a.Schifrin, B.S.: *Workshop in Fetal Heart Rate Monitoring*, ACOG, Los Angeles, 1976.

612. Scholander, P.E., Irving, L., and Grinnell, S.W.: *J Biol Chem* **142:** 431, 1942.

613. Scholander, P.E.: In *Oxygen Supply to the Human Foetus*, J. Walks and A. Turnbull, Eds., Blackwell, Oxford, 1957.

614. Schuller, A.B., and Larsen, L.S.: Studies in Progress at Sacramento Medical Center, 1976.

615. Schulman, C.A.: *Neuropediatric* **4:** 362, 1973.

615a.Schwartz, M., and Brenner, J.: *Am J Obstet Gynecol* **131:** 18, 1978.

616. Schwartz, P.: *Birth Injuries of the Newborn*, Hafner, New York, 1961.

617. Schwartz, R.L., *et al.*: In *Perinatal Factors Affecting Human Development*, Washington, D.C., 1969.

618. Schwartz, B.E., *et al.*: *Obstet Gynecol* **48:** 685, 1976.

619. Schwartz, A., *et al.*: *J Perinat Med* **1:** 153, 1973.

620. Scott, H.: *Arch Dis Child* **51:** 712, 1976.

620a.Scott, J.: *Lancet* **1:** 78, 1976.

621. Scrimgeour, J.: In *Intrauterine Fetal Visualization*, J Kaback and C. Valenti, Eds., Excerpta Medica, Amsterdam, 1976.

622. Setchik, J., and Chatkoff, M.L.: *J Appl Physiol* **38:** 443, 1975.

623. Sejeny, S.A., *et al.*: *J Clin Pathol* **28:** 812, 1975.

624. Seller, M.: *Lancet* **2:** 984, 1977.

625. Seppala, M. *et al.*: *Acta Obstet Gynecol Scand* **54:** 209, 1975.

626. Shaw, J.A., *et al.*: *J Am Acad Child Psych* **9**: 428, 1970.
627. Sheehan, H.L., and Lynch, J.B.: *Pathology of Toxemia of Pregnancy*; Williams & Wilkins, Baltimore, 1973.
628. Shepherd, J.T.: *Circulation* **50**: 418, 1974.
629. Shinebourne, E.A., *et al.*: *Circ Res* **312**: 710, 1972.
630. Siassi, B., Blanco, C., and Martin, C.B.: *Soc Gyn Inv* **43**, 1973.
631. Siendentrof, H., and Eissner, W.: *Z Geb Gyn* **96**: 76, 1929.
632. Simmons, M.A., *et al.*: *J Pediatr* **92**: 284, 1978.
632a.Simpson, J.Y., quoated by Speer, H.: *Obstetric and Gynecologic Milestones*, Macmillian, New York, 1958.
633. Sjostedt, S., Engleson, G., and Rooth, G.: *Arch Dis Child* **33**: 123, 1958.
634. Sloan, D.M.: *Female Patient* **3**: 10, 1977.
635. Smith, C.A.: *Am J Obstet Gynecol* **53**: 599, 1947.
636. Smith, C.A.: *The Physiology of the Newborn*, 2nd ed., Thomas, Springfield, 1952.
637. Smith, T.W.: *Am J Obstet Gynecol* **107**: 983, 1970.
638. Smyth, C.N.: *Lancet* **2**: 1124, 1953.
639. Smyth, C.N., and Farrow, J.L.: *Br Med J* **2**: 1005, 1958.
640. Smyth, C.N.: *J Obstet Gynecol Brit Cwlth* **79**: 920, 1965.
641. Synder, F.: *Obstetrics, Analtesia and Anesthesia*, Saunders, Philadelphia, 1949.
642. Sobin, S.S., *et al.*: *JAMA* **170**: 1546, 1959.
643. Solberg, D.A., *et al.*: *N Engl Med J* **288**: 1098, 1973.
644. Sontag, L.W., and Wallace, R.F.: *Am J Dis Child* **48**: 1050, 1934.
645. Sontag, L.W., and Wallace, R.F.: *Child Dev* **6**: 253, 1935.
646. Sontag, L.W., and Wallace, R.F.: *Am J Obstet Gynecol* **29**: 77, 1935.
647. Sontag, L.W., and Newberry, H.: *Am J Obstet Gynecol* **40**: 449, 1940.
648. Sontag, L.W.: *Am J Obstet Gynecol* **42**: 906, 1941.
649. Sontag, L.W.: In *26th Ross Pediatric Research Conf*, 1957, pp. 21.
650. Sontag, L.W., *et al.*: *Human Dev* **12**: 1, 1969.
651. Sontag, L.W.: *Physiologic Effects of Noise*, Plenum Press, New York, 1970.
652. Sophian, J.: *Pregnancy Nephropathy*, Appleton-Century-Crofts, New York, 1972.
653. Southern, E.M.: *Am J Obstet Gynecol* **73**: 233, 1957.
654. Spellacy, W.N., *et al.*: *Am J Obstet Gynecol* **121**: 835, 1975.
655. Spellacy, W.N.: *Management of High Risk Prgnancy*, University Park Press, Baltimore, 1976.
656. Spellacy, W.N., Buhi, W., and Birk, S.: *Am J Obstet Gynecol* **127**: 599, 1977.
657. Stander, H.J.: *Williams' Obstetrics*, 9th ed., Appleton-Century-Crofts, New York, 1945.
658. Steer, C., and Petrie, R.: *Am J Obstet Gynecol* **129**: 1, 1977.
659. Stehbens, J., Baker, G.L., and Kitchell, X.: *Am J Obstet Gynecol* **127**: 408, 1977.
660. Stein, Z., *et al.*: *Science* **178**: 708, 1972.
661. Stein, Z., Susser, M., Saenger, G., and Morolla, F.: *Famine and Human Development: The Dutch Hunger Winter of 1944–1945*, Oxford University Press, New York, 1975.
662. Stembera, Z.K.: In *Perinatal Medicine*, Z.K. Stembera *et al.*, Eds., 4th European Congress of Perinatal Med; Georg Thieme, Stuttgart, 1975.
663. Stephens, J.D., and Birnholz, J.C.: *ACOG*, May 11, 1977.
664. Sterman, M.B.: *Ex Neurol* **19**: 98, 1967.
665. Sterman, M.B.: *Sleep and the Maturing Nervous System*, Academic Press, New York, 1972.
666. Stewart, A.L., *et al.*: *Arch Dis Child* **52**: 97, 1977.
667. Stolte, L.A.M., personal communication.
668. Stott, D.H.: *New Society* **19**: 329, 1977.
669. Stott, D.H.: *J Am Acad Child Psych* **15**: 1, 1976.
670. Strang, L., *et al.*: *Acta Obstet Gynecol Scand* **56**: 205, 1977.
671. Sureau, C.L.: *Gynec Obstet* **55**: 21, 1956.
672. Sureau, C.L.: In *Perinatal Medizin*, Verlag, Stuttgart, 1972.
673. Sureau, C.L.: In *Perinatal Med*; Z.K. Stembera *et al.*; Eds. Georg Theime, Stuttgart, 1975.
674. Susser, M., and Stein, Z.: *Lancet* **2**: 664, 1975.
675. Susser, M., and Stein, Z.: *The Epidemiology of Prematurity*, D.M. Reed and F.J. Stanley, Eds. Urban & Schwarzenberg, Baltimore, 1977.
676. Taeusch, H.W.: *J Pediatr* **87**: 617, 1975.
677. Tatum, H.J., and Niles, J.G.: *Am J Obstet Gynecol* **93**: 767, 1965.
678. Taussig, F.J.: *Am J Obstet Gynecol* **14**: 505, 1927.
678. Taylor, A.B.W.: *Br J Obstet Gynecol* **84**: 281, 1977.
690. Tchobroutsky, C., Merlet, C., and Rey, D.: *Resp Physiol* **8**: 108, 1969.
691. ten Bensel, R.W., *et al.*: *J Pediatr* **90**: 490, 1977.
692. Teramo, K., Benowitz, N., Heymann, M.A., and Rudolph, A.M.: *Am J Obstet Gynecol* **118**: 935, 1974.
693. Territo, M., *et al.*: *Obstet Gynecol* **41**: 803, 1973.
694. Tew, M.: *New Society*, January 20, 1977 p. 120.
695. Thibeault, D.W., and Emmanouildes, G.C.: *Am J Obstet Gynecol* **129**: 43, 1977.
696. Thomas, C.R., *et al.*: *Obstet Gynecol* **22**: 335, 1963.
697. Thomas, I.T., and Smith, D.W.: *J Pediatr* **84**: 811, 1974.
698. Thoms, H.: *Classical Contributions to Obstetrics and Gynecology*, Thomas, Springfield, 1935.
699. Timor-Tritsch, I., *et al.*: *Obstet Gynecol* **48**: 292, 1976.
700. Tipton, R.H., and Chang, A.M.: *J Obstet Gynecol Common* **28**: 901, 1971.
700a.Tooley, M.: *Philosophy and Public Affairs* **2**: 37, 1972.
701. Torpin, R.: *Fetal Malformations caused by Amnion Rupture During Gestation*, Thomas, Springfield, 1968.
701a.Toubas, P.L., *et al.*: *Coeur Med Interne* **12**: 457,

1973.

702. Toubas, P.L., and Monset-Couchard, M.: *Am J Obstet Gynecol* **127:** 505, 1977.

703. Towbin, A.: *The Pathology of Cerebral Palsy*, Thomas, Springfield, 1960.

704. Towbin, A.: *Am J Dis Child* **119:** 529, 1970.

705. Trudinger, B.J.: *Br J Obstet Gynecol* **83:** 284, 1976.

705a.Treusch, X.: *Br J Pediatr* **87:** 221, 1975.

706. Truex, R.C.: In *Cardiac Arrhythmias*: W. Likoff, Ed., Grune & Stratton, New York, 1973.

707. Tuchmann-Duplessis, H.: *Drug Effects on the Fetus*, Addis, Sydney, 1975.

708. Tullis, J.L.: *JAMA* **237:** 355, 1977.

709. Tyson, J.E., *et al.*: In *The Placenta*, K.S. Moghessi and E.S.E. Hafez, Eds., Thomas, Springfield, 1974.

710. Tyson, J.E., *et al.*: *Am J Obstet Gynecol* **125:** 1073, 1976.

711. Urbach, J.R., *et al.*: *Am J Obstet Gynecol* **93:** 965, 1965.

712. Vasicka, A.: *Am J Obstet Gynec* **88:** 530, 1964.

713. Van den Berg, B.J., and Yerushalmy, J.: *J Pediatr* **69:** 531, 1966.

713a.van Wagenen, G., and Newton, W.: *Surg Gynec Obstet* **77:** 539, 1943.

714. Venge, O.: *Acta Zool* **31:** 1, 1950.

715. von Friesen, B.: *Acta Obstet Gynecol Scand Suppl* **70:** 1972.

716. von Steinbuchel, H.: *Zentral Gynak* **26:** 1304, 1902.

717. von Winkle, F.: *Handbook der geburtschulfe*, Bergmann, Weisbaden, 1903.

718. Vorherr, H.: In *Pathophysiology of Gestation*, N.S. Assali, Ed., Academic Press, New York, 1972.

719. Vosburgh, G.J., *et al.*: *Am J Obstet Gynecol* **56:** 1156, 1948.

720. Vrbanic, D., *et al.*: In *4th European Congress of Perinatal Medicine*, Z.K. Stembera *et al.*, Ed. Georg Thieme, Stuttgart, 1975.

721. Wagner, N., *et al.*: *Fert Sterl* **27:** 911, 1976.

722. Walker, A., *et al.*: *J Obstet Gynecol Brit Cwlth* **78:** 1, 1971.

723. Walker, N.: *Br Med J* **2:** 1221, 1959.

724. Walker, W., *et al.*: *J Obstet Gynaecol Brit Emp* **64:** 573, 1957.

725. Wallerstein, H.: *Science* **103:** 583, 1946.

726. Walley, P.J.: *Am J Obstet Gynecol* **97:** 723, 1967.

727. Walters, C.E.: *Child Dev* **35:** 1249, 1964.

728. Walton, A., and Hammond, J.: *Proc Roy Soc Lond B* **125:** 311, 1938.

729. Ward, J.N., and Kennedy, J.A.: *Am Heart J* **23:** 64, 1942.

730. Ward, C.V., and MacArthur, J.L.: *Am J Obstet Gynecol* **55:** 606, 1918.

731. Warkany, J.: *Am J Dis Child* **66:** 511, 1943.

732. Warnekros, K., and Gessner, X.: *Zbl Gynak* **40:** 897, 1919.

733. Warner, H.R., and Russel, R.O.: *Circ Res* **24:** 567, 1969.

734. Weeks, A.R.I., *et al.*: *Br J Obstet Gynecol* **84:** 161, 1977.

735. Wegman, M.E.: *Pediatrics* **54:** 677, 1974.

736. Weil, M.H., *et al.*: *Crit Care Med* **2:** 229, 1974.

737. Weinberger, M.M., *et al.*: *Am J Dis Child* **120:** 125, 1970.

738. Weiner, G.: *J Pediatr* **76:** 694, 1970.

739. Weinstein, L.: *Ob Gyn Surv* **31:** 581, 1976.

740. Weinstein, J., and Davidson, B.: *Lancet* **2:** 625, 1965.

741. Weissler, A.M., Harris, W.S., and Schoenfeld, C.D.: *Circulation* **37:** 149, 1968.

742. Weissler, A.M.: *Noninvasive Cardiology*, Grune & Stratton, New York, 1974.

743. Wender, P.H.: *Arch Gen Psych* **30:** 121, 1974.

744. Werner, E., *et al.*: *Pediatrics* **39:** 490, 1968.

744a.Westrom, L. *et al.*: *Am J Obstet Gynecol* **121:** 707, 1975.

745. Whetham, J., Muggah, H., and Davidson, S.: *Am J Obstet Gynecol* **125:** 577, 1976.

746. White, P.: In *Joslin's Diabetes Mellitus*, 11th ed., A. Mabel *et al.*, Eds. Lea & Fibiger, Philadelphia, 1971.

747. Whitaker, A.N., *et al.*: *Am J Path* **56:** 166, 1969.

748. Widdowson, E., and Cowen, J.: *Br J Nutr* **27:** 85, 1972.

749. Widrow, B., *et al.*: *Proc IEEE* **63:** 1692, 1975.

750. Wiggers, C.J.: *Am J Physiol* **56:** 459, 1921.

750a.Williams, E.A.: *J Obstet Gynaecol Br Emp* **59:** 635, 1952.

751. Williams, E.A., and Stallworthy, J.: *Lancet* **1:** 331, 1952.

752. Williams, J., and Whitridge, X.: *Obstetrics*, 6th ed. Appleton-Century-Crofts, New York, 1931.

753. Williams, R.L., Hof, R.P., Heymann, M.A., and Rudolph, A.M.: *Pediatr Res* **10:** 42, 1976.

754. Williams, R.L., Hof, R.P., Heymann, M.A., and Rudolph, A.M.: *Circulation* **46:** 11, 1974.

755. Williams, S.M.K.: *Midwife, Health Visitor and Community Nurses* **12:** 387, 1976.

756. Williams, T.J.: *Am J Obstet Gynecol* **55:** 169, 1948.

757. Winckel, A.: *Die Entwicklung der Sauglingsinkubatoren*, Verlag Siering, Bonn, 1880.

758. Windle, W.F.: *Physiology of the Fetus*, Saunders, Philadelphia, 1940.

759. Windle, W.F.: *JAMA* **206:** 1967, 1968.

760. Winick, M.: *Pediat Res* **2:** 352, 1968.

761. Winick, M., Rosso, P., and Waterlow, J.: *Exp Neurol* **26:** 393, 1970.

762. Winkel, C.A.: *Am J Obstet Gynecol* **126:** 720, 1976.

763. Wolfs, W.: *Zbl Gynak* **64:** 311, 1940.

764. Wolfson, R.N., *et al.*: *AM J Obstet Gynecol* **129:** 203, 1977.

765. Wynn, M., and Wynn, A.: *Prevention of Handicap of Perinatal Origin*, London Foundation for Education and Research on Child-Bearing, 1976.

765a.Yeh, S., *et al.*: *Obstet Gynecol* **41:** 365, 1973.

765b.Yeh, S., *et al.*: *Am J Obstet Gynecol* **127:** 50, 1977.

766. Yeh, M., Morishimo, H.O., and Nieman, W.H.: *Am J Obstet Gynecol* **121:** 951, 1975.

766a.Ylostalo, P., and Ylikorkala, O.: *Ann Chir Gynaecol*

Fenn **64:** 123, 1975.

766b.Young, B., and Weinstein, A.: *Am J Obstet Gynecol* **126:** 271, 1976.

767. Zangmeister, W.: *Z Geburtsh Gynak* **50:** 385, 1903.

767a.Zangmeister, W.: *Z Geburtsh Gynak* **78:** 325, 1916.

768. Zilianti, M., *et al.*: *Obstet Gynec* **42:** 831, 1973.

768a.Zlatnik, F., and Fuchs, F.: *Am J Obstet Gynecol* **112:** 610, 1972.

769. Zuckermann, H., Reiss, H., and Rubinstein, I.: *Obstet Gynecol* **44:** 787, 1977.

INDEX

Protocols

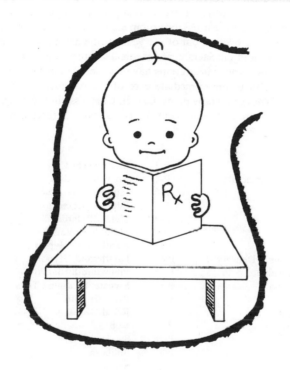

High-Risk Protocols

These protocols are intended as a quick reference to the various fetal problems as seen in our high-risk gravida. In no way are they intended to substitute for the standard obstetrical texts such as *Medical Complications During Pregnancy,* edited by G. N. Burrow and T. F. Ferris (W. B. Saunders) or *Surgical Disease in Pregnancy,* edited by H. R. K. Barber and E. A. Graber (W. B. Saunders). When protocols differ from the usual recommendations, a reference is supplied as a guide to further reading.

The intrapartum protocols are for entire labor room staffs, both physician and nonphysician. As with all of these protocols, they have evolved out of my years at the Stanford University Hospital, the Santa Clara Valley Medical Center, and the Sacramento Medical Center. Consultants, nurses, medical students, house staff, and faculty of the various institutions have all contributed to their make-up.

I find such protocols useful in the immediate care of the patient and to arrive at least a minimal consistency in the various types of therapy plans. Drs. H. C. Haesslein (Sacramento Medical Center) and R. Olson (California State Board of Health) contributed to many of these protocols.

Contents

Abortion (Habitual)

Fetal Risks:
1. Repeated miscarriages
2. CNS defects in term infants

A. Initial Dx: Procedures
1. Strict attention to specifics of past obstetrical history, including paternity of each pregnancy, sex of fetus, fetal malformations
2. Genetic counseling—history of CNS defects, male abortuses, autosomal dominant disease, cytogenetic studies of patient and husband
3. BUN, FBS, total T_4, serum progesterone, ANA
4. Cervical cultures for listerosis, mycoplasma T
5. Hysterosalpingogram or hysteroscopy

B. Studies During Pregnancy
1. Real-time sonography at 6–8 weeks
2. Immunoassay monitoring of serum estrogen, HCG, progesterone
3. Instructions to patient for collecting abortus material

C. Therapy
1. Progesterone if serum levels low
2. Abstinence (avoid orgasm)
3. Cerclage (if defect)

D. Post-abortion Studies
1. Accurate description of product of conception
2. Genetic evaluation of abortus (karyotype)
3. Instrumental examination of uterus at time of abortion

References

Behrman, S. J., and Kistner, R. W.: *Progress in Infertility.* Little, Brown & Co., Boston, Mass., 1975.
Horta, J. L. H., *et al.*: *Obstet Gynecol* **49:** 705, 1977.

Adrenocortical Insufficiency (Maternal)

Fetal Risks:
1. Death
2. IUGR

A. Initial Dx
1. Shock, nausea, vomiting
2. Plasma cortisol levels

B. Therapy
1. Prednisone
2. 9-Alpha fluorohydrocortisone

Reference

Osler, M.: *Acta Endocrinol* **41:** 67, 1962.

Anemia (Maternal)

Fetal Risks:
1. IUGR
2. Premature labor
3. Abruptio

A. Initial Dx: Procedures
1. Prior records
2. Red blood cell indices
3. Peripheral smear
4. Iron and iron binding capacity
5. Stool guiac
6. Hemoglobin electrophoresis
7. Haptoglobin (serum)
8. Bone marrow studies
9. Coombs
10. Folic acid activity (serum)
11. B-12 (serum)
12. Retic count
13. Neutrophil hypersegmentation
14. Bilirubin (serum)
15. G_6 PD assay
16. Cervix cytology (atypical morphology in folic acid deficiency)

B. Prenatal Care
1. Iron deficiency anemia: Oral iron ferrous sulfate 300 mg t.i.d. with meals, and ascorbic acid if diet deficient—500 mg t.i.d. with iron
2. High-protein diet
3. Parenteral iron, if indicated
4. Folic acid deficiency: folic acid, 1 mg
5. Ask about pica

References

Desforges, J. J.: *Reprod Med* **10**: 111, 1973.
Hall, M. H.: *Br Med J* **2**: 661, 1974.
Kitay, D. Z.: *Contrib Gynecol Obstet* **10**: 30, 1977.

Bleeding (Vaginal)

Fetal Risks:
1. Premature delivery
2. Asphyxia (cerebral palsy)
3. Anemia
4. Death

A. Initial Dx: Procedures
1. Sonogram for placental localization and identification of abruptio
2. Careful speculum exam if not recently performed
3. Four units whole blood available
4. Platelet count, PT, PTT, fibrinogen, FSP (abruptio)
5. Amniocentesis for determination of fetal maturity

B. Therapeutic Procedures
1. *Placenta Previa*
   a. Amniotic fluid L/S <2. or gestational age 36–37 weeks
      (1) No vaginal examination
      (2) Observe in hospital until bleeding stops (MgSO₄ to "inhibit" labor)
      (3) Attempt to "mature" fetus (see protocol)
      (4) Keep HCT > 32% by transfusion
      (5) Elective double setup after amniocentesis demonstrates lung maturity— cesarean section if previa confirmed
      (6) Emergency double setup exam at any time if blood loss severe—cesarean section if previa
   b. Amniotic fluid L/S > 2 or gestational age > 37 weeks
      (1) Immediate double setup exam— cesarean section if previa
2. *Placental Abruption*
   a. Maternal monitoring of HCT, coagulation, BUN, urine output, CVP, fundal height, vaginal bleeding
   b. Grade III—expedite delivery—AROM, oxytocin
   c. Grade II—cesarean section
   d. Grade I —if fetal maturity
      (1) Continuous fetal monitoring (inaccurate as regards fetal welfare)
      (2) Anticipate vaginal delivery—cesarean section for uncontrolled bleeding or failure to deliver in 4 hr
      (3) Keep up with blood loss

Cardiovascular Disease

Fetal Risks:
1. Fetal loss
2. Congenital heart lesion
3. IUGR

A. **Initial Dx: Procedures**
1. Cardiology evaluation
2. ECG, Echocardiogram
3. Chest roentgenograms
4. BUN

B. **Prenatal Care**
1. Frequent visits—evaluate weight and evidence of edema
2. Vital capacity measurement at each visit
3. Cardiac and chest auscultation at each visit
4. Search for infectious processes
5. Observation for premature labor if P_{O_2} saturation below 80 torr
6. Bed rest
7. Fetal movement record
8. Cardiac flow sheet

C. **Therapeutic Procedures**
1. Avoidance of contagious diseases
2. Cardioscope (continuous ECG monitoring) in labor
3. Antibiotic prophylaxis (low dose) throughout pregnancy (if rheumatic disease etiology)
4. Antibiotic prophylaxis for SBE in labor for all valvular lesions
5. Anticoagulation with heparin (for all prosthetic valves or Coumadin with control)
6. Blood available in labor and delivery suite—with avoidance of sudden blood volume changes
7. Anesthesiology consultation (avoid apprehension)
8. Avoidance of Valsalva maneuver
9. Semifowler or left lateral decubitus position in labor
10. Continuous O_2 by mask if cyanotic disease or failure
11. Low forceps delivery
12. Epidural anesthesia preferred

Reference

Burch, G. E.: *Am Heart J* **93:** 104, 1977.

Cardiac Disease Protocol

I. Antepartum

A. Auscultate heart of all gravida and define etiology and pathophysiology of the lesion—*if*

any diastolic murmur heard
any systolic murmur Gr. III/VI
any major cardiac complaints
any arrhythmia

} Cardiac Consult

B. Cardiology consult should include chest roentgenogram, EKG, and echocardiogram (rarely will cardiac catheterization be indicated—remember radiation danger to fetus)

C. Classification of Lesion and Outcome in Pregnancy:

		Usually do well	Moderate risk	High risk
Congenital	ASD		x[1]	x[3]
(36%)	PDA		x[1]	x[3]
	VSD	x		x[3]
	Pulmonic stenosis	x		
	Coarctation		x[2]	
	Tetralogy		x[1]	

[1] Congenital failure, arrhythmias
[2] Aortic rupture
[3] Eisenmenger's syndrome—R-L shunt and pulmonary hypertension

		Usually do well	Moderate risk	High risk
Rheumatic	M.S.		x[1]	
(61%)	M.I.	x		
	A.S.	x		
	A.I.		x	

[1] Most common cause of CHF in pregnancy

D. Classification of function:

Class 1. No symptoms and no change with ordinary physical activity

Class 2. Comfortable at rest but symptoms with ordinary physical activity

Class 3. Comfortable at rest but symptoms with *less* than ordinary physical activity

Class 4. Symptoms at rest

Symptoms to look for are: fatigue, palpitations, dyspnea, anginal pain

E. General considerations:

(1) *Physical activity* should generally be restricted (especially with M.S. and A.S.); elastic stockings should be prescribed; abdominal compression avoided; and continuous $FeSO_4$ therapy given. Since class III and IV cardiac patients may have fetuses with IUGR, severe salt (2 g Na^+) restriction and diuretics should be used only when maternal risks of CHF exceed risk of placental hypoperfusion.

(2) *Digitalization* may be helpful in patients with M.S.—they can have sudden decompensation and CHF if atrial fibrillation occurs.

DOSE: (a) Digitalize with 0.25 mg Digoxin daily for 5 days, then check dig. level.

(b) Maintenance dose 0.25–0.5 mg qd. Always check K^+, Ca^+, Mg^+ levels. Digitalis toxicity causes—anorexia, nausea, vomiting, diarrhea, fatigue, visual symptoms, headaches, delerium, dizziness, and somnolence.

(3) *Abortion* (as with Eisenmenger's syndrome and primary pulmonary hypertension) should be done prior to 16th week—after this, abortion risk nearly equal to risk of continuing pregnancy and delivery of labor. Method of choice is suction TAB or intraamniotic $F_{2\alpha}$.

(4) Valve prosthesis patients should be on continuous anticoagulation via heparin–coumadin–heparin sequence—see Anticoagulation Protocol.

(5) *Cardiac surgery* should be done prior to the 16th week if medical management of classes III or IV not adequate—the definitive procedure should usually be performed.

(6) *Rheumatic fever prophylaxis*:
200,000 U penicillin G (125 mg) p.o. b.i.d. for *all* patients with rheumatic heart lesions *or* erythromycin stearate 250 mg p.o. b.i.d. Best prophylaxis is probably Benzathine penicillin G (Bicillin) 1.2 million U a month.

II. Intrapartum

A. *At term* the cardiac rate is about 15 bpm greater than unpregnant levels and the stroke volume is normal at term—together this gives a 15% increase in cardiac output.

B. *In labor* the situation becomes complex—maternal cardiac output is increased (less so if patient is on her side and good conduction anesthesia is used), mean arterial blood pressure rises, and the heart rate drops with each contraction. These changes are variably influenced by maternal position, pain, and anesthesia.* In the second stage, the CVP also rises with each bearing-down effort, reflecting increased venous return (dangerous with M.S.). It is *most* important to avoid prolonged labor.

---

* Should sudden hypotension occur, L to R shunts may reverse and R to L shunts may worsen—both may be disastrous.

CARDIAC PATIENT MANAGEMENT

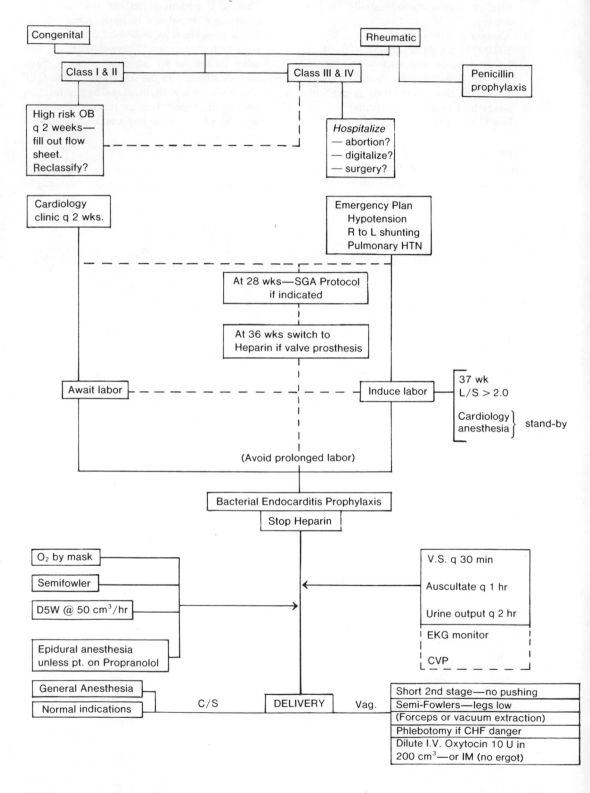

Cesarean Section (Elective)

Fetal Risks:
1. Prematurity

A. Initial Dx: Procedures
1. Records of prior cesarean section
2. Careful assessment of menstrual history for dating of pregnancy
3. FHT with Doppler before 12 weeks
4. Plan for sonogram at 18–22 weeks if *any* question of dates
5. Careful assessment of uterine size

6. If prior lower segment cesarean section and if pelvis is adequate, offer patient a vaginal delivery

B. Prenatal Care
1. If pregnancy dates confirmed by ultrasound, cesarean section at 39 weeks
2. Amniocentesis for documentation of fetal lung maturity at 37–39 weeks (preferably when cervical change is noted) if patient elects repeat cesarean section or if section is indicated

Prior Cesarean Section
(Vaginal Delivery)

A. Initial Dx: Procedures
1. Discuss relative risks (probably less, but no greater than repeat section)
2. Obtain records of prior cesarean section (must be transverse incision in lower uterine segment, uncomplicated postpartum course)
3. Pelvis must be adequate as shown by x-ray pelvimetry
4. Patient must desire vaginal delivery

B. Intrapartum Care
1. Patient prepared for immediate cesarean section
2. Epidural anesthesia useful in order to palpate uterine scar during course of labor
3. Foley catheter (to prevent bladder distention and check for hematuria)
4. Repeat cesarean section if abnormality of labor occurs (use intravenous oxytocin very cautiously)

C. Postpartum Care
1. Palpate lower segment scar and describe in delivery note; if abnormal, schedule a hysterogram
2. Caution patient that successful vaginal delivery does not necessarily indicate that subsequent delivery problems will not occur

References

Riva, H. L., and Breen, J. L.: *Am J Obstet Gynecol* **76:** 192, 1958.

Case B. D., *et al.*: *J Obstet Br Cwlth* **78:** 203, 1971.

Evard, J. R., and Gold, E. M.: *Obstet Gynecol* **50:** 594, 1977.

CNS Disease, Prior Infant with

Fetal Risks:
1. Repeat CNS lesion
2. Miscarriage
3. Meningocele

A. Initial Dx:
1. Prior records, particularly regarding specific fetal lesion (i.e., hydrocephalus due to Arnold–Chiari syndrome, medulloblastoma, toxoplasmosis, etc.), or anencephaly with or without meningocele
2. Genetic counseling (anencephaly 5% emperic risk); hydrocephalus occasionally a cross-linked or autosomal recessive; subsequent spontaneous abortion due to genetic defect at increased rate with all prior CNS lesions
3. Family studies of head size
4. Toxoplasmosis and cytomegalovirus studies

B. Prenatal Care
1. Amniocentesis for alpha-fetoprotein (even with hydrocephalus) during 2nd trimester
2. Sonogram for head size, head–thorax ratio, and size of cortical mantle (also fetal pneumoencephalogram) with suspected hydrocephalus; R. O. meningocele.
3. Confirm sonogram diagnosis of either anencephaly or hydrocephaly with roentgenograms

C. Delivery
1. Amniocentesis for hydroamnios
2. Decompression of hydrocephalus prior to vaginal delivery
3. With vaginal delivery, sharp, bony margins may cause maternal lacerations
4. Cesarean section for hydrocephalus with adequate fetal cortical mantle (low vertical incision)

References:

Fraser, F. C.: *Pediat Clin N Am* **5:** 475, 1958.
Pernoll, M. L., *et al.*: *Obstet Gynecol* **44:** 773, 1974.
Milunsky, A.: *Obstet Gynecol* **59:** 782, 1977.

Cushing's Syndrome

Fetal Risks:
1. Fetal loss
2. Premature labor
3. Adrenal insufficiency

A. Initial Dx: Procedures
1. Obtain previous records

    2. Plasma cortisol
    3. Dexamethasone suppression

B. Therapy
1. Surgical exploration

Reference

Kreines, K., and DeVaux, W.: *Pediatrics* **47**: 516, 1971.

Class A Diabetes (Gestational)

Fetal Risks: (Doubtful unless postmature)
1. Macrosomia (?)
2. Fetal loss (?)
3. Increased rate of anomalies (?)

A. Initial Dx: Procedures
1. Oral or intravenous glucose tolerance test for all patients with
   (a) family history of diabetes
   (b) glycosuria × 2 (2nd AM urine)
   (c) weight > 200 lbs
   (d) poor reproductive history, i.e., recurrent abortions and fetal death, unexplained neonatal death, fetal malformation, repeated prematurity, congenital anomaly
   (e) prior infant > 4300 g
   (f) polyhydramnios
   (g) chronic hypertension
   (h) recurrent preeclampsia

Critical values: Oral (Up to 28-week gestation)

FBS	Class A if	Do:
100–120 mg%	any 2 exceed these values	Urinalysis and culture
1 hr 200 mg%		Fundoscopic exam
2 hr 150 mg%		BUN or serum creatinine,
3 hr 130 mg%		creatinine clearance
Critical value IV: K < 1.2		Total urinary protein

B. Ongoing Assessments
1. Periodic blood sugars
2. Urine for sugar and acetone as clinically indicated
3. Sonography to determine gestational age at 18–24 weeks
4. Combination of fetal surveillance techniques beginning 36–38 weeks, sooner if pregnancy complicated by preeclampsia hydramnios, macrosomia, (e.g., OCT, estriols, amniocentesis)

C. Non-routine Assessment
1. If glucose tolerance test is ambiguous, repeat at 30–34 weeks, EKG, electrolytes

D. Therapeutic Procedures
1. See frequently (avoid excessive weight gain, postmaturity)
2. Diet: 1800–2200 calories (30 cal/kg ideal weight) 200–225 g CHO minimum 1.5 g/kg protein minimum } in six feedings
3. If, with this diet, FBS remains above 120 or 2-hr postprandial blood sugar exceeds 180, consideration of insulin therapy is necessary
4. Vitamin B_6 100 mg/day
5. Vaginal delivery at term with fetal monitoring unless evidence of fetal deterioration indicates preterm delivery

References

Gabbe, S. G., Mestman, J. *et al.*: *Am J Obstet Gynecol* **127**: 565, 1977.

Spellacy, W. N., *et al.*: *Am J Obstet Gynecol* **127**: 599, 1977.

Insulin Diabetic or Class A with Previous Stillbirth

Fetal Risks:
1. Fetal loss
2. Increased rate of anomalies
3. Macrosomia
4. Newborn hypoglycemia

A. Initial Dx: Procedures
1. Careful dating of pregnancy
2. Documentation of retinal findings
3. Hospitalize to determine control, renal threshold, and diet
4. Obtain records from all previous pregnancies
5. Sonogram
6. Nutritional consultation
7. Creatinine clearance, urine culture
8. Prenatal visits q 2 weeks

B. Prenatal Tests
1. Every 2 weeks to 28 weeks; every week thereafter
2. Blood sugar as indicated (fasting and/or postprandial)
3. Urine sugar and acetone (double voided) q.i.d.—AC & HS
4. Plasma estriol every day after 33 weeks
5. Nonstress FHR test or oxytocin challenge test (OCT) weekly after 32 weeks
6. Fetal movement record
7. Decreasing insulin levels require special fetal surveillance
8. Plasma estriol and OCT to begin earlier if hypertension or evidence of IUGR
9. L/S ratio at 35 weeks
10. Amniogram for fetal anomalies if hydramnios present

C. Therapeutic Procedures
1. Maintain FBS < 120 mg%
2. Premature delivery if fetal jeopardy indicated by estriol and OCT and L/S ratio < 2.0
3. Elective delivery at 38 weeks if L/S > 2.5 (cesarean section if fetal macrosomia present)
4. Encourage rest after 28 weeks
5. Hospitalize and treat any infections vigorously
6. Hospitalize if out of control (avoid ketoacidosis)

Reference

Gabbe, S. G., *et al.*: *Am J Obstet Gynecol* **129:** 723, 1977.

Drug Addiction (including alcohol)

Fetal Risks:
1. IUGR
2. Withdrawal symptoms
3. Increased rate of congenital malformations, mental retardation
4. Premature labor and infections
5. Gonorrhea, syphilis, and hepatitis

A. Initial Dx: Procedures
1. Identification by history of drug abuse, searching for history of multiple drugs being abused; i.e., hallucinogens (marijuana, hashish, LSD), CNS stimulants (amphetamines, cocaine), CNS depressants (barbiturates, alcohol), narcotics (heroin, methadone), and alcohol
2. Urine or blood for drug levels if clinically indicated
3. Serum Fe, iron binding capacity, folic acid, B_{12} levels, and liver enzymes

B. Prenatal Care
1. Nutritional status
2. Psychosocial analysis or social service support
3. Sonography at 18–24 weeks and repeat 26–28 weeks
4. Premature labor precautions
5. Combination of fetal surveillance techniques from 30 weeks onward (HPL, OCT, estriol, amniocentesis, fetal movements)
6. Repeat VDRL, G. C. culture, and liver enzymes

C. Therapeutic Procedures
1. Repeat dietary advice and consultation
2. Encourage discontinuation of drug abuse
3. For narcotic addiction at time of hospitalization possible methadone detoxification over 6 days or methadone maintenance program for patients refusing narcotic detoxification
4. Close neonatal evaluations

Reference

Pelosi, M. A., et al.: Obstet Gynecol **45:** 512, 1975.

Elderly Primigravida (35 or over)

Fetal Risks:
1. Increase incidence of chromosome and other anomalies
2. Fetal death and IUGR (chronic fetal distress)

A. Initial Dx: Procedures
1. BUN, FBS and 2 hr PPBS
2. Amniocentesis for cell culture and alpha fetal protein before 16 weeks
3. Early assessments of fetal growth and status
4. Ultrasound BPD at 28–30 weeks and repeat after 33 weeks

B. Prenatal Care
1. Estriol and/or HPL determinations if evidence of poor intrauterine growth
2. Amniocentesis for L/S ratio and meconium in third trimester
3. Weekly OCT from 35th week
4. Fetal movement record

C. Therapeutic Procedures
1. Rest, high protein caloric diets
2. Do not allow to go beyond term—induce labor or cesarean section
3. Do not allow long labor—after 20 hr, cesarean section
4. Do not allow long period of ruptured membranes

Reference

Morrison, I.: *Am J Obstet Gynecol* **121:** 465, 1975.

Epilepsy

Fetal Risks:
1. Coagulation abnormalities
2. Congenital abnormalities

A. Initial Dx: Procedures
1. Identify by history
2. Electroencephalogram
3. Determine need for anticonvulsants!

B. Prenatal care
1. Therapeutic procedures
2. No folic acid supplement (not proven)
3. Vitamin K near term
4. No scalp electrode (fetal bleeding)

C. Fetal risks of anticonvulsant drugs:
1. Hydantoins = 10% serious, 30% nonserious malformation
2. Trimethadone = 80% teratogenicity, 50% fetal loss
3. Barbiturates = ? decreased brain growth

References

Fedrick, J.: *Br Med J* **2:** 442, 1973.
Smith, D. W.: *Am J Dis Child* **131:** 1337, 1977.

Growth-Retarded Fetus

Fetal Risks:
1. Death
2. CNS dysfunction

A. Initial Dx: Procedures
1. High level of suspicion in gravidas with poor nutrition or decreased rate of weight gain, with toxemia, drug addiction, or prior history of GRF or small-for-dates infant
2. Rule out maternal diseases, i.e., renal or cardiovascular diseases, systemic lupus, and so forth; studies for drug addiction (BUN, FBS, ANA, drug screen)
3. Sonography, hopefully, during second trimester (fetal growth, amount of amniotic fluid)
4. Fetal surveillance tests (fetal movements may appear normal up to time of fetal death) HPL, E_3, OCT (worrisome if abrupt fetal bradycardia)

5. Maternal serum—alpha fetoprotein

B. Studies During Pregnancy
1. Repeat fetal surveillance tests
2. Repeat fetal sonography
3. Amniocentesis for fluid color, L/S, urea

C. Therapy
1. Bedrest
2. High caloric protein diet with increased fluid intake
3. Delivery if mature A/F, or abnormal fetal surveillance tests

D. Postdelivery Studies
1. Hysterogram to rule out uterine anomalies
2. Newborn chromosome studies (especially if a "funny looking kid")

Reference

Wald, N., *et al.: Lancet* **2:** 268, 1977.

Hepatitis

Fetal Risks:
1. Increased risk of congenital malformation (first trimester)
2. Hepatitis

A. Initial Dx: Procedures
1. Obtain history of exposure
2. Liver function studies
3. Australian antigen assay
4. Mononucleosis titer
5. Gastroenterology consultation

B. Prenatal Care
1. Rest with instructions
2. Nutritional counseling
3. Repeat abnormal liver function studies
4. Observation for premature labor
5. Gamma globulin to household

C. Therapy
1. Avoid hepatotoxic drugs (i.e., alcohol, halothane, phenothiazines, tetracycline, etc.)
2. Cholestryamine if pruritis severe
3. Isolation of newborn until Australian antigen negative.

Reference

Davidson, C.S.: *J Reprod Med* **10:** 107, 1973.

Herpes Genitalis

Fetal Risks:
1. TORCH complex
2. Fetal loss

A. **Initial Dx: Procedures**
1. Tissue culture using fibroblasts
2. Pap smear of lesion
3. Serum antibodies

B. **Prenatal Procedure**
1. Amniotic fluid culture for herpes
2. Condom during coitus

C. **Therapy**
1. No highly effective Rx known
2. Corticosteroids contraindicated
3. C/S of women in active labor or with ruptured membranes 4 hr or less if lesions are present or have been present within 8 weeks of delivery
4. Photoinactivation unproved but widely used
5. Symptomatic Rx with topical anesthetics
6. Local application of diethyl ether—repeat p.r.n. until symptoms subside

Alternative Therapy (Chang, T., and O'Keefe, P.: *N Engl J Med* **296:** 573, 1977)
Recurrent genital herpes is associated with brief viral excretion, is excreted in smaller amounts than primary infection and because of maternal antibodies, "it is unlikely that a liberal use of cesarean section will be beneficial to women with recurrent genital herpes starting before pregnancy."
1. Lesions on progenital area from recurrent herpes should be treated with Betadine and vaginal delivery allowed
2. Lesions on maternal cervix at time of delivery necessitates cesarean section

References
Chang, T.: *JAMA* **238:** 155, 1977.
Nahmios, A. J.: *Clin Obstet Gynecol* **15:** 929, 1972.
St. Geme, J. W.: *Am J Dis Child* **129:** 342, 1975.

Hydramnios

Fetal Risks:
1. Anomalies
2. Premature labor
3. Infection

A. Initial Dx: Procedures
1. Ultrasound
2. Glucose tolerance tests
3. Antibody screen, hemoglobin electrophoresis, TORCH titers
4. Amniography with follow-up films (fetal risk of hypothyroidism)
5. Serum proteins

B. Prenatal Care
1. Serial ultrasound exam for fetal head and abdominal growth
2. Serial measurement of maternal abdominal girth
3. Premature labor precautions
4. Bedrest
5. Amniocentesis for α-fetoprotein, L/S, bile salts, and creatinine
6. Fetal movement record

C. Therapy
1. Hospitalize at onset of rapid abdominal enlargement
2. Amniocentesis to keep hydramnios consistent with patient tolerance
3. Premature labor protocol if no fetal abnormalities

Reference

Pitkin, R. M.: *Obstet Gynecol* **48:** 425, 1976.

Hyperemesis After 19 Weeks

Fetal Risks:
1. Prematurity
2. IUGR

A. Initial Dx: Procedures
1. Amylase
2. Urine acetone
3. Liver function studies (bilirubin, alkaline phosphatase, SGOT, SGPT)
4. Sonogram for gestational age to rule out degeneration, hydatid mole
5. Nutritional assessment
6. Consider psychiatric consultation

B. Prenatal Care
1. Serial CBC and liver function
2. Periodic weight

3. Serial sonography
4. Psychiatric counseling
5. Fetal movement record
6. Hyperalimentation—only for prolonged severe cases

C. Therapy
1. I.V. fluids
2. Antiemetics (Bendectin, Dramamine)
3. Frequent feedings
4. Consider termination of pregnancy only for cases with *progressive* and *marked* deterioration of liver function
5. Consider tranquilizers

Reference

Corlett, R. C.: *Contrib Gynecol Obstet* **9**: 25, 1977.

Hypertension (Chronic)

Fetal Risks:
1. Increased fetal loss (especially midtrimester)
2. IUGR
3. Abruptio

A. Initial Dx: Procedures
1. Urinalysis and culture, renal function tests, serum creatinine clearance and 24-hr urine protein, FBS.
2. Fundoscopic exam.
3. Family history.

B. Prenatal Tests
1. Assess B/P, proteinuria, and renal function at frequent intervals, with increasing frequency in third trimester.
2. Fundoscopic exam if clinical deterioration.
3. Sonogram at 18–24 weeks to confirm gestational age; repeat at 28 weeks.
4. Combination of antenatal fetal surveillance techniques from 28 weeks onward as clinically indicated (e.g., HPL, OCT, estriols, amnio., etc.).
5. Electrolytes, IVP (if obstructive uropathy) and urinary catecholamines, EKG, chest film).

C. Therapy
1. Bedrest (not proven in controlled studies).
2. Antihypertensive Rx, attempting to maintain diastolic pressure less than 100 torr. Thiazides acceptable.
   Furosemides for sodium retention. Phenobarbital for sedation.
   Because of potential fetal effects, reserpine, propranolol,[*] diazoxide, and nitroprusside[+] are relatively contraindicated.
   Methyldopa works well (Redman).
3. Termination of pregnancy should be considered if hypertension cannot be controlled or if there is deterioration of renal function or evidence of severe fetal compromise.
4. Terminate pregnancy when amniotic fluid L/S is greater than 2.0.

[*] Associated with high incidence of newborn respiratory distress even with mature L/S.
[+] Cyanide poisoning of fetus in laboratory animals.

References

Finnerty, F. A.: *Clin Obstet Gynecol* **18:** 145, 1975.
Redman, C. W. G.: *Lancet* **2:** 753, 1976.

Immunologic Thrombotic Thrombocytopenia Purpura

Fetal Risks:
1. Thrombocytopenia
2. Death
3. Cerebral hemorrhage

A. Initial Procedures
1. Platelet counts
2. R. O. other causes (drug exposure)

B. Prenatal Care
1. Maintain platelet count above 70,000
2. Use steroids that cross placenta
3. Maintain Hct above 32%

4. Toxemia and premature labor precautions

C. Therapeutic Procedures
1. Splenectomy with caution
2. Avoid delivery during thrombocytopenia
3. Possible cesarean section to avoid fetal trauma (not proven)

References

Laros, R. K., and Sweet, R. L.: *Am J Obstet Gynecol* **122:** 182, 1975.

O'Reilly, R. A., and Taber, B.: *Obstet Gynec* **51:** 590, 1978

Incompetent Cervix (elective)

Fetal Risks:
1. Immature and premature births
2. Infections

A. Initial Dx: Procedures
1. Careful dating of pregnancy
2. Document history with old records
3. Carefully assess cervix
4. Sonography to rule out multiple gestation and document pregnancy, otherwise, thinning of lower segment

B. Prenatal Care
1. No cerclage if labor, ruptured membranes, fever
2. Cerclage at 14–18 weeks if FHT present; antibiotics at time of cerclage
3. Pelvic exam with visits (q week 14–24 weeks) if no cerclage done

C. Therapeutic Procedures
1. Minimal physical activity
2. Delalutin 250 mg IM after procedure immediately and q week for 2 weeks
3. If patient labors after 36 weeks, cut band and deliver; if at 37 weeks without labor, obtain L/S ratio; if over 2.0, cut band and observe for labor or induction
4. If premature labor ensues, attempt to stop (See Protocols IV and V)

D. Special Tests
1. Plasma estriol if hypertension or evidence of IUGR
2. L/S ratio if premature intervention
3. Serial sonography if size date discrepancy
4. Amniocentesis if premature labor 28–36 weeks for L/S ratio

Reference

Novy, M.: *Contrib Gynecol Obstet* **10:** 633, 1977.

Prevention of Isoimmunization

Women are still being sensitized by their fetuses despite routine Rh typing and use of Rh immunoglobulin. These sensitizations occur through a variety of mechanisms.

1. Errors in recording blood type
2. Non-Rh-D+ antigens (table D--88-D-90)
3. Unrecognized pregnancies with miscarriage
4. Significant fetomaternal bleeding even minimal amounts at delivery or even minimal amounts during course of complicated pregnancy (vaginal bleeding, threatened abortions, attempted versions, ectopic pregnancy, amniocentesis, etc.)
5. Patients who are D−, D^{u+} (and not given Rh immunoglobulin)

Comments[1]

The term D−, D^{u+} is applied to an individual whose red cells are not agglutinated by incomplete anti-D sera after incubation at 37°C in a high protein medium but can be demonstrated to have reacted with the antibody by a positive indirect anti-human globulin (Coomb's) test. By this definition about 1% of Caucasians and 9% of Negroes are D−, D^{u+}. These figures are composites of several different genetic factors. Among Negroes the commonest cause is simply a suppressed or weakened D antigen. Such persons cannot be stimulated to make anti-D. However, a small minority of all D−, D^{u+} individuals are, in fact, persons who lack one or more of the partial antigens that together make up the D antigen. Such persons appear to be very good producers of antibody to the missing part of the D antigen and instances of hemolytic disease of the newborn (HDN) due to this cause have been reported.

The administration of Rh immunoglobulin to all D^{u+} women who otherwise fill the criteria would result in a minimal reduction of Rh D sensitization. Those susceptible to the D sensitization amount to less than 1 per 1000 of the population. Nevertheless, total prevention of Rh immunization requires that these be identified and at present there is no practical way other than giving Rh immunoglobulin to the total D^{u+} group.

The initial purpose of the crossmatch when giving Rh immunoglobulin was to prevent its administration to a D^+ individual and also to prevent the administration of antibody present unintentionally with the anti-D to an antigen other than the D on the recipient's red cells. This fear has been shown to be overcautious. Rh immunoglobulin contains insufficient of any antibody other than anti-D to be recognized by present methods. The occasional unintentional administration of 300 μg Rh immunoglobulin to D^+ individuals has caused no harmful effect.

On the other hand, a weakly positive crossmatch may be due to greater than usual amounts of fetomaternal hemorrhage. Thus, immunosuppression may be denied to the few women most at risk. However, the almost universal practice of microscopic reading of the crossmatch allows competent technologists to distinguish between (MF) mixed field agglutination (evidence of two cell populations) and weak general agglutinations. Moreover, in most laboratories the finding of a MF alerts the physician to the need for additional dose of Rh immunoglobulin.

Fetomaternal hemorrhage can be relatively easily quantitated by the Kleihauer et al.[6] staining method as modified by Harwood.[5] If this method can be instituted, then compatibility testing could be safely dropped. Ortho Diagnostics markets Fetaldex, a quality control modification of the Kleihauer technique.

The volume of Rh positive red cells that can be eliminated by Rh immunoglobulin is 1 ml per 25 μg. Robertson[3] showed that 5% of Rh-negative women developed Rh sensitization after abortion if prevention was not given. At 4 weeks gestation (6 weeks from LMP) the risk is negligible, but at 8 weeks is 2% and at 3 months 9%. A dose of 50 μg would prevent immunization with up to 4 ml of whole blood which is the fetal blood volume at about 16 weeks gestation. Using this dose, Crispen prevented sensitization of male Rh-negative volunteers given 2.5 ml of Rh-positive red cells. It would seem reasonable, therefore, to use 50 μg Rh immunoglobulin for prevention if gestation is not more than 16 weeks.

Fetomaternal bleeding does occur following amniocentesis after 20 weeks gestation used to monitor amniotic fluid, bilirubin levels. Bowman[2] states that greater than 0.1 ml of fetal cells enter the maternal circulation in 11% of amniocentesis procedures. Using increases in maternal alpha FP, Lachman et al.[7] report greater than 0.03 ml of fetal red cells in maternal circulation following 15% diagnostic amniocentesis procedures performed at 11–17 weeks gestation (range 0.03–3.1 ml).

There seems, therefore, every reason to give Rh immunoglobulin to Rh-negative women subjected to amniocentesis. Although there is no reason to suppose that Rh-positive fetus is significantly affected by 300 μg anti-D, it is evident that 50 μg is an adequate and probably safer dose.

Ortho Diagnostics are the original producers of Rh immunoglobulin which is marketed under the trade name, Rhogam. In 1973, other pharmaceutical houses entered the market with the same generic product. These other companies priced their products about $5 below that of Ortho (#35 to UCD/SMC). There is no evidence that these products are any different in safety or therapeutic effect from Rhogam.

Summary:
1. D−, D^{u+} individuals should be given Rh immunoglobulin on the same indications as those who are D−, D^{u-} if fetomaternal hemorrhage occurs.
2. The Rh immunoglobulin crossmatch should be replaced by semiquantitated evaluation of fetomaternal hemorrhage.
3. 50 μg doses of Rh immunoglobulin are adequate for the prevention of D sensitization induced by fetomaternal bleeding from a single fetus of less than 16 weeks gestation.
4. Rh immunoglobulin should be administered to all Rh D^- women undergoing amniocentesis (unless there is certainty that the father of the fetus is also D−, D^{u-}).

References

1. Watson-Williams, E. J., Chairman, Transfusion Committee, SMC, June 14, 1977.
2. Bowman, R.: *Hematology* **12:** 189, 1975.
3. Robertson, J. G.: Ortho Research Scientific Symposium. Rh antibody mediated immunosuppression. Published, Ortho Diagnostics, Raritan, N.J., 1975, p. 33.
4. Crispen, J.: *ibid.,* p. 51.
5. Harwood, L. M.: *J Med Lab Tech* **19:** 19, 1975.
6. Kleihauer, E., Braun, H., and Betke, K.: *Klin Wochenschr* **35:** 637, 1957.
7. Lachman, E., *et al.*: *Br Med J* **1:** 1377, 1977.

Flow Sheet I: Assessment of Risk of Isoimmune Disease

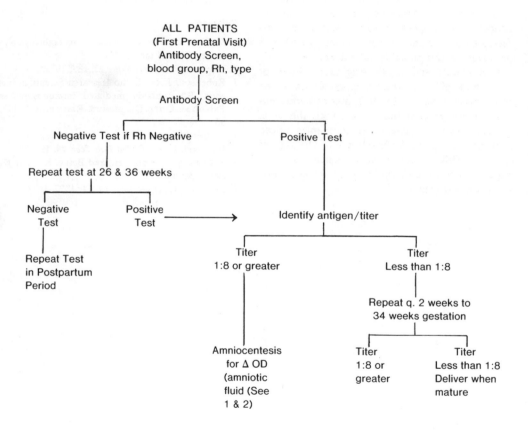

ALL PATIENTS
(First Prenatal Visit)
Antibody Screen,
blood group, Rh, type

Antibody Screen

Negative Test if Rh Negative

Positive Test

Repeat test at 26 & 36 weeks

Negative Test

Positive Test

Repeat Test in Postpartum Period

Identify antigen/titer

Titer 1:8 or greater

Titer Less than 1:8

Repeat q. 2 weeks to 34 weeks gestation

Amniocentesis for Δ OD (amniotic fluid (See 1 & 2)

Titer 1:8 or greater

Titer Less than 1:8 Deliver when mature

1. Amniocentesis should be done as soon as the titer is noted to be 1:8 or greater, but no sooner than 24 weeks gestation as fetal transfusion before this date is not practical.
2. Fetal maturity tests should be done on fluid obtained after 32 weeks gestation.

Flow Sheet II: Management of Isoimmune Disease

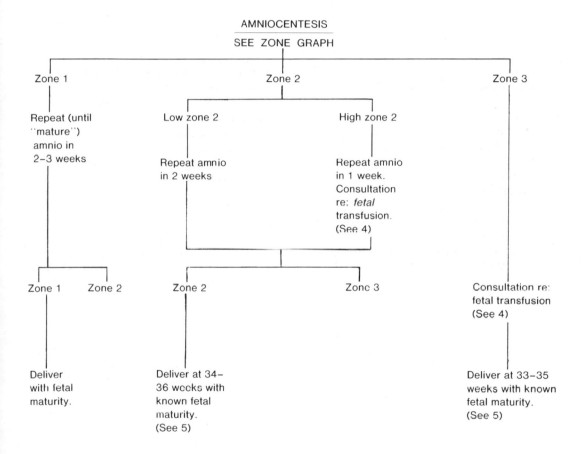

AMNIOCENTESIS

SEE ZONE GRAPH

Zone 1 → Repeat (until "mature") amnio in 2–3 weeks → Zone 1, Zone 2 → Deliver with fetal maturity.

Zone 2 → Low zone 2 → Repeat amnio in 2 weeks → Zone 2 → Deliver at 34–36 weeks with known fetal maturity. (See 5)

High zone 2 → Repeat amnio in 1 week. Consultation re: *fetal* transfusion. (See 4) → Zone 3

Zone 3 → Consultation re: fetal transfusion (See 4) → Deliver at 33–35 weeks with known fetal maturity. (See 5)

4. Intrauterine fetal transfusion has been demonstrated to improve the chance of fetal neonatal survival in severe cases if done early *before* hydrops fetalis develops.

5. There is developing experience with lecithin/sphingomyelin ratios that *suggests* that the amniotic fluid L/S ratio may be normal or inappropriately high in these patients.

Jaundice, Cholestasis of Pregnancy, Itching (Incidence 0.02–14%)

Fetal Risks:
1. Death
2. Prematurity

A. **Procedures**
 1. Liver function tests including bile acid levels
 2. Past obstetrical history (recurs with each pregnancy)
 3. Pruritus (with normal liver tests)

B. **Prenatal Care**
 1. Avoid hepatotoxic drugs (chlorpromazine, phenothiozines, sulfonomides, tetracycline, halothane)
 2. Fetal surveillance tests (E_3, HPL, OCT, fetal movement records) for fetal growth retardation

 3. Prothrombin level
 4. Watch for preeclampsia (24–33%), urinary tract infection (24%)
 5. Premature labor more common

C. **Therapeutic**
 1. Cholestyramine
 2. Tranquilizer
 3. Check possible drug reaction, especially sulfa (for UTI)

References

Steel, R., and Parker, M.: *Med J Aust* **1:** 461, 1973.
Ylostalo, P., *et al.*: *Gynaec Fenn* **64:** 123, 1975.
Espinoza, J.: *Perinatal Intensive Care.* Edited by S. Aladjem and A. Brown, Mosby, St. Louis, 1977.

Lupus Erythematosus

Fetal Risks:
1. IUGR
2. Death
3. Abruptio
4. Prematurity
5. Congenital heart disease

A. Initial Dx: Procedures
1. Lab tests: ANA, LE prep, BUN, creatinine clearance
2. Sonogram

B. Prenatal Care
1. Steroid therapy
2. Fetal surveillance (E_3, HPL, OCT, fetal movements records)
3. Bed rest
4. Premature labor, toxemia precautions

C. Therapeutic Procedures
1. Deliver when controlled and when amniotic fluid L/S > 2.0
2. Observe newborn for steroid withdrawal and lupus

Reference
Fraga, A., *et al.: Med J Aust* **1:** 749, 1973.
Chameides, L., *et al.: N Engl J Med* **297:** 1204, 1977.

Mental Retardation

Fetal Risks:
1. IUGR
2. Mental retardation

A. Initial Diagnosis
1. Records
2. Social service or psychiatric referral (mentally deficient gravida seldom have normal sexual partners)
3. Serum phenylalanine level
4. Genetic counseling

B. Prenatal Care
1. Nutritional support
2. Family planning counsel
3. Sonogram for fetal age and/or development

Multiple Gestation

Fetal Risks:
1. Prematurity
2. IUGR
3. Anomalies
4. Twin transfusion
5. Cerebral palsy with death of other twin

A. Initial Dx: Procedures
1. Careful dating of pregnancy
2. Sonogram

B. Prenatal Care
1. High protein diet, iron, folates, force fluids
2. Bed rest
3. Serial sonograms

4. Nonstress tests of all fetuses
5. Premature labor and toxemia precautions

C. Therapy
1. Premature delivery if fetal jeopardy by non-stress test and L/S ratio > 2.0.
2. Supplement folate in addition to iron and vitamin preps
3. Bed rest on side (not proven).
4. Consider cesarean section if breech, triplets premature, or acute hydramnios

Reference

Durkin, M. V.: *Eur J Pediat* **123:** 67, 1976.

Parathyroid (Hyper)

Fetal Risks:
1. Fetal loss
2. Neonatal morbidity (tetany)
3. Premature labor

A. Initial Dx: Procedures
1. Previous records
2. Serum calcium, phosphate

3. Renal function

B. Prenatal care
1. Surgical exploration

Reference

Johnstone, R. E., II, Kreindler, T., and Johnstone, R. E.: *Obstet Gynecol* **40:** 580, 1972.

Parathyroid (Hypo)

Fetal Risks:
1. Vitamin D toxicity
2. Neonatal hyperparathyroidism

A. Initial Dx: Procedures
1. Previous records
2. Serum calcium (ionized), phosphate
3. Chvostek's sign

B. Prenatal Care
1. Vitamin D, calcium

Reference

Bolen, J. W.: *Am J Obstet Gynecol* **117:** 178, 1973.

Premature Birth (Prior)

Fetal Risks:
1. Premature delivery
2. Fetal loss
3. Anomalies
4. IUGR

A. Initial Dx: Procedures
1. Prior records
2. Hysterogram (nonpregnant)
3. Urine culture
4. Thyroid index, FBS, BUN
5. Cervical evaluation

B. Prenatal Care
1. Bedrest
2. Avoid orgasm
3. Treat severe cervicitis
4. Frequent cervical examinations
5. Tranquilizers (?), alcohol (?)
6. Urine cultures
7. Sonograms
8. Delalutin (?)

References

Goodlin, R. C., *Obstet Gynecol* **38:** 916, 1971.
Viski, S., *et al.: 4th European Congress of Perinatal Medicine*, edited by Z. Stembera *et al.*, Thieme, Stuttgart, 1975.

Prenatal Screening Tests*

General

Assessments for maternal anemia or blood dyscrasia, blood group and Rh, presence of atypical antibodies, bacteriuria, chronic renal or bladder disease, syphilis, cervical carcinoma, and previous exposure to rubella are done on *all* patients when *first* evaluated and found to be or planning to become pregnant. Certain patients, as noted below, are screened for diabetes. In addition, cultures for *N. gonococcus* are obtained on many patients. At 28–35 weeks gestation, many of the screening tests are repeated.

Pregnancy should be viewed as an optimal opportunity for preventive health maintenance and patient education. Most often the patient has not had a complete screening history, physical examination, or screening laboratory assessment since childhood. Further, she often has little insight into the myriad problems of nutrition, pregnancy, sexuality, family planning, or motherhood. Nutritionists, social workers, and public health nurses are in clinic for counseling when acceptable by the gravida.

Guidelines and Specific Rationale for Screening Tests

1. Complete blood count is obtained because it is offered at a unit cost. "Anemia" in pregnancy (HCT < 28) is almost always of the iron deficient type, is not a disease of indigent patients only and is treatable with iron supplementation and high protein diet. Patients who are anemic when *first* seen or who become anemic while taking oral iron should be further investigated (Hb, indices, repeat smear evaluation, serum Fe content).

The definition of anemia is set lower in pregnancy than in the nonpregnant state because the red blood cell mass increases at a slower rate than the plasma volume particularly from 20–30 weeks gestation. Failure to decrease HCT at 28 weeks may mean decreased blood volume. Patients taking their oral iron supplements with a HCT > 30 in the late second trimester will almost never develop anemia subsequently. The check at 36–37 weeks and upon admission is done to detect hidden bleeding, malabsorption, or failure to take the prescribed iron. Even with severe maternal anemia, the fetus is almost never anemic due to iron deficiency. Also the fetus tends to tolerate labor well if the maternal anemia is chronic rather than acute.

White Blood Cell Count and Differential—These tests are done as in any new patient to detect rare abnormalities such as leukemia. It is important to note that the WBC exhibits a neutrophilia in pregnancy with total counts to 12,000 before labor and as high as 20,000–25,000 in labor and the immediate postpartum period.

2. Hemoglobin electrophoresis in all black gravida to rule out hemoglobinopathies (state law).

3. *Blood Group, Rh*—Determination of the blood group permits the detection of the more rare groups. Rh is determined *only* to advise the patient that she is or is not a potential candidate for Rh-immune globulin after delivery.

4. *Atypical Antibody Screen*—BEFORE THE WIDESPREAD USE OF SCREENING TITERS, NEARLY 30% OF *FIRST SUSPECTED PREGNANCIES* WITH ERYTHROBLASTOSIS RESULTED IN A STILLBORN. Except for the discovery of those patients who are potential candidates for Rho(D) globulin, the physician should not be concerned with whether or not his patient is Rh positive or negative. Rather it is perhaps more important to assess whether antibodies are present to *any* of the clinically significant isoantibodies involved in erythroblastosis. This test checks for anti-D antibodies as well.

5. *Bacteriuria* (Optional)—The prevalence of bacteriuria is population dependent but varies from 2–8%. Almost all patients who will have bacteriuria in pregnancy *have* bacteriuria at the initial examination. Nearly 25% of women with asymptomatic bacteriuria will develop

pyelonephritis. Pyelonephritis has an associated increased risk of premature labor and can be *prevented* in over 90% of bacteruric patients by early and appropriate antibacterial therapy.

6. *Urinalysis*—for albumin and sugar. Complete urinalysis if (5) not done. The routine urinalysis is not appreciably altered in pregnancy except for glucosuria in many patients due to increased glomerular filtration rate without concomitant increase in tubular reabsorption of glucose. Significant WBC or bacteria indicates culture.

7. *Serology*—This test is done to detect and treat syphilis before it affects the fetus. Fetal infection does not usually occur *before* 16–18 weeks gestation. The test is almost always positive within 4–6 weeks after infection. False positives (FTA negative) occur in a variety of diseases (drug abuse, lupus) which should be ruled out.

8. *Papanicolaou Smear*—Squamous cell cancer of the cervix in child-bearing years occurs as frequently as 1 in 500 women of this age. It is increasing in the younger age groups. Age of onset of coitus and number of sexual partners are influencing factors. Annual cervical cancer screening can easily be initiated at the first prenatal visit. If the smear is abnormal, colposcopy should be performed.

9. *Rubella Screen*—All patients should be screened except those who have had a previous *positive* screening test. Ten to twenty percent of adult women are negative on rubella screening tests. History taking for rubella as a childhood disease approaches worthlessness since many exanthems may be confused with rubella. Immunization against rubella *must* be followed up with a screening titer before pregnancy as lot differences and individual response variations do not result in 100% protection. Immunizations should *NOT* be done if the patient is pregnant. When immunizations are given pregnancy should be prevented for at least two months. Rubella vaccine is given to all negative (titer < 1:8) postpartum patients upon discharge.

10. *Two-hour Postprandial Blood Sugar* (Optional)—Unfortunately, the most frequent indication for investigation of the pregnant female for diabetes is *AFTER* an unexplained stillbirth. Patients with a positive family history of diabetes, obesity (20% overweight, particularly if combined with positive family history), glycosuria, reactive hypoglycemia, hydramnios, hypertensive disease of pregnancy (toxemia), recurrent infections, large for gestational age baby (> 4300 g), fetal congenital anomalies, unexplained prematurity, unexplained intrauterine or neonatal death, repeated late abortions, or infertility should all be screened. With this awesome list—combined with the shortcomings of historical notations—the physician may decide to screen all of his patients at the initial visit. In any event, all patients with a negative screen at the initial visit and all patients not previously screened should have a 2-hr postprandial blood sugar in the late second trimester. Values under 140 mg/100 cm^3 (true blood sugar) at 28–30 weeks gestation and similar values AFTER a 100 g carbohydrate meal are considered normal and need not be further evaluated. There is essentially *NO* value in performing random blood sugars which are not controlled as to type and time of meal.

11. *Cervical Culture for N. gonococcus*—This infection is a community health problem of major proportions which in some environments may be as frequent as the common cold. Important features are the frequency of 5–15% positive cultures in some prenatal populations, the lack of social distinction in prevalence, the frequency of asymptomatic carriers in both females *and* males, and the emergence of penicillin resistant strains. All positive cultures should be followed in four weeks with a repeat VDRL.

12. *Cervical Culture—Group B Streptococcus* (Optional)—Approximately 5% of women harbor this organism in the cervix and vagina and are completely asymptomatic. Infection may be sexually transmitted. This organism is a *frequent* cause of neonatal sepsis. Almost all cases of the neonatal disease have an acute onset and usually fulminate course.

13. Doppler detection of FHT prior 12 weeks—Repeat at 2-week intervals until positive. Essential for determination of EDC.

14. Ultrasonic B scanning—Whenever uterus inappropriate for size (hopefully before 28 weeks) or prior to amniocentesis.

Test	Initial visit	28 weeks	36 weeks	Approximate cost (Sacramento Medical Center, 1978)
HCT	—	X	X	$ 3.00
Complete blood count	X	—	—	11.00
Blood group, Rh	X	—	—	8.00
Atypical antibody screen	X	X	—	10.00
Bacteruria screen	(X)	(X)	—	18.00
Urinalysis	X	—	—	6.00
Serology (VDRL)	X	—	(X)	9.20
Pap Smear	X	—	—	10.50
Rubella screen (HI)	X	—	—	14.00
2-hr PPBS	—	X	—	8.00
Cervical culture				
N. Gonococcus	(X)	—	(X)	18.00
Group B *Streptococcus*	—	—	(X)	8.00 ($60)
Ultrasonic B Scanning	(X)	(X)	(X)	105.00

(X) = elective in low risk pregnancies

* Modified from Wisconsin Perinatal Center (Jack Schneider, M.D.) 1973.

Pyelonephritis

Fetal Risks:
1. Premature labor
2. IUGR

A. Initial Dx: Procedures
1. Prior records
2. Urine culture with immunofluorescence for antibody-coated bacteria
3. BUN, creatinine clearance
4. Hemoglobin electrophoresis

B. Prenatal Care
1. Serial urine cultures for remainder of pregnancy
2. Close observation for premature labor
3. Renal sonogram

4. Renal scan
5. Selected retrograde pyelogram

C. Therapeutic Procedures
If this is initial episode: Antibiotic Rx for 2 weeks and follow-up cultures. If recurrent episode or underlying renal disease, maintain on continuous suppressive antibiotic therapy for the duration of pregnancy

Dietl's position (extend ureter) for severe pain

Excess fluid intake

Reference

Harris, R. E., and Gilstrap, L. D : *Obstet Gynecol* **44:** 637, 1974.

Renal Disease

Fetal Risks:
1. Fetal loss
2. IUGR
3. Premature labor
4. Increased rate of malformations

A. Initial Dx: Procedures
1. Prior record
2. Urinalysis and culture
3. Serum creatinine and/or BUN
4. 24-hr urine for creatinine clearance and total protein.
5. Protein electrophoresis
6. ASO, cholesterol, C^3 complement
7. Renal sonograph

B. Prenatal Care
1. Serial BUN and/or creatinine clearance
2. Serial cultures if infectious etiology suspected
3. Sonographic determination of gestational age at 18–24 weeks
4. OCT, HPL, amniocentesis for L/S and meconium
5. Close observation for signs of premature labor
6. Fetal movement records

C. Therapy
1. Bed rest and increased fluids
2. Close control of hypertension, if present
3. Termination of pregnancy if marked deterioration of renal function or renal dialysis
4. TAB considered if BUN above 50 mg%

Reference

Bear, R. A.: *Obstet Gynecol* **48:** 13, 1976.

Rubella

Fetal Risks:
1. TORCH syndrome
2. Fetal loss

A. Initial Dx: Procedures
1. Rubella titer on all patients at initial visit

B. Prenatal Tests
1. Repeat titer for known exposure/or undiagnosed rash any time in gestation. Titer to be repeated 2–3 weeks after rash or possible exposure and to be run paired with first specimen
2. Rubella IgM titer

C. Therapy
1. Offer termination of pregnancy if prior to 20 weeks with documentation of infection by titer
2. If 2nd or 3rd trimester infection, sonographic assessment of growth
3. Viral studies on placenta and newborn
4. Avoidance of contact between neonate and other pregnant women until neonate negative for viral excretion
5. Immunize in immediate postpartum period if rubella titers indicate lack of previous infection
6. Gamma globulin (high titer) if exposed and wishes to continue pregnancy

Reference

Cooper, I. Z., and Krugman, S.: *Disease-a-month Year Book*, 1969.

Sickle Cell Disease

Fetal Risks:
1. IUGR
2. Abruptio
3. Fetal loss
4. Toxemia

A. Initial Dx: Procedures

1. Hemoglobin electrophoresis on all black gravida and all patients with unexplained anemia, or abnormal peripheral blood smear
2. Blood counts
3. SED rates to distinguish between pain of infection and sickling, cultures of urine/sputum as indicated for suspicion of infection, monthly urine culture

B. Therapeutic Procedures

1. Frequent visits
2. Hospitalization for crisis (average antepartum 36 days, postpartum 10.6 days)
3. Folic acid, but no iron
4. If hemoglobin drops sharply, transfuse
5. For repeated infection or crisis, over-transfusion with fresh washed packed cells (to HCT > 37%) to replace 75–80% of HbS with HbA (or exchange transfusion)
6. Treat fever and infection vigorously
7. Crisis: Bed rest, increased atmospheric O_2, hydration and analgesics; heparin for acute bone pain in last month, intrapartum and puerperally (for preventing death from marrow embol.), antibiotics
8. Consider exchange transfusion at 32 weeks

Reference

Harger, R.: *Clin Obstet Gynecol* **17:** 136, 1974.

Stillbirth (Previous)

Fetal Risks:
1. Repeat stillborn
2. Increased incidence of anomalies

A. Initial Dx: Procedures
1. Careful dating of pregnancy
2. Attempt to determine cause of previous still-birth
3. 2Hr PP blood sugar
4. Obtain records from all previous pregnancies
5. Titers for toxoplasmosis, cytomegalic disease
6. Rule out lupus (ANA) renal disease (BUN, creatinine clearance)
7. Antibody screen, hemoglobin electrophoresis
8. Hysterosalpingogram (nonpregnant)

B. Prenatal Tests
1. Sonogram
2. Fetal movement record
3. Plasma estriol 2 × week after 30 weeks
4. Oxytocin challenge test, (OCT) weekly after 30 weeks
5. Serial sonography
6. Plasma estriol and OCT to begin earlier if hypertension or evidence of IUGR
7. L/S ratio if premature intervention

C. Therapy
1. Reduced physical activity
2. Premature delivery if fetal jeopardy indicated by estriol or OCT and L/S ratio >2.0
3. Nutritional counseling if anemic, low weight or low weight gain

Syphilis

Fetal Risks:
1. Late abortion
2. Stillborn
3. Premature
4. Neonatal syphilis

A. Initial Dx: Procedures
1. Past records
2. Cutaneous lesions—dark-field examination
3. Positive VDRL plus positive FTA-ABS = syphilis

B. Prenatal Care
1. Follow quantitative STS
2. Treat active syphilis at any stage
3. Treat if previous therapy inadequate or presumed reinfection
4. Treat if prior delivery of syphilitic infant
5. If FTA-ABS negative, rule out causes of false positive VDRL, i.e., lupus, hyperglobulinemia, narcotic addiction, infections, etc.

C. Therapy During Pregnancy:

	Benzathine Penicillin G (Bicillin) (Parenteral)	Aqueous Procaine Penicillin G (Parenteral)	Cephaloridine (Parenteral)	Erythromycin (Oral)
Acquired syphilis, early stages: primary, secondary, and early latent	2.4 million U at 2-wk intervals; total dose, 4.8 million units	600,000 U per day for 8 days; total dose, 4.8 million U	0.5–1.0 g/day for 10 days	2–3 g/day for 10–15 days; total dose, 30 g
Acquired syphilis, late stages: late latent, gumma, cardiovascular, and neurosyphilis	2.4 million U at 1-week intervals; total dose 6 to 20 million U	600,000 to 2 million U per day for 10 to 15 days; total dose, 6 to 20 million U	Unknown	Total dose 80 g (?)

Reference

Lee, R.: in *Medical Complications of Pregnancy.* G. N. Burrow and T. F. Ferris, Eds., Saunders, Philadelphia, 1975.

Thyroid (Hyperthyroidism)

Fetal Risks:
1. Premature labor
2. Increased fetal loss
3. Fetal goiter (over treatment)
4. Fetal hyperthyroidism

A. Initial Dx: Procedures
1. T_4—measure of circulating thyroxin
2. RT_3U—measure of thyroid binding sites
3. FT_4I (index)—measure of total circulating thyroxin
4. T_4, T_3, alone can be misleading

B. Prenatal Care
1. FT_4I and patient's clinical status
2. LATS or LATS protector
3. TSH (?)
4. Thyroid scan only under extreme circumstances
5. Fetal surveillance (E_3, HPL, OCT)—fetal tachycardia may indicate fetal hyperthyroidism.
6. Severe thyrotoxicosis: Propylthiouracil up to 100 mg q 6 hr to obtain remission, then decrease dose as clinically indicated, attempting to reach 100 mg daily. Propranolol orally or intravenously for severe symptoms or storm, along with sodium iodide.
7. If control not possible, consider subtotal thyroidectomy

Reference

Herbst, A. L., and Selenkow, H. A.: *N Engl J Med* **273:** 627, 1965.
Burrow, G. N. *N Engl J Med* **298:** 150, 1978

Thyroid (Hypothyroidism)

Fetal Risks:
1. Fetal loss
2. Mental retardation

A. Initial Dx: Procedures
1. T_4, T_3, FT_4 index, TSH
2. Thyroid antibodies

B. Prenatal Care
1. T_4 and evaluate patient's clinical status
2. Maintain normal pregnancy thyroid levels

Reference

Man, E. B., *et al.: Am J Obstet Gynecol* **109**: 12, 1971.

Ulcerative Colitis

Fetal Risks:
1. Death
2. Prematurity

A. Initial Dx: Procedure
1. Previous records
2. Genetic counseling

B. Prenatal Care
1. Keep HCT > 32 mg%
2. Stop any sulfa agent (Azulfidine) prior to delivery
3. Prematurity and toxemia protocols

4. Bowel stoma care
5. Exclude milk?

C. Therapeutic Procedures
1. Even after rectal resection, vaginal delivery is possible, although soft tissue dystocia may occur

Reference

Meyer, J. H.: In *Gastrointestinal Disease*. M. H. Sleisinger, and J. S. Fordtran, Eds., Saunders, Philadelphia, 1973.

Urinary Tract Infection

Fetal Risks:
1. IUGR
2. Premature labor
3. Infection

A. Initial Diagnostic Procedure
1. Records
2. Urine culture and sensitivity
3. Fluorescent antibody test (? renal origin)

B. Prenatal Care
1. After repeated episode (or after 30 weeks) prophylactic antibiotic (Penicillin VK)
2. Force fluids
3. Review coital positions

C. Postpartum Care
1. IVP
2. Repeat urine culture with biannual follow-up

Reference

Harris, R. E., *et al.*: *Am J Obstet Gynecol* **126**: 20, 1976.

Prenatal Risk Index*

BASELINE DATA

Age 35+	+1
Age 40+	+2
Age < 16	+1
Para 0	+1
Para 6+	+1
Pregnancy interval < 2 years	+1
Serious illness	+1 to +3
as diabetes B, C, D, E	+2
Renal disease	+3
Repeated UTI	+1
Liver alone	+1 to +3
Unwanted pregnancy	+3
Abnormal glucose tolerance curve	+1
Heart disease	+2 to +3
Obesity > 250 lbs.	+1
Small pelvis	+1 to +3

OBSTETRICAL HISTORY

Stillborn	+1 to +3
Neonatal death	+1 to +3
Prior premature	<32 wks. +2
	<36 wks. +1
Prior Ab's. (>2)	+1

Toxemia

Preeclampsia	+1 to +3
Normal pregnancy in interim	−1
Toxemia unclassified	+3
Eclampsia	+1
Difficult labor or delivery	Cesarean section
	+3
	+1 to +3
Prior birth defect	+1 to +3
Prior infant 9+ lbs	+1 to +3
Isoimmunization	+3
One or more uneventful pregnancies	−1
Prior postpartum hemorrhage	+1 to +3

PRESENT PREGNANCY

Bleeding < 20 weeks (more than menses or more than 2X)	+1 to +3
with uterine cramps	+2
Bleeding 20+ weeks	
negative B-scan	−1
questionable B-scan	+3
Premature rupture of membranes	
at term	+1
latent period > 24 hr	+3
Anemia	
<10 g	+1
< 8 g	+3
No prenatal care	+3
after 34 weeks	+1

Blood Pressure 140 +/90+	+2
with proteinuria	+3
Hydramnios	+3
Pleural pregnancies	+3
Repeated pyrexia	+1

LABOR

Premature	+2
<36 wks.	+3
< 32 wks.	+2
>42½ wks.	

* Modified from Goodwin, et al.: Canad Med Assoc J
  101: 459, 1969.

Social Risks

Conditions and situations requiring comprehensive team prenatal care involving obstetrician, social worker, nutritionist, and public health nurse, and not necessarily special medical consultation.

1. Women under 16 years of age (refer to special teen-age prenatal clinic)
2. Illiteracy (arrange for special prenatal instructions)
3. Illegitimacy (social service to determine plans for newborn)
4. Racial or cultural minority (arrange for special interpreter)
5. Unwanted pregnancy, especially those not keeping therapeutic abortion clinic appointments (arrange for special social service and public health nurse consultation)
6. Poor dietary history (nutritionist to see gravida at every visit).
7. Severe social economic problems (social service and public health nurse consultation)
8. Pregnancy interval less than 12 months (arrange for Family Planning consultation)

In-Hospital Protocols

Contents

Diabetes in Pregnancy

The goal of management is

(a) to detect all gravida with diabetes

(b) to provide them with a tight control of their blood sugars, i.e., fasting blood sugars under 120 mg%

In the detection of diabetes, it should be recalled that the normal fasting blood sugar in the third trimester is decreased and at the same time, those with diabetes or potential diabetes, are much more likely to manifest their abnormal fasting blood sugars during the third trimester. While the third trimester is an interval which is popular for those investigators whose interests are the development of diabetes, it is less useful to the obstetrician who obviously would prefer to identify the patient at risk early in her pregnancy. A glucose tolerance test or a fasting blood sugar and blood glucose 2 hr after 100 g oral load should be done under the following conditions:

a. Two fasting glycosuria (second fasting specimen)

b. Frank diabetes in a first degree maternal relative

c. An unexplained perinatal death or severe fetal abnormality in any pregnancy (especially caudal agenesis)

d. A heavy-for-dates baby (greater than 4.3 kg)

e. Maternal weight preconception at 20% greater than expected for height and age or greater than 91 kg

f. Acute hydramnios

g. Previous gestational diabetes

h. Abnormalities of pregnancy, including hydramnios or small-for-dates babies.

Interpretation of the glucose tolerance test is really based on the first and second trimester according to O'Sullivan, who demonstrated that if two or more of the following blood levels after 100 g oral glucose load occurs in apparently normal pregnant women, that at least 25% of them will have full-blown diabetes in two years (*Diabetes* **13:** 278, 1964):

Glucose	Fasting	Hours (mg%)		
		1	2	3
Blood	90	165	145	125
Plasma	105	190	165	145

If the intravenous glucose tolerance test is used, the lower limits of normal K (absolute glucose disappearance rate) as described by Adden: First trimester 1.37, second trimester 1.18, third trimester 1.13, first week postpartum 0.93. Any K values below these levels indicates probable diabetes mellitus.

Data which support the tight control of blood sugars during pregnancy in diabetic women for optimal fetal outcome are Karlsson and Kjellmer, 1972; Gabbe et al., 1977; Essex, 1976; and Persson and Lunell, 1975. They recommended that an ideal metabolic control in pregnancy requires a mean blood sugar of less than 100 ml%. In the Karlsson series of 96 pregnant diabetics (83 of whom were insulin dependent) the perinatal mortality rate was 23.6% when the mean blood sugar was greater than 150 mg%, 15.3% between 100 and 150 mg% and 3.8% in those cases below 100 mg%. This paper has been criticized because of the difficulties in defining the mean blood sugar rate. (Obviously, it depends on how often the blood sugar is determined in any 24-hr period.) However, Persson and Lunell have produced similar good results. Gabbe et al.[3] and Essex[4] good results are reported. They also reflect tight blood sugar control (and not the fetal surveillance test).

History Taking

In case of frank diabetes, history should include: Age of onset and duration of diabetes, amounts of insulin, diet, complications of diabetes (including the presence or absence of retinopathy, neuropathy, hypertension, renal disease). Her diabetes should be classified according to White. Also include the Prognostically Bad Signs during Pregnancy (PBSP) or pyelonephritis with fever, precoma, or severe diabetic ketosis, preeclampsia, eclampsia, and neglecters of clinical follow-up (Pedersen and Pedersen).

The management at the time of delivery requires cooperation. The time and mode of delivery is the choice of the obstetrician. Depot insulin should be stopped the day before delivery if possible, because the insulin requirement changes rapidly after delivery, and depot insulin is too cumbersome. Regular insulin has a peak action in about 4 hr and lasts 12. Semi-lente is about 2 hr longer. NPH, Lente, and Globin reach peaks in about 8–12 hr and last 48 hr, thus taking 48 hr to get the full effect of a change of dose.

Reverse 5-hr Management[7, 8]

(Dr. Walworth of Santa Clara Valley Medical Center, San Jose)

The reverse or 5-hr management for determination of insulin requirements is an easy technique, readily mastered by physicians, regardless of their sophistication as regards diabetes and appears to be fairly precise. The reverse "concept" is that one always looks back over the last 5-hr period as indicative of how much insulin will be required for the next 5-hr period.

Reverse Management

I. Indications—uncontrolled diabetes, e.g.:
   A. following initial treatment of ketoacidosis
   B. during infections, operations, trauma, or deliveries
   C. occasionally for determining insulin requirement in a gravida with poor control
II. Rationale
   A. Equivalent feedings are given at equal intervals, so that the insulin dose is the only variable. Using Semi-lente insulin to cover the 9-hr interval from 10 PM to 7 AM makes this interval "equivalent" to the 5-hr intervals during the day.
   B. A 50 G diet is used because this is equal to 1 L of 5% D/W which is an ordinary substitute (do not use both I.V.'s and oral feedings without adding them together). A G equals: grams of carbohydrate × 1
   grams of protein × 0.58
   grams of fat × 0.1
   A 50 G feeding does not necessarily contain 200 calories.
   The usual 200 G diet used here contains about 1400+ calories.
III. Technique
   A. 200 g ADA diet in approximately four equal feedings.
   B. Clinitest urine before each feeding and call MD for insulin dose.
   C. Daily FBS: the lab should be alerted to those patients on 5-hr management so that their blood can be drawn first. Under no circumstances should breakfast be delayed beyond 7:30. If the blood has not been drawn, get it at noon.
   D. If the patient is receiving a depot dose of insulin to which you expect the patient to return, maintain it while on "5-hr man-

agement." If the dose is large, split it between a 7 AM and 5 PM time. After delivery, the gravida may require no insulin for up to 36 hr.

E. Before the first feeding, select a dose of insulin. The subsequent urine test will indicate that:
1. If the patient still has glycosuria, the dose was too small.
2. If the patient has hypoglycemic reaction, the dose was too large. Decrease it!
3. If the urine is negative and the patient has not had a reaction, the dose was correct. Repeat it or cautiously lower it.

HELPFUL HINTS:

1. The most common errors are
   (a) decreasing the dose too rapidly or too much, or worst of all, omitting a dose just because the urine is negative
   (b) stopping 5-hr management too soon while the insulin requirement is still changing or has not been established
   (c) giving oral feedings while receiving I.V. feedings, too

(d) Delaying breakfast to wait for the lab, the urine test, or the insulin order
2. The only times to lower the insulin dose are
   (a) following a hypoglycemic reaction
   (b) if the FBS is too low
   (c) acetonuria clears
   (d) the patient is clinically improved, for example, no longer febrile
3. To return to a single dose, add up the entire amount of regular given in 24 hr and give that amount in a single or two doses.

References

1. Karlsson, and Kjellmer: *Am J Obstet Gynecol* **112:** 213, 1972.
2. Persson, and Lunell: *Am J Obstet Gynecol* **122:** 737, 1975.
3. Gabbe, S., *et al.: Am J Obstet Gynecol* **129:** 723, 1977.
4. Essex, N., *Br J Hosp Med* **15:** 333, 1976.
5. White, P.: *Med Clin N Am* **49:** 1015, 1965.
6. Pedersen, D., and Pedersen, H.: *Acta Endocrin* **50:** 70, 1965.
7. Sutherland, H. W., and Stowers, X.: *Carbohydrate Metabolism in Pregnancy in the Newborn,* Churchill Livenston, New York, 1975.
8. Stowers, J. M., *J. R Coll Phys* **7:** 69, 1972.

Diabetic Control Utilizing Continuous Insulin Infusion*

I. Purpose: To control blood sugar in diabetic obstetric patients using a continuous infusion of insulin.

This is the initial guideline for continuous infusion of insulin for diabetic obstetric patients who require maximum control of blood sugar to meet stressful situations (i.e., induction of labor, surgery, etc.) and should be individualized based on patient response.

* Terry L. Hutton, Pharm. D., Memorial Hospital

II. Method
   A. Prior to infusion—determine the approximate ratio of total daily dose of insulin per total daily caloric uptake (i.e., 2000 cal. diet in a patient controlled on 40 U NPH: ratio—1 unit/50 cal).
   B. Use above ratio to determine initial rate of insulin infusion based on estimated caloric intake. (i.e., patient is receiving 3 liters dextrose solution per day and not eating = patient is receiving 600 cal/day. 600 cal x 1 unit/50 cal = 12 U/day.)
   C. The initial infusion rate is then deter-

mined by dividing total units/day by 24 hr (i.e., 12 U/day = 0.5 U/hr = 8.3 mil U/min.)

D. A separate peripheral 5% glucose solution should be maintained for adequate hydration, caloric, and potassium supplementation, and to provide a route for other parenteral medication when necessary. (Suggested solution is 5% dextrose in Lactated Ringers at 125 cc/hr.)

E. Insulin infusion should be decreased during night shift (2400–0800) to prevent hypoglycemia (i.e., 0.5 U/hr from 2400–0800).

III. Preparation of Solution
A. Formula (add insulin *last*):
500 cc Normal Saline
7 cc Salt Poor Albumin (1.7 g)
50 U Regular Insulin (CZI)
This yields a solution containing: 1 U insulin/10 cc

B. Infusion by IVAC Pump
Using a *"Microdrip tubing"* (60 gtts/cc) infusion rates will be as follows:
0.5 U/hr = 5 gtts/min
1.0 U/hr = 10 gtts/min
2.0 U/hr = 20 gtts/min
5.0 U/hr = 50 gtts/min

C. Infusion by Razal Pump
(CAUTION: This solution is 5 times the usual concentration of oxytocin)

Withdraw from above 500 cc bottle—30 cc in a 30 cc plastipak syringe (Razal pump infuses 0.014 cc/min/dial number):

U/hr	mU/min	Dial setting
0.25 U/hr	4.16	3
0.5 U/hr	8.33	6
0.75 U/hr	12.5	9
1 U/hr	16.7	12
2 U/hr	33.3	24

IV. Monitoring Patients While on Infusion
A. If multiple daily blood sugars are necessary to keep blood sugar below 150 mg% (and this is suggested for the first 24 hr), then an intravenous catheter maintained by a heparin lock is suggested for patient comfort.

B. Record daily
1. Urinary sugars and acetone with each specimen or every 4 hr
2. Fasting blood sugar, and probably another blood sugar in the evening (i.e., every 12 hr)
3. Hypoglycemic reactions (if they occur)
4. Caloric intake
5. Patient weight and intake and output

C. Record frequently (every 2–3 days) patient's electrolytes (especially K+) and pH.

Breech Protocol

I. *Evaluation*

(1) Roentgenogram—Obtain *flat plate* of abdomen to determine position of fetus. Rule out "stargaze" position, associated with 25% spinal cord injury. Rule out gross fetal anomalies, interlocking twins.

(2) EFW—Have as many experienced observers as possible try to estimate fetal weight.

(3) B-scan—if multiple gestation, ascertain if there is any discrepancy in size of fetal heads.

(4) Vaginal exam with clinical pelvimetry and evaluation of presenting parts and cervix.

(5) Maternal weight (if >180 lbs. there is increased risk to fetus).

II. *Risk Factors*

(1) EFW <2500 g or >3800 g

(2) Borderline pelvimetry

(3) Footling or complete breech (prolapsed cord)

(4) Abnormal labor progression

(5) Maternal weight >180 lbs

(6) "Stargazing" fetus (cervical spine injury in 25%)

(7) Multigravida may *not* have much decreased risk over primigravida and therefore previous normal vertex delivery does *not* mean a breech delivery will therefore be without complication.

III. *Delivery Mode for Low-Risk Breeches*

(1) Gestation >36 weeks

a) 2500–3800 g—Allow vaginal delivery, if parents wish.

b) >3800 g—recommend cesarean section (CS).

(2) 33–36 weeks, 1300–2500 g—recommend CS because of risk of entrappment of head by cervix, especially with PROM.

(3) 28–32 weeks, 1000–1300 g—offer a CS; requires a classical incision and repeat CS in the future; benefits currently unknown.

(4) Current Overall Survival Rate for Prematures—See Premature Delivery Protocol.

(5) Discuss relative risks with patient and husband (and document discussion in the chart).

a) Perinatal mortality >36 weeks is 3× vertex (18/1000 vs 6/1000).

b) Perinatal morbidity is 12× (1.2% vs. 0.1%), i.e., neurological problems, broken clavicles, etc. One study with a morbidity of 2.8% had 1% intracranial hemorrhage, 0.6% fractures, 0.6% paralysis, 0.6% dislocation.

c) If not frank breech, higher incidence of cord prolapse.

IV. *Intrapartum Management*

(1) Notify chief resident and attending.

(2) T&C for 2 units whole blood; alert O.R.

(3) PT, PTT, and platelet count.

(4) Pelvimetry and flat plate of abdomen ASAP.

(5) DO NOT RUPTURE MEMBRANES—monitor externally until SROM occurs.

(6) Vaginal exam q 30 min.

(7) Plot FRIEDMAN CURVE—labor should *not* exceed 18 hr, active phase slope should be >1.5 cm/hr.

(8) Anesthesiologists should be constantly available—may use epidural anesthesia if patient requests.

V. *Delivery*

(1) Most experienced obstetrician should follow the vertex.

(2) AVOID MANIPULATIVE PROCEDURES—i.e., decomposition and extraction, let fetus deliver spontaneously to umbilicus.

(3) Use *only* fetal pelvis for traction—not abdomen or thorax.

(4) Routinely apply Piper's forceps to the after-coming head.

(5) Right-angle retractors available for "vaginal breathing."

Heart Disease—Intrapartum

Fetal Risks:
1. Abruptio
2. Hypoxia

A. Initial Dx: Procedures

Amniocentesis for L/S ratio until 2+

B. Intrapartum Surveillance

Ongoing Assessments
1. B/P, pulse, respiration rate q 30 min
2. Auscultation of chest q 1–2 hours, oftener if indicated
3. Temp q 2 hr
4. Urine output q hour
5. Vital capacity q 2 hr
6. Fetal–maternal monitor; externàl until ROM, then internal
7. Cardioscope for patients with arrhythmia

C. Therapeutic Procedures
1. Induce labor during period of maximal medical coverage after 38 w, when cervix ripe and L/S ratio greater than 2.0. Start with dilute oxytocin; amniotomy after regular labor established and dilation and effacement started.
2. If labor prolonged, fails to progress—operative intervention.

Coagulants: If on heparin, stop at onset of labor. On coumadin (should switch to heparin by 37 w) give Vit K IM.

3. To forestall bacterial endocarditis, use broad spectrum antibiotic for 3 days beginning with onset of labor (penicillin and streptomycin).

1st Stage: Resume oxytocin during 1st stage of labor if necesary to decrease amount of work of patient. Semi-Fowler position (unless interferes with uterine blood I.V. infusion 5% DW at 50 ml/hr.

4. *2nd Stage*: Well anesthetized (specialist in perinatal anesthesia) to avoid urge to push. If no progress in ½–1 hr—operative intervention with midforceps or vacuum. Choice of cesarean section no different than other patients. Deliver in semi-Fowler position O_2 by face mask.

5. *3rd Stage*: Oxytocin diluted 10–20 U/1000 cc I.V. No undiluted oxytocin, no ergot derivatives. Specially careful observation postpartum—phlebotomy if failure.

6. 1–2 day postpartum—careful observation for failure until diuresis occurs.

EPH Gestosis (Preeclampsia) Protocol

A. Principles of Therapy

1. It is a disease of primigravida between the 22nd week of pregnancy and 3 days postpartum. (If it occurs in other gravida, consider underlying vascular disease, overdistention of the uterus, hydatid mole, different mate, and so forth.)
2. Most cases are "pseudo" preeclampsia (or EPH gestosis).
3. Severe preeclampsia is characterized by:
   (a) a reduced blood volume.
   (b) a rise in mean arterial blood pressure and a degree of vasoconstriction with a reduced blood flow to vital organs, i.e., placenta, liver, kidneys, eyes, brain.
   (c) a frequent dysfunction of liver, kidney and sometimes brain, heart, GI tract, etc.
   (d) thrombocytopenia and other signs of DIC such as microangiopathic disorders.
4. Therapy of severe EPH gestosis should be limited to a single or a few drugs, the lateral position, a high protein diet, and termination of pregnancy. Unless the patient has been salt depleted, excessive intravenous salt can exacerbate symptoms, especially in combination with oxytocin. Albumin, on the other hand, fulfills a need in the intravascular blood volume constricted patient. (Only heart failure is a risk.)
5. While termination of pregnancy is the cure for severe EPH gestosis, most cases of eclampsia in registered patients occur postpartum (especially if epidural anesthesia has been used).
6. If vascular complications can be avoided, there is no residual effect postpartum.

B. Antepartum care for cases of severe preeclampsia should include

1. Bed rest.
2. High-protein diet and force fluids.
3. In addition to the usual vital sign recordings, the following should be included: Blood pressure every 4 hr, urine output and protein content, presence or absence of headaches, abdominal pain, visual symptoms.
4. Sedation according to size and symptoms, (phenobarbital 300 mg b.i.d.; paraldehyde 10 ml in 20–25 ml rectally q.i.d.; diazepam 10 mg q.i.d.).
5. Anticonvulsants according to size and reflexes:
   (a) Magnesium sulfate 10 g outer gluteal IM, then 5 g q 4 hr; or 4 g initially IV and 1 g IV q 4 hr; check knee jerks and urine output q 4 hr and keep serum Mg^{++} below 8 meq/liter.
   (b) Diazepam 10 mg IM and repeat up to 50 mg/day.
6. Antihypertensives [hydralazine, cautiously intravenously if BP > 160/110; 10–20 mg or cryptenamine (Unitensen) 0.3 ml and hydralazine 10 mg in 500 cc 10% dextrose in water].
7. Fetal monitoring (E_3, HPL, OCT, B-scan and patient log of fetal activity).
8. Laboratory (check for liver, renal function; hemoconcentration and microangiopathic disorders) CBC, platelet count (? if < 100,-000), panel 12, prothrombin time, UA and total 24-hr urinary protein.

C. Intrapartum care for severe preeclampsia—In addition to the above (B)

1. Pain relief, sedation, and anticonvulsants are usually indicated.
2. Avoid marked decrease of mean blood pressure (>25%).
3. Expand blood volume prior to epidural anesthesia.
4. Expand blood volume if evidence of he-

moconcentration, to decrease the Hct. by at least 15%.*

* We use albumin, Plasmanate (plasma protein fraction), or whole blood at the rate of 2–3 "units" per day. If volume expansion is the correct therapy, a profound diuresis will occur. Heart failure is the only danger! If a CVP line is used, remember that a "normal pressure" (6–8 cmH$_2$O) can be heart failure in a severe preeclamptic. (Severe preeclamptic's CVP pressures are often zero or below.) Most studies of severe preeclampsia recognize that reduced blood volume is inherent to its basic pathophysiology.[1-4] The debate concerns whether the reduced blood volume is the result or the etiology of preeclampsia. While some believe that reduced blood volume in preeclampsia is secondary to the hypertension resulting from increased vascular reactivity to pressors[5-7] or from defective prostaglandin synthesis[8,9] others hold that the reduced blood volume, or more correctly, the failure to adequately increase blood volume as seen in normal pregnancy is at least part of the fundamental etiology of preeclampsia. According to this latter concept of reduced blood volume, if the gravida fails to expand her blood volume for any reason, there occurs a hypoperfusion or "chronic shock" like state as evidenced by a high hematocrit, a central venous pressure of −7 to 0 cmH$_2$O without hypotension or tachycardia.[10-13] This results in the compensatory vasoconstriction leading to hypertension, organ ischemia and perhaps microangiopathic disorders. If diuresis does not occur after two units of albumin, restudy the patient and discontinue the expander.

5. Cross-match for blood.
D. Postpartum care—Patient's course is often unrelated to prepartum course; i.e., mild may be severe or vice versa
   1. Use minimal amounts of oxytocin and avoid ergot preparations.
   2. Maintain anticonvulsant therapy until diuresis occurs.
   3. Arrange hypertensive workup if not typical preeclampsia.

References

1. Freis, E., and Kenney, J. F.: *J Clin Invest* **27**: 288, 1948.
2. Blekta, M., *et al.*: *Am J Obstet Gynecol* **106**: 10, 1970.
3. Smith, T. W.: *Am J Obstet Gynecol* **107**: 983, 1970.
4. Hytten, E.: *Diagnostic Indices of Pregnancy.* 1973. pp. 36–37.
5. Page, E. W.: *J Obstet Gynaecol Br Cwlth* **79**: 883, 1972.
6. Gant, N. F., *et al.*: *J Clin Invest* **52**: 2682, 1973.
7. Vorne, M. S., *et al.*: *Am J Obstet Gynecol* **119**: 610, 1974.
8. Speroff, L.: *Am J Cardiol* **32**: 582, 1973.
9. Rankin, J. H.: *Obstet Gynecol Survey* **31**: 710, 1976.
10. Cloeren, S., and Lippertt, *N Engl J Med* **287**: 1356, 1972.
11. Cloeren, S. E., Lippertt, H., and Hinselmann, M.: *Arch Gynakol* **215**: 129, 1973.
12. Hay, D.: *J Obstet Gynaecol Cwlth* **80**: 280, 1974.
13. Goodlin, R. C.: *Am J Obstet Gynecol* **125**: 747, 1976.

Inhibition of Preterm Labor Protocol

I. *Evaluation*
1) No maternal contraindications such as: heart disease, moderate–severe hypertension, preeclampsia, fever.
2) No fetal contraindications such as: erythroblastosis, IUGR, hydramnios, fetal death, abruptio, infection, placental insufficiency.
3) The patient must have contractions <10 min apart and >30 sec duration, with a cervix <4 cm dilated (if multip. <50% effaced).
4) Do Tocolysis score; record in chart.

II. *Short-Term Inhibition—<48 hr, EFW >1000-<1500 g*
1) Bed rest in lateral position.
2) I.V. fluids—1000 cc Ringers at 200 cc/hr (to decrease ADH).
3) Sedation; Phenobarbital 60 mg
             Valium   10 mg   I.M.
4) Start prophylactic antibiotics (Ampicillin 1 g q 6 hr)—to reduce chorioamnionitis.
5) Avoid Demerol, morphine, vasoconstrictors, antihistamines.
6) Limit cervical exams! (Ferguson reflex and infection).
7) Consider Dexamethasone Protocol if patient 28–33 weeks pregnant.
8) External monitoring of FHR and uterine activity.
9) DRUG THERAPY [OBTAIN INFORMED CONSENT FOR ALL DRUGS—NONE ARE APPROVED]
   a) *I.V. Alcohol* (9½%), inhibits oxytocin release—maternal and fetal side effects may be severe.
   Loading dose: 7.5 ml/kg/hr for 2 hr
   Maintenance dose: 1.5 ml/kg/hr for 10 hr or more.
   b) May *consider* beta mimetic therapy— see below.

III. *LONG-TERM INHIBITION (>48 hr)*
EFW <1000 g or after cerclage.
1) Follow procedures in Section II above, but delete steroid therapy.
2) Get Tocolysis score. If >7, *do not use* inhibitors.
3) DRUG THERAPY
   a) *Alcohol* poor choice for inhibition of labor on a long-term basis.
   b) *Beta mimetic drugs* (inhibit uterine contractions and increase uterine blood flow.)
     (1) Isoxsuprine (Vasodilan) (80 mgm isoxsuprine in 500 cc of D5.2NS)
       (a) Prehydrate the patient with 500 cc of crystalloid solution over 30–45 min.
       (b) Initial dose—0.25–0.5 mg/min (1.5–3 cc/min).
       (c) Dosage may be increased every 10–15 min up to 0.75–1.0 mg/min.
       (d) After 2 hr of desired response, wean patient from isoxsuprine by gradually decreasing intravenous infusion.
       (e) Then give 10 mg IM q 3–6 hr for next 12–24 hr.
       (f) Then give 10–20 mg, orally q.i.d. for next 72 hr. If no further irritability or contractions, the drug may be discontinued.
       (g) Maternal BP and pulse q 15 min during infusion. This drug may cause maternal hypotension and maternal and fetal tachycardia. Subjective maternal increase in heart rate almost always occurs in dosages over 0.5 mg/min.

The fetal heart rate increase of 10–20 bpm is less predictable.

Severe hypotension, requiring cessation of the drug, will occur in less than 2% of patients *if* the mother is well-hydrated before and during the infusion, if there is no antecedent hypertension and if the mother is kept on her side. If severe hypotension occurs, the FHR may *decrease*. If severe hypotension occurs, stop infusion, rapidly infuse additional fluid, and place patient in the lateral decubitus position.

Propranolol given by very slow intravenous infusion is an immediate antagonist in patients with severe complications.

(2) Terbutaline (Bricanyl)
  (a) Prehydrate patient with 500 cc crystalloid over 30–45 min prior to injection of terbutaline.
  (b) 250 μg subcutaneously q 6 hr.
  (c) Simultaneous oral terbutaline 5 mg t.i.d.
  (d) Oral dose may be maintained until 35 weeks of pregnancy.
  (e) Record maternal blood pressure every 15 min for the first hour and every hour for 8 hr after starting therapy. This drug causes maternal and fetal tachycardia (both a 30% increase approximately). Occasionally, maternal hypotension may occur. These symptoms have not necessitated discontinuing terbutaline (Ingemarsson, *Am J Obstet Gynecol* **125:** 520, 1976) but propranolol given very slowly intravenously is an immediate antagonist in patients with severe complications.

(3) 12–80 μg/min—average 30 μg/min (max. 150 μg/min) as aerosol. The usual single dose is two to three inhalations. With repetitive dosing, inhalation should usually not be repeated more often than about every 3–4 hours. Total dosage per day should not exceed *12 inhalations*. Side effects and overdose treatment as in (1) above.

IV. *STOP INHIBITION OF LABOR IF:*
  1) Cx >5 cm.
  2) Contractions continue or increase.
  3) Excessive maternal–fetal side effects occur.
  4) PROM with fetus <800 g or 26 weeks.

Reference

Chez, R. A.: In *Intrauterine Asphyxia and the Developing Fetal Brain*, L. Gluck, Ed. Year Book, Chicago, 1977.

Tocolysis Score

	0	1	2	3	4
Contraction	—	Irreg.	Regular	—	—
PROM	—	—	High or ?	—	Low
Bleeding	—	Spotting, Mod. Bleed	Severe bleed	—	—
Cervical dilation	—	1	2	3	≥4

Probability of stopping labor 1 week with betamimetics

Score	1	2	3	4	5	6	≥7
% Labor stopped	100%	90%	84%	38%	11%	7%	Never

Baumgarten—*4th Perinatal Congress*, 1975.

VI. *Current Overall Survival Rate for Prematures*

Survival	Rare	50%	82%	94%	99+	99+
g	<900	901–1000	1001–1500	1501–2000	2001–2500	>2500
weeks	<26	20–27	28–31	32–34	35–36	>36

VII. *Cesarean Section of Prematures*
   1) CS for premies less than 33 weeks—requires classical vertical or high transverse incision. (There is no lower uterine segment.) This mandates a recommendation for repeat CS in the future.
   2) PROM more than 24 hr increases CS morbidity. If patient *afebrile*, should use prophylactic antibiotic treatment (see PROM PROTOCOL). If patient *febrile*, CS contraindicated for prematurity *alone*.
   3) CS complications:
      Anesthesia
      Hemorrhage—about 20%
      Infection
   4) Vaginal delivery indicated for poor surgical risks or inability to give informed consent.

VIII. *Vaginal Delivery of Prematures*
   1) The current concept of utilizing conduction anesthesia and low outlet forceps has been disputed, although it is our present recommendation.
   2) Watch for early fetal distress (*poorly* tolerated)—use scalp pH freely.

Premature Delivery Protocol

I. *Evaluate pregnancy on the following criteria:*
 (A) Estimated gestational age—LMP (oral contraceptive use?)
 (B) Fundal size (+/− PROM)
 (C) B-scan for BPD
 (D) Evidence for IUGR—hypertension, previous small infants, severe diabetes mellitus

II. *Obtain these studies:*
 (A) B-scan
 (B) Or Fetogram to rule out multiple gestation, gross congenital anomalies, malpresentation, oligohydramnios
 (C) Abdominal or vaginal amniotic fluid sample—L/S ratio, creatinine, amylase, leukocyte count
 (D) If PROM—follow *PROTOCOL*
 (E) If premature labor—follow *PROTOCOL*

III. *Delivery mode of Singleton Vertex:*
 (A) Less than 28 weeks—DELIVER WITH CONDUCTION ANESTHESIA
 (B) 28–32 weeks (1000–1300 g)—give parents informed consent re: *possibility* of increased survival with a cesarean section (CS) versus need for classical type scar + repeat CS. See Section VI
 (C) 33–36 weeks (1300–2500 g)—deliver vaginally with epidural
 (D) More than 36 weeks—treat as term delivery (except for Class A–C D.M.)

IV. *Delivery mode Singleton Breech*—follow *BREECH PROTOCOL*

V. *Delivery mode Multiple Gestations:*
 (A) If first infant breech—get B-scan to check equality of BPD's and follow *BREECH PROTOCOL*
 (B) If first infant vertex—follow *SINGLETON VERTEX PROTOCOL*

Premature Rupture of the Membranes Protocol

Evaluation

1. Patients between 28–34 weeks or EFW 1000–1800 g.
2. Time of rupture by history.
3. Forewaters present—consider as threatened premature.
4. Do sterile vaginal exam—*ONE TIME ONLY*
   (a) Ferning test
   (b) Culture of cervix
   (c) Vaginal fluid for L/S ratio, Cr. amylase—repeat 24 hr after corticosteroids last given.

Therapy

1. Inhibit labor—See "Inhibition of Pre-term Labor" Protocol.

2. Antibiotics—Give broad-spectrum coverage—Ampicillin (Ancef), 1 g I.V. q 6 hr. (Attempt to inhibit deciduitis, fetal pneumonia.)
3. Corticosteroids—obtain patient consent for experimental use (long- and short-range fetal effects not known). Dexamethasone 12 mg I.M. every 12 hr apart X2 doses, or Betamethasone 6 mgm. I.M. every 12 hr ×2 doses. Contraindicated in toxemia, infection. Repeat L/S ratio 24 hr after last dose of steroids.

Delivery

1. Deliver if L/S mature, patient febrile, amnionitis or fetal distress occur.
2. If vertex—"Premature Delivery" Protocol.
3. If breech—"Premature Breech" Protocol.

Prolonged Pregnancy

General: Certain characteristics of pregnancies in excess of 42½ weeks' menstrual age, if present, should alert the clinician to the need to intercede by induction of labor or cesarean section. Studies should be initiated in patients after the 14th to 16th day post due date to define those patients at risk. Pregnancies exceeding 43 weeks' gestation are at increased risk for fetal or neonatal death. (R/O fetal anomalies, i.e., anencephaly.)

Definitions:

1. *Prolonged pregnancy*—pregnancy in excess of 17 days beyond EDC.
2. *Post-datism*—Same as 1.

3. *Postmaturity*—a syndrome occurring in a *small* percentage of prolonged pregnancies. Characteristics: scant and/or meconium-stained amniotic fluid; an infant with long nails, desquamating epidermis, abundant scalp hair with decreased or absent lanugo hair, and alert (wide-eyed stare) appearance. In severe cases, the skin, cord, and nails are stained a yellowish-brown color.
4. *Dysmaturity*—Same as 3, except that fetus shows symptoms anytime after 35 weeks.

Incidence: Variably reported between 3.5 and 14% of sample. *Prospective* study of Beischer *et al.* (*Am J Obstet Gynecol* **103:** 467–504) which was very carefully structured, gave an incidence of 11.4%.

FLOW SHEET FOR ACTION OF AT-RISK GROUP FOR DYSMATURITY OR POSTMATURITY

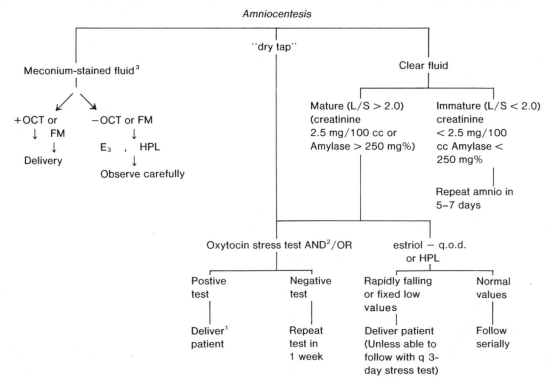

Selection of Potential Risk Group: Careful determination of EDC and Doppler FHR before 12 weeks. (a) Correlation of LMP with uterine size may be helpful in early weeks (but there is much variation). (b) Withdrawal bleed from oral contraceptives in the "last menstrual period" will frequently overestimate the gestational age of the pregnancy:

1. Cases of prolonged pregnancy (17 days or over).
2. Cases of intrauterine growth retardation with no apparent cause (dysmature).
3. Cases of suspected oversized (macrosomia) fetus (> 4000 g) post-EDC.
4. Cases of elderly primagravida at 7 days post-EDC.
5. Cases of chronic hypertension, "mild" preeclampsia, or chronic renal disease (This latter group is ideally delivered at 37–40 weeks if the cervix is favorable.)

Tests [(Begin whenever suspect "dysmaturity" or postdatism (42 weeks)]:

1. HPL
2. Estriol
3. Amnioscopy or amniocentesis
4. Oxytocin stress test. (With the dysmature fetus, "variable" FHR decelerations are probably ominous.)
5. Fetal movements (give patient flow sheet).
6. If possible (i.e., diabetics, hypertensives) do B-scan in second trimester and repeat at six weeks.

Notations:

1. Induction of labor should only be done with a "favorable" cervix *and* availability of continuous fetal heart rate monitoring and fetal acid–base studies. Cesarean section is the safest approach as concerns the fetus if unable to provide continuous monitoring.
2. With estriol and HPL determinations in dysmature fetuses, the correlation with fetal distress in labor has been a significant one. The oxytocin challenge test (or attempted induction) is an appropriate approach. The greatest risk to the postdate fetus is in labor. The oxytocin stress test is repeated every three days in rapidly falling or fixed low estriol or HPL values, and the stress test is used as the final criterion for interruption of the pregnancy.
3. Some clinicians favor cesarean section with meconium-stained fluid to preclude meconium aspiration pneumonitis.

Intrapartum Fetal Distress

I. PURPOSE

Labor room personnel should be able to:

A. Recognize by review of the prenatal record mothers who are at high risk of having complications of labor and delivery.

B. Use electronic fetal monitoring equipment.

C. Recognize labor patterns, FHR changes, and other signs indicating possible fetal distress.

D. Initiate immediate steps in management of fetal distress as outlined below.

II. PREPARATION

A. Review of Prenatal Record.

The labor room personnel should review the Prenatal Record and note on the Obstetrical Labor Admission Record high risk factors such as the following (hopefully these factors will have been recognized by the prenatal staff):

1. Antepartum.

a. Maternal factors of importance in the obstetrical population, rather than to the individual:

(1) Height under 5 ft. 2 in. (whites).

(2) Weight <100, >200 lbs.

(3) Age: Primigravida <16, >30 years.
Multipara >35 years.

(4) Parity >5.

b. Maternal factors that are specific for this patient:

(1) Medical complications.

(a) Anemia-Hg <9.5 g.

(b) Addiction to drugs.*

(c) Diabetes.*

(d) Hyperthyroidism.*

(e) Hypertensive disease including preeclampsia.

(f) Renal disease.*

(g) Heart disease.*

(h) Severe pulmonary disease.*

(i) Other.

(2) Past obstetrical history.

(a) Infertility.

(b) Previous stillborn.

(c) Previous neonatal death.

(d) Previous abruptio or placenta previa.*

(e) Previous cesarean section.

(f) Other.

(3) Obstetrical problems in this pregnancy.

(a) Bleeding (note weeks of gestation when bleeding occurred).*

(b) Abnormal clinical or x-ray pelvimetry.

(c) Other.

c. Fetal.

(1) Prematurity (Labor before 36 weeks).

(2) Small-for-dates infant.

(3) Post-dates (labor after 42 weeks).

(4) Excessive size infant.*

(5) Rh isoimmunization.*

(6) Multiple pregnancy.*

(7) Malpresentation.*

(8) Hydramnios.*

(9) Prolonged rupture of membranes (over 12 hr before labor).

(10) Antepartum monitoring abnormalities.

(a) Estriol, − values 50%.*

(b) Human placental lactogen, − values <4.

(c) Oxytocin stress test, positive or suspicious test.

(d) Amniotic fluid.

* Of particular concern.

     i. L/S ratio <2.
     ii. Meconium, especially before 36 weeks.
     iii. Creatinine <2 mg%.
  (11) Other.

B. Preparation for Electronic Monitoring.

If the patient is in active labor, the nurse should start external fetal monitoring as soon as possible. The physician may order "no monitoring" in instances in which the inconvenience or risks are judged to outweigh the benefits.

If there are more patients in active labor than can be monitored using all available equipment, priority should be given to mothers with:

1. Medical and obstetrical high-risk factors (see above).
2. Fetal high-risk factors (see above).
3. Regional or paracervical block anesthesia.
4. Oxytocin infusions.
5. Active labor (versus early labor).

III. PROCEDURE

A. Recognition of Intrapartum High-Risk Factors.
1. Maternal.
   a. Labor onset <36 weeks or >42 weeks.
   b. Vaginal bleeding of more than a "bloody show"
   c. Fever (over 37.5°C).
   d. Abnormal labor pattern (Obstetrical Labor Graphic Record).

	Nullipara	*Multipara*
(1) Prolonged latent phase.	>20 hr	>15 hr
(2) Protracted active phase.	<1.2 cm/hr	<1.5 cm/hr
(3) Secondary arrest of dilatation (no progress in active phase).	>2 hr	>2 hr
(4) Prolonged deceleration phase.	>3 hr	>1 hr
(5) Prolonged descent.	<1 cm/hr	<2 cm/hr

	Nullipara	*Multipara*
(6) Arrest of descent (2nd stage).	>1 hr	>1 hr

2. Fetal
   a. Meconium in amniotic fluid.
   b. Fetal heart rate abnormalities detected by auscultation during and after contraction.

B. Use of Electronic Fetal Monitor.
1. Starting Monitoring:

Labor room personnel should be familiar with the use of the Hewlett Packard, Berkeley, Corometrics, and other monitoring equipment used in the delivery suite.

External monitoring (abdominal pressure and ultrasound) should be used unless the fetal signals are unsatisfactory. Labor room personnel who have received special instruction and have been observed by the Director may apply scalp electrodes upon order by the responsible physician.

Baseline tracings should be obtained before oxytocin and before regional or paracervical anesthesia when possible.

2. Recognition of Abnormalities.

Many abnormal FHR patterns are iatrogenic (supine position, oxytocin, PCB or epidural block). Parturients without anesthesia, on their sides and without oxytocin have very few FHR abnormalities.

a. Abnormal Baseline.
   (1) Beat-to-beat variability (normal 7–14 bpm)
       (a) Increased—>15 bpm.
       (b) Decreased—<5 bpm (may be sleep, sedation or mild depression).
       (c) Absent (may be sedation, asleep or severe depression).
   (2) Rate (normal 120–160 bpm)
       (a) Tachycardia—>160.
       (b) Bradycardia—<100.
b. Acute bradycardia
   (1) Delayed recovery, gradual onset (late deceleration or type II).
   (2) Acute, severe (variable).
3. Immediate management of fetal heart rate abnormalities.
   a. Always check for prolapsed umbilical cord.

* Of particular concern.

b. Position patient on her side. If already on side, then change to other side.
c. Stop oxytocin.
d. Give oxygen by mask.
e. Check maternal BP and P.
f. Notify responsible physician.
    (1) Ask physician for order to start electronic fetal monitoring if not being done.
    (2) Prepare for fetal scalp pH determination.
    (3) Prepare for a potential cesarean section. (2 units of blood, CBC, permits, abdominal prep).

If responsible physician is not immediately available and placenta previa has not been suspected, do vaginal examination to check for umbilical cord prolapse, meconium, or blood. If umbilical cord is palpable, hold fetal presenting part out of pelvis adequately to allow cord pulsation. Continue to do this until relieved of the responsibility.

IV. CHARTING
  A. Nursing Responsibility.
     On the tracing from the monitor, attach a gummed label stamped with the patient's card (name, record number, etc.). Note the date and time of starting tracing, type of monitor (HP, Corometric, etc.), type of FHR recorder (abdominal, scalp), contraction recorder (abdominal, catheter), paper speed. Note any change in these conditions and any conditions which affect tracing such as position change, amniotomy, drugs, oxytocin, anesthetics, full dilation, pushing, transfer to delivery room. Note bleeding or meconium.
  B. On the Fetal Monitoring Report, check the indications for monitoring and initial this entry.
  C. An ignored or improperly functioning fetal monitor is worse than no monitor. The FHR record should be initialed every 30 min by the responsible nurse. FHR monitoring paper is expensive and difficult to store. The slow paper speeds are therefore preferred if the FHR recordings are normal. Most of the FHR recordings may be discarded so that all notating "for the record" should also be made on labor progress record.

V. PRINCIPLES OF MONITORING
  A. With maximum interference of labor, most FHR abnormalities will be iatrogenic.
  B. Most fetuses with anomalies incompatible with extrauterine life will have signs of fetal distress during labor.
  C. True fetal distress is rare (FHR abnormalities plus acidemia), about 4/1000 deliveries. Monitoring should, therefore, be without complications.
  D. Except for "terminal" FHR patterns (prolonged bradycardia and loss of B-B variability) or cord prolapse, *no* FHR pattern by itself is diagnostic of fetal distress.
  E. All cases of suspected fetal distress should be confirmed by scalp pH.
  F. When performing scalp pH, two samples should be obtained within 15 min. A maternal pH (dorsum of hand or anticubical vein) should be done simultaneously. If abnormal FHR persists, scalp pH should be repeated every 20 min as long as above 7.25. With a normal maternal pH and a scalp pH below 7.20 × 2, fetal distress is presumably present and the fetus should be delivered as soon as possible. (Modified from Stanford University Hospital Protocol, R. Cauwet, M.D., 1975.)

Protocol for Prevention of Meconium Aspiration

In order to prevent substantial meconium aspiration of the neonate, there has been some evidence that suction of the naso-oral pharynx prior to delivery of the shoulder can eliminate the presence of meconium below the vocal cords.

Proposal:

All fetuses that exhibit meconium stained amniotic fluid will have their nasal and oropharynx suctioned by a soft, polyethylene catheter once the head has been delivered *prior* to delivery of the anterior shoulder.

Method:

A floor suction unit will be situated next to the delivery table and connected to a small pediatric suction catheter which will be given to the obstetrician over the patient's draped leg in a sterile manner. The suction catheter will then be gently inserted in the fetus's mouth and nose and gentle suction accomplished prior to delivery of the shoulder. Not more than 30 seconds should be spent on this procedure.

Follow-up:

The newborn should be given immediately to the pediatrician in the labor and delivery room, who will then proceed with normal intubation and with documentation of presence of meconium below the vocal cords.

References

Gregory, G. A., *et al.*: *J Pediat* **85:** 848, 1974.
Carson, V. S., *et al.*: *Am J Obstet Gynecol* **126:** 712, 1976.

IV Oxytocin for Induction or Augmentation of Labor

I. PURPOSE

The intravenous route for administration of an oxytocic medication is used to induce or augment labor. IM or buccal routes for oxytocin are not permitted.

On the order of a physician, the nurse in the delivery room may initiate, monitor and adjust the flow rate of intavenous oxytocin for induction or augmentation of labor.

II. EQUIPMENT

A. IV tray (includes oxytocic medication).
B. IV stand.
C. IV solution—5% dextrose in Ringer's lactate, 1000 ml.
D. Electronic infusion pump.
E. Labor record.

III. PROCEDURE

A. Oxytocin infusion may be initiated only on the order of a member of the obstetrical staff. Before starting the infusion, be certain the responsible physician has examined the patient, has filled out the Admission Examination section of the Obstetrical Labor Admission Record. Record on the Progress of Labor Record the responsible physician or his designated substitute who must be immediately available to manage any complications.

B. Start the IV infusion with an intravenous catheter and then add the correct dosage of oxytocin to the bottle. The concentration should be 1.0 ml (10 U) of oxytocin/1000 of 5% dextrose in lactated Ringer's unless otherwise specifically ordered. Shake bottle gently to mix solution evenly. Keep the patient on her side.

C. Attach electronic pump or flow control meter to IV apparatus. Regulate so that oxytocin solution is begun at 1 mU/min or at the rate ordered by the responsible physician.

D. Fill out and attach to IV bottle a label which states:
1. Name and amount of oxytocic agent and the amount of fluid in the bottle to which it was added (concentration).
2. Date and time started.
3. Initials of person who prepared solution.
4. Number of IV bottle (1st, 2nd, etc., given to patient).

E. Remain with the patient for at least 15 min to evaluate labor pattern and FHR. Every 10 min thereafter, note the following on the Obstetrical Labor Graphic Record:
1. Strength, duration, and frequency of contractions.
2. FHR by auscultation or electronic monitor. FHR monitoring by auscultation should be done only if electronic monitoring is not feasible or not acceptable to the patient.
3. Any change in rate of oxytocin infusion in milliunits per minute.

F. Change in infusion rate or concentration: The rate of IV infusion should be adjusted to establish a progressive labor pattern at approximate 15 min intervals by doubling the dosage. Once labor is established, reduce the amount to approximately ⅔ or ½ of highest rate. If contractions then are insufficient, return to higher rate. For most elective inductions or augmentations, it will not be necessary to exceed 10 milliunits of oxytocin per minute. If the drip rate reaches 8 mU/min, notify the responsible physician.

G. The infusion should be decreased to the slowest possible rate or discontinued and the physician notified by the charge nurse under the following conditions:

1. Excessive uterine response: Increase in baseline tonus, peak contraction duration 60 sec, contraction frequency <2 min.
2. Precipitate labor.
3. FHR abnormalities (See Fetal Distress).
4. Apparent overdosage (decreasing uterine activity with increasing dosage).

IV. CHARTING

A. On the Intake and Output Record, chart the IV solution and amount as well as the name and dosage of oxytocic drug added.

B. On the Obstetrical Vital Signs Record, record FHR every 15 min during the first stage and every 5 min during the second stage if FHR is not electronically monitored.

C. On the Obstetrical Labor Graphic Record, record every 15 min the frequency and duration of contractions. Record any change in rate of oxytocic agent infusion in milliunits of oxytocin per minute and any vaginal exams for dilatation of cervix. This form is to be kept at the bedside.

Oxytocin Stress Test
(Oxytocin Contraction Test)

General: The oxytocin fetal stress test is yet another test for assessment of the utero–placental–fetal unit. Simultaneous recording of uterine contractions and fetal heart-rate pattern are made while Syntocinon is given intravenously to stimulate the stress of labor. Thus the reponse of the fetus to this stress helps to evaluate the function of the utero–placental–fetal unit and the fetus' ability to tolerate labor and/or continuation of the intrauterine environment.

Specifically, the test is being used to aid in the selection of the optimal delivery time and the route of delivery. The test itself is simple, the length of time the test required is over 2 hr average and a physician should be in attendance.

A. *Objective*: To test the respiratory reserve of the fetus, i.e., whether abnormal fetal heart rate patterns occur after minimal fetal stimuli.

B. *Current Clinical Application*: Assessment of fetal–placental well-being in
  1. Toxemias
    a. Chronic hypertension
    b. Chronic renal disease
    c. Diabetes mellitus
    d. Hypertensive disease of pregnancy (preeclampsia)
    e. Severe isoimmune sensitization
  2. Postdatism (over 42 weeks). Particularly important if associated with intra-uterine growth retardation.
  3. Intrauterine growth retardation—small for gestational age (SFD).
  4. Maternal hypoxia syndromes:
    a. Maternal cyanotic heart disease
    b. Sickle cell anemia
    c. Maternal chronic lung disease

Indications: Selection of optimal delivery time in above conditions (see interpretation of results, below).

Complications: Those attendant with any intravenous infusion of an oxytocic. The onset of labor may be precipitated with a responsive uterus, bleeding, amnionitis, and so forth.

Procedure:

1. Consultation guidelines
  a. The test is to be performed ONLY after evaluation of the patient's history and physical findings by a staff member.
2. Materials and Equipment
  a. Butterfly needle—catheter (#19 Ga.)
  b. Infusion pump with one ampule of oxytocin in 1000 0.9% NaCl (NS) or equivalent to prime the pump.
  c. External fetal heart rate monitor equipment. Abdominal ECG (best) for microphone or Doppler (least desirable).

C. *Technique:*

1. Using external monitor (ECG, microphone or Doppler), obtain FHR with best beat to beat detection that is possible. This is most important!
2. Observe recordings for at least 30 min to determine whether spontaneous uterine activity is occurring. If uterine contractions occur at rate of 2–3 per 10 min, this is adequate and NO OXYTOCIN is required.
3. If inadequate uterine activity is occurring spontaneously, begin IV oxytocin infusion; start at 1 mU per 5 minutes and double dose every 15 minutes (*maximum* is 8 mU) until contractions occur. *Consult with staff* if oxytocin infusion must go above 8 mU. Once contractions have occurred at desired frequency, stop the infusion.

D. *Interpretations:*

1. a. If FHR transducer can be adequately applied, then a beat-to-beat variability of 6+% over 1 min time, or if bouts of

acceleration of FHR occur, no stress test is probably required.

   b. If no decelerations of FHR occur, the test is negative.

   c. If severe type II (late, delayed recovery, etc.) occur after more than 50% of uterine contractions, test is positive. If occur less than 50%, test is suspicious. With type II, the minimal but prolonged recovery of FHR is considered the most ominous.

2. a. If test is negative, it can be repeated in 1 week.

   b. If test is suspicious, repeat next day or so.

   c. If test is positive, test amniotic fluid, E_3, HPL, fetal movement, etc. The majority of positive tests in the absence of other abnormal findings, will be negative when repeated.

Pitfalls to Avoid:

1. Maternal position—some fetuses will have a positive test if their mother is forced to maintain the flat, supine position over a prolonged period of time. In other words, avoid the maternal, supine, flat position.

3. Despite claims from Los Angeles, most every other institution has had high-risk fetuses die soon after a "negative" OCT test. It may be that we cannot duplicate the expertise available at USC, or whatever; but never assume that all will be well for the fetus for the next week because its OCT test was "negative."

4. Do not induce labor prematurely, cause a placenta previa to bleed or otherwise compromise the health of the fetus with an OCT. The gravida must always be examined and evaluated prior to beginning and after terminating an OCT.

5. An extended OCT is an attempt at elective induction and a decision must be made at 4–5 hr (after uterine contractions have begun) as to whether the gravida will be delivered that day. If delivery does not seem likely, discontinue the oxytocin infusion. Do not continue oxytocin infusions over prolonged periods (6–8 hr plus) without indications for delivery.

Records to be Kept: Record in high-risk pregnancy book and in prenatal chart.

1. Indication for test
2. Pertinent physical findings
3. Date of test and weeks' gestation of pregnancy
4. Notation as to whether test was read as negative or positive *and who read the tracing.*

Exercise Stress Test

A. *Purpose*

This is a technique which may uncover marginal maternal–placental perfusion by stressing the mother via a standardized exercise test. It is believed that especially the patient with vascular disease (toxemia, hypertension), post-term dysmaturity, and intrauterine growth retardation (SGA) may have marginal placental perfusion which will be revealed by maternal exercise (Hon, E. H.: *Am J Obstet Gynecol* **87:** 814, 1963).

B. *Method*

Patients selected for the EST will have a *standard NST performed* for 30 min.
1. Blood presure and pulse on admission
2. Semi-Fowler or lateral position
3. Best external monitor for FHR variability possible
4. Recording of fetal movement
Then the patient is asked to perform a *3-min* exercise test (modified from Masters, 1968) and have the number of trips *recorded*.
1. The steps will be placed near a wall (for patient security).
2. The patient will turn *toward* the EST nurse after each trip to avoid dizziness.
3. After 3 min, the patient will return to the bed, fetal heart monitor will be placed, and maternal heart rate and pulse will be recorded.
4. If the postexercise FHR is *different* from the pre-exercise rate (change in absolute rate or variability) the staff will be notified *immediately*. Monitoring will continue for 20 min *or* until all abnormality has disappeared.

Use of Fetal Scalp Capillary Blood pH in Assessment of Fetal Distress in Labor

Goals

1. Aid in the detection of fetal distress and selection of mode of delivery.
2. Reduce number of "unnecessary cesarean sections" or difficult forceps for "fetal distress."

Basic Assumptions

1. No single parameter now available is 100% reliable as an indicator of fetal distress.
2. Electronic fetal heart rate monitors have increased our ability to detect fetal distress, but have a high incidence of "false positive" results.
3. Fetal scalp blood sampling is reasonably safe, technically simple and inexpensive.
4. The combination of electronic FHR monitoring as a screening procedure and fetal capillary pH as a "confirmatory test" will result in fewer immediate terminations of lab.

History of Fetal Scalp Blood pH Determination

First proven practical by Saling in 1961.
Flurry of clinical papers late 1960s.
   Proved impractical as a screening procedure.
   "Distress" FHR >160 or <120 or meconium 77% of patient's pH >7.26; however, pH <7.26 statistically related to Apgar <6.
Scalp pH and umbilical vein pH were very closely related.
pH <7.20 53% required vigorous resuscitation.
pH >7.20 8% required vigorous resuscitation.
Most of these were traumatic deliveries.

Important Points

pH in early labor is almost invariably normal.
pH only reflects fetal condition at the time it is obtained.
pH naturally falls slightly during labor and especially during 2nd stage.

Procedure for Obtaining Fetal Blood Sample

1. Examine patient and determine that membranes are ruptured and cervix is at least 2 cm dilated.
2. Insert largest endoscope which will fit the cervix and hold firmly against fetal presenting part (not so tight as to cause stasis).
3. Attach light to endoscope. (For convenience, place light at top of endoscope.)
4. Clean scalp with sponge. (Vigorous cleansing helps produce hyperemia.)
5. Spray scalp with ethyl chloride to produce blanching.
6. Swab scalp with mineral oil or silicone grease.
7. Puncture scalp with blade. Single, clean puncture is best, preferably at upper area of visible scalp. If multiple punctures necessary to produce adequate bleeding, make them close together and to a point.
8. Using glass capillary with attached mouthpiece, collect sample of fetal blood from drop on scalp. Avoid air. If air bubble occurs, expel it against scalp and then resume sampling.
9. When approximately 10 cm sample of blood obtained, placed stirrer inside capillary, seal with clay and mix with magnet.
10. After sample obtained, hold pressure on puncture site with sponge through one contraction. Observe for bleeding through two more contractions.

Normal Values

pH >7.25 is normal
pH <7.20 indicates fetal acidemia
pH <7.25 and >7.20 is "preacidosis" and must be followed with repeat samples.
OBTAIN SIMULTANEOUS MATERNAL pH to eliminate maternal acidemia as an etiology.

Complications

Scalp abscess 3/687 infants (1200 sample)
Significant hemorrhage 3/687 infants (1200 sample)
Blade breakage—if twisted during sampling (2 cases reported)

Sources of Error

Slow drop formation. Slow loss of CO_2 with rise in pH.
If formation in <5 seconds; no significant loss of CO_2
Caput: if severe, may lead to false low pH.

Fetal Scalp Blood Tray, Contents:

1 175 mm Endoscope (Rocket of London)
1 130 mm Endoscope (Rocket of London)
1 blade holder (Rocket of London)
1 ring forceps
2 towels
4 "cherry" sponges
1 vial of mineral oil (pharmacy)
1 medium glass—for mineral oil

Small Tray for Light–Cold Sterilizing Solution

Supply Tray, Contents:

List of tray contents
Copy of procedure for fetal scalp blood sampling
Battery box (Rocket of London)
Supply of capillary tubes (Rocket of London)
Mouth piece
Metal stirrers (Rocket of London)
Magnet (Rocket of London)
Bottle of ethyl chloride (hospital pharmacy)
Crito-o-Seal

Protocol for Home-style Delivery System

Requirements for Enrollment in Homestyle Delivery Program

1. Patient should request this type of delivery and do so prior to her 22nd week of pregnancy.
2. She should be in excellent health.
3. She and her "mate" must be advised that this form of delivery may have increased risks and complications to both herself and her infant, including death.
4. If the gravida is followed by the obstetrical service, she should enroll in the Family Practice Clinic prior to delivery for continuing care of the infant.
5. All gravida must enroll in and complete classes for childbirth preparation, nutritional counseling and care of newborns, in addition to regular prenatal care.
6. At least one home visit by the program's nurse practitioner or the physician following the gravida shall be made prior to delivery to assure adequate home preparation.
7. The gravida must be of low risk (antenatal Goodwin score of one or less) or be approved by the obstetrical staff.
8. She shall sign forms requesting this program and which state that she does not want intravenous therapy, electronic fetal monitoring, or significant pain relief unless absolutely necessary and that such would require removal from the home-style delivery program.
9. It must be understood that at any point in the prenatal course or during labor the attending physician or the obstetrical staff have the right to refuse the gravida home-style delivery if, in their judgment, she is no longer in a low-risk category.

Requirements Concerning Conduct of Labor and Delivery in the Homestyle Delivery Program

1. There will be available on a 24-hr basis obstetrical and nursery consultation services and facilities.
2. Labor and delivery will proceed in a specially prepared homestyle delivery room. If this room is unavailable, every attempt will be made to allow homestyle delivery in a regular labor room. However, no guarantee can be made that every patient will be able to use the home-style delivery room.
3. Hospital gowns may be worn by the physician and all others in attendance during labor and delivery. During the delivery itself, the physician and any assistants in the actual delivery will be gowned and scrubbed.
4. Vital signs will be taken and recorded in the usual fashion by the responsible physician or a nurse practitioner or a labor nurse if she is available as follows: temperature, pressure, and respirations q 4 hr; blood pressure q 2 hr; fetal heart tones q 30 min and q 5 min for 15 min when membranes rupture. Fetal heart tones should be checked more frequently during second stage and as otherwise indicated. The physician following the patient is ultimately responsible that these vital signs be recorded and taken as above.
5. The gravida must remain at low risk (see Goodwin score) during labor.
6. Clear liquids may be taken during labor.
7. The nursery and the OB service shall be notified when the gravida is admitted and again after delivery. If the patient is followed by the obstetrical service, the Family Practice resident on-call shall be notified prior to delivery.
8. Positions for labor and delivery are optional and shall be determined by the physician, nurse practitioner, and mother.
9. Analgesia shall be limited to a total of 150 mg Demerol or its equivalent. Anesthesia for delivery shall be restricted to local block.

Medication or anesthesia in addition to the above will require management in the regular labor and delivery room.

10. Use of oxytocin for augmentation or induction shall be managed in the regular labor room. Electronic fetal monitoring, if necessary, shall be done in the regular labor room.

11. Factors requiring removal from the home-style delivery technique include:
    (a) Blood pressure greater than 140/90 mmHg between contractions.
    (b) Inadequate progress of labor as defined by:
        (1) Second stage greater than 2 hr.
        (2) Active stage (primigravida) greater than 20 hr or active stage (multigravida) greater than 18 hr.
    (c) Maternal temperature greater than 38°C or evidence of infection.
    (d) Prolonged rupture of membranes.
    (e) Fetal heart rate abnormalities as determined with the fetoscope such as,
        (1) Tachycardia greater than 170 bpm.
        (2) Sustained bradycardia less than 90 beats per minute for greater than 60 sec.
        (3) Failure of fetal heart tones to return to the baseline 30 sec after the end of the contraction.
    (f) Episiotomy or a tear greater than second degree and/or significant vaginal wall or cervical tear shall be repaired in the delivery room, but do not necessarily require removal from rooming-in status.
    (g) Any presentation other than vertex.
    (h) Any delivery which is other than low forceps or spontaneous vaginal delivery will be acomplished in the delivery room.

12. Other factors such as excessive apprehension, fear, or inappropriate reactions on the part of visitors or the mother may, in the judgment of the physician or mother, require management in the regular labor room.

13. Resuscitation equipment for both the mother and the newborn must be available in or near the home-style delivery room.

Requirements for Care and Monitoring of the Newborn

1. A physician who has SMC nursery experience and/or who is approved by the director of the nursery shall perform a newborn physical examination within 2 hr of birth.

2. There shall be an infant record kept which includes the infant's physical examination, vital signs, and note of procedures done to the infant which can then become a part of the permanent infant record.

3. The infant shall have:
    (a) An Apgar score greater than or equal to 7 at 1 min and greater than or equal to 8 at 5 min.
    (b) Birth weight greater than 2500 g or less than 4300 g.
    (c) Normal physical examination as above.

4. The nursery shall be notified of the condition of the infant.

5. Vital signs to include temperature, heart rate, and respirations will be taken q hour times 4 or until stable and then q 6 hr. These are to be done by a physician or a nurse practitioner or other qualified nurses approved by the nursery staff. Stable vital signs are defined as temperature between 36.5 and 37.5, heart rate 100 to 160, respirations 30 to 60.

6. Blood type, Rh, and Coombs on cord blood is to be done if mother is type O or Rh negative.

7. NG suction is to be done at the time of the newborn physical examination to check for amount of gastric contents and continuity of the esophagus.

8. Hematocrit and dextrostix are to be done if the infant is symptomatic, pale, or plethoric.

9. Breast feeding may be initiated at delivery. If the infant is not breast fed, water and glucose shall be offered at 4 hr of age and formula may be offered at 8 hr of age. If mother is breast feeding, the breast must be cleaned in the usual fashion prior to suckling.

10. Silver nitrate eye drops and Vitamin K injections are to be given.

11. An OB nurse or a nurse practitioner must be in attendance at the delivery.

12. If maternal and infant vital signs are stable and the above criteria are met, rooming in the home-style delivery room or other available room will be continued.

Discharge Criteria for the Infant (Less than 24 hours)

1. Normal physical examination at the time of discharge to be done by nursery approved physician or nurse practitioner.

2. Vital signs stable for at least 4 hr with:

(a)temperature greater than 36.5, less than 37.5°C,
(b)heart rate 100–160,
(c)respirations 30–60,
(d)no excessive jaundice or central cyanosis,
(e)weight greater than 2500 g or less than 4300 g.
3. No evidence of blood type incompatibility.
4. At least one water feeding must have been tolerated well by the infant or the infant must be suckling well if breast fed.
5. The infant must void prior to discharge.
6. The mother must demonstrate ability to handle and care for the infant to the satisfaction of the nurse practitioner or physician.
7. Birth certificate signed.

Discharge Criteria for the Mother

1. Stable vital signs with:
   (a)temperature less than 38°C,
   (b)pulse less than 100,
   (c)blood pressure greater than 90/60 and less than 140/90.
2. Fundus firm with no excessive bleeding.
3. Ambulating well and able to care for infant.
4. Has voided.
5. Rhogam requirement has been determined and therapy instituted.

Requirements for Continuing Care

1. At least one home visit prior to delivery.
2. Daily checks on the mother's and child's status are to be done for the subsequent 72 hr by program approved nurse practitioner at home or in the Family Practice Clinic. At these times, whether at home or in the Clinic, appropriate tests will be performed and the responsible physician notified of the results. These will include PKU testing and routine laboratory tests in addition to vital signs and weights. A physician will be available for problems which arise on a 24-hr continuous basis.
3. Upon discharge, the mother will receive a checklist for observations on the infant. This will include instructions on observing the infant for respiratory patterns, cyanosis, jaundice, feeding problems, stooling (meconium must be passed within 36 hours or physician notified), voiding, and general activity.
4. There must be someone at home in addition to the mother who will be available on a live-in basis to manage the routine household activities and assist with care of the infant. There must be access to a telephone and immediate transportation.
5. Well-child care and postpartum checks will be arranged in the usual fashion.

SECTION THREE

Obstetrical Data

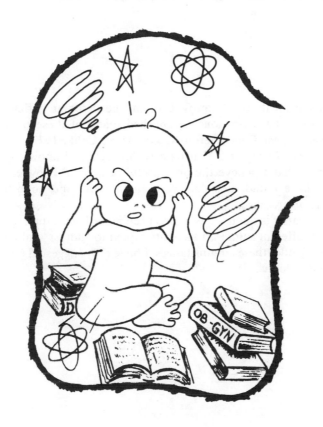

Preface to Obstetrical Data

The data section represents the outgrowth of my need for an efficient filing system of obstetrical information. I have previously published many of these tables in *Handbook of Obstetrical and Gynecological Data* (Geron-X, Los Altos, Calif., 1972). My past efforts have been criticized; it has been suggested that data without clinical knowledge are dangerous. I hope that it is obvious that I believe the only useful obstetrical knowledge is that based on data. At any rate, I have found such data collections useful and hope that the reader will likewise appreciate their presence.

Only when a single paper is quoted has a direct reference been supplied. Many times, when combining data from different sources, I have attempted to "adjust" values reported from the different laboratories. Under these circumstances, I have only suggested ("see") an outstanding paper for that particular topic.

Contents

Fetal Surveillance Tests

Some of the many fetal surveillance tests are provided on pages D-6–D-17. For most, a 50% decrease in value is considered ominous as regards fetal welfare. Obviously, one must know his or her own laboratory values for "normal" values.

I enclose Dr. Bissonnette's description of FHR patterns. It is obviously different from mine (Chapter 9), but its logic (and not the terms) has much to recommend it for widespread use.

Criteria for classification of FHR patterns

FHR pattern	Criteria
Normal	Rate in the range 120 to 160 bpm; no change in rate throughout uterine contract. beat-to-beat variation greater than 5 bpm
Uncomplicated baseline tachycardia	FHR between contractions of 160 or more bpm; no change in rate throughout contract. the beat-to-beat variation greater than 5 bpm
Uncomplicated baseline bradycardia	FHR between contractions of 120 or more bpm; no change in rate throughout contract.; the beat-to-beat variation greater than 5 bpm
Uncomplicated loss of beat-to-beat variation	Variation in FHR of five or less bpm; rate of 160 or more or rate of 120 or less bpm
Acceleration	FHR increases above the baseline rate during uterine contract.; rate in the range of 120 to 160; beat-to-beat variation greater than 5 bpm
Early deceleration	FHR decreases below baseline as the intrauterine pressure is rising and returns to base line before end of contract. amplituae of the deceleration does not exceed 40 bpm

FETAL SURVEILLANCE TESTS

Criteria for Classification of FHR Patterns

FHR pattern	Criteria
Late deceleration	FHR decelerations character-ized by a lag time of at least 18 seconds; failure of FHR to return to baseline well after the end of the con-traction' amp. of decelera-tion rarely exceeds 30 bpm
Variable deceleration with normal baseline	FHR deceleration is variable in onset relative to uterine contraction and variable in its shape; FHR deceleration abrupt with sharp return to baseline; base line rate be-tween 120-160 bpm; beat-to-beat variability greater than 5 bpm
Variable deceleration with abnormal baseline	Baseline rate 160 or more, or 120 or less bpm; variation in FHR of 5 bpm or less

See Bissonnette, J.M.: Brit J Obstet Gynecol 82: 24, 1975

FETAL SURVEILLANCE TESTS

Metabolic Clearance Rates

	Non-Preg.	1st Trim.	2nd Trim.	3rd Trim.
Dehydroisoandrosterone sulfate				
L/24 hours	8.0±5.0		30±2.0	49±3.0
Pregnenoione				
L/24 hours		2670±389		4250±502
Progesterone				
L/24 hours				2292±210

mean ± SD

See Gant, N.F., Hutchinson, H.T., Siiteri, P.K., et al:
     Am J Obstet Gynecol 111: 555, 1971.

     Little, B., Billiar, R.B., Halla, M., et al:
     Am J Obstet Gynecol 111: 505, 1971.

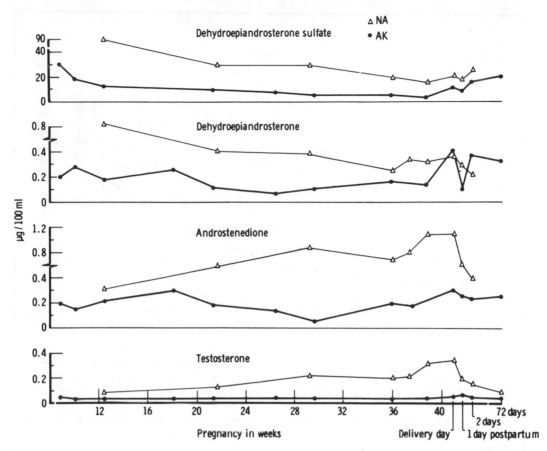

Fig. D-1. C$_{19}$ steroids in two gravidu. (From Gandy, H. M.: In *Endocrinology of Pregnancy,* F. Fuchs and A. Klopper, Eds., Harper & Row, Hagerstown, Md., 1971. Reproduced with permission.)

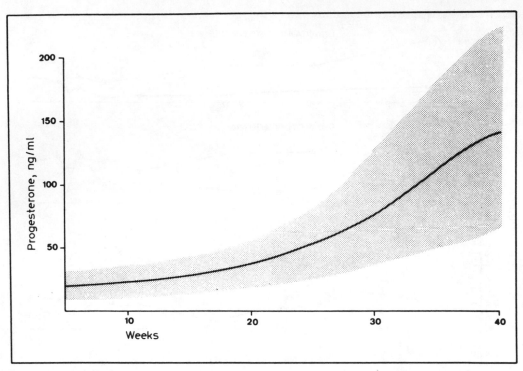

Fig. D-2. Serum progesterone in normal pregnancies. Mean values and 95% confidence limit. (From Keller, P. J.: *Contrib Gynecol Obstet* **2:** 101, 1977. Reproduced with permission of the author and S. Karger AG, Basel, publisher.)

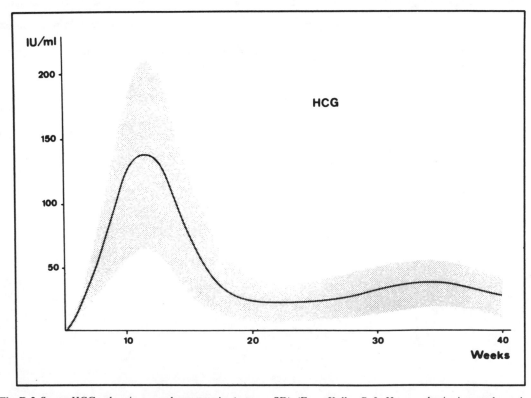

Fig. D-3. Serum HCG values in normal pregnancies (mean ± SD). (From Keller, P. J.: Human chorionic gonadotropin. *Contrib Gynecol Obstet* **2:** 121, 1977. Reproduced with permission of the author and S. Karger AG, Basel, publisher.)

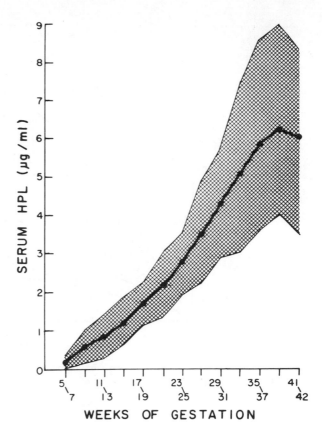

Fig. D-4. Human placental lactogen (mean ± SD). (From Varma, K.: *Obstet Gynecol* **38:** 487, 1971. Reproduced with permission.)

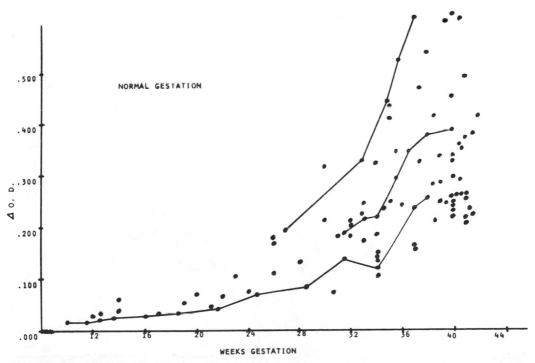

Fig. D-5. Serum CAP activity in normal pregnancy. (From Spellacy, W. N.: *Management of High Risk Pregnancy,* University Park Press, Baltimore, 1976. Reproduced with permission.)

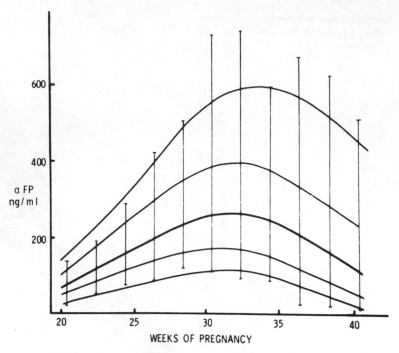

Fig. D-6a. Maternal serum AFP levels during normal pregnancies (mean ± 2 SD). (From Seppala, M.: *Int J Obstet Gynecol* **14:** 310, 1977. Reproduced with permission.)

Fig. D-6b. Leukocyte alkaline phosphate values during pregnancy. (From Polishuk, W. Z., *et al.*: *Am J Obstet Gynecol* **107:** 604, 1970. Reproduced with permission.)

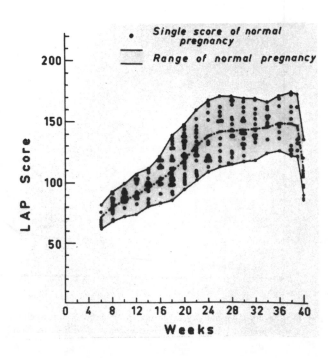

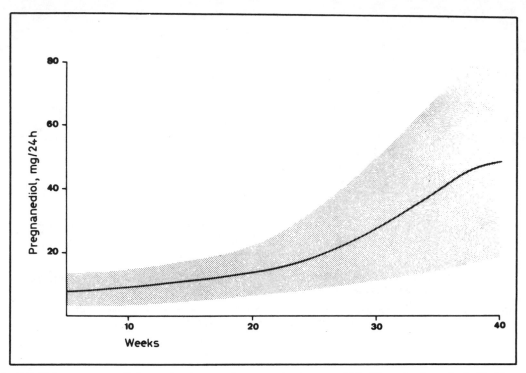

Fig. D-7. Urinary pregnanediol excretion in normal pregnancies (mean ± SD). (From Letchworth, A. T.: Human placental lactogen. *Contrib Gynecol Obstet* **2:** 121, 1977. Reproduced with permission of the author and S. Karger AG, Basel, publisher.)

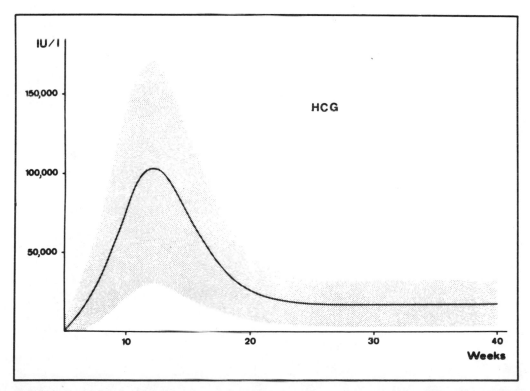

Fig. D-8. Urinary excretion of human chorionic gonadotropin in normal pregnancies (mean ± SD). (From Keller, P. J.: Human chorionic gonadotropin. *Contrib Gynecol Obstet* **2:** 121, 1977. Reproduced with permission of the author and S. Karger AG, Basel, publisher.)

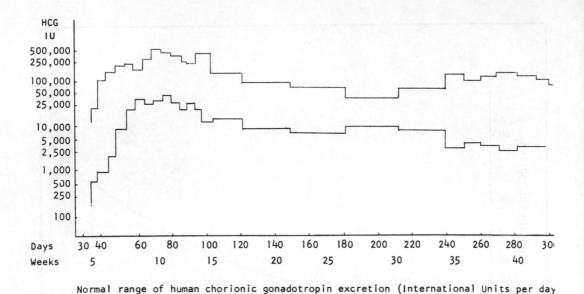

Normal range of human chorionic gonadotropin excretion (International Units per day during pregnancy (Wide, Acta Endocrinologica, Supplement 70).

Fig. D-9. Urinary excretion of human chorionic gonadotropin (normal range in International Units per day during pregnancy). (Reproduced with permission of *Wide Acta Endocrinol Suppl* **70**.)

Fetal Surveillance Tests

Scoring system for each of the four parameters of the
"Lautitzen" DHEA-S test*

Parameters	Points						
	0	1	2	3	4	6	8
Init. estriol value (mg +20%)	0.5	0.5 -0.9	1 -1.4	1.5 -1.9	2 -2.4	2.5 -2.9	3 -3.4
Time of peak estriol elim. (hrs)	0	8	6	4	2		
Height peak(mg)	0	0.1 -0.4	0.5 -0.9	1 -1.4	1.5 -1.9	2 -2.4	2.5 -2.9
Total estriol recovery (mg)	0	0.1 -0.4	0.5 -0.9	1 -1.4	1.5 -1.9	2 -2.4	2.5 -2.9

	10	12	14	16	18	20
Initial estriol value (mg+20%)	3.5 -3.9	4 -4.4	4.5 -4.9	5 -5.4	5.5 -5.9	6 -6.4
Height peak (mg)	3 -3.4	3.5 -3.9	4 -4.4	4.5 -4.9	5 -5.4	5.5 -5.9
Total estriol recovery (mg)	3 -3.4	3.5 -3.9	4 -4.4	4.5 -4.9	5 -5.4	5.5 -5.9

*After 30 mg DHEA-S I.V.

15+ points = healthy fetus

7 points or less = sick fetus

See Stembera et al, High Risk Pregnancy and Child,
1976

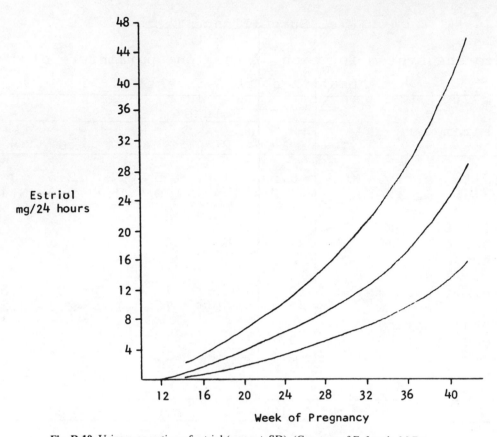

Fig. D-10. Urinary excretion of estriol (mean ± SD). (Courtesy of E. Lamb, M.D.)

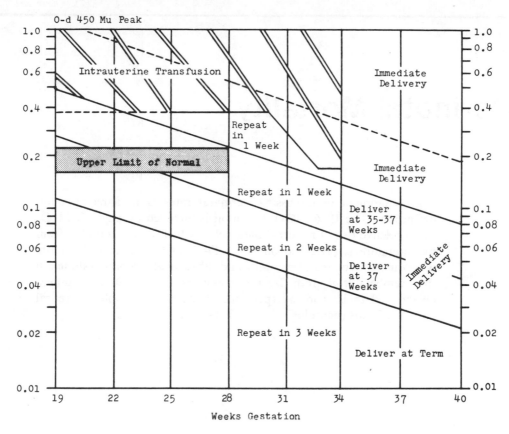

Fig. D-11. Modified Liley graph of 450 (After Liley, A.: Liquor amnii analysis in the management of the pregnancy complicated by rhesus sensitization. *Am J Obstet Gynecol* **82:** 1359, 1961.) Note that 1 IU = ~1 ng; for example, at 16 weeks gestation, 50% of normal amniotic fluids have an AFP concentration of 20,000 IU/ml.

Perinatal Mortality

One problem in discussing perinatal rates is in agreeing upon definitions. The 1976 FIGO definition is included on pages D-21–D-31. A relative risk of maternal parameters which I have collected from the literature is presented on pages D-32–D-36. Another risk score which includes perinatal mortality and subsequent cerebral dysfunction (by Stembera *et al.* from Czechoslovakia) is on page D-36. Stembera determined their score by (perinatal mortality) × 2, plus (cerebral palsy) × 2 plus (neurological deviations) × 11.

PERINATAL MORTALITY

Causes of Perinatal Death per 1,000 Births

	Still-Births	Age, Days 0-7	Days 7.1-28	Total cases (%)
Amniotic fluid infection	2.00	4.05	0.11	6.16 (16.7)
Abruptio placentae	2.57	1.31	0	3.88 (10.5)
Premature rupture of membranes	1.06	2.44	0.23	3.73 (10.1)
Congenital anomalies	1.13	1.78	0.52	3.43 (9.3)
Large placental infarcts	2.00	0.26	0	2.26 (6.1)
Rhesus erythroblastosis fetalis	1.12	0.42	0.02	1.56 (4.2)
Umbilical cord compression	1.1-	0.17	0	1.27 (3.4)
Placenta markedly growth retarded	0.56	0.29	0	0.85 (2.3)
Placenta previa	0.27	0.46	0	0.73 (2.0)
Birth Trauma	0.11	0.44	0.06	0.61 (1.17)
Postnatal respiratory tract infections	0	0.35	0.17	0.52 (1.4)
Umbilical cord knots, stenosis	0.44	0.06	0	0.50 (1.4)
Thrombosis, placental vessels	0.33	0.13	0	0.46 (1.2)
Other acute infections	0.04	0.15	0.21	0.40 (1.1)
Cesarean Section	0	0.33	0	0.33 (0.9)
Extensive fibrosis of placental villi	0.26	0.06	0	0.32 (0.9)

	Still-Births	Age, Days		Total cases (%)
		0-7	7.1-28	
Intervillous thrombi	0.19	0.11	0	0.30 (0.8)
Monovular twin trans. syndrome	0.13	0.13	0	0.26 (0.7)
Incompetent cervix	0.11	0.13	0	0.24 (0.7)
Hydramnion	0.04	0.19	0.02	0.25 (0.7)
Uterine rupture	0.13	0.04	0	0.17 (0.5)
Marginal sinus rupture	0.08	0.09	0	0.17 (0.5)
Therapeutic abortion	0.09	0.02	0	0.11 (0.3)
Trauma to gravida	0.09	0.02	0	0.11 (0.3)
Congenital syphilis	0.06	0.02	0	0.08 (0.2)
Postmaturity	0.04	0.02	0	0.06 (0.2)
Ectopic pregnancy	0.04	0.02	0	0.06 (0.2)
Congenital rubella	0.04	0	0.02	0.06 (0.2)
Severe fetal under-nutrition	0.02	0.02	0	0.04 (0.1)
Other disorders	0.15	0.29	0.10	0.54 (1.5)
Diagnosis unknown	4.89	2.26	0.32	7.47 (20.3)
Total	19.09	16.06	1.78	36.93 (100.4)

See   Naeye, R.L. JAMA 238: 227, 1977.

D-20

WHO: Recommended Definitions, Terminology and Format for Statistical Tables Related to the Perinatal Period and use of a new Certificate for Cause of Perinatal Deaths
(Modifications Recommended by FIGO as Amended October 14, 1976)

1.0 The following limits for the inclusion of birth and perinatal death in statistics are recommended:

1.1 That all fetuses and infants delivered weighing 500 g or more be reported in the country's statistic whether or not they are alive or dead. It is recognized that legal requirements in many countries may set different criteria for registrations purposes, but is hoped that the countries will arrange the registration or reporting procedures in such a way that the events required for inclusion in the statistics can be identified easily. (WHO- Approved by FIGO)

1.2 That mortality statistics reported for purposes of international comparison should include only those born, weighing 1000 g or more. (WHO- Approved by FIGO)

2.0 Perinatal Statistics

2.1 Birth Weight

The first weight of the fetus or newborn obtained after birth. This weight should be measured preferably within one hour of life before significant post-natal weight loss has occurred. (WHO- Approved by FIGO)

22. Low Birth weight

Less than 2500 g (WHO- Modified by FIGO by deleting the words: "up to and including 2499 g".)

2.3 Gestational Age

The duration of gestation as measured from the first day of the last normal menstrual period. Gestational age is expressed in completed days or completed

weeks (e.g. events occurring 280 to less than 287 days after the onset of the last menstrual period are considered to have occurred at 40 weeks of gestation)
    Measures of fetal growth, as they represent continuous variables are expressed in relation to a specific week of gestation (e.g. the mean birth wght. for 40 weeks is the one obtained at 280 days- less than 287 days of gestation on a wght-for gestational age curve). (WHO- Accepted by FIGO)

2.4 Perinatal Period

The perinatal period is the one extending from the gestational age at which the fetus attains the wght. of 1000 g (equivalent to 28 completed weeks of gestation) to the end of the seventh completed day (168 completed hours) of life. (WHO- Approved by FIGO is the work "completed" is included where underscored).

2.5 Pre-Term

Less than 37 completed weeks (less than 259 completed days). (WHO- Accepted by FIGO)

2.6 Term

From 37 completed weeks to less than 42 completed weeks. (259 to 293 days). (WHO- Accepted by FIGO)

2.7 Post-Term

Forty-two completed weeks or more. (WHO- Approved by FIGO)

2.8 Birth

Complete expulsion or extraction from its mother, of a fetus irrespective of whether or not the umbilical cord has been cut or the placenta is attached. Fetuses weighing less than 500 g are not viable and are therefore not considered as births for the purposes of perinatal statistics. In the absence of a measured birth weight, a gestational age of (20) to 22 completed weeks is considered equivalent to 500 g. When neither birth weight nor gestational age of (20) to 22 completed weeks is available, a body length of 25 cm (crown-heel) is considered equivalent to 500 g. (WHO- Approved by FIGO)

2.9 Life at Birth

Life is considered to be present at birth when the infant breathes or shows any other evidence of life, such as beating of the heart, pulsation of the um- bilical cord, or definite movement of the voluntary muscles. (WHO- Approved by FIGO)

2.10 Live Birth

The process of birth when there is evidence of life after birth.(WHO- Approved by FIGO)

2.11 Live-born infant

The product of a live birth (WHO - Approved by FIGO)

2.12 Stillbirth

The process of birth of a fetus weighing more than 500 g when there is no evidence of life after birth. For the purposes of calculation of standard peri- natal mortality rates for international comparison (6.3) only stillbirths with a stillborn infant birth weight of 1000 g or more are included. (WHO- Approved by FIGO, with the suggested italicized modifications)

2.13 Stillborn Infant

The product of a stillbirth (WHO- Approved by FIGO)

2.14 Early Neonatal Death

Death of a live-born infant during the first seven completed days (168 hours) of life. (WHO- Approved by FIGO)

2.15 Late Neonatal Death

Death of a live-born infant after 7 completed days but before 28 completed days of life. (WHO- Approved by FIGO with the above suggested italicized modifi- cation of "completed days".)

3.1 Stillbirth Rate

Is the number of stillborn infants weighing 1000 g or more per 1000 total births (stillborn infants plus live-born infants) at birth weighing 1000 g or more over a given period. (WHO- Accepted by FIGO with the suggested underscored modification)

3.2 Early Neonatal Mortality Rate

Is the number of early neonatal deaths of infants weighing 1000 g or more occurring less than 7 completed days (168 completed hours) from the time of birth per 1000 live-births of infants weighing 1000 g or more. (WHO- Accepted by FIGO with the suggested italicized modification).

3.3 The calculation of these rates for international comparison calls for inclusion of births of infants weighing 1000 g and over. If the birth weight of a fetus or infant is not known, a gestational age of 28 completed weeks should be taken as equivalent to 1000 g birth weight. If neither birth weight nor gestational age is known, a body length (crown-heel) at birth of 35 cm should be taken as equivalent to 1000 g birth weight. (WHO- Approved by FIGO)

4.0 Recommendations for Uniform Minimal Statistical Tables

For the foreseeable future, mortality statistics for infants should be restricted to those weighing 1000 g and over and are intended to provide comparable information for all countries. They should also provide minimal data for those countries which are, at this time, unable to produce a more detailed analysis. It is recommended that all countries provide the following minimal uniform statistics as soon as possible. (WHO- Approved by FIGO)

4.1 Perinatal Mortality Rate

Stillborn infants weighing 1000 g and over + early neonatal deaths of infants weighing 1000 g and over
_____ X 1000

Live-born infants weighing 1000 g and over
(WHO-Approved by FIGO)

4.3 Stillbirth Rate

Stillborn infants weighing 1000 g and over

_____ X 1000

Stillborn infants weighing 1000 g and over + live-
born infants weighing 1000 g and over at birth.
(WHO- Approved by FIGO with the suggested modification of adding the italicized words "at birth")

5.0 Recommendations for Further Analysis

For more detailed analysis of data on the perinatal
period concerned with birth weight and gestational
age, statistics should be presented in a uniform
way which allows comparisons to be made easily.

    Detailed tables should be given, where appropri-
ate, related to the total number of infants born,
identifying separately those stillborn, those live-
born, but dying in the first 7 days, and those surviving 7 days.

5.1 By Birthweight

The weight interval of 500 g is accepted by FIGO but
not the method of designation, i.e. 1000-1499 g,
1500-1999 g., etc. Because some confusion might
occur for an infant weighing 1499.5 g FIGO prefers
the following techniques of designation: From 1000
g to less than 1500 g to less than 2000 g, and so on.

5.2 By Gestational Age[1]

The weekly intervals are accepted by FIGO but not
the technique of designation, because it is felt
that there is some margin for error. Because a
weekly interval does not gain a numerical designation until the 7 days of that interval have been

---

[1]The duration of gestation is measured from the 1st
day of last normal period. Gestational age is expressed in completed days or completed weeks (e.g.:

completed, i.e., week no. 1 is so designated when the
first 7 days have been completed, the 2nd week when 14
days have been completed, and so on. FIGO suggests
the following technique for designating weekly intervals.

Gestational Age[1]

28 weeks to less than 32 completed weeks
(196 days to less than 224 completed days)

32 weeks to less than 36 completed weeks
(224 days to less than 252 completed days)

36 weeks to less than 38 completed weeks
(252 days to less than 266 completed days)

38 weeks to less than 42 completed weeks
(266 days to less than 294 completed days)

42 completed weeks (294 days) and over

5.3 For early neonatal deaths, by age of death, using
the following intervals:

Birth to less than 60 completed minutes
1 hour to less than 12 completed hours
12 hours to less than 24 completed hours
24 hours to less than 48 completed hours
48 hours to less than 72 completed hours
72 hours to less than 168 completed hours

Where detailed information is not available, data
on age at death should be provided as follows:

Birth to less than 60 completed minutes
1-less than 24 completed hours
24-less than 168 completed hours
(WHO - Modified by FIGO)

In each table, appropriate totals and subtotals
should be given (for example, all infants with birth
weight 1000 up to less than 1500 g, or all infants
of 28 to less than 38 completed weeks gestation, etc.

---

[1] events occurring 280 to less than 287 days after onset
of last period are considered to occur at 40 weeks gest.

(together with appropriate percentages. If more detailed breakdowns are tabulated, it should be possible
to aggregate them into the above groupings).
(WHO - Approved by FIGO with the italicized suggested
modifications)

6.0 Mortality Statistics

These should be presented in relation to different
groups of infants, using the definitions of rates
given below:

6.1 Stillbirth and Perinatal Death Rates

(a) all infants 1000 g or more
(b) all infants 1000 g or more in 500 g groups
(c) all infants weighing 1000 up to less than 2500 g
(d) all infnats weighing 2500 up to less than 4000 g
(e) infants weighing 4000 g or more
(f) gestational age groups
(WHO - Approved by FIGO with the suggested italicized
modifications)

7.0 Cause of Death

Mortality statistics (numbers and rates) should be
presented according to the appropriate ICD list,
separately for stillbirths, early neonatal death, and
perinatal deaths. These should be given for all infants
weighing 1000 g or more as well as in the appropriate
sub-groups of weight, gestational age, and age at death.
(WHO - Approved by FIGO)

8.0 Other Variables

Whenever possible, the above statistical tabulations
should also be produced separately, for the group of
infants weighing 500 up to less than 1000 g at birth,
using the corresponding denominators restricted to
infants of 500 up to less than 1000 g.
(WHO - Approved FIGO with the suggested italicized
modifications)

10.0 Maternal Mortality

Maternal death is defined as death of any woman

while pregnant or within 42 completed days of termination or pregnancy, irrespective of the duration
and the site of the pregnancy, from any cause related to or aggravated by the pregnancy or its management but not from accidental or incidental causes.
(WHO- Approved by FIGO with the addition of the
italicized modification)

10.2 Maternal deaths are subdivided into two groups.
(WHO- Accepted by FIGO)

10.2.1 Direct obstetric deaths: those resulting from
obstetric complications of the pregnancy state (pregnancy state (pregnancy, labour and puerperium), from
interventions, omissions, incorrect treatment, or
from a chain of events resulting from any of the
above. (WHO- Approved by FIGO)

10.2.2 Indirect obstetric deaths: those resulting
from previous existing diesase or disease that developed during pregnancy and which was not due to
direct obstetric causes, but which was aggravated
by the physiological effects of pregnancy. (WHO-
Approved by FIGO)

10.3 The maternal mortality rate, the direct obstetrical death rate and the indirect obstetric death
rate should be expressed as rates per 1000 total
births, the latter defined as the births of infants
born live or dead, weighting 1000 g or more at birth.
(WHO- Approved by FIGO)

11.0 Special Certificate of Cause of Perinatal Death

11.1 A separate certificate of perinatal death
should be adopted, in which the causes are set out
in the following manner.

(a) Main disease or conditions in fetus or infant
(b) Other diseases or conditions in fetus or infant
(c) Main maternal disease or maternal condition
    affecting fetus or infant
(d) Other maternal diseases or maternal conditions
    affecting fetus or infant
(e) Other relevant circumstances
    (WHO- Approved by FIGO)

11.2 In addition, the following items were considered to be an integral part of any medical certificate of causes of perinatal death: (i) identifying particulars including relevant dates and times; (ii) a statement as to whether the baby was born alive or dead; (iii) information about autopsy. (WHO- Approved by FIGO)

11.3 While the supplementary information to be collected at death or stillbirth may be varied in accordance with the wishes of the individual countries, it is recommended that consideration be given to the collection of the following items as a minimum:

    MOTHER
    Date of Birth:
    Previous History:
    Number of previous pregnancies; live births/ stillbirths/ abortions
    Outcome of previous pregnancies; live births/ stillbirths/ abortions and date
    (WHO- Approved by FIGO)

GYNECOLOGICAL TERMS AND DEFINITIONS

2.1 Postmenstrual phase
(Menstrual period, Menstruation, Menses)

The postmenstrual phase is the phase that includes the 4-5 days following the menstrual phase. The endometrium is thin, measuring ordinarily only 1 or 2 mm in thickness. The surface epithelium and the epithelium lining the glands is of cuboidal type. The endometrial glands are straight, narrow, and collapsed; the stroma is dense and compact.

2.2 Proliferative Phase

The proliferative phase is the growth phase of the endometrium. The endometrium is stimulated by estrogen. The endometrial glands are straight and short, and the glandular epithelium is cuboidal and shows no evidence of secretory activity. The stromal cells multiply, and the spiral arteries begin to grow.

2.3 Secretory Phase

The secretory phase is the postovulatory phase of the endometrium. The endometrium is stimulated by estrogen and progesterone. The endometrial glands are long and tortuous. The glandular epithelium is columnar and filled with secretion. The stromal cells are large, and the spiral arteries are long and tortuous.

2.4 Premenstrual Phase

The premenstrual phase is the phase that includes the 2-3 days prior to the menstrual phase and corresponds to the regression of the corpus luteum. The chief histologic characteristic of the phase is the infiltration of the stroma by polymorphonuclear or mononuclear leukocytes, producing a pseudoinflammatory appearance. Concurrently, the reticular framework of the stroma in the superficial zone disintegrates. As a result of the loss of tissue fluid and secretion, the thickness of the endometrium often decreases significantly during the 2 days before the menstrual phase. In the process of reduction, the glands and arteries collapse.

2.5 Menstrual Phase-Menstrual Period

The menstrual phase is the period of desquamation of the endometrium. There are increased numbers of polymorphonuclear leukocytes, plasmatocytes, and other wandering blood cells in the tissue.

2.6 Amenorrhea

Amenorrhea is the absence of menstruation. It may be primary or secondary, physiologic or pathologic. It is a subjective, but not a reliable sign of pregnancy.

2.7 Amenorrhea, Pathologic

Pathologic amenorrhea is the cessation of menstruation for at least 3 months at any time after puberty, other than during pregnancy and lactation, and before the onset of menopause. It can be either primary or secondary and caused by any of the following factors: congenital abnormalities, systemic conditions, ovarian disturbances, central nervous system lesions, and uterine trauma.

2.8 Amenorrhea, Physiologic

Physiologic amenorrhea is the normal absence of menstruation before the menarche, during pregnancy and lactation, and after the menopause.

2.9 Anovular Menstruation
    (Anovular Bleeding)

Anobular menstruation is menstrual bleeding without discharge of an ovum.

2.10 Dysmenorrhea

Dysmenorrhea is a symptom characterized by painful menstruation.

2.11 Mechanical Dysmenorrhea

Mechanical dysmenorrhea is a menstrual pain due to cervical stenosis or other obstruction to menstrual flow.

See Acta Obstet Gynecol Scand 56:247-253, 1977

PERINATAL MORBIDITY AND MORTALITY

Maternal Parameters and Fetal Prognosis
(mean figure adjusted to 1)

Maternal Parameter	Prematurity	Congenital Malform.	Perinatal Mort. Rate
All births	1.0 (6.9%)	1.0 (3.2%)	1.0(2.65%)
Age			
<20	1.3	1.1	1.0
35-39	1.0	1.0	1.2
>40	1.4	1.5	1.6
Height			
<62"	1.2		0.9
>68"	0.7		1.0
Weight			
Overweight	0.8		
Underweight	2.0		
Genetic history			
Menses <25 days	0.6		1.5
Menses irregular	1.5		1.6
Menarche <11 years	1.1		1.3
Uterine anom.	3.5		5.0

PERINATAL MORTALITY

Maternal Parameters and Fetal Prognosis

	Prematurity	Congenital Malform.	Perinatal Mortality
Parity 0	1.1	1.1	1.0
Parity 4+	1.0	0.9	1.3
Birth intervals 12 months	2.1		4.0
Previous infertility			1.3
Previous curettage			1.8
Previous abortion	2.8		1.7
Previous stillborn			3.0
Previous neonatal death	2.8		3.5
Previous premature	2.5		

Prenatal history

	Prematurity	Congenital Malform.	Perinatal Mortality
Drugs			
Adrenal steroids			0.8
Diuretics			0.8
Estrogens			4.7
Hypotensive agents			1.4
Insulin			9.8
Progestins			4.0
Thyroid			2.0
Tranquilizers			1.3
Vitamins			0.85
Maternal anemia			
$<$8 gm%	1.2		3.1
8-11 gm%	1.0		1.1
Chronic renal disease	2.8		
Congenital heart disease	3.0	4.0	
Maternal infection			
"Virus"	1.2	1.0	1.6
"Vaginal"	1.3	1.2	1.1

Maternal Parameters and Fetal Prognosis

Maternal surgical operation (abdominal or pelvic)	2.9		
Maternal shock or fright	1.4	1.0	2.2
Maternal physical injury	1.5		2.8
Maternal psych. care	1.4		
Maternal hyperemesis	1.3	1.5	
Maternal preeclampsia			1.1
Maternal hydramnios	2.9	4.3	7.9
Oligohydramnios	4.7	2.1	7.5
Maternal leg edema	0.6		1.0
Maternal generalized edema	1.0		1.1
Hemorrhage			
Early	2.1	1.2	2.4
Painless	2.0	1.4	2.2
Cramping	3.0	1.3	4.0
Late	4.0	1.6	5.5
Abruptio			12.1
Premature rupture membrane	4.0		11.1

Social History

Single			1.4
Non-sedentary employment	1.3		1.4
Smoking			
None	0.7	1.0	0.9
< pack/day	1.1	0.9	1.0
> pack/day	1.8	0.9	1.4
Low family income	2.0		1.5

PERINATAL MORTALITY

Live Birth Rates by Altitude

Altitude Interval (feet)	Mean Altitude	Atmos. Pressure (mmHg)	Percent Live Births 2500g or less
0-500	263	753	6.57
501-1,000	633	743	6.66
1,001-1,500	1,118	729	6.17
1,501-2,000	1,786	713	7.97
2,001-2,500	2,286	699	7.78
2,501-3,000	2,864	684	7.14
3,001-3,500	3,256	674	8.24
3,501-4,000	3,756	662	8.46
4,001-4,500	4,287	649	8.67
4,501-5,000	4,824	636	9.47
5,001-5,500	5,237	627	10.37
5,501-6,000	5,661	617	9.80
6,001-6,500	6,149	605	10.74
6,501-7,000	6,767	591	11.54
7,001-7,500	7,213	582	11.17
7,501-8,000	7,721	570	13.04
8,001-9,000	8,519	553	12.93
9,001-10,000	9,568	532	16.57
10,001-11,000	10,410	513	23.70

See Grahn, D. and Kratchman, J.: Am J Human Genetics 15: 329, 1963.

PERINATAL MORTALITY

Risk Factors According to Event During Pregnancy
(relative risks)

History	Score	Pregnancy	Score
Diabetes before Pregnancy	21	Diabetes only in Pregnancy	22
Sterility	15	Rh isoimmunization	21
Obesity	15	Breech Presentation	18
Unmarried	15	Weight gain 7 kg	15
Age 30 years	12	Bleeding in 1st Trim.	13
Height 155 cm	11	Twins	9
Legal Abortion before Preg.	5	EPH gestosis 4 pts.	7
Perinatal death in history	4	Transverse position	7
Low education	3	EPH gestosis 2-3 pts	5

Labor	Score	Newborn	Score
Prolapse of the cord	21	Birth wt. 1500 g	130
Stained amnio. fluid 5hr	12	Path. signs 3 days	123
FHR 100/min. in 1st stage	11	Birth wt. 1501-2000g	65
FHR 120-100 min 1st Stage	8	Apgar score 9/10 min	35
FHR 100/min 2nd stage	8	Twin B	+25
High forceps	5	Path. signs 3 days	10
Low forceps	3	Birth wt. 2001-2500g	9
Partial breech	3	Apgar score 8/5 min	4
2nd stage labor 1 hr	3	Small-for-dates	4

MOD FROM Steinberg Z.K. et al Euro Cong Perinatal Med

Risk Score Indices

Score indices represents tables developed by many different investigators to determine various risk factors. They cover a wide range of topics.

S.I. (international) Conversion Factors

Substance	Old Unit	New Unit	Factor	Sig. Change
Albumin	g/dl	g/l	10	3/gl
Bilirubin	mg/dl	μmol/l	17.1	5μmol/l
Cholestrol	mg/dl	mmol/l	0.026	0.5 mmol/l
Creatinine	mg/dl	mmol/l	0.088	0.02 mmol/l
Fibrinogen	g/dl	g/l	10	1 g/l
Glucose	mg/dl	mmol/l	0.056	0.5mmol/l
Iron	μg/dl	μmol/l	0.179	3.0μmol/l
Magnesium	mg/dl	mmol/l	0.411	0.1 mmol/l
Phosphate, inorganic	mg/dl	mmol/l	0.323	0.1 mmol/l
PCO_2, PO_2	mmHg (torr)	kPa	0.133	0.5 kPa
Total Protein	g/dl	g/l	10	3 g/l
Uric Acid	mg/dl	mmol/l	0.06	0.02 mmol/l
Urea nitrogen	mg/dl	mmol/l	0.167	0.05 mmol/l
Calcium	mg/dl	mmol/l	0.25	0.05 mmol/l

See   Lynch's Medical Laboratory Technology Third Edition, Philadelphia, Saunders and Co., 1976

Criteria for Scoring
Breech Presentation

	Points		
	0	1	2
Parity	Primigravida	Multipara	
Gest. age	39 wk or more	38 weeks	37 weeks or less
Weight (est. fetal)	more than 8lb. (3630 g)	7 lb.-7 lb. 15 oz. (3629-3176 g)	less than 7 lb.(3175g)
Previous Breech (Greater than 2500g)	None	1	2 or more
Dilation *	2 cm	3 cm	4 cm or more
Station *	-3 or higher	-2	-1 or lower

* Determined by vaginal examination on admission
Score of 3 or less should be delivered by cesarean
section

See Zatuchni, G.I. and Andros, G.J.: Am J Obstet
     Gynecol 93: 237, 1965.

SCORE INDICES

Criteria for Gestational Age Assessment of Newborns

	Gestational Age		
	To 36 weeks	37-38 wks	39+ weeks
Sole creases	Anterior transverse crease	Occipital crease anterior 2/3	Sole cover w/ creases
Breast nodule diam.	2 mm	4 mm	7 mm
Scalp hair	fine, fuzzy	fine, fuzzy	coarse, silky
Earlobe	pliable. no cart.	some cartilage	stiffened thick cart.
Testes	testes in lower canal	intermed.	testes pendulous
scrotum	small, few rugae		full, extensive rugae

See Hellman, L.M. and Pritchard, J.A.: Williams
     Obstetrics, 14th Edition, Appleton-Century-Crofts
     New York, 1971, p. 1030.

SCORE INDICES

Obstetrics
Fetal Maturity Score

Observation	Score		
	0	1	2
Creatinine (mg%)	1.5	1.5-1.9	1.9
Distal Femoral epiphysis	Absent	Equivocal	Present
Estimated fetal weight (lb)	5	5-6	6
Fetal Fat Cells (%)	10	10-19	19
Spectrophoto-metric scan (OD 450 mu)	0.04	0.04-0.02	0.02

Maturity = Score 6 or more

Prematurity = Score 5 or less

See O'Leary, J.A. and Bezjian, A.A. Obstet. Gynec. 38: 375, 1971

SCORE INDICES

Fetal Maturity (36 weeks)

Test	Technique	S/S of Maturity
Contrast media (Ethiodan)[1]	Intra-amniotic injection	Spotty skin absorption
Creatinine[2]		2 mg
450 MU Peak[3]	Spectral analysis	Disappears 36 weeks
Fat Stain[4]	Stain sediment	10% cells stain 36 weeks
Lecithin: sphingomyelin[5] ratio	Thin layer chromatography	Ratio 2 after lung maturity about 36 weeks
Phosphatidyl inositol[6]		+
Foam (shake) test[7]	95% ethanol	foam persists
Thromboplastic activity[8]		113 seconds
650 mm absorption[9]		OD 0.15

1 Brosens, I., Gordon, H. , Baert, A.J. Obstet Gynaec Brit Cwlth 76:20-26, January 1969
2 Pitkin, R. in Spellancy, W. Management of High Risk Pregnancy Baltimore University, Park, 1975
3 Mandelbaum, B., LaCroix, G.C., Robinson, A.R. Obstet Gynec 29:471, April 1967
4 Floyd, D. et al Obstet Gynec 34: 583, 1970
5 Gluck, L. et al Amer J. Obstet Gynec 109:440-445, 1971
6 Gluck, L. Intrauterine Asphyxia of the Developing Brain, Year Book, 1977
7 Clements, J.A. et al NEJM 286: 1077, 1972
8 Yaffe, H. Brit J. Obstet Gynec 84: 354, 1977
9 Sbarra, A.J. et al, Obstet Gynec. 50: 723, 1977

SCORE INDICES

Criteria for Apgar Score

Sign	Score		
	0	1	2
Heart rate	Absent	Slow (<100)	>100
Respiratory effort	Absent	Slow, irreg.	Good cry
Muscle Tone	Flaccid	Some flexion of extrem.	Active motion
Reflex irritability	No response	Grimace	Cry
Color	Blue, pale	Body pink, extrem. blue	Complete pink

Obstetrics
Pelvic Score for elective induction

	Score			
	0	1	2	3
Dilatation (cm)	0	1-2	3-4	5-6
Effacement (%)	0-30	40-50	60-70	80+
Station	-3	-2	-1,0	+1,+2
Cervical consistency	Firm	Medium	Soft	
Cervical position	Posterior	Mid	Anterior	

Elective induction with score of 9+

See Bishop, E.H. Obstet. Gynec. 24: 266, 1964

SCORE INDICES

Premature Labor Risks

Increased when:

Past History

1) Age=<17 or >38 years
2) Height = short stature
3) Non gravid wt. = 110 lbs.

4) No or many pregnancies
5) Therapeutic or spon. abortions
6) Short interval between pregnancies
7) Uterine malformations

Current Pregnancy

1) Poor nutrition
2) Anemia
3) Infections, esp. urinary tract
4) EPG gestosis
5) Cardiopathies

6) Plural pregnancies

7) Placental abnorm.
8) Smoking
9) Poor social or working conditions

Cervical examination

Risk score of premature labor >8 points

Points	0	1	2
Length	normal	short.	1.5 cm
Passage	external or closed	open part or finger	open for whole finger
Position	in pos. vaginal vault	middle of vault	anteriorly
Consistency	tough	semi-tough	soft
Presenting part	vaginal vault empty	engaging	lower segment dilating

Modified from Stembera, Z., Znamenacek, K. and Polacek, K.; High risk pregnancy and child; The Hague, Martinus, 1976

SCORE INDICES

Fetal Anemia Due to Erythroblastosis

Lab Test	Technique	Positive Sign
Antibody titer		titer indicates progressive dis.
Bilirubin[1]	1.35 (OD454-OD574) = mg%	0.000-0.035=mild 0.035-0.060=mild, moderate 0.060-0.160= moderate >0.160=severe
Conjugated Bilirubin		Positive (+) indicates fetal anemia
Δ450	Spectral analysis	See Lilley chart p.
Estriol[3]		Weeks ug% 26-32=39.7+7.8 33-36= 57+10 37-40=135+40 (all above ind. normal pattern) Decrease=anemia
Ovenstone factor[4]	2.3(OD480-OD500)	0-10=unaffected 11-20= mild 21-30=moderate 31-40=severe > 41= too late
Protein[5]		>0.35 gm%=anemia
Ratio[6]	520MU Transmission / 490MU Transmission	31-33 weeks: 1.04=mild <1.04-1.1 =mod. > 1.1 =severe

1 Stewart, A.G., Taylor, W.C. J. Obstet Gynaed. Brit Cwlth. 71:604-608, 1964
2 Kopecky, P. Geburtsh Frauenheilk(ger) 29: 818-826, Sept. 1969
3 Aleem, F.R., Pinkerton, J.H.M., Neill, D.W. J. Obstet Gynaec Brit. Cwlth 76:200, March 1969
4 Connon, A.F. Obstet, Gynec. 33: 72-78, January, 1969
5. Walker, W. Landon, MJ, Oxley, A. Brit Med J. 1:605, March 1969
6. Savage, R.D. et al Lancet 2: 816, October 1966

SCORE INDICES

Tocolysis Score

	0	1	2	3	4
Temperature	-	-	-	-	+
Contractions	miss.	irreg.	reg.	-	-
Rupture of membranes	miss.	-	high or uncert.	-	low
Bleeding	miss.	mod. (spot)	severe	-	-
Cervical dilatation	miss.	1 cm	2 cm	3 cm	4 cm or more

Modified from Gruber, W. and Baumgarten, K.: in 4th European
Congress of Perinatal Medicine, Stuttgaart,
1975, George Thieme Verlag

SCORE INDICES

Per Cent Deviation from Calculated EDC Using
Naegele's Rule of Term-Size Infants

Deviation(days)	Early Delivery	Late Delivery
1-5	18%	17%
6-10	13	12
11-20	15	10
21-30	5	3
31+	2	1

See Burger, K. and Korompai, I. Zbl Gynaek. 63:
1290, 1939.

Cerebral Dysfunction Scores

This is a list of various perinatal factors associated with subsequent cerebral palsy. Most such scores, unfortunately, ignore *in utero* events such as viral infections or growth retardation, which, as noted in Chapter 23, are very important.

Relationship between Neonatal Symptoms and Later Condition in Presence of One Specific, Plus One or More Other Symptoms

Neonatal Symptoms	Followup Groups (%) Birth Weight >2500gm			
	Severe	Moderate	Mild	Normal
Convulsion				
+ cyanosis	44%	19%	%	37%
+ flaccidity	45	10		45
+ respiratory abnormality	33	22		45
Irritability				
+ cyanosis	64	9	9	18
+ flaccidity	67	8	8	17
+ respiratory abnormality	50	10		40
Rigidity				
+ cyanosis	47	20		33
+ flaccidity	70			30
+ respiratory abnormality	44	12		44
Tremor				
+ cyanosis	44	19	12	25
+ flaccidity	55	18	9	18
+ respiratory abnormality	36	18	10	36
	40-60%			20-40%

CEREBRAL DYSFUNCTION

Neonatal Symptoms	Followup Groups (%) Birth Weight <2500g			
	Severe	Moderate	Mild	Normal
Convulsion				
+ cyanosis	%	50%	%	50%
+ flaccidity				100
+ respiratory abnormality				
Irritability				
+ cyanosis	50		50	
+ flaccidity				
+ respiratory abnormality				
Rigidity				
+ cyanosis				
+ flaccidity	100			
+ respiratory abnormality	100			
Tremor				
+ cyanosis		34	33	33
+ flaccidity				100
+ respiratory abnormality			50	50

See Thorne, I, Acta Paed. Scand. Supp. 195: 1969

CEREBRAL DYSFUNCTION

Relationship of Maternal and Pregnancy Factors to Signs of Minimal Cerebral Dysfunction at 7 Years

	A	B	C	D	E	F	G	H
Pre-term	*	***	***	***	***	***		ns
Small for dates	ns	**	**	***	***	***		ns
Smoker	ns	ns	ns	ns	**	ns	***	ns
Severe EPH gestosis	ns	ns	ns	ns	**	ns	ns	*
Vag. bleeding	ns	ns	ns	ns	ns	ns	ns	*
Antepartum hemorrhage	ns	ns	ns	ns	ns	ns	ns	ns
unskilled fam.	***	***	**	***	***	**		ns
5th + child	***	***	**	***	***	**		ns

A. 'Clumsiness'
C. Poor coord. legs
E. Poor speech
G. Enuretic

B. 'Fidgety'
D. Poor Coord. arms
F. Poor visuo-motor (copy-designs)
H. Left or mixed-handed

$*p < .05$
$**p < .01$
$***p < .001$
ns = not significant

Modified from Butler, M. in Perinatal Medicine. Stembera, Z.K. et al ED: Stuttgart, Thieme, 1975

Neurological Followup of Apgar Score at 1 Year of Age

	Abnormal (%) 1.9% of all scores		
Apgar scores @ Birth	0-3	4-6	7-10
Newborn weight =			
1001 - 2000 g (10.4% of all scores)	18.8	14.3	8.8
2001 - 2500 g (4.1% of all scores)	12.5	4.6	4.0
2501 + g (1.5% of all scores)	4.3	4.2	1.4

Source: Hammer, D.J. et al: Exhibit Am Acad Pediat Chicago, 1971

Relationship of Type of Delivery to Physical and Educational Disability at 7 years of Age

	Disability		Poor Ed.		Progress		Ears/Eyes	
	A	B	C	D	E	F	G	H
Fetal Distress	ns	ns	ns	ns	ns	ns	ns	ns
D.L. (24 hrs)	ns	[*]	ns	ns	ns	ns	ns	ns
Breech	ns	ns	**	**	**	ns	ns	ns
Nonelec. CS	ns	ns	ns	[*]	ns	ns	ns	ns
Elective CS	ns	ns	ns	ns	ns	ns	ns	ns
Forceps	ns	ns	***	**	ns	ns	ns	ns
Unattended	***	***	***	***	***	*	ns	ns

A. Severe handicap	B. Educ. disability	*p <.05
C. Poor reading	D. Poor expression	**p <.01
E. Poor numbers	F. 'Maladjustment'	***p <.001
G. Subopt. hearing	H. Subopt. vision	ns = not
D.L. Duration of labor [*] = neg. corr.		significant

Congenital Malformations

The reported incidence of congenital malformations is dependent on many factors. For instance, the high incidence of neural tube defects in England and Wales is decreasing markedly for unknown reasons (*Lancet* **1:** 164, 1978). The tables presented here are intended only to indicate the relative incidence of the various anomalies. A more complete reference is my book, *Handbook of Obstetrical and Gynecological Data* (Geron-X), or better is the monumental *Birth Defects,* D. Bergsma, Ed., published by the National Foundation.

CONGENITAL MALFORMATION

Time of Occurrence of Human Malformation

Malformation	Fetal Age (weeks since conception)
Agnathia	6
Arms deformity (Thalidomide)	5-6
Brachycephaly	7
Carpal or pedal ablation	5-6
Cataract lenticular	6
Cataract nuclear	5
Cleft Palate	7
Congenital Heart Disease	6-8
Interventricular septal defect	7
Pulmonary stenosis	7
Septal and aortic anomalies	6
Cranial nerve defects (Thalidomide)	4-5
Digital ablation	7
Ear	
External (Thalidomide)	4
Internal (Thalidomide)	4-5
Ectopia cordia	3
Ectromilia	3-4
Epicanthus	7-8
Harelip	6
Hemivertebrae	4-5
Leg abnormalities (Thalidomide)	5-6
Microphthalmia	5
Rectal Stenosis (Thalidomide)	7
Thumbs deleted (Thalidomide)	4

See Lenz, W.: Proc 2nd Int Conf Congenital Malform
    Johns Hopkins Press, Baltimore, 1963.

CONGENITAL MALFORMATION

Congenital Malformations- Incidence per 1000 Births

Malformation	Race White	Black
Anencephaly	14.0	4.1
Cleft gum, uvula	14.6	37.7
Cleft palate	4.8	4.1
Harelip ± cleft palate	13.4	4.1
Hypospadias	30.5	19.5
Meningomyelocele, meningocele, and encephalocele	5.5	5.3
Metatarsus varus	12.2	13.6
Polydactyly	14.0	128.0
Specific cardiovascular disease	20.1	18.3
Syndactyly	17.7	5.9
Talipes calcaneovalgus	7.9	2.4
Talipes equinovarus	23.2	12.4
TOTAL	178.2	255.3
Total minus polydactyly	164.2	127.4

Sex Chromosome Abnormalities per 10,000 Births

Chromosome	No. of Abnormalities
XXY	13
XO	3
XYY	10

See Mikamo, K. and deWatteville, H. Int. J. Fertility 14: 95-100, 1969

CONGENITAL MALFORMATIONS

Maternal age (years)	Parity				All Parities
	0	1	2-3	4+	
20	3.9%	4.4%	%	3.9%	
25-29	3.2	2.7	2.8	2.8	2.9
35-39	4.6	3.7	3.8	2.3	3.4
40	8.3		4.5	4.7	4.8

Frequency of Malformations per 10,000 Births
for Whites and Blacks

	Whites	Blacks
Anencephaly	14.0	4.1
Meningocele, encephalocele, meningomyelocele	5.5	5.3
Cleft gum, uvula	14.6	37.7
Harelip ± cleft palate	13.4	4.1
Specific cardiovascular diseases	20.1	18.3
Hypospadias	30.5	19.5
Polydactyly	14.0	128.0
Syndactyly	17.7	5.9
Metatarsus varus	12.2	13.6
Talipes calcaneovalgus	7.9	2.4
Talipes equinovarus	23.2	12.4
TOTAL	178.2	255.3
Total minus polydactyly	164.2	127.4

CONGENITAL MALFORMATION

Incidence of Selected Malformations by Mother's Age
(mean figure adjusted to 1)

	All Ages /10,000	15-19	Maternal Age (yrs) 20-24	25-29
All malform.	10.7	1.1	1.0	0.9
Achondroplasia	0.4		1.0	1.0
Cleft lip/ palate	10.8	1.0	1.0	1.0
Club Foot	12.4	1.2	1.1	0.9
Down's syn.	3.9	0.6	0.5	0.6
Heart malform.	18.1	0.9	0.9	0.8
Hydrocephalus	7.7	2.0	1.0	0.9
Imperforate anus	1.5	1.0	1.0	1.0
Microcephalus	0.9	1.2	0.9	0.9
Spina bifida	10.7	1.1	1.1	0.9

	30-34	35-39	40-44	45+
All malform.	1.0	1.2	1.5	2.0
Achondroplasia	0.5	1.8	3.0	
Cleft lip/ palate	1.0	0.9	1.2	1.5
Club Foot	0.9	1.0	1.2	1.5
Down's syn.	1.0	3.0	10.0	20.0
Heart Malform.	0.8	1.3	1.6	3.0
Hydrocephalus	1.0	1.3	2.1	3.1
Imperforate anus	1.0	1.1	1.0	
Microcephalus	1.0	1.2	15.0	
Spina bifida	1.0	1.1	1.1	1.6

See Milham, S, and Gittelsohn, A. Human Biol 37:13, 1965

Congenital Anomalies- Incidence and Inheritance

Anomaly and Location	Incidence	Comments
Breasts		
Supernumerary	10:1000	Inheritance?
Endocrine Organs		
Adrenal, agenesis	1:1600	Assoc. w/ anencephaly, pituitary defects and cyclopia
Adrenal hyperplasia, (adreno- genital syndrome)		Four enzymatic defects, all recessive: test amniotic fluid 1) 21-hydroxylase defic. overprod. androgens w/ 1/3 adrenal insuff. both mild and severe (Have increased 17-ketosteroids and pregnanetriol) 2) 11-hydroxylase defic. hypertension and viril-ization. (Have increase in 17-ketosteroid, 17-hydroxysteroid and tetrahydro-s) 3) 3-B hydroxysteroid dehydrogenase defic. are salt-losers, early mortality. Females w/ virilization and males crypt. orchidism (Increase tetrahydroiso-androsterone) 4) 17-hydroxylase defic. Hypogonadism in female lack sexual hair. Not reported in males.(Increase pregnanediol; decrease 17-ketoster. hydroxysteroids)
Adrenal hypo.	1:5000	Inheritance? Test amni. fluid DHS test-Mater. E_3 Placental Sulfatase defic.

CONGENITAL MALFORMATION

Anomaly and Location	Incidence	Comments
Thyroid, agenesis		Associated w/ deafness probably recessive
Face and eye		
Cataracts		Part of many syndromes, metabolic disorders, viral infection, pure genetic factors
Cleft lip (with or w/o cleft palate)	1:1000	Empiric w/cleft lip 4-7% cleft palate has no empiric risk w/siblings, more orientals, assoc. w/hydramnios.
Macrocephaly		Rare, more in males
Meningocele		About 10% spina bifida cystica; fetoprotein
Microcephaly	0.5:1	Sometimes asso. w/ X-ray during embryonic life
Micrognethia, severe	1:1000	Part of several syndromes hydramnios
Mongolism, (London-Down's synd. Tristomy 21 anomaly)		If mother under 26 years 2% assoc. w/ translocation where risk is 25-30% for subsequent siblings
Maternal Age:		
25	1:2000	
-30 - 34	1:1000	
-35 - 39	1:357	
-40 - 44	1:141	
-45 - 49	1:36	
Myelomeningocele		90% of spina bifida, rare feto protein
Natal teeth	4:1000	Small caps enamel, not in
Nystagmus	1:1000	All modes inheritance
Retinoblastoma Strabismus, congenital	1:25000	Frequently dominant Common frequently domin.

CONGENITAL MALFORMATIONS

Gastrointestinal Tract

Anus, imperforate	1:5,000	In females usually ass. w/ external fistula
Asplenia or hyposplenia		Rare/ Assoc. w/ cardiac anomalies. Depends on side of truncus invol. Hereditary factors unkn. recurrence rate 2%
Biliary atresia		Rare. 25% live longer than 1 year
Diaphragmatic hernia	1:2,200	? Inherited factors. Fetal D_x w/ ultrasound
Esophageal atresia	1:2,500	Usually assoc. w/ hydramnios
Fibrocystic disease of pancreas	1:1,000	Recessive. 5% white pop. are carriers
Intestine, atresia	1:10,000	Usually assoc. w/hydramnios
Kartagener's syndrome		Dextrocardia w/ sinus inversion
Megacolon (Hirschsprung's)	1:25,000	90% are males, empiric risk in males 20%
Mechel's diverticulum	20:1,000	
Meconium ileus		Assoc. w/ cystic fibrosis
Omphalocele	1:6,600	Assoc. w/ abnormalities of bowel. ? Hereditary factors; signs of fetal distress in labor
Pyloric stenosis hypertrophic	3:1,000	Males five times females
Umbilical artery, single	2-13:1,000	Associated with other abnorm, particularly renal; no deleterious effect other than other anomalies

CONGENITAL MALFORMATION

Anomaly and Location	Incidence	Comments
Nervous System		
Anencephaly	1:1000	3/4 female. Empiric risk of 3-5% subsequent child having Anenceph. or myelomenigocele; 25% risk abortion
Arnold-Chiari malformation	1:1000	Assoc. w/ other nervous system anomalies
Craniostenosis		Rare. 85% male. Occas. seen as dominant.
Encephalocele	1:2000	3% recurrance in future siblings. Prog. guarded
Hydrocephalus congenital, internal	2:1000	Empiric risk for sibling 1%. Occas. inherited as recessive. X-linked. Many etiol. Dx w/ultrasound.
Neurofibrometosis (von Recklinghausen disease)		Autosomal dominant
Phenylketonuria		Rare. Autosomal recess. Mothers may produce mentally defective fetus who themselves do not have disease
Porencephaly		Rare
Rachischisis		Rare, probably fatal
Spina bifida	1:1000	38% Male. Empiric risk for sub. child 4%. Gen. uncertain
Sturge-Weber syndrome. (Encephalotregeminal Angiomatosis, Nevoid Amentia)		Port-wine stain along course trigeminal nerve convulsions and mental deficiency. Rare.

CONGENITAL MALFORMATIONS

Skeletal System	Incidence	Comments
Achrondrophasia (fetal rickets)	1:10,000	? Dominant;hydramnios
Hypophosphatosia		Rare. Low serum alkaline phosphatase. Fetal skull may be decalcified.
Osteogenesis imperfecta(brittle bone- part of Van der Hoeve's syndrome)	1:50,000	Dominant. XRay Dx inutero.
Osteopetrosis (marble bones)		Rare. Assoc. w/ optic atrophy. Recessive.

Urogenital System		
Bladder, exstrophy of.	1 :50,000	No apparent genetic factors.
Bonnevie-Ullrich syndrome		Part of gonadal dysgenesis. Redundancy of neck skin. Perhaps recessive.
Clitoris, congenital hypertrophy		As part of adrenal cortical hyperplasia is autosomal recess. Sporatic or reflect maternal medications.
Epispadas		Rare. Females more than males. No known genetic factors.
Hematocolpos		Rare. Sometimes is recessive.
Hydrocolpos		Rare. Sometimes is recessive
Hymen imperforate	1:2000	Sometimes dominant
Hypospadias, male	1:160-2000	May be intersex prob. chromosome abnorm., sporadic or dominant
Kidney, agenesis (Potter's syndrome)	1:6000	Assoc. w/ typical faces. Inheritance?

CONGENITAL MALFORMATION

Anomaly and location	Incidence	Comments
Urogenital Anomalies		
Megaloureter (prune belly)		Assoc. w/megacolon bladder atony. Rare- genetic?
Micropenia		Rare. Part of several hypogenital syndromes Not usually genetic
Pseudohermaphroditism (female) (gonads are ovaries)		Results from fetal mascu. such as maternal drugs, fetal adrenal hyperplasia Adrenal anom. recessive
Pseudohermaphroditism (male) (gonads are testes)		Rare wide variation from testicular feminization to apparent "males" w/ uteri. Usually inherited consist. family patterns
Testicle, improperly descended(cryptochism)		Usually inherited
Testicular feminization (testes with vagina but no uterus)		Rare. Is end organ failure to testosterone
Ureter, ectopy of		3/4 female. Rare. Apparently not genetic.
Ureter, reduplication of (double ureter)	1:161	Males 2 times females
Ureter, stricure		2/3 female. Not familial
Urogenital sinus		Often part adrenal hyperplasia syndrome
Uterus, absence of	1:1000	Inheritance?
Uterus, anomalies all (from duplication (didelphys) to bicornus)	2% all patients	Are common 2-3% Perhaps assoc. w/ multiple birth Both patient and children more likely to be twins

CONGENITAL MALFORMATION

Uterus, didelphys	1:30000
Vagina, absence of	1:1000
Vagina, septum of	Rare. Has been reported as recessive and also as dominant

Estimates for Spontaneous Mutation Rates at Some Autosomal Gene Loci

Dominant Conditions	Rate per million gene loci per generation	Country
Achondroplasia	45	Denmark
Aniridia	5	Denmark
Marfan's Syndrome	5	Ulster
Multiple polyposis of colon	13	U.S.A.
Neurofibromatosis	100	U.S.A.
Retinoblastoma	4	Germany
Tuberous sclerosis	8	England
Waardenburg's Syndrome	4	Holland

See Carter, C.O. Lancet 1: 1203-1206, 1969

CONGENITAL MALFORMATIONS

Incidence of Selected Malformations by Father's Age
(New York State)

	Paternal Age (years)			
	15-19	20-24	25-29	30-34
Anencephalus	0.2	0.5	0.7	1.0
Cleft lip	0.25	0.3	0.7	0.9
Club Foot	0.15	0.5	0.7	1.0
Down's Syndrome	0.2	0.5	0.6	0.5
Heart malformation	0.1	0.5	0.7	0.9
Hydrocephalus	0.05	0.3	0.7	1.0
Imperforate anus	0.01	0.3	0.8	1.0
Microcephalus	0.6	0.3	0.6	0.8
Spina bifida	0.2	0.5	0.7	1.0
	35-39	40-44	45-49	50+
Anencephalus	1.2	2.0	3.0	7.0
Cleft lip	1.3	2.0	3.0	6.0
Club foot	1.3	2.0	2.9	7.0
Down's Syndrome	0.6	1.2	2.0	4.0
Heart malformation	1.2	1.8	2.5	6.0
Hydrocephalus	1.2	1.8	3.0	5.0
Imperforate anus	1.2	2.1	3.1	5.8
Microcephalus	1.1	2.0	2.7	5.0
Spina bifida	1.3	2.0	3.0	6.0

Mean figure adjusted to 1

See Milham, S. and Gittelsohn, A.: Human Biol. 37: 13, 1965.

CONGENITAL MALFORMATIONS

Relationship of Common Malformations and Various
Parameters   Correlation Coefficients

	All Malformations	Talipes Equinovarus	Hypospadias
Age, maternal	0.0063	-0.0014	0.0221
Age, paternal	0.0297	-0.0024	-0.0051
Diseases	-0.0006	-0.0122	-0.0153
Education, father's	0.0070	-0.0020	0.0024
Education, mother's	-0.0119	-0.0004	-0.0017
Housing density	-0.0009	-0.0007	-0.00004
Hypertension, previous	0.1131	0.0280	-0.0188
Income	-0.0014	0.0009	-0.0005
Marital status	-0.0586	0.0095	-0.0144
Medication	-0.0131	0.0060	0.0004
Pregnancies, previous	-0.0371	-0.0023	0.0022
Radiologic examinations	0.0350	-0.0047	0.0139

	Cardio-vascular disease	Polydactyly
Age, maternal	-0.0456	0.0115
Age, paternal	0.0064	-0.0079
Diseases	0.0056	-0.0040
Education, father's	-0.0006	-0.0035
Education, mother's	0.0050	-0.0014

CONGENITAL MALFORMATION

	Cardio-vascular diseases	Polydactyly
Housing density	-0.0012	0.0020
Hypertension, previous	-0.0031	0.0942
Income	0.0005	-0.0010
Marital status	0.0289	-0.0865
Medication	-0.0152	-0.0004
Pregnancies, previous	0.0171	-0.0155
Radiologic examinations	0.0229	-0.0018

Dermoglyphic Patterns Associated With Congenital Anomalies

Area	Normal	Rare	Condition
Axial triradius	Proximal	Distal	Mongolism (Down's syndrome); Dl trisomy; congen. heart disease; rubella syndrome; Turner's syndrome
Bilateral Simian crease	Absent	Present	Mongolism; Dl trisomy; trisomy 18; rubella
Clinodactyly	Absent	Present	Mongolism
4th and 5th fingers	Ulnar loop or whorl	Radial loop	Mongolism; rubella
Hallucal area	loop or whorl	Arch tibial	Mongolism
Hypothenar	Pattern-less	Loop or whorl	Mongolism; Turner's syndrome; XXXY Kleinfelter's syndrome
Same pattern on 7 or more digits	Rare	Arches; ulnar loops	Trisomy 18; mongolism
Thenar and 1st interdigital	Pattern-less	Loop or whorl	Cri-du-chat syndrome

CONGENITAL MALFORMATIONS

Empiric Incidence for Recurrence of Some Common
Single Malformations (not due to single gene)

Defect	Subsequent Sibling With:		
	Unaffected Parents(%)	Affected Parents(%)	Gen. Pop.
Anencephaly or meningomyelocele	3.4		2/1000
Cleft lip ± cleft palate	4.9	4.3	1/1000
Cleft palate alone	2.0	6.0	
Clubfoot (talipes equinovarus)	2.8		1/1000
Dislocation of hip	3.5 (brothers 0.5 sisters 6.3)		1/1000
Heart disease			
Atrial-septal defect		2.6	
Ventricular- septal defect		3.7	
Pyloric stenosis	3.2 (brothers 4.0 sisters 2.4)	(with affect fathers 4.6, affected mothers 16.2)	2/1000

CONGENITAL MALFORMATION

Defect	1st Degree	Relative 2nd Degree	3rd Degree
Anencephaly or meningomyelocele	8x		2x
Cleft lip + cleft palate	35x	7x	3x
Cleft palate alone			
Clubfoot (talipes equinovarus)	20x	5x	2x
Dislocation of hip	40x	4x	1.5x
Heart disease	-	-	-
Atrial-septal	-	-	-
Ventricular-septal	-	-	-
Pyloric stenosis	20x	5x	2x

See   Smith, D.W, et al J. Pediat. 76: 653, 1970

The Disorders (inborn errors) which can be diagnosed
from cultured amniotic cells

Mucopolysaccharidoses

Hurler disease
Hunter disease
Sanfilippo A

Lipid storage diseases

Fabry's disease
Gaucher's disease
GM_1 gangliosidosis, Type 1 and Type 2

Tay-Sachs disease
Sandhoff's disease
Krabbe's disease
Metachromatic leukodystrophy
Nieman-Pick disease type A
Wolman's disease

Glycogen storage and carbohydrate metabolism

Pompe's disease (Glycogen storage type II)
Galactosemia

Amino acid and organic acid disorders

Maple syrup urine disease (Infantile form)
Cystinosis
Argininosuccinic aciduria
Methylmalonic aciduria (Vitamin B_{12} responsive)
Methylmalonic aciduria
Propionic acidemia (ketotic hyperglycinemia)
Citrullinemia

Other disorders

Thalassemia and sickle cell anemia
Mucolipidosis II (I Cell disease)
Mucolipidoses IV
Lesch-Nyhan syndrome
Combined immune deficiency
Lysosomal acid phosphate deficiency
Hypophosphatasia
Xeroderma pigmentosum

(Matalon, R., Int J Gynecol Obstet 14:301,
1976)

Disorders of Amino Acid Metabolism and Related Disorders That Can Be
Diagnosed Prenatally

Disease	Genetics	Deficiency Enzyme
*Maple syrup urine disease (severe infantile form)	A.R.	branched-chain ketoacid decarboxylase
*Maple syrup urine disease (intermittent form)	A.R.	branched-chain ketoacid decarboxylase
+Methylmalonicaciduria I (vitamin B_{12} unresponsive)	A.R.	methylmalonic-CoA isomerase
*Methylmalonicaciduria II (vitamin B_{12} responsive)	A.R.	partial defect in vitamin B_{12} coenzyme
+Methylmalonicaciduria III	A.R.	methylmalonic-CoA racemase
+Methyltetrahydrofolate methyltransferase deficiency	A.R.	N^5-methyltetrahydro-folate methyltrans-ferase
+Ornithinemia	A.R.	ornithine α-ketoacid transaminase
+Phenylketonuria	A.R.	phenylalanine hydroxy-lase
+Propionicacidemia	A.R.	propionyl-CoA carboxy-lase
+Vitamin B_{12} metabolic defect	A.R.	vitamin B_{12} coenzyme defect

A.R. = Autosomal recessive, X.L.R. = X-linked recessive

*Prenatal diagnosis made

+Prenatal diagnosis possible

(modified from Rhine, S.A., Clin Obstet Gynec 19:855, 1977)

Inborn Errors of Glycogen Storage Carbohydrate Metabolism That Can Be
Diagnosed Prenatally

Disease	Genetics	Deficient Enzyme
*Glycogen storage disease type II (Pompe's disease)	A.R.	α-1,4-glucosidase
+Glycogen storage disease type III	A.R.	amylo-1,6-glucosidase (debrancher enzyme)
*Glycogen storage disease type IV	A.R.	amylo-1,4-to 1,6-trans-glucosidase
+Glycogen storage disease type VIII	X.L.R.	phosphorylase kinase
*Galactosemia	A.R.	galactose 1-phosphate uridyl transferase
+Galactokinase deficiency	A.R.	galactokinase
+Glucose 6-phosphate dehydrogenase deficiency	X.L.R.	glucose 6-phosphate dehydrogenase
+Fucosidosis	A.R.	α-fucosidase
+Mannosidosis	A.R.	α-mannosidase
+Phosphohexose isomerase deficiency	A.D.	Phosphohexose isomerase
+Pyruvate decarboxylase deficiency	A.R.	Pyruvate decarboxylase
+Pyruvate dehydrogenase deficiency	A.R.	Pyruvate dehydrogenase
Pyruvate carboxylase deficiency		Pyruvate carboxylase

A.D. = Autosomal dominant, A.R. = Autosomal recessive, X.L.R. = X-linked
recessive

*Prenatal diagnosis made

+Prenatal diagnosis possible

(modified from Rhine, S.A., Clin Obstet Gynec 19:855, 1977)

Mucopolysaccharidoses (MPS) That Can Be Diagnosed Prenatally

Disease	Genetics	Deficient Enzyme
*Hurler's syndrome (MPS I H;gargoylism)	A.R.	α-L-iduronidase
+Scheie's syndrome (MPS I S; formerly MPS V)	A.R.	α-L-iduronidase
+Hurler-Scheie compound (MPS I H/S)	A.R.	α-L-iduronidase
*Hunter's syndrome (severe) (MPS II A)	X.L.R.	sulfoiduronide sulfatase
+Hunter's syndrome (mild) (MPS II B)	X.L.R.	sulfoiduronide sulfatase
*Sanfilippo's syndrome A (MPS III A)	A.R.	heparin sulfate sulfatase
+Sanfilippo's syndrome B (MPS III B)	A.R.	N-acetyl-α-D glucosaminidase
+Morquio's syndrome (MPS IV)	A.R.	? chondroitin sulfate sulfatase
+Maroteaux-Lamy syndrome (severe) (MPS VI A)	A.R.	arylsulfatase B
+Maroteaux-Lamy syndrome (mild) (MPS VI B)	A.R.	arylsulfatase B
+ -Gluronidase deficiency (MPS VII)	A.R.	β-glucuronidase

A.R. = Autosomal recessive, X.L.R. = X-linked recessive

*Prenatal diagnosis made

+Prenatal diagnosis possible

(Rhine, S.A., Clin Obstet Gynec 19:855, 1977)

Lipidoses That Can Be Diagnosed Prenatally

Disease	Genetics	Deficient Enzyme
*Generalized gangliosidosis (GM_1 gangliosidosis type 1)	A.R.	β-galactosidase A & B
*Juvenile GM_1 gangliosidosis (GM_1 gangliosidosis type 2)	A.R.	β-galactosidase A & B
*Tay-Sachs disease GM_2 gangliosidosis type 1)	A.R.	hexosaminidase A
*Sandhoff's disease (GM_2 gangliosidosis type 2)	A.R.	hexosaminidase A & B
+Juvenile GM_2 gangliosidosis (GM_2 gangliosidosis type 3)	A.R.	hexosaminidase A (partial)
+GM_3 Sphingolipodystrophy	A.R.	GM_3-UDP-N-acetyl-galactosaminyl transferase
*Gaucher's disease (3 types)	A.R.	β-glucosidase
*Niemann-Pick disease type A	A.R.	sphingomyelinase
+Niemann-Pick disease type B	A.R.	sphingomyelinase
*Krabbe's disease (globoid cell leukodystrophy)	A.R.	galactocerebroside β-galactosidase
+Lactosyl ceramidosis	A.R.	lactosyl ceramidase
*Metachromatic leukodystrophy	A.R.	arylsulfatase A
*Fabry's disease	X.L.R.	ceramide trihexoside galactosidase
+Farber's disease	A.R.	ceramidase
+Refsum's disease	A.R.	phytanic acid α-hydroxylase
+Wolman's disease	A.R.	acid lipase
+Cholesterol ester storage disease	A.R.	acid lipase
Hypercholesterolemia (familia)	A.R.	

A.R. = Autosomal recessive, X.L.R. = X-linked recessive
*Prenatal diagnosis made
+Prenatal diagnosis possible

(modified from Rhine, S.A., Clin Obstet Gynec 19:855, 1977)

Disorders of Amino Acid Metabolism and Related Disorders That Can Be
Diagnosed Prenatally

Disease	Genetics	Deficiency Enzyme
Arginase deficiency	A.R.	arginase
*Argininosuccinicaciduria	A.R.	argininosuccinase
+Aspartylglucosaminuria	A.R.	-aspartyl-β-glyco-aminidase
*Citrullinemia	A.R.	argininosuccinic acid synthetase
+Cystathioninuria	A.R.	cystathioninase
*Cystinosis	A.R.	
*Cystinuria	A.R.	transport enzyme
+Hartnup disease	A.R.	transport enzyme
+Histidinemia	A.R.	histidase
+Homocystinuria (due to cystathionine synthetase deficiency)	A.R.	cystathionine synthetase
+Homocystinuria (due to methylene-tetrahydrofolate reductase deficiency)	A.R.	$N^{5,10}$-methylene-tetra-hydrofolate reductase
+Hyperammonemia I	A.R.	ornithine transcar-bamylase
	X.L.R.	ornithine transcar-bamylase
+Hyperammonemia II	A.R.	carbamyl phosphate synthetase
+Hyperargininemia	A.R.	arginase
+Hyperlysinemia	A.R.	lysine ketoglutarate reductase
+Hypervalinemia	A.R.	valine transaminase
*Iminoglycinuria	A.R.	transport enzyme
+Isoleucine catabolism disorder	A.R.	defect in isoleucine oxidation
+Isovalericacidemia	A.R.	isovaleric acid dehy-drogenase

GENETIC AMNIOTIC FLUID DIAGNOSIS

Miscellaneous Disorders That May
Be Diagnosed Prenatally

Disease	Genetics	Basis of Diagnosis
*Acatalasemia	A.R.	catalase
+Acute inter- mittent porphyria	A.D.	porphobilinogen deaminase
*Adenosine deaminase deficiency	A.R, (A.D.)	adenosine deaminase
*Adrenogenital syndrome	A.R.	↑17-ketosteroids in amniotic fluid
+Carnitine deficiency	A.R.	
+Chediak-Higashi syndrome	A.R,	cellular inclusions
+Congenital erythro- poietic porphyria	A.R.	uroporphyrinogen III cosynthetase
*Congenital nephrosis	A.R.	↑α-fetoprotein in amniotic fluid
+Cystic fibrosis	A.R.	various possibil- ities
*Cystinosis	A.R.	↑cystine in fibro- blasts
*Duodenal atresia	A.R.	amniography
+Ehlers-Danlos syndrome VI	A.R.	protocollagen lysyl hydroxylase
+Familial hyper- lipoproteinemia	A.D.	defective reductase deficiency
*Hemoglobinopathies	A.D.	blood sampling by fetoscopy or pla- cental aspiration
*Hypophosphatasia	A.R.	alkaline phosphatase

A.D. = Autosomal dominant; A.R.=Autosomal recessive
* = Prenatal diagnosis made
+ = Prenatal diagnosis possible

GENETIC AMNIOTIC FLUID DIAGNOSIS

Diagnosis	Genetics	Basis of Diagnosis
+Hypothyroidism	A.R.	T_3-T_4 in amniotic fluid
+Leigh's encephalopathy	A.R.	Phosphotransferase inhibitor
*Lesch-Nyhan syndrome	X.L.R.	hypoxanthine-quanine phosphoribosyltrans-ferase
*Lysosomal acid phosphate deficiency	A.R.	lysosomal acid phosphatase
+Marfan's syndrome	A.D.	excess hyaluronic acid skin fibroblasts
*Mucolipidosis II (I-cell disease)	A.R.	$^{35}SO_4$ accumulation and enzyme deficiency
+Mucolipidosis III	A.R.	glycosyltransferase
+Muscular dystrophy	X.L.R.	muscle biopsy
*Myotonic dystrophy	A.D.	linkage with secretor locus
+Nail-patella syndrome	A.D.	linkage with ABO locus
+Oroticaciduria (2 types) Orotic aciduria	A.R.	orotidylic pyrophos-phorylase orotidylic decarboxylase
*Osteopetrosis	A.R.	radiography
+Progeria	A.R.	decreased cell life span in vitro
+Pseudovaginal perineoscrotal hypospadias	A.R.	5-α-reductase

A.D. = Autosomal dominant; A.R. = Autosomal recessive
X.L.R. = X-linked recessive
* = Prenatal diagnosis made
+ = Prenatal diagnosis possible

GENETIC AMNIOTIC FLUID DIAGNOSIS

Disease	Genetics	Basis of Diagnosis
+Saccharopinuria	A.R.	enzyme analysis
+Saldino-Noonan dwarfism	A.R.	radiography
+Testicular feminization	X.L.R.	decrease in intra-cellular binding of testosterone
+Thrombocytopenia-absent radius (TAR) syndrome	A.R.	radiography

Disease	McKusick No.	Genetics	Basis of Diagnosis
+Vogt-Spielmeyer disease	20420	A.R.	peroxidase
*Xeroderma pigmentation	27870	A.R.	absence of DNA repair in cells
+Xylosidase deficiency	27890	A.R.	xylosidase

A.R. = Autosomal recessive; X.L.R. = X-linked recessive
  * = Prenatal diagnosis made
  + = Prenatal diagnosis possible

modified from Rhine, S.A.: Clin Obstet Gynecol
        19: 855, 1977.

Chromosome Anomalies

Since the various bonding techniques have become available, the number of different syndromes associated with chromosome anomalies has grown enormously. Included here are some of the more common and older anomalies.

CHROMOSOMES

Risk of Occurrence of Chromosome Abnormalities

Prior History	Literature Survey No. Invest.	No. Abnorm.	%
Familial translocation	91	13	14
X-linked diseases	149	75	50
High maternal age[a]	1 404	41	2.8
Earlier chromosome abnormality	630	11	1.7
Other indications	776	12	1.5

Prior History	German Survey No. Invest.	No. Abnorm.	%
Familial translocation	36	4	11
X-linked diseases	16	7	43
High maternal age[a]	728	22	3.6
Earlier chromosome abnormality	295	6	2.9
Other indications	193	(1)	0.5

Prior History	European Survey No. Invest.	No. Abnorm.	%
Familial translocation	179	12	6.7
X-linked diseases	280	124	44
High maternal age[a]	1 293 (2 296)	63	2.8
Earlier chromosome abnormality	1 047	14	1.3
Other indications	-	-	-

[a] 35 or 40

See Philip, J. & Bang, J., Acta Obstet. Gynecol Scand. 56: 239, 1977

CHROMOSOMES

Chromosome Nomenclature Symbols

A - G	Chromosome Groups
1 - 22	Autosome numbers (Denver System)
X,Y	Sex Chromosomes
Diagonal (/)	Separates cell lines in describing mosaicism
Plus sign (+) or minus sign (-)	When placed immediately after the autosome number or group letter, designates that partucular chromosome as extra or missing; placed immediately after the arm or structural symbol, designates that particular arm or structure as larger or smaller than normal.
Question mark (?)	Indicates questionable identification of chromosome or chromosome structure.
Asterisk (*)	Designates a chromosome or chromosome structure explained in text or footnote.
Repeated symbols	Duplication of chromosome structure
ace	Acentric
cen	Centromere
dic	Dicentric
end	Endoreduplication
h	Secondary constriction or negatively staining region.
i	Isochromosome
inv	Inversion
inv(p+q-) or inv(p-q+)	Pericentric inversion

CHROMOSOMES

mar	Marker chromosome
mat	Maternal origin
p	Short arm of chromosome
pat	Paternal origin
q	Long arm of chromosome
r	Ring chromosome
s	Satellite
t	Translocation
tri	Tricentric

Incidence of Chromosome Anomalies per 1000 Births

	Spontaneous Abortions	Liveborns
XO (Turner's)	8.25	0.10
Trisomy 21 (Down's)	3.74	1.45
Trisomy 13	4.5	0.05
Trisomy 16	4.5	-
Trisomy 18	0.75	0.15
Other Trisomy	3.0	-
XXY	-	0.85
XXX	-	0.60

CHROMOSOMES

Sex Chromosome Abnormalities

Female phenotypes	Disease	Comments
Aneuploidy	Turner's	Short stature, streak gonads, sexual infantilism
	Noonan's Syndrome	46,XY or 46,XX (Broad forehead, hypertelorism, flat nasal bridge, congenital heart disease, webbing of neck, short stature, cubitus valgus, mental retardation) is an autosomal dominant unrelated to Turner's syndrome. Gonadal function is variable

Karotypes in Turner's Syndrome

Karotypes	Barr Bodies	Comments
Monosomy X		
45,X	0	Short-full syndrome
Mosaicism		
46,XX/45,X	1	
47,XXX/45,X	2	Tall, Variable
47,XXX/46,XX,45,X	2	stigmata
Isochromosome X		
46,X,i(Xq)	1	Short, full syndrome
46,X,i(Xq)/45,X	1	Short, full syndrome
47,X,i(Xq),i(Xq)/ 46,X,i(Xq)45,X	2	Short, full syndrome
46,X,i(Xq)	1	Tall, few stigmata
46,X,i(Xp)/45,X	1	Tall, few stigmata

CHROMOSOMES

Karotypes in Turner's Syndrome

Karotypes	Barr Bodies	Comments
Deletion of X		
46,X,del(Xp)	1	Tall, few stigmata
46,X,del(Xq)	1	
46,X,del(Xp)/45,X	1	
46,X,del(Xq)/45,X	1	
X ring		
46,X,r(X)/45,X	1	Tall, few stigmata
Y Chromosome		
46,XY	0	Variable stigmata
46,XY/45,X	0	
46,XXY/45,X	0	
46,X,del(Yq)45,X	0	
46,X,i(Yq)	0	
46,X,dic(Y)	0	
Normal karyotype		
46,XX	1	Rare
47,XXX	1	Frequent (0.8/1000 females) often normal secondary anomalies
48,XXXX	1	Rare, some with mental deficiency. Others "like" 21 trisomy
49,XXXXX	1	Rare, "like" 21 trisomy with heavy-set face

Modified from Grouchy, J. and Turleau, C. Clinical Atlas of
Human Chromosomes, New York, Wiley, 1977

Karyotypes in Gonadal Dysgenesis

Pure G. D.	Mixed G. D.
46, XY	46,XY/45,X
46,XY/45,X	45,X
47,XYY/46,XY/45,X	46,XY
46,XX/46,XY	46,XX/46,XY/45,X
46,XX	48,XXXY/45,X
46,XX/45,X	47,XXY/46,XX/46,XY/45,X
46,X,del (Xq)	46,X,del(Yq)/46,X,del (Yq)/ 48,XXX,del(Yq)/46,X,del (Yq)/ 45,X

Modified from Grouchy, J. and Turleau, C.: Clinical Atlas of Human Chromosomes, New York, 1977, Wiley.

CHROMOSOMES

Male Phenotypes

Type	Disease	Comments
47,XXY	Klinefelter's	Tall, aspermic, eunuchoid
48,XXXˇ	Klinefelter's	Tall, aspermic, eunuchoid, perhaps mental deficiency
49,XX⌣Y	Klinefelter's	Mental deficiency; ambiguous external genitalia, bone lesions, oval face
47,XYY	Double Y male	Tall, agressive, antisocial behavior fertile
46,XY	Incomplete testicular feminization	Uteri, virilization to variable degree

Male Karyotypes (pseudohermaphrodism)

Type	Disease	Comments
46,XY	Testicular feminization	Voluptuous females w/absent uteri, pubic and axillary hair, often inguinal testes; familial
46,XY	Gonadal dysgenesis w/ gonadoblastoma	Virilization; Turner's stigmata

Karyotypes in Male Pseudohermaphroditism Due to Chromosomal Rearrangement

In most cases:

46,XY/45,X

Exceptionally:
46,X,del(Yq)/45,X
46,X/46,XY/45,X
47,XY,i(Yq)/46,X,i(Yq)/45,X
47,XXY/46,XX/46,XY/45,X
47,XXY
47,XXY/47,XYY/46,XY
46,XX/45,X
46,XX
45,X

Karyotype	Frequency
46,XX	50
46,XY	20
46,XY/45,X	20
46,XX/46,XY	20
47,XXY/46,XX	10
47,XXY/46,XY/46,XX	10
48,XXYY/46,XX	10
49,XXYYY/47,XXY/46,XX	10
47,XX,i(Yq)46,XX/45,X	10
47,XXX,46,XX	10

From Grouchy, J. and Turleau, C.: Clinical Atlas of Human Chromosomes New York, 1977, Wiley.

CHROMOSOME SYNDROME

Chromosome Abnormality

Mean birth weight:
* lower than 2500g   r(1), del 4 , tri 11q del 11$_q$, del 13^p, r(15)

*higher than 3500g   tri 12p

Small crown-heel
length at birth
(46cm)   del 4p, tri 6p, del 11q, 45, X

Hypotonia   del 5p, tri 10p, tri 12p, del 18q, tri 21, r(22)

Severe hypotrophy   r(1), del 4p, tri 10q, tri 10p, del 11q, tri 14, tri 18, del 18q, tri 22

Corpulent infants   tri 12p

Peculiar cry   del 5p

Cranium

Microcephaly   del 4p, tri 4q, del 5p, tri 10q, del 11p, del 12p, del 13, tri 21, r(21), tri 22, r(23)

Dolichocephaly   del 4p, tri 9q, tri 9, tri 10p, tri 18, r(21)

Brachycephaly   tri 6p, tri 9p, tri 10q, tri 21, tri 22

Eyes

Palpebral fissures
slanted:
* upwards/outwards   del 9p, tri 21, 48, XXXX, 49,XXXXX, 49,XXXXY

* downwards/outwards   tri 10q, r(21), 45.X

Hypertelorism   del 4p, de; 5p, tri 12p, del 13, 49,XXXXY

Hypotelorism   tri 5p, tri 6p, tri 14, r(22)

Epicanthus   del, 4p, del 5p, tri 12p, del 13, tri 21, r(22), 45 X, 48, XXXX

Nose

Nosebridge:
*protruding   tri 4q, tri 5q, tri 6p, tri 10p, tri 18, r(21)

*flat   del 5p, del 9p, tri 10q del 10q, tri 12p, tri 21, 49,XXXXX, 49,XXXXY

*wide   del 4p

Upper Lip

Long upper lip   tri 4p, del 9p, tri 10q, tri 11q, tri 14, r(21), tri 22.

Harelip   tri 13

Mouth

Cleft palate   del 4p, tri 10p, tri 11q, tri 13, tri 14, tri 22,

High arched palate   45,X

Small mouth   tri 6p, tri 9q, del 9p, tri 21, r(21)

Wide mouth   tri 4p, tri 10q, del 11q, tri 12p, del 18p

Chin

Micrognathia   del 4p, tri 4q, del 5p, tri 8, tri 9q, tri 9, tri 10q, tri 11q, tri 18, r(21) tri 22,45,X

Protruding chin   tri 10p, del 18q

Ears

Low set   tri 4p, tri 4q, tri 6p, tri 8, tri 9, del 9p, tri 10q, tri 10p, tri 11q, del 12p, tri 13, tri 18, del 18p, tri 22,45,X

Posteriorly rotated	tri 4q, tri 10q, tri 10p, tri 11q, del 18p, tri 22

Neck, Thorax, Abdomen

Wide-spaced nipples	tri 4p, 45,X
Supernumerary nipples	tri 12p

Genitalia

Minor anomalies in male (crypto-torchidism, micro-penis)	del 4p, tri 4p, tri 4q, tri 9, tri 10q, tri 10p tri 11q, del 12p, tri 13, del 13, tri 18, del 18q, r(21), tri 22
Testicular atrophy	47,XXY, 46,XX, 48,XXYY, 49,XXXXY
Hypospadias	del 4p, del 18q, r(21)
Hyperplasia of labia minora	del 9p
Hypoplasia of labia minora	tri 9p, del 18q
Streak gonads	45,X
Abnormal uterus	tri 13
Anal atresia and perineal malform.	del 13, tri 18
Primary amenorrhea	45,X
Absence of puberty	45,X

Malformations

Cardiac	del 4p, tri 9, del 9p, tri 10p, tri 11q, tri 13, del 13, tri 18, tri 21, r(21). tri 22, 45,X
Renal and urinary tract	tri 4q, tri 10p, tri 11q, tri 13, del 13, tri 18, tri 21, r(21), tri 22, 45,X
Digestive	tri 13, tri 18, tri 21, r(21)

Cerebral (arrhin-encephaly, cebo-cephaly, etc.)	tri 13, del 13, del 18p
Osteoarticular, minor	del 4p, tri 4p, tri 10q, tri 10p, tri 11q, tri 13, del 13, tri 14, del 18q, tri 21, r(21), tri 22, 45,X, 48,XXXX, 49 XXXXX, 49,XXXXY

Dermatoglyphics

Abnormal palmar creases	tri 4p, del 5p, tri 9p, tri 13, tri 18, tri 21,
Immature ridges	del 4p, tri 21
Hypermature ridges	r(21)
Axial triradius t'	del 5p, tri 9p
t"	del 9p, tri 18, tri 21
t"'	tri 13
Absence of triradii b and c	tri 9p
Excess of arches	del 4p, tri 9p, tri 13, tri 18
Excess of whorls	tri 4p, del 9p, del 18q
Excess of ulnar loops	tri 21
Supernumerary flexion creases on fingers	del 9p

Modified from   Grouchy, J. and Turleau, C.: Clinical Atlas of
Human Chromosomes. New York Wiley, 1977

Twinning Pregnancies

There is reason to believe that these reported rates are partially underestimated because of the high fetal loss and perinatal mortality associated with such pregnancies.

Rates of Twinning

	Total	Incidence/1000 Births	
		Dizygous	Monozygous
Africa			
Gambia	16.6	9.9	6.7
Nigeria	44.9	39.9	5.0
England/Wales	12.3	8.8	3.5
Europe	12.0	8.6	3.4
India	16.8	8.5	8.3
Japan	6.8	2.9	3.9
United States			
White	11.3	7.1	4.2
Black	15.8	11.1	4.7

See   Strong, S.J. and Corney, G. The Placenta in Twin Pregnancy Pergamon Press, New York, 1967

TWIN PREGNANCIES

Monozygotic Twinning

Membrane	Separation Time
Dichorionic placentae (separate or fused)	Separation of early blastomeres within 24 hr of conception
Monochorionic diamniotic	Dup. of inner cell mass between days 4 and 7
Monochorionic monoamniotic	Dup. of germ disc between implantation (day 7) and day 15
Conjoined twins	Asso. w/ incomplete dup. of germ disc.

See Corner, G.W. Am J. Obstet. Gynec. 70: 933, 1955

TWIN TRANSFUSION SYNDROME
(15% of Monochorional twins)

Anemic Twin	Plethoric Twin
Decreased hemoglobin	Increased hemoglobin (at least 5 gm% greater)
Small body and organs	Large body and organs
Oligoamnios	Hydramnios
Small Heart	Large Heart (with hyperplasia)
Hypotension	Hypertension Hyperbilirubinemia

See Naeye, R.L. New Eng. J. Med. 268: 804, 1963

Drugs: Deleterious Effects

It is almost a universal policy that medical journals have double standards when reporting drug effects (*Lancet* editorial, Jan. 21, 1978). They require rigorous proof of the efficiency of a drug, but only a flimsy suggestion that the drug may be harmful in order that its effects be published.

While they defend such policies as necessary to protect us from ourselves, it means that obstetricians must evaluate each adverse report with the journals' views in mind. The adverse drug list presented here is a collection of such reports available in 1978.

Drugs Adversely Affecting the Human Fetus
(? before = doubtful occurrence, ? after = very rare)

Drug	Adverse Effect	Stage of Pregnancy
Analgesic		
Heroin	SGA, chromosome abnormalities Withdrawal symptoms, respiratory depression	Near term
Morphine	Depressed newborn for up to 30 days	Labor
Meperidine (Demerol)	Loss of BBV, late depressive effects in newborns	Labor
Salicylates	Neonatal bleeding, coagulation defects, patent ductus (not teratogenic).	Near term
Talwin	Withdrawal (newborn)	
Anesthetic		
Halothane	? Abortion	Early
Mepivacaine (Carbocaine)	Fetal bradycardia (?), stillborn with PCB	Labor
Lidocain	" " " " "	"
Nitrous oxide	Fetal anomalies (?)	1st trimester
Tetracaine	Neonatal depression	Labor
Antibiotic		
Chloroquine	Auditory nerve, CNS damage	1st & 2nd trimester
Chloramphenicol (Chloromycetin)	"Gray syndrome", death, thrombocytopenia	Term & labor
INH (Isoniazid)	? embryotoxic, retarded psychomotor activity	Near term
Kanamycin	? ototoxicity	
Metronidazole	? embryotoxic	1st trimester
Nitrofurantoin (Furadantin)	Hemolysis with G-6 PD deficiency	Near term
Novobiocin (Albamycin)	Hyperbilirubinemia (?)	Near term
Streptomycin	8th nerve damage (?), micromelia, hearing loss, multiple skeletal anomalies - slight danger	All stages

Drug	Adverse Effect	Stage of Pregnancy
Antibiotic		
Sulfonamides (long-acting)	Hyperbilirubinemia, kernicterus, thrombocytopenia	Near term
Tetracyclines	Inhibition of bone growth, discoloration of teeth, micromelia, syndactyly	2nd and 3rd trimesters
Anticarcinogen		
Amethopterin (Methotrexate)	Cleft palate, ocular teratogen, abortion	1st trimester
Aminopterin	" " " " "	1st trimester
Azathioprine (Imuran)	Alone not teratogenic	
Busulfan (Myleran)	Cleft palate (?)	1st trimester
Chlorambucil	? Cleft palate	1st trimester
Cyclophosphamide (Cytoxan)	Severe stunting, fetal death, extremity defects (Also normal infants born)	1st trimester
Mercaptopurine	Malformations, hemolytic disease	1st trimester
Anticoagulant		
Dicumarol	Fetal death, fetal anomalies, hemorrhage	All stages
Sodium warfarin (Coumadin)	50% nasal hypoplasia, optic atrophy, mental retardation, chondrodysplasia punctata	1st trimester
	Fetal death (16%), hemorrhage (No deaths with good control)	All stages
Anticonvulsant		
Dilantin (Phenytoin)	Cleft palate, "typical" syndrome with heart lesions	Entire pregnancy
Paramethadione	Growth retardation	" "
Trimethadione	Multiple anomalies	" "
Phenobarbital	Bleeding (Vitamin K dependent)	" "
Antidiabetic		
Chlorpropamide (Diabinese)	Respiratory distress; prolonged neonatal hypoglycemia (?)	All stages
Insulin	? Caudal regression	1st trimester
Phenformin (DBl)	? Lactic acidosis, neonatal hypoglycemia	All stages
Tolbutamide (Orinase)	? Congenital anomalies, neonatal hypoglycemia	All stages
Antihypertensive		
Hexamethonium bromide	Neonatal ileus	
Reserpine	Nasal block	
Anti-inflammatory		
Cortisone	? Cleft palate, (?) newborn shock	All stages
Antimalarial		
Chloroquine	Auditory and retinal damage (?)	All stages
Quinine	? Deafness, thrombocytopenia, CNS abnormalities	All stages
Antimitotic		
Podophyllum	Fetal resorption, (?) multiple deformities	1st trimester
Antithyroid		
Methimazole (Tapazole)	Goiter, mental retardation	14th week on
Potassium iodide	" " "	14th week on
Prophylthiouracil	" " "	14th week on
Radioactive iodine	Congenital hypothyroidism, cretinism	14th week on
Depressant or Sedative		
Lithium	? Dysmorphogenic (Ebstein's anomaly, other heart anomalies)	1st trimester
Phenobarbital	Neonatal bleeding, coagulation defects, thrombocytopenia	Near term
Reserpine	Nasal block	Near term
Meprobamate	Newborn flaccidity, thrombocytopenia	Near term
Thalidomide	Phocomelia, hearing defect	28th–42nd days
Diuretic		
Ammonium chloride	Acidosis (?)	Late
Thiazides (Chlorothiazide, Hydrochlorothiazide, Methyclothiazide)	Thrombocytopenia, neonatal death, fetal ascites	Late

Drug	Adverse Effect	Stage of Pregnancy

Cardiac

Diazoxide	? Newborn depression	All stages
Digitoxin	Fetal death with overdose	" "
Propranolol	Hypoglycemia, SFD, (?) respiratory bradycardia	" "

Sex Steroid

Androgens	Masculinization, labial fusion, clitoris enlargement	All stages
Estrogens (Stilbestrol, dienstrol, hexestrol)	" " Adenocarcinoma of vagina, masculinization (?), labial fusion (?), clitoris enlargement (?)	All stages All stages
Oral contraceptives	? Pierre-Robin syndrome, (?) limb and heart abnormalities, Vactrel syndrome.	All stages
Oral progestogens	Masculinization, labial fusion, clitoris enlargement Cardiac anomalies	All stages

Steroid

Cortisone Dexamethasone Hydrocortisone Prednisone Prednisolone	? Cleft palate ? Newborn adrenal failure ? Placental insufficiency	Early Late Late

Stimulant

Dextroamphetamine sulfate (Dexedrine)	Transposition of great vessels	
Phenmetrazine (Preludin)	Skeletal and visceral anomalies	4th-12th weeks
Serotonin	Multiple anomalies of skeleton and organs	

Tranquilizer

Chlorpromazine (high doses)	Retinal changes	
Meprobamate Diazopam	Fetal inactivity, newborn flaccidity, cardiac anomalies.	All stages

Vaccine

Influenza	Increased regular antibodies (?), abortion	
Pertussis	Abortion	
Polio	Fetal loss (?)	Early
Rubella	Rubella syndrome (?)	
Smallpox	Vaccinia	All stages

Vitamin

Vitamin A	Congenital anomalies, cleft palate, eye damage, syndactyly	All stages
Vitamin D	Excessive blood calcium, mental retardation Supravalvular, aortic syndrome	All stages
Vitamin K analogues	Hyperbilirubinemia, kernicterus	Near term

Miscellaneous

Acetophenetidin	Methemoglobinemia	
Cholinesterase inhibitors	Transient muscular weakness	All stages
Alcohol	Fetal alcohol syndrome (mental deficiency, micro-cephaly, short palpebral fissure)	All stages
Intravenous fluids	Electrolyte abnormalities	
Intravenous potassium	Fetal flaccidity	Labor
Lysergic acid diethylamide (LSD)	Chromosomal damage (?), stunted offspring (?)	1st trimester
Mercury	Cerebral palsy, mental retardation	
Nicotine and smoking	Small babies (Reduced maternal blood volume, decreased oxygen supply, decreased tranquility)	All stages
Penicillamine	Fetal collagen tissue	All stages

DRUGS

Antibiotics in Serum of Patients
Maternal-Fetal Effects

Antibiotic	Gen. toxicity in pregnancy	Cord Blood Level (%)	Amn. Fluid level (%)	Rec.(%) in urine
Ampho-tericin B	Nephrotoxic hemolytic anemia	?	?	5-40
Ampicillin	Cross react. to penicillin elevated SGOT	80	120	40
Bacitracin	Nephrotoxic			9-31
Carbeni-cillin	Elevated SGOT and SGPT	?	?	-
Cefazolin	no known adverse effect	high	-	-
Cephalexin	no known adverse effect	low	low	?
Cephacetrile	Requires 12g/ 24 hr.	low	low	-
Chloroquin	Fetal CNS damage	-	-	-
Cephalori-dine	Cross Sensi-tivity with penicillin; occasional di-rect Coomb's +, increased SGOT, alkaline phosphatase	90	60	70
Chloram-phenicol	Bone marrow depression, Gray syndrome in newborns	60	5	5-15

Antibodies in Serum of Patients
Maternal-Fetal Effects

Antibiotic	Gen. toxicity to pregnancy	Cord Blood Level (%)	Amn. Fluid level (%)	Rec.(%) urine
Chlortetra-cycline	Phototoxicity, contraindicated in pregnancy (tooth dis-coloration)	60	5	18
Clindamycin	Concentrated in fetal liver. No ill effects	high	high	-
Cloxacillin	-	-	-	40
Colistin	Nephrotoxic, neurotoxicity	-	-	40-80
Cycloserine	Mental symptom, seizures, neph-rotoxic	?	?	15-20 oral
Dimethyl-chlortetra-cycline	Liver toxicity, nephrotoxic	80	5	42
Dicloxa-cillin	Same as methicillin, elevated SGOT	20	15	40
Erythromycin	-	?	?	15
Gentamicin	Same as Kanamycin, ototoxicity, nephrotoxic	?	?	86-100
Isoiazid	-	?	?	5-27 oral
Kanamycin	Nephrotoxic ototoxic	80	5	52-90

Antibiotics in Serum of Patients
Maternal-Fetal Effects

Antibiotic	Gen. toxicity in pregnancy	Cord Blood level (%)	Amn. Fluid level (%)	Rec(%) in urine
Limecycline	Tooth staining	80	60	80
Lincomycin	Diarrhea elevated SGOT	80	60	10-15
Mebendazole	Avoid during pregnancy	-	-	-
Methacycline	Liver toxicity nephrotoxic	80	5	60
Methicillin	Staphylo-coccilis resistance only, cross to penicillin	85	110	71
Nitrofurantoin	Newborn anemia, hemolytic anemia in prima-quine sensitive	-	-	-
Novobiocin	Fetal anemia? liver toxicity skin lesions blood dyscrasia	-	-	1.5-3.3
Oxacillin	-	-	-	40
Oxytetra-cycline	Liver toxicity nephrotoxic	80	5	70
p-amnio-salicylic	-	?	?	80 oral

Antibiotics in Serum of Patients
Maternal-Fetal Effects

Antibiotic	Gen. toxicity in pregnancy	Cord Blood Level (%)	Amn.Fluid level (%)	Rec(%) in urine
Penicillin G	Increased fetal loss? potential fetal sensitization, each 15×10^6 contain 25mEq	80	110	58-85
Phosphomycin	no untoward effect	high	high	-
Polymyxin	Nephrotoxic, Neurotoxic	-	-	large
Rifampin	? multiple anomalies	60	?	-
Ristocetin	-	-	-	79.4 dog
Streptomycin	Dermatitis nephrotoxic VIII nerve damage, bone marrow depress.	80	5	30-80
Tetracycline	Contraindicated in pregnancy (fetal tooth and bone stain)	-	-	60
Tobramycin	teratogin in mice	-	-	-
Vancomycin	Nephrotoxic ototoxic	?	?	30-100

See Kunin, C.M. Ann. Int. Med. 67: 151, 1967

Amniotic Fluid

Many of these tables contain figures from different laboratories. I have attempted to list a representative source for each set of data, however.

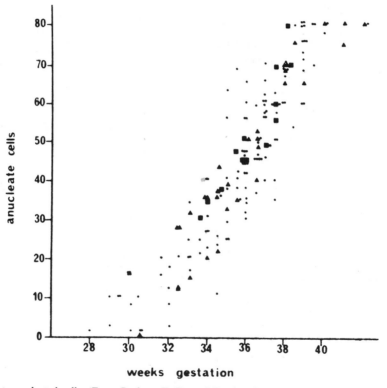

Fig. D-12. Percent anucleated cells. (From Baskett, T. F., and Dunbar, L. M.: *Int J Gynaecol Obstet* **14:** 335, 1976. Reproduced with permission.)

AMNIOTIC FLUID

Creatine Levels (mg%)

Menstrual Weeks	Normal Pregnancy	Pre-eclampic Toxemia
35	1.21 ± 0.56	2.06 ± 1.02
36	1.46 ± 0.56	2.30 ± 0.97
37	1.72 ± 0.56	2.53 ± 0.93
38	1.97 ± 0.55	2.76 ± 0.91
39	2.33 ± 0.55	2.99 ± 0.91
40	2.48 ± 0.55	3.23 ± 0.93
41	2.74 ± 0.55	3.46 ± 0.96
42	2.99 + 0.56	3.69 + 1.01

Roopnarinesingh, S., J. Obstet. Gynaec. Brit. Cwith 77: 785-790, September 1970.

Amniotic Fluid Volume
(mean with range)

Menstrual weeks	Amniotic fluid volume (ml)	Rate of increase per week (ml)
8	7 (1-11)	
10	32 (2-46)	
12	50 (5-90)	25
14	100 (50-220)	25
16	180 (150-290)	50
18	320 (200-480)	50
20	400 (210-540)	50
24	540 (300-700)	50
28	610 (340-1000)	50
32	850 (360-1100)	25
36	1000 (380-1500)	-50
40	800 (320-1200)	-100
43	420 (100-600)	

See Ostergard, D.R. Obstet. Gynec. Survey 25: 297, 1970

Amniotic Fluid Amino Acids and Related Compounds

	1st Tri.	2nd Tri.	3rd Tri.
Alinine	0.387+0.072 (0.30$\overline{1}$-.498)	0.267+0.072 (.186$\overline{-}$.353)	.121+.042 (.061$\overline{-}$.214)
α-amino-N-butyric acid	.017+ .006 (.01$\overline{1}$-.027)	.009+.002 (.00$\overline{7}$-.012)	.006+.004 (.002$\overline{-}$.015)
Arginine	.064+.018 (.0$\overline{3}$3-.089)	.045 +.026 (.029$\overline{-}$.076)	.014+.003 (.010$\overline{-}$.019)
Asparagine*	.200 (.040-.410)	.200 (.060-.660)	.070 (.040-.120)
Aspartic acid*	.120 (.000-.550)	.140 (.000-.540)	.040 (.000-.060)
Citrulline	.012+.005 (.00$\overline{5}$-.017)	.009+.003 (.00$\overline{5}$-.012)	.004+.005 (tra$\overline{c}$e-.017)
Cystathionine	.002+.001 (tra$\overline{c}$e-.005)	.002+.001 (tra$\overline{c}$e-.004)	trace (.000-.003)
Cysteic acid*	.110 (.050-.180)	.140 (.100-.210)	.170 (.080-.260)
Cystine	.045+.011 (.02$\overline{6}$-.059)	.052+ .009 (.04$\overline{4}$-.063)	.042+.010 (.02$\overline{9}$-.057)
Ethanolamine	.010+.006 (.003$\overline{-}$.006)	.012+ .005) (.00$\overline{7}$-.018)	.020+.008 (.00$\overline{9}$-.039)
Glutamic acid	.227+.111 (.12$\overline{6}$-.468)	.091+.070 (.01$\overline{3}$-.199)	.074+ .076 (.00$\overline{9}$-.271)
Glutamine	.091+.079 (.00$\overline{7}$-.272)	.190+.066 (.08$\overline{5}$-.258)	.094+.039 (.01$\overline{5}$-.172)
Glycine	.170+ .032 (.13$\overline{6}$-.228)	.172+ .023 (.14$\overline{6}$-.203)	.130+ .046 .059$\overline{-}$.192
Histidine	.117+.026 (.090-.176)	.089+.023 (.06$\overline{6}$-.128)	.038+.014 (.01$\overline{8}$-.068)
Hydroxy-proline	.052+ .014 (.02$\overline{9}$-.078)	.040+.002 (.03$\overline{4}$-.042)	.034+.013 (.01$\overline{3}$-.054)
Isoleucine	.044+.014 (.02$\overline{7}$-.062)	.018+ .008 (.01$\overline{0}$-.031)	.010+.004 (.00$\overline{5}$-.017)
Leucine	.109+.041 (.05$\overline{8}$-.181)	.042+.022 (.02$\overline{0}$-.082)	.022+ .010 (.01$\overline{1}$-.045)

	1st Tri.	2nd Tri.	3rd Tri.
Lysine	.338+ .091 (.245-.473)	.200+.046 (.136-.256)	.125+ .049 (.081-.232)
Methionine	.028+.007 (.016-.044)	.015+.006 (.010-.025)	.007+ .003 (.003-.014)
Orinthine	.057+.017 (.035-.088)	.025+.005 (.021-.033)	.021+ .010 (.008-.040)
Phenyla-lanine	.070+ .018 (.049- .103)	.043+ .018 (.028-.073)	.018+ .008 (.007-.032)
Phosphoe-thanolamine*	.060 (.000-.280)	.130 (.000-.440)	.220 (.000-.270)
Proline	.192+.038 (.130-.247)	.143+ .031 (.113-.186)	.083+.027 (.047-.131)
Serine	.070+.019 (.048-.107)	.060+.016 (.045-.077)	.049+.020 (.019-.089)
Taurine	.059+.023 (.037-.105)	.049+.010 .042-.066	.088+ .045 (.024-.175)
Threonine	.218+.070 (.124-.344)	.164+.023 (.142-.193)	.096+.036 (.045-.154)
Tryptophan*	.120 (.000-.280)	.110 (.000-.400)	.010 (.000-.050)
Tyrosine	.067+.019 (.044-.102)	.044+.014 (.030-.061)	.017+.008 (.005-.034)
Valine	.195+.057 (.111-.266)	.100+.043 (.057-.162)	.046+ .017 (.023-.078)

---

*levels shown in mg%. Other levels shown in uM/ml

See   Emery, A.E.H. et al. Lancet 1: 1307-1308, June 1970
      O'Neil, R.T. et al. Obstet. Gynec. 37: 550-554, April 1971

AMNIOTIC FLUID

Amniotic Fluid Chemistry

	1st Trim.	2nd Trimester	3rd. Trimester
Acetone bodies			< 1
Bilirubin (△450mu peak)		0.06	0.01
Calcium (mEq/L) [0.25]	7	7	5 (3.1-6.1)
Carbohydrates Fructose (mg%)			3.5
Glucose (mg%) [0.056]	51		33 (23-40)
Lactic acid (mEq/L)	10.9		8.3
Pyrurate (mg%)			1.0 (0.8-13.5)
Chloride (mEq/L)	109 (104-111)	106	102 (99-107)
Copper (ug%)			
Creatinine (mg%)	0.4 (0.2-1.0)	0.6 (0.4-0.8)	2.4 (1.8-3.4)
Enzymes (Mu/ml) Alkaline phosphatase		0.2 (0.1-0.4)	0.4 (0.1-2.0)
LDH		50	64
SGOT		14	44
Gases CO_2 (mM/L)	21.7		16.2 (14.0-16.6)

AMNIOTIC FLUID

Amniotic Fluid Chemistry

	1st Trim.	2nd Trimester	3rd Trimester
pCO_2 (torr)	45		57.1 (55.0-63.5)
pO_2 (torr)	37		20 (1-55)
pH (units)	7.28		7.04 (6.96-7.20)
Immunoglobulins (mg%)			
α_1 antitrypsin			< 30
Ceruloplasmin			< 12 (< 5-21)
Complement C'3			29
Haptoglobin			2
Immunoglobin A (lgA)			< 10
Immunoglobin G (lgG)			91±14
Immunoglobin M (lgM)			< 10
β lipoprotein			5
α_2 macroglobulin			< 10
Orosomucoid			16
Transferrin			17 (13-22)
Lipids (total mg%)			48
Cholesterol		15	25
Fatty acids			24
Phospholipids			3 (3.0-4.5)
Magnesium (mEq/L)	3.8	4.1	4
NPN (mg%)	25 (20-28)	26	28 (23-32)
Osmolality (m)sm/kg/H_2O)	285 (280-293)	272 (260-280)	260 (251-271)
Phosphorous (mEq/L)	4	3	2.9
Potassium (mEq/L)	4.0 (3.0-4.2)	4.0 (3.7-4.5)	4.1 (3.7-4.2)
Proteins (total) (mg%)	0.5 (0.20-0.61)	0.25	0.36 (0.22-0.48)

AMNIOTIC FLUID

	1st Tri.	2nd Tri.	3rd Tri.
Albumin (%)			60(51.8-73.4)
α1 globulin			7.3(6.0-10.7)
α2 globulin			6.5(4.6-9.7)
α1 and 2 globulin (%)			12.3(8.7-16.2)
β globulin (%)			15.5(11.0-23.6)
Gamma Glob. (%)			12.2(8.8-20.0)
Sodium (mEg/L)	136 (130-139)	137 130-142)	
Steroid (ug/L)			
17-oxo-steroids			
Total	29	74	120
Free(%)		13.7	10.0
Glucuronide(%)		49	50
Sulfate		30	46
17-hydroxy-corticosteroid			
Total(ug/L)	52	145	240
Free (%)		26	17
Glucuronide(%)		44	47
Sulfate		29	35
Estriol(ug%)		36±7	135.2± 40
Pregnanediol (ug/L)			145(21-436)
Strontium(UG/L)			39
Urea(mg%)	18(16-30)	29(26-40)	34(29-44)
Uric Acid(mg%)	2.8	3.6	8.5(5-15)

see Mendenhall, H.W. Am J Obstet Gynecol 106: 581, 1970
      Schindler, A., Ratanasopa,V.: Acta Endo. 59: 239, 1968.

AMNIOTIC FLUID

Clinical Interpretation

Objective	Technique	Application
Fetal well-being		
ph	"Blood-gas" analysis	Indirect eval. of uterine anoxia
pO_2		
pCO_2		
pCO_3		
Pigment	Visual Inspection	Heavy Strain (tobacco juice)= fetal death
		Yellow (old meconium)= fetal anemia
		fetal gut obstruction lack of swallow.
Genetic Counseling		
Chromosome analysis	Fetal karyotype determination from sediment	Chromosome abnorm. or Mongolism
Sex determination	Female fetus - stain sediment for Barr body (inactive X)	X- linked hereditary disease
	Male fetus - fluorescent stain for Y chromosome	

HUMAN BLOOD ANTIGENS AND ANTIBODIES

Systems	Common red cell antigens (symbol)	Antibody Name	Antibody Symbol	Serum antibody immunoglobulin in vivo role of antibody Hemolytic transfusion reaction	Hemolytic disease of the newborn
ABO	A	Anti-A	Anti-A	Yes-Common	Yes-Common
	B	Anti-B	Anti-B	Yes-Common	Yes-Fairly frequent
Diego	Di^a	Anti-Diego	Anti-Di^a	Unknown-unreported	Very rare
Duffy	Fy^a	Anti-Duffy	Anti-Fy^a	Infrequent	*Rare
	Fy^b	Anti-Duffy	Anti-Fy^b	Rare	Rare
I	I	Anti-I	Anti-I*	Very rare	No
Kell	K (K_1)	Anti-Kell K_1	Anti-K	Fairly common	Rare
	k (K_2)	Anti-Cellano K_2	Anti-k	Very rare	Very rare
	Kp^a	Anti-Penny,K_3	Anti-Kp^a	Very rare	Rare
	Kp^b	Anti-Rautenberg K_4	Anti-Kp^b	Very rare	Rare
	Js^a	Anti-Sutter,K_6	Anti-KJs^a	Very rare	Rare
	Js^b	Anti-Matthews,K_7	Anti-Js^b	Very rare	Rare
Kidd	Jk^a	Anti-Kidd	Anti-Jk^a	Infrequent	*Rare
	Jk^b	Anti-Kidd	Anti-Jk^b	Rare	Rare
Lewis	Le^a	Anti-Lewis	Anti-Le^a*	Rare	None
	Le^b	Anti-Lewis	Anti-Le^b*	Rare	None
Lutheran	Lu^a	Anti-Lutheran	Anti-Lu^a*	Very rare	None
	Lu^b	Anti-Lutheran	Anti-Lu^b*	Extremely rare	None
MN	M	Anti-M	Anti-M*	Rare	*Very rare
	N	Anti-N	Anti-N*	Unlikely	Unreported-unlikely
	S	Anti-S	Anti-S	Very rare	*Rare
	s	Anti-s	Anti-s	Unreported	Extremely rare
P	P_1	Anti-P_{1a}	Anti-P_{1a}*+	Very rare	None
	P (Tj^a)	Anti-Tj	Anti-Tj*+	Rare	None
Rh	c (hr^1)	Anti-c	Anti-c (hr^1)	Yes-infrequent	*Yes-fairly common
	D (Rh_o)	Anti-Rh_o	Anti-D (Rh_o)	Yes-common	*Yes-common
	Du	Anti-Du	Anti-Du	Yes-rare	*Yes-rare
	E (Rh'')	Anti-E	Anti-E (Rh'')	Yes-fairly common	*Yes-infrequent
Xg	Xg^a	Anti-Xg^a		Rare	Mild

Public antigens					
Yt^a					*Moderate to severe
Lan					Mild only
Ge					Mild only
Co^a					*Severe

Private antigens					
Batty					Mild only
Becker					Mild only
Berrens					Mild only
Biles					Moderate
Evans					Mild only
Gonzales					Mild only
Good					*Severe
Heibel					Moderate
Hunt					Mild only
Jobbins					Mild only
Radin					Moderate
Rm					Mild only
Ven					
Wright					*Severe
Zd					Moderate

+*May be naturally occurring antibodies, without proved immunizations.
* Amniotic fluid bilirubin studies
  Modified from Bowman, H.S. Am. J. Obstet. Gynec. 101:614-622, 1968 and Weinstein, L. Ob/Gyn Sur.

In addition to bacterial infections acquired with amnionitis, the following have been described as <u>agents responsible for transplacental fetal infection.</u>*

Agent (Maternal Effect)	Fetal Defect	Trimester

Bacteria

Group B Streptococci (GBS)   Early = fulminating disease   3rd
                                                Late = mild to meningitis

    See Baker, C.J.et al.J. Pediat.82:724, 1973.

Listeria monocytogenes   Abortion (early), infection and   All
  (Listerosis)   death (late)
  See Rendinh, G.et al. Clin Gyn. 10:441, 1968 and Ahlfors, C.E. et al.
  Amer. J. Dis. Child. 131:405, 1977.

Treponema pallidum   Abortion, death, anomalies   All

V. cholerae   Acidosis   All
  (maternal acidosis)
  See Hirschhorn, N. et al. Lancet 1:1230-1232, June, 1969.

Fungi

  Candida albicans   Infection
    See Kozinn, P.J. et al. Pediatrics 21:421, 1958.

  Histoplasma capsulatus

Mycoplasma

  Mycoplasma hominis   Abortions, newborn infection
    See Boe, O., et al. Scand. J. Inf. Dis. 5:283, 1973.

Protozoa

  Toxoplasma gondii   If antibodies before pregnancy,
  (toxoplasmosis)   no fetal infection!
  See Sever, J.L. Hosp. Prac.   Abortion (early), repeat abortion (?),   All
  5:75-83, April, 1970.   mental retardation (late), hepato-
  Desmonts, G. & Couvreur, J.   splenomegaly (late) TORCH
  NEJM 290:1110, 1974.

<u>Viruses</u>   See Hardy, J.B., Arch. Otolaryngol. 98:218, 1973,
              Sever, J.L. Int'l. J. Gynaec. Obstet. 8:763-769, September, 1970.

  Arboviruses   Newborn seizures, encephalitis   3rd
  (equine encephalomyelitis)

  Chickenpox - Shingles   Abortion (early), infection of newborn   1st,3rd
  (maternal pleurodynia)

  Coxsackie   Congenital heart (12%), myocarditis,   2nd
    See Brown, J. Med. World News 11:17,1970. encephalitis

  Cytomegalovirus   Microcephaly   2nd
  (3% gravida excrete virus; 2/3 above   Chorioetinitis, deafness, mental retard-3rd
   excrete in milk)   ation, CP, jaundice, petechia, TORCH.
  See Diosi, P. et al. Lancet 2:1063-1066, November, 1967

  Echo virus
    See Sever, J.L. Hosp. Prac. 5:75-83, April, 1970.

  Enteroviruses

  Hepatitis   Hepatitis, hydrocephalus   3rd
  (maternal death)
  See D'Cruz, I.A. et al. Obstet. Gynec. 31:449-455, April, 1968.
  Garty, R. et al. Lancet 2:434, August, 1971.

  Herpes simplex (Type II)   Microcephaly, microphthalmos, retinal   1st
                                  damage (early)
                                  Herpes, encephalitis, death (late)(TORCH) 3rd
  See Nahmias, A.J. et al. Am. J. Obstet. Gynec. 110:825-837, July, 1971.
  Naib, Z.M. et al. Obstet. Gynec. 35:260-263, February 1970.

  Herpes Zoster   ?

  Influenza   Abortion (?), stillbirth (?), malformation   ?
    See Harty, J. et al. J Public Health 51:1182, 1961.
  Wilson, M.G. and Stein, A.M. JAMA 210:336-337, October 1969.

Agent	Fetal Effect	Trimester
Measles (Rubeola) See Jespersen, C.S. et al. ACTA Pediat. 66:367, 1977.	Abortion, stillbirth, TORCH	1st

Mumps
  See Siegel, M. et al.
    New Eng. J. Med. 274:768-771, April,1966.
	Fetal death
	Endocardial fibroelastosis (?),
	cardiac malformation(?)
		1st

Poliomyelitis	Abortion (early) (?) Polio	1st 3rd

Rubella
  See Aase, J.M. et al. NEJM 286:1379, 1972,
    Hardy, J.B. et al. JAMA 207:2414-2420,
    March, 1969.
	Congenital heart
	Cataracts, deafness, microcephaly,
	mental retardation, newborn hepato-
	splenomegaly, hepatitis, TORCH
	School-age growth retardation, hearing,
	reading problem
		1st
		
		2nd

Rubeola (See Measles)		
Smallpox	Abortion Stillbirth, smallpox, hydrops fetalis, cataracts	1st 3rd

Vaccina
  See Table D-95
    Levine, M.M. Lancet 2:34, 197
    Liebeschuetz, H.J. J. Obstet. Gynaec. Brit. Cwlth. 71:132-134, 1964.
	Abortion, premature delivery
	Generalized vaccinia
		1st
		3rd

Varicella See Srabstein, J.C. et al. J. Ped. 84:239, 1974.	Multiple defects, CNS, microphthalmia	1st
Virus pneumonia	Pneumonitis	3rd

*See Infectious Diseases of Fetus & Newborn, editor Remington, J. & Klein, J. Philadelphia, Saunders, 1976.

Clinical Interpretation: 5% of pregnancies are complicated by infections (excluding colds). IgM cord blood levels usually are elevated after fetal infection.

FETAL INFECTION

Percentage of Mothers with Clinical Symptoms or Signs of Infection With TORCH Agents

Agent	Symptom	Mother	Percentage Newborn (within 1 mo)
Toxoplasma	Mononucleosis or rash	<10	≈ 25
Rubella	Rash	<50	≈ 35
Cytomegalo-virus	Mononucleosis	<1	<5(intra-uterine)
	Genital	<1	<1(intra-partum)
Herpes simplex	Genital	≈ 20	>95

From Nahmias, A.J.: The TORCH complex, Hosp. Prac. 9:65, 1974

Outcome and Clinical Findings in Fetus and Newborn Infected with TORCH Agents

Outcome or Finding	Agent			
	T	R	C	H
Abortions and stillbirths	+	+	+	+
Prematurity and/or intrauterine growth retardation	+	+	+	+
Constitutional signs- lethargy, poor feeding	+	+	+	+
Disseminated intravascular coagulation	?	?	?	+
Reticuloendothelial System				
Hepatosplenomegaly	+	+	+	+
Liver calcification	+	?	+	+
Jaundice	+	+	+	+
Hemolytic and other anemias	+	+	+	+
Petechiae-ecchymoses	+	+	+	+

FETAL INFECTION

Immunization during Pregnancy

	Smallpox	Yellow Fever	Cholera
Risk from Dis. to preg female	Mortality in. to 90% during preg.	Significant morb., mort. rate, not altered by pregnancy	Sig. morb. mortality rate, not altered by pregnancy
Risk from disease to fetus or neonate	Possible increase abort. rate Congenital smallpox reported	Unknown	Unknown
Vaccine	Live vacc., virus vacc.	Live, attenuated virus vaccine	Killed bact. vaccine
Risk from Vaccine to Fetus	Rare cases of congen. vaccinia	Unknown	Unknown
Indications for Vaccination during pregnancy	Not recommended in USA except at risk pop. (hosp., public health workers) Avoid, exc. in cases of prob. exposure	Contraind. except for unavoid. exposure	Only to meet internat. travel req.
Dose/Schedule	Give VIG(0.3cc kg) w/primary vaccination, when avail. Revacc. w/o VIG.	Single inj. per 10 yrs.	2 inject. 4-8 week apart
Comments	**	Postpone. travel pref. to vaccination	Vaccine of low efficacy

FETAL INFECTION

	Agent			
Outcome or Finding	T	R	C	H
Mucocutaneous vesicular or ulcerative lesions	0	0	0	+
Lungs- pneumonitis	+	+	+	+
Heart				
Myocarditis	+	+	+	+
Congenital heart disease	?	+	+	?
Bone Lesions	+	+	+	?
Central Nervous System				
Encephalitis	+	+	+	+
Microcephaly	+	+	+	+
Hydrocephaly	+	+	+	+
Intracranial calcification	+	+	+	+
Psychomotor retardation	+	+	+	+
Hearing loss	+	+	+	?
Eye				
Chorioretinitis	+	0	+	+
Pigmented retina	0	+	0?	0
Keratoconjunctivitis	0	0	0	+
Cataracts	0	+	0	+
Glaucoma	0	+	0	0
Visual impairment	+	+	+	+
Immunologic abnormalities, humoral, and/or cell-mediated	+	+	?	?

From Nahmias, A.J. The TORCH complex. Hosp. Prac. 9:65, 1974

FETAL INFECTION

Immunization during Pregnancy

	Plague	Rabies
Risk from Dis. to pregnant female	Significant morbidity and mortality, not altered by pregnancy	Near 100% fatality not altered by preg.
Risk from Disease to Fetus or Neonate	Unknown	Determined by Maternal disease
Vaccine	Killed bacterial vaccine	Unknown
Risk from Vaccine to Fetus	None reported	Unknown
Indications for Vaccin. during Preg.	Very selective vaccin. of exposed person	Pregnancy does not alter indic. for prophylaxis. Each case individually considered
Dose/Schedule	Consult public health authority for indic. and doseage	Consult public health authority for indications and doseage
Comments	---	----

Immunization during Pregnancy

	Hepatitis-A (infectious)	Varicella Zoster
Risk from Disease to Pregnant Female	Significant morbidity, low mortality, not altered by pregnancy	Low morbidity and mortality not altered by pregnancy
Risk from Disease to Fetus or Neonate	Transmission to fetus and possibility of neonatal hepa.	Possible increased risk of severe dis. to neonate, especially if premature
Vaccine	Pooled immune serum globulin	Zoster immune globulin or convalescent zoster plasma.
Risk from Vaccine to fetus	None reported	None reported
Indications for Vaccine during preg.	Household or institutional exposure. Travel in dev. countries	Experimental drug. NO PHS recommend. for use in pregnancy
Dose/Sched.	2 ccIM for adult for exposure of short-term travel	---
Comments	Not recommend. as protection against hepatitis (B)	CDC is maintaining surveillance for varicella during pregnancy

**Though congenital vaccinia and abortion following smallpox vaccination are not unknown, they are certainly rare. The safest procedure for primary smallpox vaccination during pregnancy is to give simultaneous, separate preparation of vaccinia immune globulin. When not available, vaccine must be given during epidemics or travel in epidemic areas.

From Amer College of Obstet. and Gynec. Tech. Bulletin No 20, March 1973

FETAL HEMATOLOGY

Blood Values in the Human Fetus

Weeks	Weight (gm)	RBC x10^6)	Hemogl. (ml)	Ht. (ml*)	MCV (u^3)	MCH (uug)
11	9.2	0.88	-	25	285	-
14	44	1.96	9.1	26.2	134	47
16	86	2.94	13.1	44	150	45
17	185	3.00	10.5	34	113	35
18	-	2.59	10.8	36	138	42
19	255	2,24	11.3	32	139	51
20	290	2.30	8.7	30	130	38
21	362	2.91	12.8	36.1	125	40
22	411	2.76	11	34.6	125	40
23	450	3.25	14.6	44.5	136	45
24	626	3.86	14.7	48.1	124	42
25	960	3.51	14 1	41.2	116	40

MCHC (%)	Icterus Index	Fresh (u)	Stained (u)	NRC(%)	Retic. (%)	WBC (x1000 mm^3)
-	-	10.96	9.18	7.6	94	-
34	7	10.64	9.37	4.0	18	2.0
30	35	8.49	7.72	-	12	15.5
31	-	7.80	8.40	1.2	18	6.6
20	7	8.55	7.96	0.4	9	-
36	-	8.30	7.90	-	-	-
29	10	9.30	8.50	0.7	22	17
35	20	8.70	7.50	0.3	10	12.2
32	8	8	7.68	0.6	18	14
33	5	8.40	8.10	0.2	6	8.6
30	16	8.81	8.05	1	7	17.4
34	-	-	7.88	0.3	-	8.8

*Ht = volume of packed cells/100 ml blood
See Wintrobe, M. Clinical Hematology 5th Edition, Lea and
     Febiger, Philadelphia, 1961.

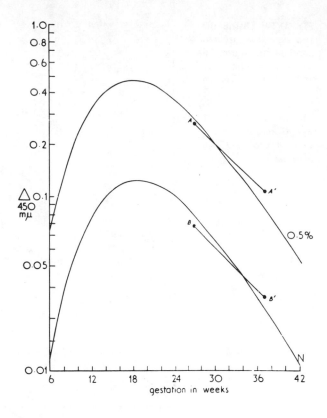

Fig. D-13a. Liley's lines for log 450 of normal (BB) and 5% confidence. (From Carlton, M. A.: *Br J Obstet Gynaecol* **77**: 221, 1970. Reproduced with permission.)

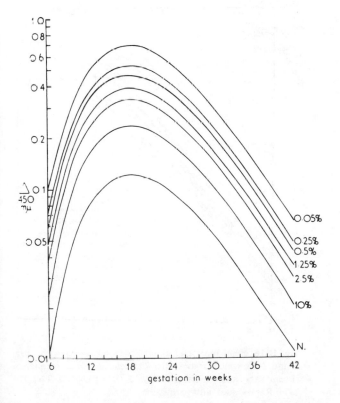

Fig. D-13b. Log 450 curves for normal pregnancies and confidence limits. (From Carlton, M. A.: *Br J Obstet Gynaecol* **77**: 211, 1970. Reproduced with permission.)

Fig. D-14. Distribution and regression curves for amniotic fluid osmolality, and sodium, urea, and creatinine concentration. (From Lind, T., Billewicz, W. Z., and Cheyne, G. A.: *Br J Obstet Gynaecol* **78:** 505, 1971. Reproduced with permission.)

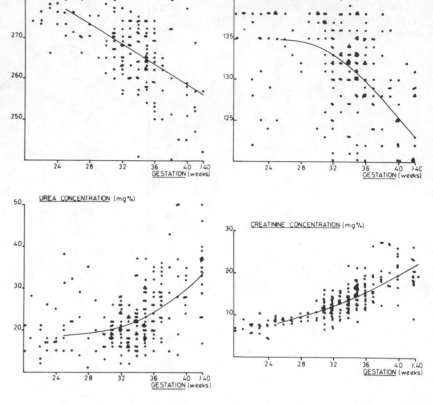

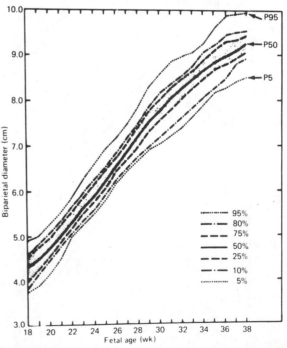

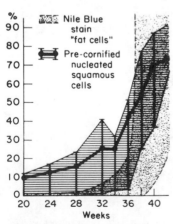

Fig. D-15. Proportion of fat cells and precornified cells in amniotic fluid of normal pregnancies. (From Floyd, W. S., Goodman, P. A., and Wilson, A.: *Obstet Gynecol* **34:** 583, 1969. Reproduced with permission.)

Fig. D-16. Fetal biparietal diameters as measured with ultrasound. Note wide variation after 28 weeks of normal pregnancy. (From Sabbagha, R. E., *et al.*: *Am J Obstet Gynecol* **126:** 479, 1976. Reproduced with permission.)

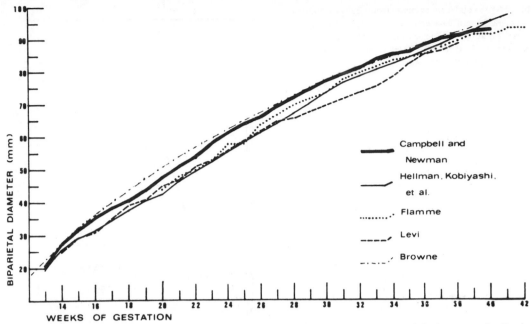

Fig. D-17. Results of different surveys of the correlations between biparietal diameters and fetal age, standardized at the speed of sound at 1540 sec. (From Bartolucci, L. and Sanders, R.: In *Ultrasound in Obstetrics and Gynecology*, R. C. Sanders and A. E. James, Eds., Appleton-Century-Crofts, New York, 1977. Reproduced with permission.)

Fig. D-18. Biparietal fetal diameter according to Campbell and Newman. (From *Br J Obstet Gynecol* **78:** 513, 1971. Reproduced with permission.)

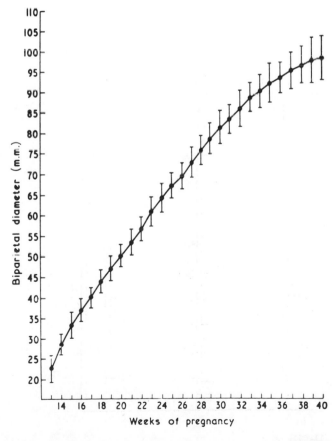

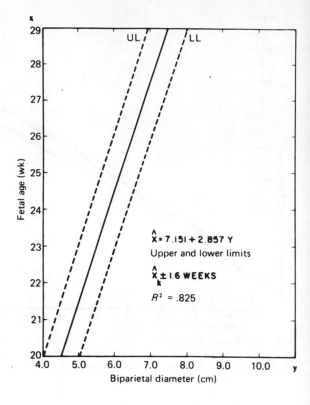

Fig. D-19. Fetal age estimate from BPDs obtained between 20 and 28 weeks. Note that the maximum variation about the mean value is ± 11 days. (From Sabbagha, R. E. *et al.*: *Obstet Gynecol* **43**: 7, 1974. Reproduced with permission.)

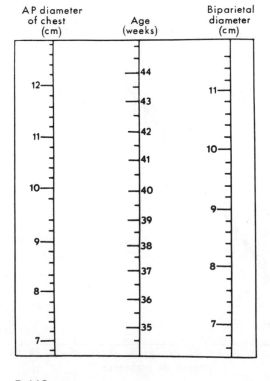

Fig. D-20. Estimation of fetal gestational age by biparietal and AP chest diameters. (To obtain estimated gestational age, place a straight edge across the nomogram bisecting both the anteroposterior chest diameter and the biparietal diameter. The estimated gestational age is then read from the point where the straight edge crosses the gestational age line.) (From Thompson, H. E. and Makowski, E. L.: *Obstet Gynecol* **37**: 44, 1971. Reproduced with permission.)

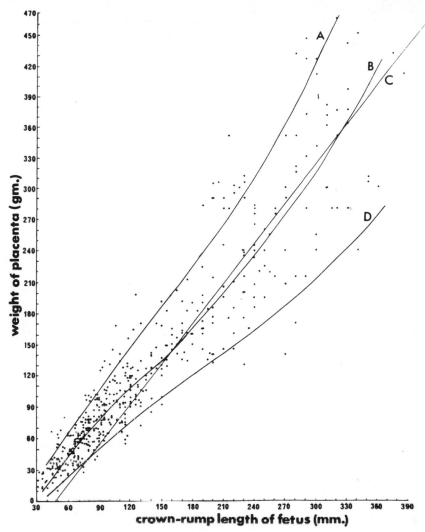

Fig. D-21. Relationship between human fetal crown-rump length and weight of placenta. A = 10%; B = regression line; C = 50%; D = 90%. (From Grimes, D. H. and Hamilton, W. J.: *Br J Obstet Gynecol* **78**: 620, 1971. Reproduced with permission.)

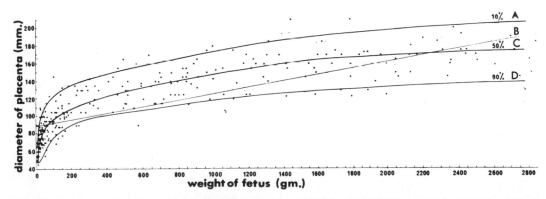

Fig. D-22. Relationship between human fetal weight and placental weight. A = 10%; B = regression line; C = 50%; D = 90%. (From Grimes, D. H. and Hamilton, W. J.: *Br J Obstet Gynecol* **78**: 620, 1971. Reproduced with permission.)

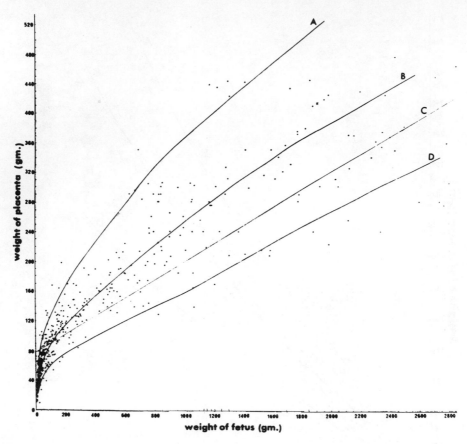

Fig. D-23. Relationship between weight of the fetus and weight of the placenta. (From Grimes, D. H., and Hamilton, W. J.: *Br J Obstet Gynecol* **78:** 620, 1971. Reproduced with permission.)

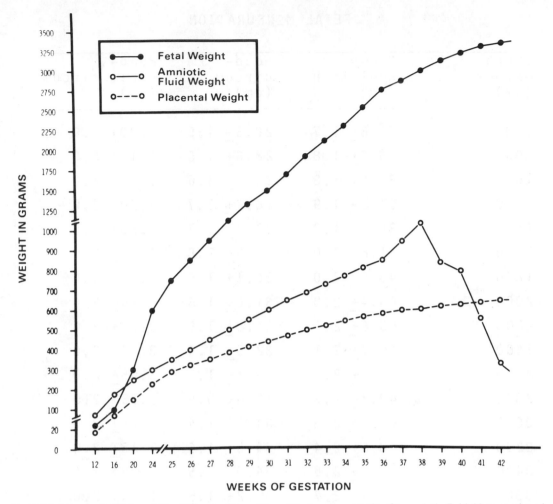

Fig. D-24. "Average" weights of (●—●) human fetus, (○— ○) placenta, and (○—○) amniotic fluid. Note continued fetal weight increase as compared with placenta and amniotic fluid. (From Hochberg, H.: Roche Medical Electronics, 1976. Reproduced with permission.)

FETAL MENSURATION

Birth weight (gm)	Crown-Heel lgth (cm)	Head-circum. (cm)	Head-chest circum. (cm)
600	31.0± 1.7	20.5± 1.5	1.80± 2.0
800	33.3± 1.8	22.6± 1.6	3.15± 2.0
1000	35.6± 1.8	24.5± 1.6	3.85± 2.0
1200	37.8± 1.9	26.2± 1.7	4.20± 2.0
1400	39.8± 1.9	27.7± 1.7	4.50± 2.0
1600	41.6± 2.0	29.0± 1.8	4.50± 2.0
1800	43.2± 2.0	30.1± 1.6	4.25± 2.0
2000	44.4± 2.0	31.0± 1.6	3.95± 2.0
2200	45.6± 2.1	31.8± 1.5	3.65± 2.0
2400	46.7± 2.1	32.5± 1.4	3.35± 2.0
2600	47.7± 2.2	33.1± 1.2	3.05± 2.0
2800	48.7± 2.3	33.6± 0.9	2.75± 2.0
3000	49.7± 2.3	34.1± 1.4	2.45± 2.0
3200	50.6± 2.4	34.5± 1.6	2.15± 2.0
3400	51.5± 2.5	34.9± 1.5	1.85± 2.0
3600	52.4± 2.7	35.2± 1.5	1.55± 2.0
3800	53.1± 2.8	35.5± 1.4	1.25± 2.0
4000	53.6± 2.8	35.8± 1.4	0.95± 2.0

See Usher, R. and McLean, F.J. Pediat. 74: 906, 1969

FETAL MENSURATION

Weight and Crown-Rump Length in Relation to Mensural Age

Mensural Age(wks)	Mensural Age(days)	Weight (gm)	Crown-Rump Length(mm)
11	80.0 (77-82)	14.8+ 6.1 (4.5- 27.5)	59.9+ 8.7 (42.5- 78)
12	86.2 (84-90)	20.8+ 14.4 (4.1- 67.3)	65.7+ 13.2 (43- 100)
13	93.7 (91-97)	72.6+ 70.3 (12.4-254.5)	94.0+ 30.2 (56- 160)
14	100.1 (98-103)	77.7+ 55.5 18.3- 264.0)	99.5+ 20.1 (66- 151)
15	107.0 (105-110)	82.5+ 32.3 (39.0- 138.0)	103.8+ 11.9 (83- 125)
16	114.0 (112-118)	117.3+ 66.8 (23.5- 267.5)	116.8+ 16.7 (73- 155)
17	121.4 (119-124)	182.3+ 97.8 (24.0- 395.0)	135.3+ 25.2 (76- 179)
18	137.0 (126- 132)	223.0+ 47.4 (152.0-303.0)	146.1+ 15.8 (128- 159)
19	137.4 (133- 145)	246.8+ 110.7 (64.0- 444.0)	147.8+ 22.3 (100- 177)
21	149.6 (147- 152)	301.7+ 152.9 (7.4- 549.0)	154.8+ 37.7 (51- 195)
22	155.7 (154- 159)	457.6+ 218.3 (78.0- 857.0)	179.0+ 28.1 (108- 230)
24	164.6 (161- 172)	613.6+ 198.8 (351.0- 957.0)	205.7+ 25.2 (165- 250)

See Hardwich, D.F., J. Reprod. Med. 2: 98, 1969

FETAL MENSURATION

(mean + SD)

Mensural Age(wks)	Birth Weight(g)	Crown-Heel(cm)	Head (cm)	Chest (cm)
25	850+ 200	34.6+3.0	23.2+2.5	19.8+2.9
26	933+ 230	35.6+3.0	24.2+2.6	20.2+2.9
27	1016+ 270	36.6+3.1	24.8+2.7	20.8+2.9
28	1113+ 300	37.6+3.1	25.6+2.7	21.3+2.9
29	1228+ 330	38.8+3.2	26.6+2.7	22.1+3.0
30	1373+ 350	39.9+3.3	27.6+2.8	23.0+3.0
31	1540+ 400	41.1+3.3	28.7+2.8	24.0+3.1
32	1727+ 450	42.4+3.4	29.6+2.8	25.1+3.1
33	1900+ 500	43.7+3.4	30.5+2.8	26.3+3.1
34	2113+ 560	45.0+3.5	31.4+2.7	27.6+3.1
35	2347+ 630	46.2+3.5	32.2+2.6	28.7+3.2
36	2589+ 700	47.4+3.6	33.0+2.5	29.8+3.2

FETAL MENSURATION

(mean + SD)

Mensural Age(wks)	Birth weight(gm)	Crown-Heel(cm)	Head (cm)	Chest (cm)
37	2868+ 750 (3270+ 440)	48.6+3.6	33.8+2.4	30.9+3.3
38	3133+ 800 (3490+ 470)	49.8+3.7	34.3+2.3	32.2+3.3
39	3360+ 860 (3710+ 500)	50.7+3.7	34.8+2.2	32.9+3.3
40	3480+ 920 (3890+ 530)	51.2+3.8	35.1+2.1	33.4+3.4
41	3567+ 950 (4150+ 555)	51.7+3.8	35.2+2.0	33.6+3.4
42	3513+ 960 (4370+ 580)	51.5+3.8	35.1+1.9	33.5+3.4
43	3416+ 970	51.3+3.8	35.0+1.8	33.2+3.5
44+	3384+ 970	51.0+3.8	34.6+1.8	33.0+3.5

Figures in parentheses indicate predicted optimal weight gain.

See Greunwald, P. Public Health Report 83: 867, 1968

See Usher, R. and McLean, F. J. Pediat. 74: 906, 1969

FETAL MENSURATION

Fetal Growth

Menstrual age (weeks)	Mean Weight* (gm)	Percentiles (gm)						
		5%	10%	25%	50%	75%	90%	95%
27	1034±217	593	687	837	1022	1193	1375	1468
28	1172±344	597	695	929	1118	1302	1691	1887
29	1322±339	871	993	1102	1275	1450	1893	2012
30	1529±474	824	1034	1255	1458	1742	2024	2381
31	1757±495	1076	1184	1408	1648	1968	2443	2818
32	1881±437	1269	1351	1578	1861	2134	2453	2734
33	2158±511	1504	1588	1812	2095	2407	2893	3145
34	2340±552	1542	1746	1986	2298	2683	3104	3424
35	2518±468	1802	1943	2245	2489	2806	3137	3329
36	2749±490	2033	2173	2406	2697	3044	3414	3661
37	2989±466	2258	2392	2657	2960	3286	3620	3793
38	3185±450	2468	2602	2875	3171	3466	3745	3958
39	3333±444	2582	2763	3044	3325	3623	3902	4090
40	3462±456	2720	2880	3150	3448	3745	4045	4246
41	3569±468	2813	3003	3254	3547	3870	4186	4392
42	3637±482	2851	3039	3306	3618	3934	4288	4478
43	3660±502	2817	3014	3309	3652	3966	4330	4499
44	3619±515	2758	2962	3278	3589	3966	4252	4517

*Mean ± standard deviation

See Babson, S.G. et al. Pediat. 45: 937, 1970.

FETAL MENSURATION

Appearance of Fetal Hormones

	Menstrual Age (weeks)
Cortisol (from Maternal progesterone)	10
Estrogen	10
FSH	11 - 14
HCG	1.5
HGH	9 - 10
Insulin	12
LH	18
Placental lactogen (HCP)	3
Placental steroid	6
Testosterone	9
Thyrocolcitonin	12
TSH	14 - 16
Thyroglobulin synthesis	4.5
Iodination of protein	11

See Gitlin, D. and Biasucci, A.J.: Clin Endocr Metab 29:926, 1969.

Villee, D.H.: New Eng J Med 281:473, 1969.

FETAL REFLEXES

Sequence of Development of Reflexes of an Avoiding
and/or Protective Nature on Stimulation of Areas
Supplied by Sensory Fibers of the Trigeminal Nerve

Age from Conception (weeks)	Area Stimulated	Reflexes Observed
5.5	Perioral	Contralateral flexion in neck region, i.e., away from stimulus (avoiding reflex)
6.5	Perioral	Contralateral flexion in neck and trunk region, i.e., away from stimulus, coupled with shoulder movement and pelvic rotation
7.5	Perioral (particularly common from midline)	Head and trunk extension (movement away from stimulus)
8-8.5	Upper eyelid (spreading to include even upper and lower lips by 11 weeks)	Orbicularis oculi contraction ("squint" type of reflex)
8.5	Bridge of nose and below eyelid	Rotation of face to contralateral side (movement away from stimulus), usually with lateral neck and trunk flexion
8.5	Lower eyelid	Contralateral trunk flexion with or without extension of brachia
9	Upper eyelid or eyebrow area	Corrugator supercilii contraction ("scowl" type reflex)
10	Upper eyelid or eyebrow area	"Squint" and "scowl" reflexes may be continued
10-10.5	Upper eyelid	Downward rotation of eyeballs

10.5	Lips, unilaterally	Head extension with mouth opening and closing
11-12	Upper lip and ala of nose	Elevation of angle of mouth and ala of nose ("sneer" type reflex)
11.5-12	Perioral face area	Contralateral rotation of face without trunk movement, sometimes with "sneer" type reflex
11-14.5	Upper eyelid and eyebrows; later, lower eyelid, cheek region, lips, inside of mouth	Local reflexes such as "squint" are combined with neck and trunk extension or with rotation of face away from stimulus
12.5	Upper lip bilaterally	Bilateral "squint" type reflex
13.5	Lips at rima oris	"Squint" may be combined with mouth closure and/or head extension
14	Nose and upper lip	"Squint", "scowl" and "sneer" combined with head extension
21.5	Use of respirator	Phonation (high-pitched cry) on establishing respiration
22	Inside of nostrils	Sneezing
23	Tapping eyelids gently	Palpebral reflex

See Humphrey, T. Prog. Brain Res. 4: 93, 1964.

FETAL REFLEXES

Developmental Sequence of Cutaneous Sensitivity

Age (wks)	Skin Area Demonstrated Sensitive to Stimulation
5.5	About the mouth (perioral-maxillary and mandibular fibers of trigeminal nerve)
6-7.5	Extension of perioral area to include alae of nose, and chin
8-8.5	Eyelids (ophthalmic division of trigeminal nerve)
8.5	Shoulder, genital area, anal area, genito-femoral sulcus
8.5-9	Soles of feet
9	Eyebrow, forehead, upper arm, forearm
9.5	Entire face now sensitive, except peripherally upper chest
9-10	Thighs, legs
11	Remaining chest areas
12	Tongue, back, side of trunk, over scapula
13	Abdomen
15	Buttocks
30	Inside of thigh

CLINICAL INTERPRETATION

Effects of Anoxia on Reflexes Elicited by Cutaneous Stim.

Reflex	First Appears (weeks)	Order of Suppression
Neck and trunk flexion to opposite side with rotation of pelvis and extension of arms at shoulders	6.5	Last to disappear
Finger closure	8.5	Third
Foot-Sole response	9	Second
Elevate angle of mouth	11-12	First

FETAL REFLEXES

Relationship of Direction of Head and Trunk Reflexes to Area of Face Stimulated

Reflex Elicited	Age When Reflex Appears (weeks)	
	Away From Stimulus	Toward Stimulus
Lateral flexion of head (neck muscle contraction) and trunk	5.5 (neck muscles only)	6
Midline head (and trunk) movements:		
Head extension (face moved away from stimulus)	7.5	
Ventral head flexion (face moved toward stimulus)		8
Rotation of face accomplished by lateral trunk flexion or head extension	8.5	9-9.5
Rotation of face alone (without lateral trunk flexion)	11.5-12	Newborn infants

FETAL REFLEXES

Fetal and Newborn Reflexes

Age (wks) since conception	Protective and/or avoiding locomotion	Feeding
5.5	Contralateral neck flexion	
6-6.5	Contralateral neck and trunk flexion	Ipsilateral neck, trunk flexion
7.5	Head and trunk extension	Mouth opening
8-8.5	Orbicularis oculi contract. ("squint") rotation of face to contralateral side, usually w/ trunk flex.	Ventral head flexion
9-9.5	Corrugator supercilli contraction ("scowl")	Ipsilateral head rotation
10-10.5	Squint and scowl combined	Lip closure, swallowing
11-14.5	Squint comb. w/ neck trunk extension, or w/ contralateral head rotation	Mouth opening, closure, swallowing, ventral head flexion, tongue movement
15-21.5		Protrusion of lips
22		Sucking
25		
30		
Premature and newborn	Primitive swim movements	Babkin reflex

FETAL REFLEXES

Age	Grasping and Plantar	Genital	Respiratory like
5.5			
6-6.5			
7.5			
8-8.5	Incomplete finger clos. plantar flexion of all toes	Bilateral flex. of thighs on pelvis	
9-9.5			
10-10.5	Principally dorsi-flexion of big toe and toe fanning; flex. at foot; knee, hip		
11-14.5	Complete finger closure, maintained finger closure		Isolated respiratory chest contractions; abdominal muscle contractions
15-21.5	Effective but weak true grasp		Temporary diaphragmatic contraction; temp. effective resp. chest contract. and phonation if delivered
22			
25	Maintained grasp to support most of body wt. momentarily		Permanent resp. est. on delivery
30		Cremasteric reflex	
Premature and new.	Grasp weak but stronger while sucking		

FETAL SCALP BLOOD VALUES

	First Stage	Second Stage	Umbilical Vein (Delivery)
PO_2 (torr)	23.7 ± 5.7	21.5 ± 4.3	29.5 ± 8.3
Oxygen saturation (%)	50.8 ±16.9	37.3 ±14.3	60.0 ±19.8
Hematocrit (%)	49.6 ± 8.7	52.3 ± 7.0	54.8 ± 6.4
pH	7.33± 0.05	7.29± 0.05	7.30± 0.07
PCO_2 (torr)	41.0 ± 8.2	47.2 ±10.1	41.8 ± 9.1
Base deficit (mEq/L)	4.8 ± 2.5	6.6 ± 2.7	6.7 ± 2.3
Lactate (m mol/L)			3.4 ± 1.3
Glucose (mg%)	66.1 ±21.4	69.0 ±22.0	92.9 ±26.2

See Paterson, P.J. et al. J. Obstet. Gynaec. Brit. Cwlth. 77:390, 1970.

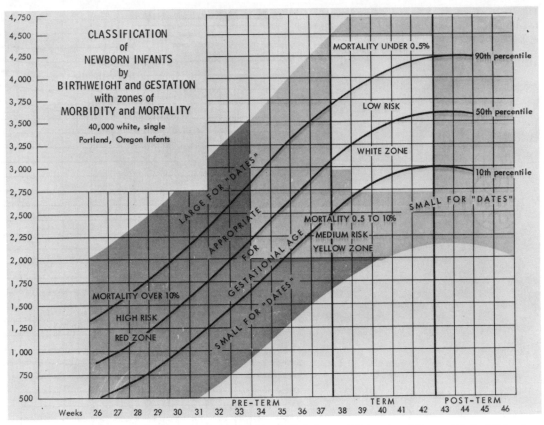

Fig. D-25. Presented at ACOG meeting in Portland by S. G. Babson of University of Oregon Medical School.

Fig. D-26. Fetal head growth, weight, and length. (From Lubchenco, L. O.: *Pediatrics* **37**: 403, 1966. Reproduced with permission.)

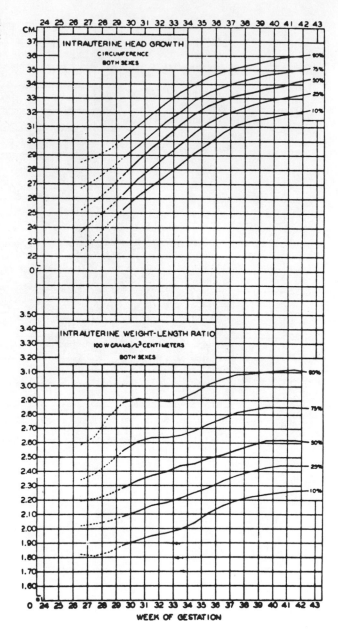

Fig. D-27. Fetal length and weight. (From Lubchenco, L. O.: *Pediatrics* **37**: 403, 1966. Reproduced with permission.)

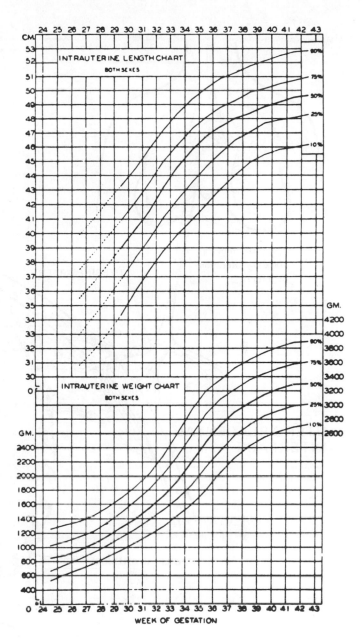

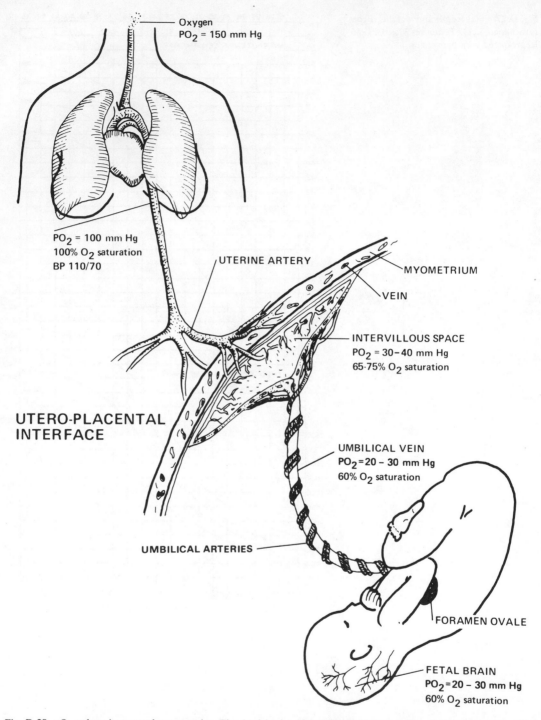

Fig. D-28. pO₂ values in normal pregnancies. The fetal brain pO₂ of 20–30 Torr is achieved through various fetal shunts. (From Hochberg, H.: Roche Medical Electronics, 1976. Reproduced with permission.)

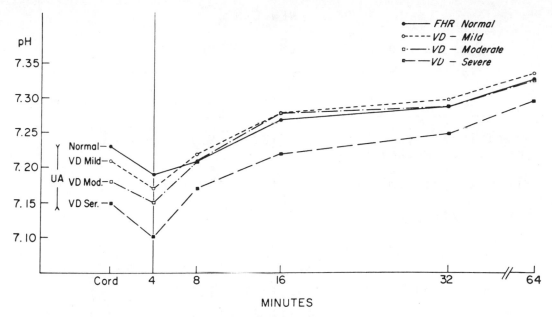

Fig. D-29. Neonatal pH values according to FHR patterns. VD = variable decelerations. (From Staisch, K., *et al.*: In *Perinatal Medicine,* Stembera, Z. K., Ed. PSE, Stuttgart, 1975. Reproduced with permission.)

HEMATOLOGIC VALUES OF NEWBORNS

	Small for Dates	Normal (full-term)	Premature
Gestational age (menstrual weeks)	39.7±0.2	39.7±0.2	35.2±0.4[1,2]
Birth weight (gm)	2257±60	3128±48	2248±84[2]
Erythrocytes			
Count (Million/mm^3)	5.3±0.1	4.5±0.2	4.4±0.1[1]
Fetal (%)	81.0±3.3	83.3±2.5	89.7±1.9
Transitional (%)	15.0±2.1	11.1±1.1	8.6±1.3
Adult (%)	4.3±1.7	5.3±1.7	2.2±0.6[1,2]
Hematocrit (%)			
Capillary	67.2±1.9	58.9±1.3	54.4±4.5[1]
Venous	59.4±1.4	52.8±1.2	49.9±1.3[1]
Hemoglobin			
Total (gm%)	19.8±0.5	17.5±0.4	16.1±0.4[1]
Fetal (% total Hgb)	77.5±2.2	66.2±1.7	75.7±0.9[2]
HgF concentration (gm%)	15.4±0.6	11.6±0.4	12.1±0.4[1]
MCV (u^3)	114.7±2.7	118.0±3.5	113.2±2.2
MCH (uug)	37.4±0.8	39.3±1.5	36.5±0.6
MCHC (%)	32.8±0.4	33.1±0.5	32.3±0.3
Reticulocyte count (/100 RBC)	2.7±0.4	5.0±0.4	4.5±0.7[1]

1 = P <0.01 when compared with full-term, small for dates infants.
2 = P <0.01 when compared with normal full-term infants.

See Humbert et al. J. Pediat. 75:812, 1969.

NEWBORN

Fetal Urine at Term

Osmolality (mOsm/L)	Na$^+$ (mEq/L)	K$^+$ (mEq/L)	Cl (mEq/L)	Urea (mg%)
137 (97-232)	44.1 (13-66.5)	4.7 (1.2-16.8)	41 (20-61)	102 (48-252)

See McCance, R.A. and Widdowson, E.M.:
     Proc Royal Soc Sec B 41: 488, 1953.

NEWBORN

Cord Blood at Delivery

	Umbilical Vein	Umbilical Artery
Acid base		
Oxygen		
pO_2 torr [0.133]	24.4 (16.1-35.1)	14.5 (0-22)
saturation %	50.3 (17-83)	20.2 (0-45)
Carbon dioxide		
pCO_2 torr [0.133]	43.4 (30-57)	56.8 (33-80)
CO_2 content (vol%)	60	
pH units		
actual	7.30 (7.15-7.45)	7.25 (7.09-7.40)
equilibrated		
(qu40)	7.24 (7.09-7.35)	7.16
Base excess mEq/L	-9-54 (-16.6 to -2.5)	

(See Saling, E. Foetal and Neonatal Hypoxia. Williams and Wilkins, Baltimore, 1968.)

Bilirubin mg%	1.6 (0.4-4)
Buffer base mEq/L	37.23 (30.8-43.7)
Standard	
mEq/L	16.62 (11.8-21.4)
Coagulation	
Bleeding time (min.)	2
Coagulation time	
(minutes)	2.5 (2-3)
Platelets x 10^3	225 (140-290)
Electrolytes mEq/L	
Bicarbonate (HCO_3)	22
Calcium (Ca^{++}) [0.25]	11.3
Chloride (Cl)	107
Phosphorous (mg%)	5.5
Potassium (K^+)	9.8
Sodium (Na^+)	144
Iron (ugm%) [0.179]	160

NEWBORN

Cord Blood at Delivery

	Umbilical Vein	Umbilical Artery
Enzymes		
Alkaline phosphate (BU)	4-10	
SGOT		
Nitrogen		
BUN mg% [0.167]	8.8 (3.7-14)	
Uric acid (mg%)	3.1 (2.4-5.0)	
Albumin gm%	3.75	
globulin gm%	1.35	
Sedimentation	100	

[S.I.] Conversion Factor

PHYSICAL MATURITY

	0	1	2	3	4	5
Skin	gelatinous red, transparent	smooth pink, visible veins	superficial peeling &/or rash, few veins	cracking pale area rare veins	parchment, deep cracking no vessels	leathery, cracked, wrinkled
Lanugo	none	abundant	thinning	bald areas	mostly bald	
Plantar creases	no crease	faint red marks	anterior transverse crease only	creases ant. 2/3	creases cover entire sole	
Breast	barely percept.	flat areola, no bud	stippled areola, 1-2 mm bud	raised areola, 3-4 mm bud	full areola, 5-10 mm bud	
Ear	pinna flat stays folded	sl. curved pinna, soft with slow recoil	well-curv. pinna, soft but ready recoil	formed & firm with instant recoil	thick cartilage, ear stiff	
Genitals Male	scrotum empty, no rugae		testes descending, few rugae	testes down, good rugae	testes down, good rugae	
Genitals Female	prominent clitoris & labia minora		majora & minora equally prominent	majora large, minora small	clitoris & minora completely covered	

Score	2	5	8	10	12	15	18	20

Weeks	26	28	30	32	34	36	38	40

From Ballard, J.L. et al. Pediat. Res. 11:374, 1977

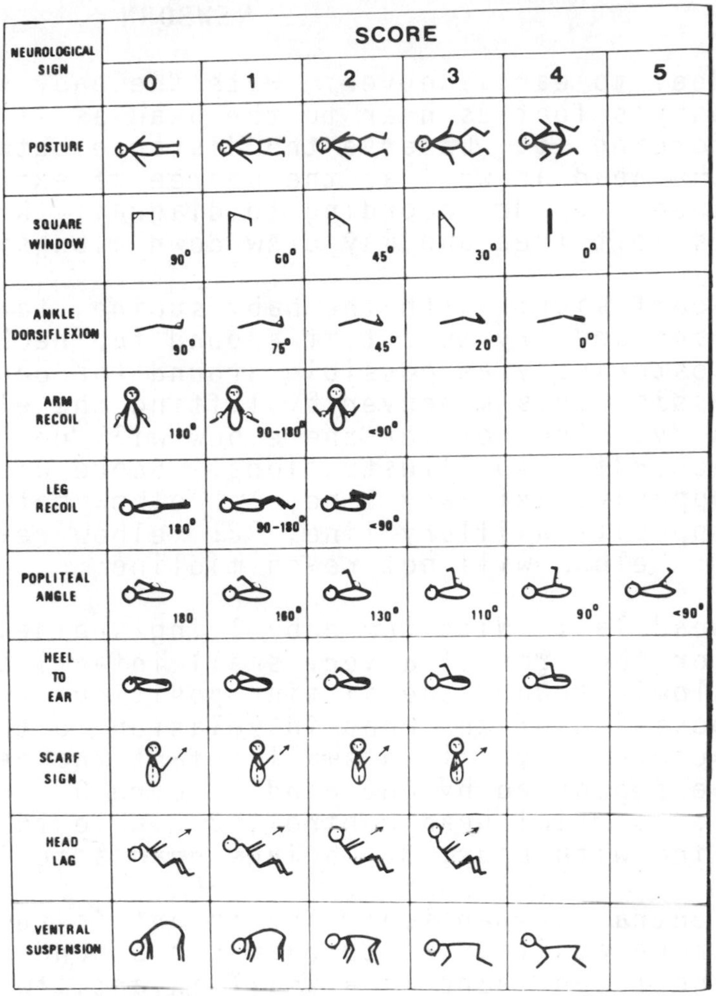

Fig. D-30. The "Dubowitz" scoring system for neurological maturity. (From Dobowitz, L., Dubowitz, V., and Goldberg, C.: *J Pediat* **77**: 1, 1970. Reproduced with permission.)

Heel to ear maneuver: With the baby supine, draw the baby's foot as near to the head as it will go without forcing it. Observe the distance between the foot and the head as well as the degree of extension at the knee. Grade according to diagram. Note that the knee is left free and may draw down alongside the abdomen.

Scarf sign: With the baby supine, take the infant's hand and try to put it around the neck and as far posteriorly as possible around the opposite shoulder. Assist this maneuver by lifting the elbow across the body. See how far the elbow will go across and grade according to illustrations. Score 0: elbow reaches opposite axillary line; 1: elbow between midline and opposite axillary line; 2: elbow reaches midline; 3: elbow will not reach midline.

Head lag: With the baby lying supine, grasp the hands (or the arms if a very small infant) and pull him slowly toward the sitting position. Observe the position of the head in relation to the trunk and grade accordingly. In a small infant the head may initially be supported by one hand. Score 0: complete lag; 1: partial head control; 2: able to maintain head in line with body; 3: brings head anterior to body.

Ventral suspension: The infant is suspended in the prone position, with examiner's hand under the infant's chest (one hand in a small infant, two in a large infant). Observe the degree of extension of the back and the amount of flexion of the arms and legs. Also note the relation of the head to the trunk. Grade according to diagrams.

If score differs on the two sides, take the mean.

Posture: Observed with infant quiet and in supine
position. Score 0: arms and legs extended; 1:
beginning of flexion of hips and knees, arms extended;
2: stronger flexion of legs, arms extended; 3: arms
slightly flexed, legs flexed and abducted; 4: full
flexion of arms and legs.

Square window: The hand is flexed on the forearm
between the thumb and index finger of the examiner.
Enough pressure is applied to get as full a flexion
as possible, and the angle between the hypothenar
eminence and the ventral aspect of the forearm is
measured and graded according to diagram. (Care is
taken not to rotate the infant's wrist while doing
this maneuver.)

Ankle dorsiflexion: The foot is dorsiflexed onto the
anterior aspect of the leg, with the examiner's thumb
on the sole of the foot and other fingers behind the
leg. Enough pressure is applied to get as full flexion
as possible, and the angle between the dorsum of the
foot and the anterior aspect of the leg is measured.

Arm recoil: With the infant in the supine position,
the forearms are first flexed for 5 seconds, then
fully extended by pulling on the hands, and then
released. The sign is fully positive if the arms
return briskly to full flexion (Score 2). If the
arms return to incomplete flexion or the response
is sluggish, it is graded as Score 1. If they remain
extended or are only followed by random movements,
the score is 0.

Leg recoil: With the infant supine, the hips and knees
are fully flexed for 5 seconds, then extended by
traction on the feet, and released. A maximal response
is one of full flexion of the hips and knees (Score 2).
A partial flexion scores 1, and minimal or no movement
scores 0.

Popliteal angle: With the infant supine and his pelvis
flat on the examining couch, the thigh is held in the
knee-chest position by the examiner's left index finger
and thumb supporting the knee. The leg is then extended
by gentle pressure from the examiner's right index
finger behing the ankle, and the popliteal angle is
measured.

PLACENTA

Placental Dimensions

	Premature	Term	Small for Dates
Birth Weight(g)	2035± 80	3313± 49	2295± 52
Placental wt (g)	330± 13	420± 8.5	311± 6.4
Decidual area (cm^2)	230± 11.7	253± 6.6	204± 6.2
Thickness (cm)	1.43± 0.04	1.64± 0.05	1.54± 0.05
Density	0.993	0.995	0.996
Cord diameter (mm)	9.5± 0.02	10.1± 0.01	7.1± 0.02

See   Younoszai, M.K. and Haworth, J.C. Am. J. Obstet. Gynec. 103: 265, 1969

PLACENTA

Maternal Antibodies That Cross the Placenta

Actinomycetes
M. tuberculosis

Allergers
Blocking
Skin sensitizing

Bacteria
Bacillary dysentary
(shigellosis)
Colon bacillus
(E. coli)
Diptheria baciillus
H. pertussis
H. influenzae
Pneumococcus
Staphlococcus
Streptococcus
Tetanus bacillus
Typhoid bacillus

Richettsia
Q. fever

Spirochetes
T. pallidum

Sporoza
Coccidodomycosis
Histoplasmosis
Toxoplasmosis

Viruses

Adenovirus
Chicken pox (varicella)
Cold agglutins
ECHO virus (types 1, 2, 8, 11, and 20)
Herpes simplex
Influenza A
Influenza B
Japanese B. encephalitis

Lympho grauloma venereum
Measles
Mumps
Poliovirus
Smallpox
St. Louis encephalitis
Vaccina
Varicella - Zoster
Western equine encephalitis

PLACENTA

Placental Transfer

Electrolytes (minerals)	Symbol	Agent	Transport	Animal
Aluminum	Al	----	?	----
Antimony	Sb	----	?	----
Arsenic	As	----	+	Mouse
Barium	Ba	----	?	----
Bismuth	Bi	----	?	----
Bromine	Br	Br^{82}	+	Mouse
Cadmium	Cd	Cd^{109}	+	Hamster
Calcium	Ca	Ca^{45}	+	Cow, guinea pig, rat
Carbon	C	----	o	----
Cesium	Cs	Cs^{137}	+	----
Chlorine	Cl	Cl^{36}	+	rabbit, sheep
Chromium	Cr	Cr^{51}	-	rat
Cobalt	Co	----	+	rat
Copper	Cu	----		----
Fluorine	F	F^{18}	+	human
Gold	Au	----	o	----
Helium	He	----	+	dog
Hydrogen	H	----	+	human
Iodine	I	I^{131}	+	human

PLACENTA

Electrolytes (minerals)	Symbol	Agent	Transport	Animal
Iron	Fe	F^{59}, F^{55}	+	human
Lead	Pb	- - - -	+	human
Lithium	Li	- - - -	+	human, rat
Magnesium	Mg	Mg^{99}	+	human
Manganese	Mn	- - - -	+	pig
Molybdenum	Mo	- - - -	?	- - - -
Mercury	Hg	- - - -	?	- - - -
Nickel	Ni	- - - -	+	human
Nitrogen	N	- - - -	+	human
Oxygen	O	- - - -	+	human
Ozone	O_3	- - - -	+	human
Phosphorus	P	P^{32}	+	human
Potassium	K	K^{42}	$\pm$	rat, guinea pig
Radium	Ra	- - - -	?	- - - -
Radon	Rn	- - - -	?	- - - -
Selenium	Se	Se^{75}	+	- - - -
Silicon	Si	- - - -	o	- - - -
Silver	Ag	- - - -	o	- - - -

PLACENTA

Electrolytes (minerals)	Symbol	Agent	Transport	Animal
Sodium	Na	Na^{125}, Na^{131}, Na^{22}, Na^{24}	+	human, rabbit
Strontium	Sr	Sr^{90}	+	rat
Sulfur	S	S^{35}	+	mouse, pig, rabbit, rat
Tin	Sn	----	o	----
Uranium	U	----	o	----
Zinc	Zn	Zn^{65}	+	mouse, rat, rabbit

+ = effective transport

? = no information

o = no transport

Labor

Most of the data reflect the studies of E. A. Friedman. These data are presented in detail because they have become so much a part of our obstetrical dogma. I believe that the concepts of C. Hendricks are perhaps more accurate, but Hendricks' data have failed to attract the attention of our specialty.

LABOR

Length of Labor (Vertex)

	Nulliparas	Multiparas
Latent phase (hr)	8.6 ± 0.27	5.3 ± 0.19
Active phase (hr)	4.9 ± 0.15	2.2 ± 0.07
Deceleration (hr)	0.9 ± 0.05	0.23 ± 0.01
Maximum slope (cm/hr)	3.0 ± 0.08	5.7 ± 0.16
Second Stage (hr)	0.95 ± 0.04	0.24 ± 0.01

See   Friedman, E.A. et al. Obstet Gynec. 6: 570, 1955
      Friedman, E.A. et al Obstet Gynec. 8: 692, 1956

Phase of Labor and Mean Station

	Nulliparas	Multiparas
Begin Labor	-0.5 ± 0.06	-1.3 ± 0.11
Terminal latent phase	+0.4 ± 0.06	-0.3 ± 0.09
Midpoint of maximum slope	+1.1 ± 0.07	+0.6 ± 0.10
Begin deceleration phase	+2.0 ± 0.09	+1.8 ± 0.14
Begin second stage	+3.4 ± 0.10	+3.4 ± 0.16

See   Friedman, E.A. Labor - Clinical Evaluation and Management
      Appleton, Century, Crofts, New York, 1967

LABOR

Statistical Limits of Labor Parameters by Parity

Dimension (hours)	Parity		
	0	1-2	3+
Latent phase	16.5(21.0)	13.7(18.0)	12.0(15.3)
Active phase	11.7(15.0)	6.9(9.5)	6.6(8.8)
Maximum slope (cm/hr)	1.08(0.84)	1.37(1.01)	1.50(1.03)
Deceleration phase	2.71(4.92)	1.22(1.92)	0.98(1.70)
First stage	24.0(30.0)	18.0(20.5)	15.5(20.0)
Second stage	2.90(4.30)	1.24(2.16)	0.88(1.60)
Total labor	25.0(30.0)	18.5(21.0)	16.5(21.0)

Statistical limits expressed as 5 percentile points on cumulative distribution curve for maximum slope and 95 percentile for all other dimensions; parentheses enclose 2 and 98 percentile limits, respectively.

See Friedman, E.A. and Kroll, B.H. J. Reprod. Med. 6:179, April, 1971

LABOR

Abnormalities and Length of Labor (Nulliparas)

	Latent Phase (hrs)	Active Phase (hrs)	Max. Slope (cm/hr)	Decel. Phase (hrs.)
Control (vertex)	8.6+ 0.27	4.9+ 0.15	3.0+ 0.08	0.90+ 0.05
Fetopelvic disproportion (inlet 25% & 75% midplane)	10.3+ 0.78	13.4+ 0.67*	0.72+ 0.07*	9.6+ 0.52*
Breech	6.7+ 0.53	5.3+ 0.47	2.9+ 0.24	0.98+ 0.11
Face	10.9+ 2.63*	4.9+ 0.50	2.6+ 0.19	1.26+ 0.69
Brow	7.5+ 0.74	4.8+ 0.50	2.6+ 0.19	0.73+ 0.11
Premature	6.6+ 0.43	3.2+ 0.19	4.4+ 0.23	0.50+ 0.04
Fetal weight (4000 + gm)	6.9+ 0.97	6.0+ 0.86	2.3+ 0.22	0.94+ 0.10
Fibroid	6.3+ 0.51	3.9+ 0.28	3.1+ 0.20	0.56+ 0.07
Premature rupture of membranes	7.1+ 0.93	4.7+ 0.62	3.1+ 0.26	1.13+ 0.36
Hydramnios with term infants	8.6+ 2.33	3.2+ 0.68	3.8+ 0.64	0.57+ 0.12
Multiple pregnancy	6.2+ 0.82*	5.4+ 0.51	3.0+ 0.40	1.26+ 0.26

* Significant differences

LABOR

X-Ray Pelvimetry Interpretations

Pelvic Diameters (cm)	Normal	Critical Value
Allen		
Inlet $\dfrac{(AP \times trans)}{4}$	130+	<105
Midplane $\dfrac{(Trans \times AP\ outlet)}{4}$	120+	<100
Kaltreider*		
Inlet		
Anterior-posterior	11.6 (9.0-13.4)	10.0
Transverse	12.5 (10.7-15.2)	11.5
Midplane		
Anterior-posterior	12.1	11.5
Transverse	10.3	9.5
Posterior sagittal	5.2	4.0
Mengerts		
Inlet (AP x trans)	145(100%)	124(85%)
Midplane (AP x trans)	126(100%)	106(85%)
Moloy		
Inlet and midplane - smallest diameter of pelvis minus biparietal diameter of fetal head should be >1.8 cm.		
Weinberg and Scadron		
Inlet (AP + trans)	24.1	<23
Midplane (posterior sagittal + interspinous)	15.0	<13.5

See Kaltrieder, D.F. Am. J. Obstet. Gynec. 62: 600, 1951
    Kaltrieder, D.F. Am. J. Obstet. Gynec. 63: 393, 1952

Pelvis

Onset of Ossification and Fusion of Female Pelvic Bones

Bone	Ossification (years)	Fusion (years)
Illium		
Crest	13.5	18
Acetabular lip	9	10
Ischium		
Epiphysic tuberosity	12	16
Sacrum		
Lateral margin epiphyses	14	18

Mean External Measurements (cm)

	White	Black	Latin
Intercristal	26.4	25.8	26.4
Interspinous	23.2	22.3	24.2
External conjugate	18.3	18.7	18.3
Biichial	7.9	8.0	7.9

Type of Pelvis (%)

	White	Black	Latin
Android	32%	15%	22%
Anthropoid	24	41	30
Gynecoid	42	42	46
Platypelloid	2	2	2

MILK

Comparison of Human Milk and Cow's Milk
(Whole and Evaporated)

	Human Milk	Cow's Milk Whole	Evap.
Bacteria	None	Present	None
Calories per fluid ounce	20	20	40
Curd	Soft, flocculent	Hard, large	Soft, flocculent
Digestion		Less rapidly	
Emptying stomach		Less rapidly	
Fat(%)	3.5-4.0 (whole olein and less of volatile fatty acids)	3.5-5.2	7.9-8.2
Minerals(%)	0.15-0.25	0.7-0.75	1.5-1.6
Calcium	0.034-0.045	0.122-0.179	
Chlorine	0.035-0.043	0.098-0.116	
Copper	0.00003	0.00002	
Iron	0.0001	0.00004	
Magnesium	0.0005-0.0006	0.013-0.019	
Phosphorus	0.015-0.040	0.090-0.196	
Potassium	0.048-0.065	0.138-0.172	
Sodium	0.011-0.019	0.051-0.060	
Sulphur	0.0035-0.0037	0.030-0.032	

MILK

Comparison of Human Milk with Cow's Milk

	Human	Cow's Whole	Evap.
Protein (%)	1.0-1.5	3.2-4.1	6.8-7.0
Casein	0.4-0.5	3.0	5.7
Lactalbumin	0.7-0.8	0.5	1.1
Reactin	Alkaline or amphoteric	Acid or amphoteric	Acid or amphoteric
Sugar (lactose) (%)	6.5-7.5	4.5-5.0	9.8-10.0
Vitamins (per 100 cc)			
A	60-500 IU	80-220 IU*	No loss
C	1.2-10.8 mg	0.9-1.4mg*	0.6 mg
D	0.4-10.0 IU	0.3-4.4 IU*	No loss
Niacin	0.10-0.20mg	0.10 mg	
Riboflavin	0.015-0.080mg	0.010-0.26 mg	No loss
Thiamine	0.002-0.36mg	0.03-0.04mg*	0.02-0.03 mg
Water (%)	87.0-88.0	83.0-88.0	73.0-74.0

* Values are for pasteurized milk

Drugs Excreted in Human Milk

Drugs	Comments
Alcohol	Non-intoxicating levels- no effect
Allergens	
Ambenonium chloride (Mytelase)	
Aminophyline (theophylline with ethylenediamine)	
Amphetamines	Usually no effect
Amphetamine sulfate (Benzedrine and numerous other trade names) and other salts of amphetamine	
Dextroamphetamine sulfate (Dexedrine and numerous other trade names) and other salts of d-amphetamine	
Analgesics (non-narcotic)	Usually doses are detectable in milk but produce no effect on infant
Acetaminophen (Amdil, Anelix, Apamide, Elixodyne, Febrolin, Fendon, Lestemp, Lyteca syrup, Metalid, Nacetyl, Mebs, Tempra, Tylenol)	
Aspirin	Concentration in milk 50% serum levels
Dextropropoxyphene hydrochloride (Darvon)	
Phenacetin	
Sodium Salicylate	

Drugs Excreted in Human Milk

Drugs	Comments
Analgesics (narcotic)	
Codeine	
Mefenamic (Ponstel)	Variable amounts secreted permissible
Methadone hydrochloride	
Adanon, Althose syrup, Dolophine	
Morphine (trace)	No effect
Heroin	Amount variable, 50% infants are symptomatic
Anesthetics	
Chloroform	
Cyclopropane	
Ether	
Antibiotics and chemotherapeutics	In general, the more basic compounds are secreted in greater amounts than acid compounds, but infant does not obtain therapeutic amounts
Chloramphenicol (Chlormycetin)	
Clindamycin	
Cycloserine (Seromycin)	
Erythromycin	
*Flagyl	
Furodanti..	
Isoniazid (more than 20 trade names)	
Mandelic acid	
Neomycin Sulfate (Mycifradin, Neobiotic)	
Nitrofurantoins	
Novobiocin (Albamycin, Cathomycin)	
Oxacillin	
Para-aminosalicylic acid and salts (many trade)	
Penicillin (G; Benzyl)	
Streptomycin	

Drugs Excreted in Human Milk

Drugs	Comments
*Ergot	
Ethyl biscoumacetate(Tromexan)	
Hexachlorobenzene	
Imipramine hydrochloride (Tofranil)	
*Iodides including ^{131}I	27% of ^{131}I dose may be secreted in milk
Iopanoic acid (Telepaque)	
Isoniazid	
Laxatives and cathartics	Variable amounts detectable; frequent held responsible for infant diarrhea; few studies reported
Aloin Calomel (mild mercurous chloride) Danthron (Dionone, Dorbane, Istizin) Rhubarb	Said either not to pass, or conversely, to purge infant
*Lithium	
Levopropoxyphene (Novrad)	
Mandelic Acid	
Mephenoxalone (Trepidone)	
Methocarbamol (Robaxin)	
Metals, salts, minerals	
Arsenic Calcium Chloride Copper Iodides Lead Magnesium *Mercurous chloride (see calomel) Phosphate	

Drugs Excreted in Human Milk

Drugs	Comments
Metals(cont)	
Potassium	
Sodium	
Sulfur	
Nicotine	10-20 cigarettes/day can produce detectable amount
Oral Contraceptives	Effect unknown, may pro-
Norethynodrel	duce jaundice in infant (progesterone-related)
Papaverine	
Phenylbutazone (Butazolidin)	
Phenylthiazides	
Phenytoin (Diphenylhydantoin (Dilantin)	Usual therapeutic dose has no effect
Propylthiouracil	
Pseudoephedrine (Sudafed)	
Pyrimethamine (Daraprim)	
Quinidine	
Quinine	
Reserpine (many trade names and preparations)	
Salicylates	
Scopolamine (Hyoscine)	
Sedatives	
Barbituates	
Bromides	
Chloralhydrate	
Ethinamate (Valmid)	
Sodium Chloride	
Thiazides	
Thiouracil	
Thyroid	
Tolbutamide	
Tranquilizers (Chloropromazine- Thorazine)	

* potentially harmful

See Drug Intelligence and Clinical Pharmacy. 11: 233, 1977.

DIET

	Pregnancy	Lactation
Energy (Kcal)	+ 300	+ 500
Protein (gm)	+ 30	+ 20
Vitamin A (I.U.)	5,000	6,000
Vitamin D (I.U.)	400	400
Vitamin E (I.U.)	15	15
Ascorbic acid (mg)	60	80
Folacin (μg)	800	600
Niacin (mg)	+ 2	+ 4
Riboflavin (mg)	+ 0.3	+ 0.5
Thiamin (mg)	+ 0.3	+ 0.3
Vitamin B_6 (mg)	2.5	2.5
Vitamin B_{12} (μg)	4	4
Calcium (mg)	1,200	1,200
Phosphorus (mg)	1,200	1,200
Iodine (μg)	125	150
Iron (mg)	‖	18
Magnesium (mg)	450	450
Zinc (mg)	20	25

*Food and Nutrition Board, National Academy of Sciences - National Research Council, Eighth Edition, 1974

‖ The increased requirements of pregnancy cannot usually be met by ordinary diets; therefore, the use of supplemental iron is recommended.

+ Minimal requirements

DIET

Maternal Daily Foods

Food	Calories	Calcium (mg)	Iron (mg)	Protein (g)	Sodium (mg)
Bread (4 slices)	260	84	2.5	8	480
Butter (2 Tbs)	200	6	--	--	300
Egg (1)	80	27	1.2	6	60
Fruit					
Citrus (1)	55	11	0.2	1	1
Other (2)	150	20	1.6	--	2
Ice Cream (¼ pt=½ c.)	145	87	0.1	3	44
Meat					
Cooked (4 oz.)	300	13	3.3	28	80
Lunch	80-113	2-5	0.5-1.1	4-16	300
Bologna (1 oz)					
Ham (1 oz)					
Tuna (2 oz)					
Milk (2 c.)	330	576	0.2	17	244
Vegetables					
Green/ yellow(½c.)	27	45	0.8	2	50
Potato (½ c.)	65	6	0.5	3	5
Other (2 serv.)	90	36	1.6	4	20
TOTAL	1647-1680 C	900 mg	12.6 mg	76-88g	1580 mg

Maternal
Data

These data were obtained from many sources and reflect a composite of results from many different laboratories. With each group, a single authoritative reference is given although the exact figures I have selected may differ from that source. Most of these tables were previously published in my *Handbook of Obstetrical and Gynecological Data*, as published with permission of Geron-X of Los Altos, California.

MATERNAL AMINO ACIDS

Maternal Blood Amino Acids

Amino Acids	Non-Pregnant	1st Trim.	2nd Trim.	3rd Trim.
Alanine	223.8+ 76.8	210.0	240.5+ 42.1	284.8+ 92.7
α- Amino -n-butyrate	22.2+ 6.9		11.7+ 5.0	21.4+ 28.9
Arginine	80+ 24	68+ 31	59+ 23	75+ 33
Asparagine	28+ 9	28+ 13	27+ 13	32+ 23
Cystine	22+ 9	37+ 24	24+ 11	33+ 21
Glutamic Acid	145+ 56	148+ 79	167+ 64	162+ 71
Glycine	161+ 37	154+ 37	132+ 44	246+ 105
Histidine	92+ 22	92+ 11	93+ 17	92+ 34
Isoleucine	58+ 19	50+ 15	49+ 11	56+ 23
Leucine	100+ 27	99+ 20	85+ 18	105+ 46
Lysine	163+ 41	170+ 31	152+ 26	212+ 99
Methionine	12+ 8	13+ 7	12+ 5	18+ 5
Ornithine	46+ 10	53+ 13	46+ 15	93+ 43
Phenyla-lanine	54+ 18	56+ 13	50+ 9	61+ 24
Proline	150+ 58	151+ 62	167+ 51	251+ 88
Serine	135+ 50	143+ 62	118+ 44	169+ 73
Taurine	80+ 34	75+ 26	62+ 15	104+ 69
Threonine	295+ 46	378+ 75	354+ 106	400+ 118
Tyrosine	47+ 18	42+ 6	45+ 6	68+ 31
Valine	186+ 45	178+ 33	156+ 33	204+ 93

mean ± SD

Modified from Hytten, F.E. and Cheyne, G.A.: J. Obstet Gynaecol Br Commonw 79: 424, 1972.

MATERNAL BLOOD GASES
(acid base)

* A - Arterial **V - Venous	Non-pregnant	1st Trim.	2nd Trim.	3rd Trim.	Post Partum
Base-excess (mEg/L blood) (A)*	-1.0± 1.2	-3.6+ 0.9	-3.4± 1.2	-2.8 1.2	
Bicarbonate, actual (mEg/L plasma) (A)	24.0+ 1.3	19.2+ 0.6	19.4+ 1.1	19.7+ 1.2	
Bicarbonate, HCO_3 (mEg/L) (A)	23.7 (23.2-24.0)	24.6 (22.0-27.0)	23.9 (21.5-27.0)	23.2 (21.5-26.5)	25.3 (25.0-28.0)
Bicarbonate, standard (mEg/L plasma) (A)	25.2+ 0.8	20.6+ 0.6	20.8+ 1.0	21.2+ 1.0	
Buffer Base (mEg/L blood) (A)	44.7+ 2.0	42.3+ 0.9	42.6+ 1.4	43.1+ 1.1	
ph (A)	7.412 (7.39-7.43)	7.400+ 0.007	7.404+ (0.14)	7.42 (7.38-7.46)	
ph (V)**	7.38 (7.35-7.39)	7.39 (7.32-7.46)	7.30 (7.30-7.46)	7.41 (7.33-7.46)	7.80 (7.34-7.46)

See Kirschbaum, T.H. and DeHaven, J.C.: 3. Maternal and fetal blood Constituents. In N.S. Assaii (ed), Biology of Gestation. Vol II. The Fetus and Neonate. Academic Press New York, 1968, pp. 143-187

MATERNAL BLOOD GASES

A- Arterial V- Venous	Non- Pregnant	1st Trim.	2nd Trim.	3rd Trim.
CO_2 dissolved (mM/L plasma)				
A	1.22			1.00
V	1.35			1.21
CO_2 dissolved (mM/L RBC)				
A	1.01			0.83
V	1.10			1.00
CO_2 combined (HCO_3- +carbonate) (mM^3/L blood)				
A	20.4			17.3
V	21.8			
CO_2 combined (mM/L plasma)				
A	0.36			0.27
V	0.36			
Oxygen capacity (ml/100 ml blood)	18.3 (16.4-23.0)			15.5 (14.5-16.8)

MATERNAL BLOOD GASES

A- Arterial V- Venous	Non- Pregnant	1st Trim.	2nd Trim.	3rd Trim.
Oxygen content **(ml/100 ml blood)**				
A	17.5 (16.0-17.9)			14.5 (13.5-16.1)
V	13.7			11.0
Oxygen dissolved **(ml/100 ml blood)**				
A	0.28			0.29
V	0.12			0.10
O_2 **combined (ml/** **100ml blood)**				
A	17.2			14.4
V	13.6			10.9
O_2 **hemoglobin** **(salt-water %)**				
A	96.0 (91.9- 99.9)			97.0 (95.2- 97.5)
pO_2 **(torr)**				
A	107.0+ 8.5−	107.7+ 8.5−	107.7+ 8.5−	104.0+ 6.2−
pCO_2 **(torr)**				
A	38.0 (37.1- 38.5)	31.9+ 1.2−	32.1+ 1.7−	32.0+ 2.3−
V	47.0 (45.0- 48.3)			39.0

See Kirschbaum, T.H. and DeHaven, J.C.: 3. Maternal and Fetal
     Blood Constituents. In N. S. Assali (ed), Biology of
     Gestation. Vol. II The Fetus and Neonate. Academic Press
     New York, 1968, pp. 143-187

MATERNAL BLOOD GROUPS

Blood Type Frequencies

Group and Type	Genotypes	Proportion	Gene Frequency White	Black
ABO Group				
A_1	A_1A_1	0.044		
	A_1A_2	0.029		
	A_1O	0.276	0.209	0.135
A_2	A_2A_2	0.005		
	A_2O	0.091	0.070	0.038
A_1B	A_1B	0.025	0.026	
A_2B	A_2B	0.009	0.009	
B	BB	0.004		
	BO	0.081	0.061	0.114
O	OO	0.436	0.660	0.713
Kell				
K+	KK	0.002	0.045	
	Kk	0.08		
K-	kk	0.91	0.954	
Lutheran				
Lu(a+)	Lu^aLu^a	0.015		
	Lu^aLu^b	0.075	0.04	0.02
Lu(a-)	Lu^bLu^b	0.92	0.96	0.980
MN Group				
MS	MS/MS	0.061	0.247	0.098
	MS/Ms	0.040		

Blood Type Frequencies

Group and Type	Genotypes	Proportion	Gene Frequency White	Black
MN Group(cont)				
Ms	Ms/Ms	0.081	0.283	0.336
MS/NS	MS/NS	0.040	0.040	
	MS/Ns	0.192		
	Ms/NS	0.045		
Ms/Ns	Ms/Ns	0.221	0.221	
NS/NS	NS/NS	0.006	0.080	0.073
	NS/Ns	0.062		
Ns/Ns	Ns/Ns	0.151	0.389	-.380
P Group				
P_1	P_1P_1	0.292		
	P_1P_2	0.497	0.540	0.836
P_2	P_2P_2	0.2115	0.460	0.164
Secretors				
Se	SeSe	0.274		
	Sese	0.499		
se	sese	0.277	0.476	

Adapted from Race, R.R. and Sanger, R. Blood Groups in Man
F. A. Davis, Co., Philadelphia, 1962

Postprandial Maternal Urine Glucose
(includes Clinistix and Clinitest)

	Non-Pregnant	3rd Trimester
Concentration (mg%)		
0 - 15	94%	49%
15 - 100	6	35
100+		16
Commercial Tests:		
<u>Clinistix</u>		
Negative		48
Light		24
Medium		18
Dark		10
<u>Clinitest</u>		
Negative		40
Trace		30
0.5%		20
0.75%		2
1.0%		2
2.0%		6
Excretion (mg/hour)		
0 - 10	98	12
10 - 100	2	56
100+		32

See Soler, N.G. and Malins, J.M.: Lancet I: 619, 621, 1971.

Maternal Blood Carbohydrate Levels
(Includes IV Glucose Tolerance Test and Insulin Levels)

	Non-Preg.	1st Trim.	2nd Trim.	3rd Trim.	Post-Partum
Fucose (mg%)	9.1+ 3.2−			8.3+ 1.9−	8.8+ 2.4−
Hexose (mg%) (protein bound)		101.5+ 4.2−		125.6+ 5.1−	
Seromucoid (mg%) (hyaluronic acid)		11.8+ 0.54−		12.1+ 0.23−	
Glucose (mg%) 0.056					
Fasting	71.5+ 8.5−		72.7+ 5.3−	77.2+ 7.2−	
30 min.	106.7+ 25.1−		104.0+ 20.01−	119.9+ 18.3−	
60 min.	82.9+ 27.2−		84.7+ 18.7−	106.0+ 20.3−	
120 min.	65.3+ 14.2−		65.6+ 10.0−	74.2+ 14.2−	
Glucose Tolerance Test (IV):					
Mean K	1.68	2.37	1.88	1.86	1.53
Low K	0.98	1.37	1.18	1.13	0.93
Insulin (mean levels):					
Fasting	11.6+ 5.4−		12.4+ 4.5−	16.2+ 9.9−	
30 min.	45.4+ 26.9−		55.2+ 25.8−	83.1+ 32.1−	
60 min.	28.8+ 15.1−		38.3+ 24.5−	70.3+ 42.1−	
120 min.	12.2+ 7.1−		19.8+ 18.4−	25.0+ 14.8−	

See Campbell, N. Pyke, D.A. and Taylor, K.W. J. Obstet. Gynaec.
     Brit. Cwlth. 78: 498-504, June, 1971
     Scandrett, F.J. Obstet. Gynaec. Brit. Cwlth. 70: 78-82 1963
     Spellacy, W.N. et al. Obstet. Gynec. 35: 39-43, January 1970

A CLINICAL INTERPRETATION

Glucose Tolerance Test (Intravenous):

A 50% solution of 25 gm glucose is injected. Blood glucose usually is determined at 10-15 minute intervals following injection (when rate of decline is constant) and the results are plotted on a semilogarithmic graph. After calculating to zero time and determining half value, the interception time (t) is used to determind the K value:

$$K = \frac{0.693}{t(min)} \ X \ 100$$

Diabetes is suggested when K = <1.0 units. Normal value for K = >1.2 units.

[ ] = S.I. conversion factor

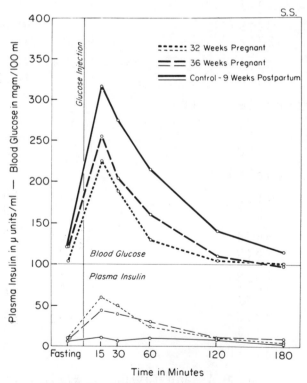

Fig. D-31. Blood glucose and insulin levels during pregnancy after oral 100-g glucose tolerance test. (From Spellacy, W. N.: In *Endocrinology of Pregnancy;* F. Fuchs and A. Klopper, Eds., Harper & Row, Hagerstown, Md., 1971. Reproduced with permission.)

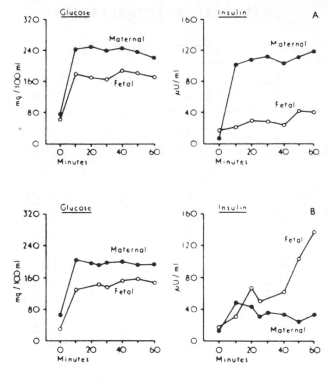

Fig. D-32. Glucose and insulin responses in (A) normal and (B) gestational diabetic pregnancy. (From Oakley, N. W., Beard, R. W., and Turner, R. C.: *Br Med J* **1**: 446, 1972. Reproduced with permission.)

Maternal Serum Electrolytes

	Non-Pregnant	1st Trim.	2nd Trim.	3rd Trim.	Post-Partum
Bicarbonate (HCO_3)(mEg/L)	23.7 (23.2-24)	24.6 (22-27)	23.9 (21.5-26.5)	23.2 (20.5-26)	25.3 (23-28)
Calcium (Ca^{++}) (mEg/L)[0.25]	4.8 (4.7-4.9)	4.94 (4.45-5.55)	4.81 (4.1-5.5)	4.69 (4.15-5.5)	4.96 (4.5-5.95)
Chloride (Cl) (mEg/L)	103.5 (102.7-107)	106.7 (98.7-112)	109.2 (96-117)	104.2 (98-108)	103.5 (92-107)
Copper (Cu) (ug%)	120 $\pm$23	242 $\pm$48	236 $\pm$50	264 $\pm$52	150 $\pm$21
Iron (Fe) (mEg/L)[0.179]		151 $\pm$63	109 $\pm$54	100 $\pm$60	90 $\pm$60
Magnesium (Mg^{++}) (mEg/L)[0.411]	2.0 (1.7-2.7)	1.57 (1.34-2.2)	1.53 (1.14-1.8)	1.47 (1.03-1.74)	1.45 (1.04-1.65)
Phosphate (HPO_4^{--}) (mEg/L)		1.95 (1.45-2.6)	1.78 (1.2-2.3)	1.82 (1.3-2.6)	2.4 (1.7-3)
Potassium (K^+) (mEg/L)	5.0 (3.5-5.2)	4.07 (3.15-5.2)	4.0 (3.15-4.65)	3.97 (3.15-4.45)	4.1 (3.1-4.55)
Sodium (Na^+) (mEg/L)	139.5 (137-142)	138.9 (135-144)	139.1 (131-144)	139.5 (132.5-143)	140.2 (135-145)
Zinc (Zn) (ug%)		270 $\pm$200	160 $\pm$101	130 $\pm$90	

[ ] SI Conversion Factor

See Kirschbaum, T.H. and DeHaven, J.C.: 3. Maternal and Fetal Blood Constituents. In N.S. Assaii (ed), Biology of Gestation. Vol. II The Fetus and Neonate, Academic Press, New York, 1968, pp. 143-187.

MATERNAL ELECTROLYTES

Osmolar Changes During Pregnancy

	Non-Preg.	1st Trim.	2nd Trim.	3rd Trim.	Post-Partum
Osmolality (mOsm/kg)					
Plasma	281.0±0.6	283.0±0.5	283.0±5.0	279.0±4.0	289.0±0.7
Serum	280.0±0.5	282.0±0.5	284.4±0.5	284.5±0.5	288.3±0.8
Colloid osmotic pressure (torr)	30.6	29.8	30.5	29.6	-

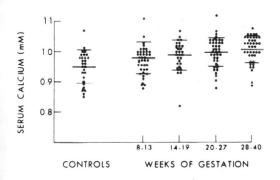

Fig. D-33. Ionized serum calcium in mM (mean ± SD) in nonpregnant females and 8–13, 14–19, 20–27, and 28–40 weeks of pregnancy. (From Reitz, R. E., Daane, T. A., *et al.: Obstet Gynecol* **50**: 701, 1977. Reproduced with permission.)

Fig. D-34. Total serum calcium in mg/dl (mean ± SD) in nonpregnant females and 8–13, 14–19, 20–27, and 28–40 weeks of pregnancy. (From Reitz, R. E., *et al.: Obstet Gynecol* **50**: 701, 1977. Reproduced with permission.)

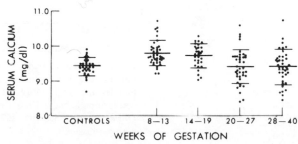

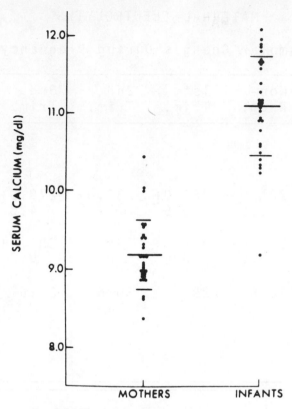

Fig. D-35. Total serum calcium in mg/dl (mean ± SD) in mothers and infants at delivery. (From Reitz, R. E., *et al.*: *Obstet Gynecol* **50**: 701, 1977. Reproduced with permission.)

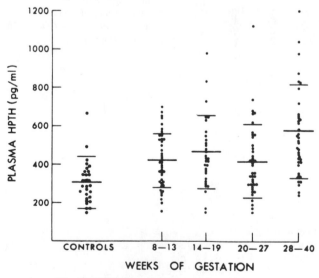

Fig. D-36. Plasma human parathyroid hormone in pg/dl (mean ± SD) in nonpregnant females and 8–13, 14–19, 20–27, and 28–40 weeks of pregnancy. (From Reitz, R. E., *et al.*: *Obstet Gynecol* **50**: 701, 1977. Reproduced with permission.)

MATERNAL ENZYMES

Maternal Serum Enzyme Activity

	Non-Preg.	1st Trim.	2nd Trim.	3rd Trim.	Post-Partum
Alkaline Phosphatase[1] (King-Armstrong)					
Units		9.0 ± 1.6	10.9 ± 5.5	24.4 ± 17.0	
Heat Stable			5.5 ± 3.5	11.0 ± 7.0	
Leukocyte (LAP units)	50 ± 4	81 ± 7	141 ± 18.1	150 ± 14.4	53 ± 2
Arylsulphatase	12	12	17.3	17.5	12
Creatinine phosphokinase (CPK)(mu/ml)	2.1 ± 0.9			6.04 ± 5.77	5.14 ± 5.33
Diamine oxidase[2]		10-60	90-210	90-240	
Glutamic oxalacetic transaminase (SGOT)(u/ml)	15.2 ± 1	17 (6-20)	16.8 (7-20)	15.8 (8.14[1])	7.6 ± 3.4
Glutamic pyruvic transaminase (SGPT)(u/ml)	17.2 ± 5.7	16 (5-19)	14 (5-17)	13.0 ± 7.3	7.4 ± 3.4
-hydroxy-butyric dyhydrogenase (HBD)(u/ml)	164 ± 62	148 ± 64	150 ± 60	164 ± 62	214.7 ± 62.5

Maternal Serum Enzyme Activity

	Non-Preg.	1st Trim.	2nd Trim.	3rd Trim.	Post-Partum
Iso-citrate dyhydrogenase (ICD)(u/ml)	11	6.2 ± 2.7	5.6 ± 2.3	5.5 ± 2.5	7.3 ± 3.1
Lactic dehydrogenase (LDH)(u/ml)	244 ± 11.9	230 ± 66	208 ± 70	234.9 ± 67	417.5 ± 266.7
Leucine-aminopeptidase (units mu)	15	18	27	75	
Oxytocinase (SCAP) OD	.10	.24	.50	200 (.50-500)	
Pseudocholin-esterase (PsChE) ($x10^3$ units)	2.2	3.96 ± 0.82	4.08 ± 0.72	4.02 ± 0.68	3.88 ± 0.94

See   Curzen, P. and Morris, J.: J Obstet Gynaec Brit Cwlth 72: 397-401, 1965.
Konttinen, A. and Pyorala, T.: Scand J Clin Lab Invest 15:429,435, 1963.
Poczekoj, J., Wenclewski, A. and Lewick, J.:Ginek Pol 34: 321, 1963.
Polishuk, W.Z. et al: Am J Obstet Gynecol 107: 604, 1970.

MATERNAL HEMATOLOGY

Hematology Changes During Pregnancy

	Non-Preg.	1st Trim.	2nd Trim.	3rd Trim.	Post Partum
Blood volume Total (ml)	3,787 (3,573-3,991)			5,026 (4,946-5,346)	
ml/kg	66.6			79.7	
Erythro-proteins (units/ml)	0.03	0.03	0.08	0.07	0.03
Folic acid					
FIGIU excre. (mg/6hrs)	18.6+ 0.6	19.3+ 3.5	22.73+ 4.7	9.8+ 1.5	16.4+ 3.3
Serum(L. casel folate) (umg/ml)	4.80+ 0.53	7.7+ 1.5	7.20+ 1.1	6.2+ 0.8	5.74+ 0.6
S. fecalis (umg/ml)	25.7+ 1.9	24.0+ 2.2	23.0+ 1.7	16.9+ 1.6	22.8+ 1.9
Urocanic acid (mm/6hrs)	1.05+ 0.5	0.85+ 0.3	0.87+ 0.4	0.84+ 0.4	0.91+ 0.8
Hematocrit(%)					
Arterial	(33-36)		35.8 (31-37)	34.0 (32-38)	
Venous	39.6 (35.1+ 46.3)	35.3 (32.3+ 37.1)	32.5 (27.5+ 36.4)	31.6 (28.6+ 38.4)	37.8 (31.5+ 42.3)
Ratio (red cell volume: plasma volume)	0.871+ 0.038	0.877+ 0.0255	0.882+ 0.023	0.873+ 0.042	0.846+ 0.023
Hemoglobin(mg%)	13.9 (11.5-16.0)	13.1	12.0 (10.8-14.4)	12.6 (11.2-15.0)	

MATERNAL HEMATOLOGY

Hematology Changes during Pregnancy

	Non-Preg.	1st Trim.	2nd Trim.	3rd Trim.	Post Partum
Iron					
Serum(mean) (Y%) 0.179	120	118	82	60	65
Binding capacity (mean)(Y%)		200	245	375	
Leukocytes ($/mm^3$)	7.4+2.4−	10.2+2.8−	10.5+2.5−	10.4+2.5−	8.2+1.8−
Basophiles	0.5	0.2	0.2	0.1	0.3
Eosinophiles	2.0	1.7	1.5	1.5	2.8
Lymphocytes	38.0	27.9	25.2	25.3	41.3
Monocytes	4.0	3.9	4.0	4.5	4.3
Neutrophiles	55.0	66.3	69.6	69.0	51.3
Plasma					
Total (ml)	2,413 (2,284-2,761)			3,503 (2,979-3,493)	
ml/kg	42.6	47.3	56.8	65.9	47.2
RBC ($/mm^3$)	4.8 (4.2-5.4)		4.0 (3.5-4.8)	4.2 (3.7-5.0)	
Protoporphyrin (mean)(Y%)		45	45	60	
Sedimentation rate (mm/hr)	22±2	24±3	45±25	52±18	45±23

Hematology Changes During Pregnancy

	Non-Preg.	1st Trim.	2nd Trim.	3rd Trim.	Post-Partum
Red Cell mass					
Total (ml)	1,368 (1,285- 1,457)			1,523 (1,453- 1,737)	
ml/kg	23.9			24.1	
Vitamin B_{12} (serum) (uug/ml)	559.5+ 23.4$^-$	573.2+ 39.5$^-$	467.1+ 26.5$^-$	357+ 31.$\overline{3}$	583+ 23.$\overline{1}$

See Edelstein, T. et al: J Obstet Gynecol Brit Cwlth
73: 197-204, April 1966·
Efrati, P.: Obstet Gynecol 23: 429-432, March 1964.
Paintin, D.B. J: Obstet Gynaecol Brit Cwlth 70:
807,810, 1963.
Retief, F.P. and Brink, A.J.: J. Obstet Gynaecol Brit
Cwlth 74: 683-693, October 1967
Spector, W.S. (ed), Handbook of Biological Data.
W.B. Saunders, Philadelphia, 1956
Sturgis, C.C. and Bethell, F.H.: Physiol Rev 23:
279-303, 1943.

MATERNAL HEMATOLOGY

Bone Marrow Differential Cell Count in Pregnancy
(cells/mm^3)

Cell Type[1]	Non-Preg.	1st Trim.	2nd Trim.	3rd Trim.
Basophiles (segmented)	53(0-184)	78(0-197)	47(0-125)	49(0-191)
Eosinophiles (segmented[2])	246(60-642)	371(48-1140)	299(18-990)	228(0-700)
Lymphocytes	3428 (1721-6520)	3975 (2894-6300)	4467 (1686-10,000)	3719 (1318-5400)
Metamyelocytes (neutrophilic)	1437 (168-4324)	2165 (259-5913)	2623 (251-10,250)	1879 (340-4900)
Monocytes	312 (32-717)	333 (40-965)	245 (0-642)	194 (0-732)
Myeloblasts	89 (0-279)	63 (0-328)	173 (0-1250)	96 (0-635)
Myelocytes				
Eosinophilic[3]	147 (0-544)	218 (28-494)	251 (0-1400)	167 (0-700)
Neutrophilic (early)	147 (0-630)	262 (0-675)	446 (0-3500)	362 (1050)
Neutrophilic	1568 (168-4140)	2267 (172-4336)	3229 (659-13,125)	2138 (391-7937)
Neutrophiles				
Band	6048 (1091-14,490)	11,659 (2189-28,251)	15,415 (3077-46,250)	11,819 (4901-29,400)
Segmented	3565 (1132-7084)	5445 (4050-8835)	5441 (1575-11,750)	4613 (394-8680)

MATERNAL HEMATOLOGY

Bone Marrow Differential Cell Count in Pregnancy
$(cells/mm^3)$

Cell Type[1]	Non Preg.	1st Trim.	2nd Trim.	3rd Trim.
Normoblasts				
Early	616 (62-1396)	749 (86-1314)	797 (251-1875)	1050 (51-3937)
Intermediate	1199 (134-2904)	1139 (259-2628)	1803 (314-7000)	1865 (51-8638)
Late	453 (43-1089)	944 (28-2700)	835 (250-2000)	836 (119-2730)
Proerythroblasts	28 (0-122)	56 (0-136)	73 (0-203)	61 (0-210)
Progranulocytes	251 (11-736)	378 (38-900)	462 (69-2500)	341 (0-1460)
Cells				
Disintegrated	3578 (1081-6534)	4684 (1382-8100)	4675 (1037-11,500)	4480 (1329-11,900)
Nucleated (total)	23,100 (7,500-46,000)	34,580 (14,400-65,700)	41,510 (15,700-125,000)	33,930 (16,900-70,000)

[1] Not tabulated but present 0.1%: basophilic myelocytes, early myelocytes, (basic, eosinophilic) plasmacytes and proplasmacytes.

[2] Includes band eosinophiles

[3] Includes eosinophilic metamyelocytes

See Pitts, H.H. and Packham, E.A.: Arch Int Med. 46: 471-482, 1939.

HEMOGLOBINOPATHY

Average Findings with Inherited Disorders of Hemoglobin Synthesis

Disease	Hemoglobin (%)	Reticulo-cytes (%)	Smear	Spleen
HbSS	710-8.5	5-15	Sickle cells; aniso., poik., NRBC, targets	Not palp., after child-hood
HbSC	9.5-12.0	0-6	Sickle cells; (rare) target	Usually enlarged
HbS-thalβ	8.5-10.5	0-8	Hypochromia; targets, sickles, stippling, microcytosis	Over 50% enlarged
HbSA	10.5-13.0	0-3	Not espec. remarkable	Normal
HbSD	7.0-10.0	15-30	Sickles, targets, hypochromia, microcytosis, NRBC	30% palp.
Thal. major	6.5-8.0	3-8	Hypochromia, targets, microcytosis	Almost always enlarged
Thal. minor	10.0-12.0	Normal	Hypochromia, microcytosis, targets, stippling	Normal
HbC-thal	9.5-9.0	to 5	Microcytosis, targets, (sometimes giant, NRBC)	usually enlarged
HbCA	nearly normal	nearly normal	Targets (+ giant) mild hypochromia	Rarely enlarged
HbCC	9-12	4-8	Same as above	almost always enlarged

HEMOGLOBINOPATHY

Disease	Urinary Tract	Bones	Icterus	Sickle Prep.	Hemo-globin %
HbSS	Rare hematuria* papillary necrosis, hyposthen-uria	Infarcts aseptic necrosis, codfish vertebrae	+++	++++	HbS=76-98 HbF= 2-24
HbSC	Same as HbSS	Same as HbSS	$\pm$	++	HbS=40 HbC=60 HbF= 0-8
HbS-thal β	Same as HbSS	Same as HbSS	+	+++	HbS=60-90* HbA=0-30* HbF=0-20* HbA_2=0-8*
HbSA	Same as HbSS	Normal w/ rare aseptic necrosis	0	++	HbS=40 HbA=60
HbSD	Hypos-thenuria	Infarcts, sclerosis	++	++	HbS=25-75 HbD=75-25
Thal. major	unre-markable	codfish vertebrae, bone cysts	+++	0	HbA usual < 25 HbF usual > 75
Thal. minor	unre-markable	Normal	0	0	HbA=78-94* HbA_2=2-6* Hb F=2-16*
HbC-thal	unre-markable	unre-markable	+	0	HbC=60-90* HbA=0-30* $HbA_2$0-7* HbF=0-20*
HbCA	rare hematuria	Dental infarcts	0	0	HbC=40 HbA=60
HbCC	rare hematuria	Same	$\pm$	0	HbC=90+ HbF=0-7

* Depends upon type of thalβ inheritance

See Perkins, R.P.: Am J Obstet Gynecol 111: 120, 1971.

Hemodynamic Parameters Throughout Pregnancy

	Non-pregnant	1st Trim.	2nd Trim.	3rd Trim.	Post Partum
Arterial pressure (mean systemic) (torr)					
Lateral		82+ 13.79	84+ 10.32	85	
Supine		81+ 12.85	86+ 10.88		
Blood volume					
Total (ml)		3,787 (3,573- 3,991)		5,026 (4,946- 5,346)	
ml/kg		66.6		79.7	
Cardiopulmonary (ml)					
Lateral		436+ 115.4	447+ 79.7		
Supine		431+ 104.1	439+ 57.0		
Cardiac output (L/min)					
Lateral		6.10+ 0.82	6.18+ 0.69	6.0+ 0.5	
Supine		6.06+ 0.76	6.12+ 0.95	5.0 (4.6-6.0)	
Cardiac stroke volume (ml)					
Lateral		76+ 12.26	75+ 14.15	76	
Supine		74+ 12.55	75+ 13.60	68	
Circulation time (sec)					
Arm to carotid	17	14	13.6	13.6	15.2
Arm to leg	16	13	11.5	15.8	15.1
Arm to lung	6.6+1.0	6.6+ 0.8	5.8+ 0.9	5.0+ 0.7	
Arm to tongue	12.8+1.4	12.4+ 1.0	11.3+ 1.3	10.2+ 1.1	
Lung to tongue	6.1+1.0	5.8+ 0.9	5.5+ 0.7	5.3+ 0.5	

Hemodynamic Parameters Throughout Pregnancy

	Non-pregnant	1st Trim.	2nd Trim.	3rd Trim.	Post Partum
Central venous pressure (cmH_2O)	8-11.2	6.5-8.2	3.6-4.6	2.0-4.4	
(Colditz, R.B. and Josey, W.E. Obstet. Gynec. 36: 769, 1970)					
Heart rate (/min)					
Lateral		81+9.78	84+8.94	85	
Supine		82+9.60	83+9.33		
Heart volume (radiography) (ml)				681±113	
Vascular resistance (mean systemic) ($dyne/sec/cm^{-5}$)					
Lateral		1,087+ 241.5	1,093+ 216.5		
Supine		1,075+ 232.8	1,143+ 212.5		
Venous pressure (cmH_2O)					
Brachial	8 (4-11)	8 (4-10)	8.5 (7-16)	10 (5-15)	8 (5-16)
Femoral	7 (3-9)	12 (8-16)	18 (16-22)	22 (16-26)	8 (4-9)
Venous tone (torr)	3.49+ 0.6	3.02+ 0.31	3.26+ 0.41	3.48+ 0.35	3.28+ 0.42

See Duncan, S.L.B. and Bernard, A.G. J.Obstet. Gynaec. Brit. Cwlth.
75: 142-150, February, 1968.
Hytten, F.E. et al. J. Obstet. Gynaec. Brit. Cwlth.
70: 817-820, October, 1963.
Kerr, M.G. Brit. Med. Bull. 24:19-24, January, 1968.
Lees, M.M. et al. J. Obstet. Gynaec. Brit. Cwlth.
74: 319-328, June, 1967.
Manchester, B. and Loube, S.D. Am. Heart J. 32: 215-221, 1946.

Hormone Levels During Pregnancy

	Non-Preg.	1st Trim.	2nd Trim.	3rd Trim.	Post-Partum
Blood					
Cortisol(ug/ml)	-	270 ± 20	360 ± 32	380 ± 40	-
Cortisone (ug/L)	10	10	9	13	-
Estradiol (ug/L)	-	-	-	30-40	-
Unconjugated estriol(ug/ml)	-	1-2	2-8	6-12	-
Estrone (ug/L)	-	-	-	40-80	-
FSH (mlu/ml plasma)		0-13	14 ± 4	13 ± 3	-
HCG (IU/ml serum)	-	150 ± 11	30 ± 4	40 ± 5	-
HCG (IU/ml serum)(ug/ml)	-	12.5 ± 0.9	2.3 ± 0.3	4.9 ± 0.4	-
HPL (ug/ml)	-	0.5 ± 0.3	2-3	6.0 ± 1.5	-
17-hydroxy - cortisone(ug/L)	22	20	18	26	-
17-ketosteroid	-	-	-	30-40	-
MSH (melanocyte stimulating hormone)(Units/ml)	1.3	-	-	200	-
PBI (protein-bound iodine)	5.0	6.2 (5.5-9.5)	6.2 (5.6-7.8)	6.4 (4.0-8.5)	5.5 (4.5-6.9)
Pregnanediol[1] (ug%)	-	-	-	100	80 (34-104)
Pregnanetriol (mg/L)	-	-	-	212	-

MATERNAL HORMONES

Hormone Levels During Pregnancy

	Non-Preg.	1st Trim.	2nd Trim.	3rd Trim.	Post Partum
Progesterone (ug/ml)	-	3	8	15-17	12 (6.8-15.0)
Testosterone (pg/ml)	-	400	500	450	-
Relaxin (GPU/ml serum)	-	0.2	-	2.0	-
Aldosterone (mg%)	12 ± 1	232	163	122	-
Renin (units/L)	24.9 ± 1.0	52	37	33	-
TSH (mu%)	-	-	-	12.4	-

Urine

	Non-Preg.	1st Trim.	2nd Trim.	3rd Trim.	Post Partum
Estradiol (mg/24 hr)	-	0.2	0.3	0.9	-
Estriol[2] (mg/24hr)	-	1	10	24	-
Estrone (mg/24hr)	-	0.2	1.5	1.9	-
6β-hydroxycortisol (ug/24 hr)	-	2.1 ± 0.2	2.5 ± 0.4	3.2 ± 0.5	-
6β-hydroxy-20α-di-hydrocortisol (ug/24 hr)	-	44 ± 8	64 ± 15	72 ± 12	-
Pregnanediol (mg/24 hr)	-	8.43 ± 1.83	14.88 ± 3.22	42.6 ± 14.4	-

[1] hourly variation. See Craft, I., Wyman, H., Sommerville, I.F. J. Obstet. Gynec. Brit. Cwlth. 76: 1080 - 1089, 1969

[2] See Chart, p.
See Saxena, B.N., Emerson, K. Jr., Selenkow, H.A. New Eng. J. Med 281: 225-231, July 1969
See Short, R.V., Elton, B.J. Endocr. 18:418-425, 1959
See Varma, K., Larrage, L., Selenkow, H.A. Obstet. Gynec. 37: 10-18, January, 1971
See Zarrow, M.X., Yochim, J. Endocr 69: 292-304, August 1961
See Spellacy, W. Management of High-Risk Pregnancy Baltimore University, Park, 1975

MATERNAL HORMONE

Thyroid Tests

	Non-Preg.	1st Trim.	2nd Trim.	3rd Trim.	Post-Partum
Plasma inorganic iodine (ug%)	0.17 ± 0.05	0.13 ± 0.02	0.06 ± 0.02	0.12 ± 0.03	0.18 ± 0.04
Thyroid clearance of iodine (ug%)	24.8 ± 5.0	48.7 ± 5.8	49.7 ± 6.2	53.1 ± 3.4	22.8 ± 4.7
Iodine uptake by gland (ug/hr)	-	3.42 ± 0.06	1.63 ± 0.20	3.82 ± 0.90	2.53 ± 0.40
BEI (ug%)	5	5	6	6	-
BMR (% changed)	0	+5	+8	+9	-
T_3 (ug%)	0.38 ± 0.12	-	-	0.41 ± 0.11	-
T_3 (free) (ug%)	1.16 ± 0.41	-	-	0.80 ± 0.30	-
T_3 (index)	1-3	1-3	1-3	1-3	1-3
TT_4 (ug%)	3.0-7.5	-	-	5.5-10.5	-
TBG (ug%)	24.0 ± 4.0	-	-	46.0 ± 6.6	-
TBPA (ug%)	195.0 ± 80.0	-	-	149.0 ± 59.0	-
RT_3 (%)	25.0-30.0	-	-	21.0	
FT_4 (ng%)	4.5-8 5	-	-	3.2-5.6	-
RT_3 uptake ratio	0.92 ± 0.019	0.84 ± 0.09	0.57 ± 0.012	0.60 ± 0.010	-
PBI (ug%)	5.52 ± 0.159	6.92 ± 0.05	8.36 ± 0.17	7.91 ± 0.220	-
FTI (PBI)	5.13 ± 0.21	5.57 ± 0.16	4.72 ± 0.10	4.74 ± 0.13	-

See   Dussault, J.et al, J. Clin. Endocrinol. Metab. 29:595, 1969
      Papapetrou, P.D. et al Int. J. Obstet. Gynec. 9:20, 1971

MATERNAL RESPIRATION

Respiratory Changes

	Non-Preg.	1st Trim.	2nd Trim.	3rd Trim.	Post-Partum
Alveolar ventilation(% changed)	0	+35	+40	+60	-
Basal metabolic rate (% changed)	0	+5	+8	+9	-
Expiratory reserve volume (L)	0.65+ 0.25−	0.65	0.61	0.55+ 0.25−	0.56
Inspiratory capacity (L)	2.6+ 0.4−	2.6	2.7	2.7+ 0.4−	2.5
Maximum breath. capacity (L/min)	102+22	97	96	96+22	92
Minute ventilation (% changed)	0	+15	+30	+45	
Minute volume (L/min)	7.3+ 3.0−	8.7	9.7	10.3+ 3.0−	9.5
Residual vol.(L)	1.0+ 0.2−	1.0	0.9	0.8+ 0.2−	1.0
Respiratory rate (breaths/min)	15+4	16	16	16+4	17
Tidal vol. (L)	0.50+ 0.3	0.56	0.61	0.7+ 0.3−	0.55
Total lung capacity (L)	4.2+ 0.6−	4.2	4.1	4.1+ 0.6−	4.1
Ventilatory equivalent (ml air/ml O_2)	3.0+ 2.0−	3.3	3.5	3.3+ 2.0−	3.4
Vital capacity(L)	3.3+ 0.5−	3.2 (2.8-3.9)	3.2 (2.8-3.9)	3.3+ 0.4−	3.1 (2.5-3.7)

See Cugell, D.W. et al. Am Rev. Tuberc. 67: 568, 1953

MATERNAL RESPIRATION

Mean Cardiorespiratory Measurements at Increasing Work Loads

	Work Load (KgM/min)	Non-Preg.	1st Trim*	2nd Trim*	3rd Trim*
Oxygen uptake (L/min)	150	0.53±0.06	-0.02±0.08	0.00±0.07	+0.04±0.05
	250	0.74±0.09	-0.03±0.09	-0.02±0.10	+0.05±0.11
	350	0.94±0.28	-0.04±0.11	-0.01±0.14	+0.03±0.15
Minute ventilation (L/min)	150	17.5±3.2	+2.0±4.1	+2.4±3.1	+4.2±2.8
	250	22.1±2.6	+2.8±3.3	+2,7±2.9	+4.7±3.3
	350	28.1±4.0	+2.2±2.3	+3.1±2.6	+4.6±3.0
Heart rate (/min)	150	103.1±12.7	+5.2±14.2	+7.8±9.7	+15.8±8.1
	250	111.8±7.3	+8.2±11.1	+7.4±9.0	+12.9±9.5
	350	123.4±7.1	+9.1±10.9	+7.3±9.0	+11.1±10.3
Cardiac Output (L/min)	150	5.2±1.6	+1.7±1.9	+0.9±1.0	+1.4±1.8
	250	6.9±1.1	+1.8±2.0	+1.4±2.0	+2.3±1.5
	350	9.1±1.4	+1.5±1.9	+1.8±2.1	+1.2±1.3

Mean (*mean change) ± standard deviation

See Guzman, C,A, and Caplan, R. Am. J. Obstet. Gynec. 108: 600 - 605, October, 1970

MATERNAL RESPIRATION

Work Studies in Pregnant Women

	Non-Preg.	1st Trim.	2nd Trim.	3rd Trim.	Post-Partum
Heart Rate		128 (118-136)	119 (100-140)	120 (116-137)	117 (104-133)
Maximum ventilator capacity (% changed)	0	+16 (-18 +44)	+11 (-18 +44)	+9 (-17 +32)	+15 (-12 +40)
Steady state ventilation	0	0.24	0.23	0.23	0.18
Maximum ventilator capacity		(0.17-0.36)	(0.14-0.30)	(0.17-0.27)	(0.12-0.28)
pCO_2 (torr)	-	34 (31-37)	35 (32-39)	36 (31-37)	39 (36-48)
V_{O_2} (% changed)	0	+5 (-5 +40)	-5 (-12 +28)	-8 (-16 +20)	+5 (-32 +40)

See Gilbert, R. and Auchincloss, J.H. Am. J. Med. Sc. 252: 270, 1966

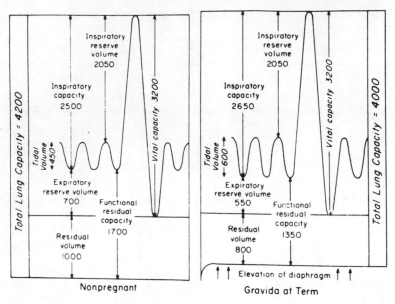

Fig. D-37. Pulmonary volumes and capacities during pregnancy, labor, and postpartum period. (From Leontic, E. A.: *Med Clin North Am* **61**: 114, 1977. Reproduced with permission.)

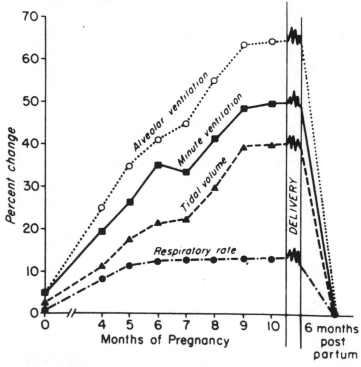

Fig. D-38. Changes in respiratory parameters during pregnancy. The curves for rate, tidal volume, and minute ventilation were developed from data of Cugell, D. W., *et al.: Am Rev Tuberc* **67**: 568, 1953. (From Leontic, E. A.: *Med Clin North Am* **61**: 113, 1977. Reproduced with permission.)

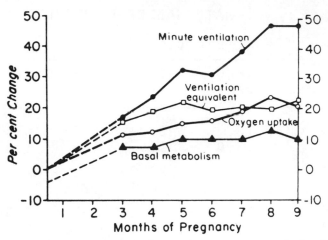

Fig. D-39. Percent change of minute ventilation, oxygen uptake, basal metabolism, and ventilation equivalent for oxygen at monthly intervals throughout pregnancy. (From Leontic, E. A.: *Med Clin North Am* **61:** 113, 1977. Reproduced with permission.)

MATERNAL RENAL

Renal Function Studies

	Non-Preg.	1st Trim.	2nd Trim.	3rd Trim.	Post-Partum
BUN (mg%) 0.167	13.1±3.0	8.2±1.5	6.0±1.3	6.4±1.4	13
NPN (mg%)		28.0±2.7	24.0±2.2	24.9±1.9	
Uric Acid (mg%) 0.06	5.0±1.2	-	3.2	3.34±0.84	3.74±0.85
Renal blood flow (/1.73m^2)	965±272	1280±161	1216±108	940±186	886±270
Mean glomerular filtration rate (Cinulin/1.73 m^2)	100.0±13.5	140±18	160±21	155±21	98±8
Clearance/1.73m^2 (ml/min)					
Creatinine	90-120	110-150	-	109-160	98±8
Diodrost	518	-	-	610	-
Inulin	100.0±13.5	140±18	150±21	145±24	-
PAH	600	680	700	625	-
Sodium	1.01±0.52	-	-	1.04±0.66	-
Uric Acid	-	-	-	18.4	13
Specific Gravity	1.001-1.035	—	—	1.022 (1.004-1.029)	1.020
Urine output(ml) (3 hour after 1 L ingestion)					
Lateral	1,295	1,355	1,310	1,101	
Supine	1,373	1,172	1,178	785	

Renal Function Studies

	Non-Preg.	1st Trim.	2nd Trim.	3rd Trim.	Post-Partum
Psp excretion (IM after 2hrs) (%)	60-85%	-	-	70-90%	-
Urine protein content					
gm/24 hrs.	0.0-0.03	0.0-0.03	0.0-0.04	0.0-0.05	-
Sulfosali-cylic acid (% positive)	20%	20%	22%	37%	-
Maximum $\frac{\text{plasma urea}}{\text{urine urea}}$	10/1	10/1	9/1	9/1	-

See Sims, E.A.H. and Krantz, K.E. J. Clin. Invest. 37: 1764, 1958

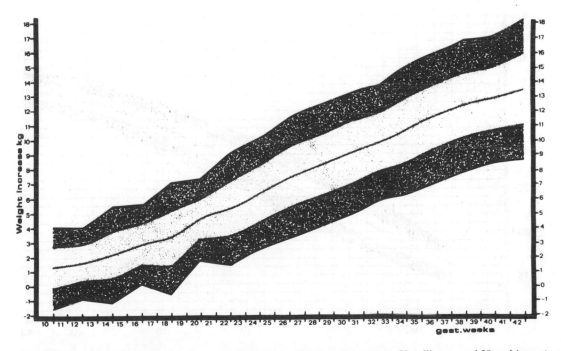

Fig. D-40. Maternal weight increase (mean ± 2 SD) in 100 healthy pregnant women (50 nulliparae and 50 multiparae). All infants were normal for date (NFD). (From Westin, B.: *Acta Obstet Gynecol Scand* **56:** 273, 1977. Reproduced with permission.)

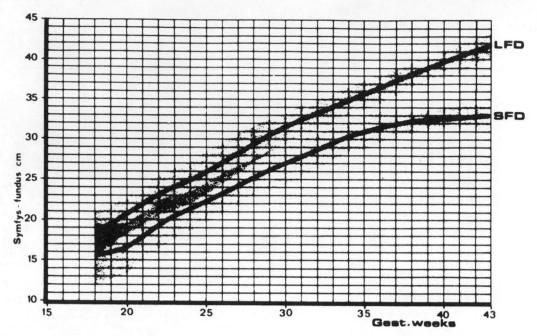

Fig. D-41. Maternal symphysis–fundus growth charts (mean ± SD) in 50 large for date (LFD) and 50 small for date (SFD) infants. (From Westin, B.: *Acta Obstet Gynecol Scand* **56:** 273, 1977. Reproduced with permission.)

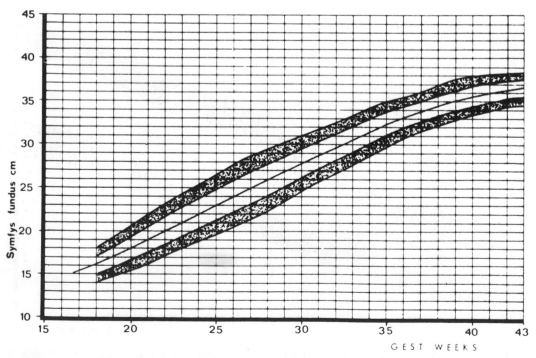

Fig. D-42. Maternal symphysis–fundus growth chart (mean ± 2 SD) in normal pregnancy. Infants were NFD. (From Westin, B.: *Acta Obstet Gynecol Scand* **56:** 273, 1977. Reproduced with permission.)

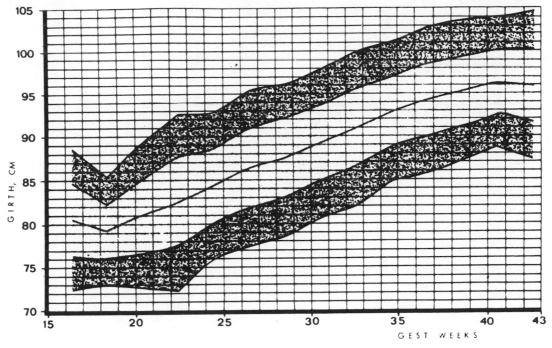

Fig. D-43. Maternal girth increase (mean ± SD) in normal pregnancy. Infants were NFD. (From Westin, B.: *Acta Obstet Gynecol Scand* **56:** 273, 1977. Reproduced with permission.)

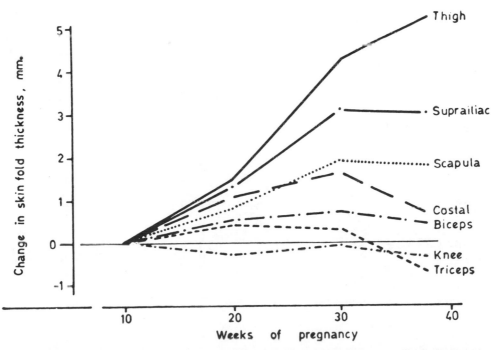

Fig. D-44. Increase in skin-fold thickness at seven sites in pregnancy. (From F. Hytten and I. Leitch: *The Physiology of Human Pregnancy* (2nd ed.), Oxford, Blackwell, 1971. Reproduced with permission.)

MATERNAL WEIGHT GAIN

Weight Gain During Pregnancy

	Non-Preg.	1st Trim.	2nd Trim.	3rd Trim.	8wk post-partum
Mammary glands (gm)					
Gross weight	-	50	200	450	-
Blood	-	5	20	45	-
Gland Tissue	-	45	180	405	-
Uterus (gm)					
Gross weight	50	200	700	1050	-
Blood	5	20	70	105	-
Increase above- non-pregnant uterus	-	135	585	900	-
Leg*					
Thigh volume (L)					
no edema	-	11.6 ± 2.7	12.1 ± 2.5	12.6 ± 2.5	12.0 ± 2.3
Leg edema	-	12.3 ± 1.8	12.9 ± 1.9	13.9 ± 2.2	13.6 ± 1.9
generalized edema	-	13.2 ± 2.8	14.2 ± 2.7	15.0 ± 2.8	14.4 ± 2.6
Thigh skinfold (mm)					
no edema	-	27.5 ± 12.9	29.7 ± 11.6	32.5 ± 10.9	30.9 ± 10.6
Leg edema	-	29.5 ± 9.8	32.7 ± 10.2	37.8 ± 8.4	35.5 ± 6.7
Generalized edema	-	37.4 ± 9.0	33.8 ± 9.2	40.8 ± 10.1	37.4 ± 8.9

MATERNAL WEIGHT GAIN

Weight Gain During Pregnancy

	Non-Preg.	1st Trim.	2nd Trim.	3rd Trim.	8wk post-Partum
Leg Volume(L)					
No edema	-	6.5± 0.9	6.5± 0.8	6.7± 0.9	6.4± 0.9
Leg edema	-	6.5± 0.6	6.6± 0.6	7.1± 0.5	6.6± 0.5
Generalized edema	-	6.7± 1.5	6.7± 1.4	7.2± 1.4	6.7± 1.3
Ankle girth (mm)					
No edema	-	205± 13.6	206± 13.1	208± 12.9	204± 12.2
Leg edema	-	212± 10.1	213± 10.3	219± 6.7	212± 8.7
Generalized edema	-	210± 18.0	211± 17.5	217± 18.9	210± 17.3
Products of Conception (gm)					
Fetus	-	5	300	3300	-
Placenta	-	20	170	650	-
Amniotic Fluid	-	30	250	800	-
Water					
Total gained (ml)	-	1500 (20 wk)	3750 (30 wk)	700 (40 wk)	-
Retention (L) (mean increase in total water)					
No edema	-	0.2	3.2	3.0	-
Ankle Edema	-	0.2	3.3	3.8	-
Generalized edema	-	0.2	4.2	6.8	-

*Mean ± standard deviation

See Hytten, F.E. and Leitch, I. Physiology of Pregnancy, F.A.
     Davis, Philadelphia, 1964, P. 271, 272, 284.
     Hytten, F.E. and Taggart, N.: J Obstet Gynaecol Brit Cwlth
     74: 663, 1967.

VITAMINS

Serum Vitamin Levels During Pregnancy

	Non-Preg.	1st Trim.	2nd Trim.	3rd Trim.	Post-Partum
Vitamin A (ug%)	30.5±25	36.0±30	28.0±64	26.0±7.2	40.5±3.0
-Carotin (ug%)	88±20	94±6	87±6	90±7	103±6
Vitamin B_1 (ug/ml)	170.8±15.6	-	-	166.7±25	-
Riboflavin					
Free (ug%)	-	-	-	0.55±0.12	-
Flavin adenine dinucleotide	-	-	-	2.48±0.18	-
Flavin mono-nucleotide	-	-	-	0.09±0.10	-
Total	-	-	-	3.07±0.20	-
Vitamin B_6					
Leukocytes (mY/million cells)	0.22 (0.14-0.30)	-	-	0.09 (0.02-0.19)	-
Plasma (ug%)	8.4±2.5	-	-	118±32.5	
Pyridoxic (muM/ml) acid	0.412±0.132	0.477±0.151	0.228±0.124	0.256±0.126	-
Pyridoxal phosphate (muM/ml)	0.62±0.018	0.092±0.017	0.044±0.024	0.044±0.020	-
Pyridoxamine phosphate (muM/ml)	1.14±0.14	1.13±0.15	0.48±0.20	0.32±31.3	-

VITAMINS

Serum Vitamin Levels During Pregnancy

	Non-Preg.	1st Trim.	2nd Trim.	3rd Trim.	Post-Partum
Vitamin B_{12} (ug/ml)	559.5± 2 3.4	573.2± 39.5	467.1± 26.5	357.0± 31.3	-
Pantothenic acid					
Bound	84.8± 28.6	56.6± 11.4	49.7± 9.1	88.1± 25.2	-
Free	11.8± 5.4	10.0± 2.7	11.2± 4.5	9.7± 3.5	-
Vitamin C (mg%) (ascorbic acid) (influenced by a patient's diet)	1.2 (0.7- 1.5)	1.1	1.04± 0.26	0.89± 0.18	0.88 (0.6- 1.2)
Vitamin E (ug%)	900± 75	1050± 100	1400± 105	1600± 90	1450± 75

See Herre, H.D., Z. Geburt u Gynek 161: 48, 1964
Teel, H. et al Am. J. Dis. Child 56: 1004, 1938
Slobody, L. et al. Am J. Dis Child 77: 736, 1949
Karlin, R. and Dumont, M, Gynec et Obstet. 62: 281, 1963
Hillman, R.W. et al Am. J. Clin. Nut. 10: 512, 1962
Coursin, D. Brown, B. Am. J. Obstet. Gynec 82: 1307, 1961
Ishiguro, K., Tohoko, K. J Exp. Med. 78: 6, 1963
Lust, J. et al J. Clin. Invest. 33: 38, 1954
Baker, H. et al Am J. Obstet Gynec. 129: 521, 1977

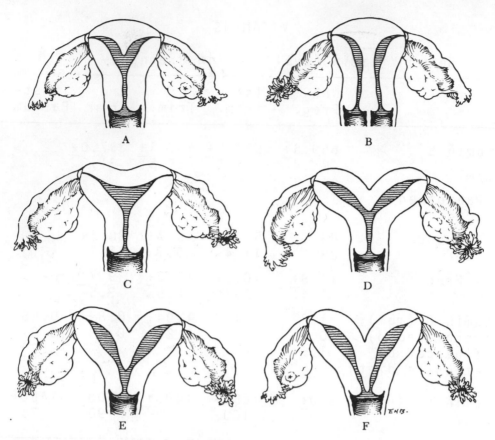

Fig. D-45. Developmental abnormalities of the uterus. (A) Uterus subseptus unicollis; (B) uterus septus duplex, double vagina; (C) uterus arcuatus; (D) uterus bicornis unicollis; (E) uterus bicornis subseptus; (F) uterus bicornis septus. (From Eastman, N. J.: *Williams Obstetrics* (11th ed.), Appleton-Century-Crofts, New York, 1956, Chap. 25. Reproduced with permission.)

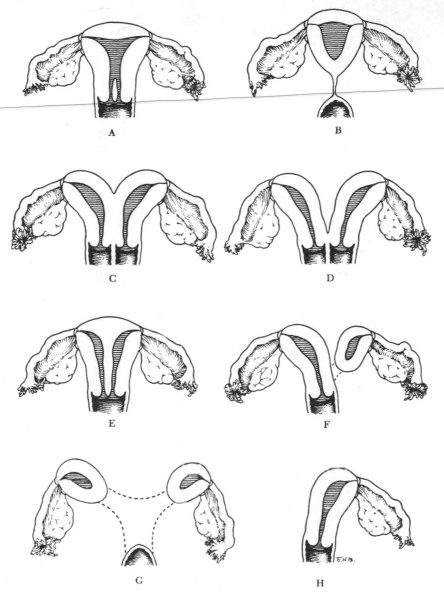

Fig. D-46. Developmental abnormalities of the uterus. (A) Uterus biforis supra simplex; (B) partial gynatresia; (C) uterus bicornis duplex, double vagina; (D) uterus didelphys, double vagina; (E) uterus septus duplex; (F) uterus bicornis unicollis, one rudimentary horn; (G) uterus didelphys, two rudimentary horns, gynatresia; (H) uterus unicornis. (From Eastman, N. J.: *Williams Obstetrics*, 11th ed., Appleton-Century-Crofts, New York, 1956, Chap. 25. Reproduced with permission.)